RESEARCH PROGRESS
IN
EPILEPSY

RESEARCH PROGRESS IN EPILEPSY

Edited by

F Clifford Rose FRCP

Physician-in-Charge
Department of Neurology
Charing Cross Hospital

and

Consultant Neurologist
Medical Ophthalmology Unit
St Thomas' Hospital
London

PITMAN

First Published 1983

Catalogue Number 21.3272.81

Pitman Books Limited
128 Long Acre
London WC2E 9AN

Associated Companies:
Pitman Publishing Pty Ltd, Melbourne
Pitman Publishing New Zealand Ltd, Wellington

British Library Cataloguing in Publication Data

Research progress in epilepsy.—(Progress in
  neurology series, ISSN 0260–0013)
  1. Epilepsy
  I. Rose, F. Clifford   II. Series
  616.8153   RC372

  ISBN 0–272–79684–0

Printed and bound in Great Britain
at The Pitman Press, Bath

FOREWORD

The challenge of epilepsy lies in the diversity of the problems which it presents. Knowledge of the epileptic process requires the most fundamental research on the neural structures of the brain. Chemotherapy is increasingly being shown to operate through the action of anticonvulsant drugs on neurotransmitters and post-synaptic receptor structures. Many different forms of epilepsy are being differentiated, and clinical investigations are required to establish an appropriate classification.

But beyond these purely scientific and medical issues, the management of epilepsy requires attention to the serious social problems of education, employment, security, and complex psychosocial interactions. The latter involve an interplay of the effects on the brain of structural damage, seizure activity, drugs, and social relations.

For this volume, Dr Clifford Rose has brought together knowledgeable experts to provide a broad overview of the evolution of knowledge in these and related fields.

The symposium on which this volume has been based was sponsored by both the World Federation of Neurology and Epilepsy International. The World Federation of Neurology is an organisation of national neurological societies involved in all aspects of neurological disorders. Epilepsy International is an association of lay and professional societies interested in the control of epilepsy and its consequences. The objective of all is to achieve a broader understanding of epilepsy.

Richard L Masland MD
President
World Federation of Neurology

PREFACE

This volume is based on the Proceedings of the International Epilepsy Symposium under the auspices of both the World Federation of Neurology and Epilepsy International held at Charing Cross Hospital in 1982. The symposium proved to be very stimulating, particularly the controversy over classification, which is fully covered in Part I and will help the reader to make up his own mind.

Parts II and III are concerned with the basic and clinical aspects respectively, whilst Part IV is a larger section because of the current interest in the psychological aspects of epilepsy. Part V is given to paediatric aspects because of the more frequent incidence of epilepsy in children, whilst Part VI reviews newer aspects in the investigation of epilepsy. By far the largest section, Part VII, is concerned with treatment, both non-drug and surgical aspects being included, and there are several chapters concerned with the new knowledge of the biochemistry of how the drugs work. The final section, Part VIII, is concerned with the still important aspects of the sociology of epilepsy.

Epilepsy is still a great problem but the recent advances resulting from the burgeoning world-wide research interests, reflected in this volume, are testimony to the greater help that people with epilepsy can now receive.

F Clifford Rose
London

CONTRIBUTORS

J Aicardi
MD

Hôpital des Enfants Malades, Rue de Sevres, Paris, France

G M Anlezark
PhD, BSc

University Department of Neurology, Institute of Psychiatry and King's College Hospital Medical School, London

J Arends

Department of Neurology, University of Nijmegen, The Netherlands

A Aynesley-Green
MA, DPhil, MRCP

Department of Paediatrics, John Radcliffe Hospital, Oxford

M Baraitser
BSc, MB, ChB, FRCP

The Hospital for Sick Children, Great Ormond Street, London

T A Betts
MB, ChB, DPM, MRCPsych

Senior Lecturer in Psychiatry, University of Birmingham, Queen Elizabeth Hospital, Birmingham

B D Bower
MD, FRCP, DCH

Consultant Paediatrician, John Radcliffe Hospital, Oxford

N R Butler
MD, FRCP, DCH

Professor of Child Health, Royal Hospital for Sick Children, Bristol

D Chadwick
MA, DM(Oxon), MRCP

Consultant Neurologist, Walton Hospital, Liverpool

A G Chapman
PhD

Institute of Psychiatry, London

A G Craig
PhD, MIHE

Head of Education and Training British Epilepsy Association, Wokingham, Berkshire

P H Crandall
MD

Division of Neurosurgery, Department of Surgery, UCLA School of Medicine, Center for the Health Sciences, Los Angeles, California, USA

R E Cull
PhD, BSc, MB, ChB, MRCP

Consultant Neurologist, Royal Infirmary, Edinburgh

J de Belleroche
PhD

Department of Neurology, Charing Cross Hospital and Department of Biochemistry, Charing Cross Hospital Medical School, London

C I Dellaportas
MD

Clinical Assistant, Epilepsy Clinic, Department of Neurology, Charing Cross Hospital, London

J Eaton SRD	Department of Paediatrics, John Radcliffe Hospital, Oxford
A Elithorn MD, FRCP, FRCPsych	Consultant Psychiatrist, Royal Free Hospital, and Institute of Neurology, London
A Elyas MLSO	Department of Chemical Pathology, Institute of Neurology, National Hospital, Queen Square, London
J Engel Jr MD, PhD	Chief of the Laboratories of Clinical Neurophysiology and Professor of Neurology and Anatomy, UCLA School of Medicine, Los Angeles, California, USA
M C Evans PhD, BSc	University Department of Neurology, Institute of Psychiatry and King's College Hospital Medical School, London
G W Fenton FRCP, FRCPsych	Professor in Mental Health, Department of Psychiatry, Belfast City Hospital, Belfast
P B C Fenwick MB, BChir, MRCPsych, DPM	Consultant Neurophysiologist, St Thomas' Hospital, London
I B Gartside PhD	Department of Physiology, Charing Cross Hospital Medical School, London
H Gastaut	Professor, Service de Neurophysiologie Clinique, WHO Collaborating Center for Research and Training in Neurological Disorders, Hôpital de la Timone, Marseille, France
V D Goldberg PhD	Department of Chemical Pathology, Institute of Neurology, National Hospital, Queen Square, London
J Golding MA, PhD	Wellcome Trust Senior Lecturer, Department of Child Health, University of Bristol
R H E Grant MB BS, DCH	Director, The David Lewis Centre for Epilepsy, Alderley Edge, Cheshire. Lately Secretary-General, The International Bureau for Epilepsy
T Griffiths PhD, BSc	University Department of Neurology, Institute of Psychiatry and King's College Hospital Medical School, London
U Heinemann	Max-Planck-Institut fur Psychiatrie, Munich, Germany
A Herxheimer MB, FRCP	Departments of Medicine and Pharmacology, Charing Cross Hospital, London
O Hommes	Department of Neurology, University of Nijmegen, The Netherlands

D Janz — Professor, Department of Neurology, Klinikum Charlottenburg, Freie Universität Berlin, Berlin

P M Jeavons
MA, FRCP, FRCPsych — Honorary Visiting Professor, Clinical Neurophysiology Unit, Department of Ophthalmic Optics, University of Aston, Birmingham

C Knott
BSc — Anaesthetic Unit, St Thomas' Hospital Medical School, London

J Kogeorgos
MD, MRCPsych — Senior Registrar in Clinical Neurophysiology, The London Hospital, London

D E Kuhl
MD — Chief of the Laboratory of Nuclear Medicine and Professor of Radiological Sciences, UCLA School of Medicine, Los Angeles, California, USA

Z Kurtz
MB, MSc, MFCM — Department of Community Medicine and General Practice, Charing Cross Hospital Medical School, London

P T Lascelles
MD, FRCPath — Department of Chemical Pathology, Institute of Neurology, National Hospital, Queen Square, London

R H Lowe
BSc — Department of Chemical Pathology, Institute of Neurology, National Hospital, Queen Square, London

H D Lux — Professor, Max-Planck-Institut für Psychiatrie, Munich, Germany

M E L McGowan
MB, BCh, MRCP(UK) — Research Registrar, Departments of Paediatrics and Neurology, King's College Hospital and Honorary Registrar in Paediatrics, Guy's Hospital, London

R L Masland
MD — President, World Federation of Neurology, Secretary-General Epilepsy International, H Houston Merritt Professor of Neurology Emeritus, College of Physicians and Surgeons, Columbia University, New York, USA

B S Meldrum
MB, PhD — University Department of Neurology, Institute of Psychiatry and King's College Hospital Medical School, London

J H D Millar
MD, FRCP — Consultant Neurologist, Royal Victoria and Claremont Street Hospitals, Belfast

A M Moffett
BSc, MA — Research Fellow, EEG Department, Section of Neurological Sciences, London Hospital, London

I F Moseley
MD, FRCR — Consultant Neuroradiologist, Lysholm Radiological Department, National Hospital, Queen Square, London

N V O'Donohoe MD, FRCPI, DCH	Professor of Paediatrics, Trinity College, Dublin and National Children's Hospital, Dublin
G Pampiglione MD, FRCP	Physician in Charge, Department of Clinical Neurophysiology, The Hospital for Sick Children, Great Ormond Street, London
M Parsonage BSc, MB, FRCP, DCH	Honorary Consultant Neurophysician to the David Lewis Centre for Epilepsy, Alderley Edge, Cheshire. Formerly Senior Consultant Physician, Neurology Department, General Infirmary, Leeds and Director of the Neuropsychiatric Unit and Special Centre for Epilepsy, Bootham Park Hospital, York
P N Patsalos PhD	Research Associate, Department of Neurobiology and Anatomy, The University of Texas Medical School at Houston, Texas, USA. Formerly Senior Clinical Lecturer, University of Leeds
C S Peckham MD, MFCM	Reader, Department of Community Medicine, Charing Cross Hospital Medical School, London
M E Phelps PhD	Chief of the Division of Biophysics and Professor of Radiological Sciences, UCLA School of Medicine, Los Angeles, California, USA
C E Polkey MD, FRCS	Consultant Neurosurgeon, Neurosurgical Unit of Guy's, Maudsley and King's College Hospitals, London
Sir Desmond Pond MD, FRCP, FRCPsych	Professor, Department of Psychiatry, The London Hospital Medical College, London
R J Porter MD	Chief, Epilepsy Branch, Neurological Disorders Program, National Institute of Neurological and Communicative Disorders and Stroke, Bethesda, USA
J Powell BA, MA	Department of Psychiatry, Royal Free Hospital, London
N Ratnaraj FIMLS	Department of Chemical Pathology, Institute of Neurology, National Hospital, Queen Square, London
R Rausch PhD	Assistant Research Psychologist, Departments of Surgery and Neurology, Center for Health Sciences, University of California, Los Angeles, USA
M D Rawlins BSc, MD, FRCP	Professor of Clinical Pharmacology, University of Newcastle upon Tyne
E H Reynolds MD, FRCP	Consultant Neurologist, King's College Hospital, London

F Reynolds
MD, FFA, RCS

Anaesthetic Unit, St Thomas' Hospital Medical School, London

F Clifford Rose
FRCP

Physician in Charge, Department of Neurology, Charing Cross Hospital, London

E M Ross
MD, FRCP, DCH

Senior Lecturer in Child Health and Community Medicine, Middlesex Hospital Medical School, London

J S Ruiz

Research Fellow, Lysholm Radiological Department, National Hospital, Queen Square, London

R H Schwartz
MRCP, DRCOG

Senior Registrar, Department of Paediatrics, Northwick Park Hospital, Middlesex

D F Scott
FRCP, DPM

Consultant in Charge, EEG Department, Section of Neurological Sciences, The London Hospital, London

T Sensky
PhD, MB

Psychiatric Registrar, Maudsley Hospital, London

S D Shorvon
MA, MB, MRCP

Registrar, University Department of Clinical Neurology, Institute of Neurology, National Hospital, Queen Square, London

A Stavrou
BA(Hons)

Department of Psychiatry, Royal Free Hospital, London

J B P Stephenson
MA, BM, FRCP, DCH

Consultant in Paediatric Neurology, Fraser of Allander Unit, Royal Hospital for Sick Children, Glasgow

G Stores
MA, MD, MRCP, FRCPsych

Consultant Neuropsychiatrist and Clinical Lecturer, National Centre for Children with Epilepsy and University Department of Psychiatry, Park Hospital for Children, Oxford

M Swash
MD, FRCP

Consultant Neurologist, The London Hospital, London

J F Taylor
MB BS, DRCOG, MFCM, DIH

Senior Medical Adviser, Department of Transport, Swansea, Wales

P J Thompson
BSc, PhD

Department of Psychology, Institute of Neurology, University of London

M R Trimble
MRCP, MRCPsych

Consultant Physician in Psychological Medicine, The National Hospital, Queen Square. Senior Lecturer in Behavioural Neurology, Institute of Psychiatry, University of London, London

D M Turnbull
MB BS, MRCP

MRC Training Fellow and Honorary Senior Research Associate, Department of Neurology, The Royal Victoria Infirmary, Newcastle upon Tyne

D Weightman   Assistant, Department of Medical Statistics,
University of Newcastle upon Tyne

A Wilson   Research Registrar, Epilepsy Clinic, Department
MRCP   of Neurology, Charing Cross Hospital, London

CONTENTS

xvi

1

HISTORY OF CLASSIFICATION IN EPILEPSY

M R Trimble

In a recently overheard conversation, a neurologist was to say that the one subject strictly forbidden on his ward rounds was philosophy. Indeed, that subject is not taught routinely as part of the medical school curriculum, and generally the knowledge of philosophical issues that doctors possess is scanty. This omission is strange. Not only were many philosophers to write on medical issues (for example Aristotle, Plato, Hume), but many well known philosophers have also been physicians (for example Locke, Schiller, and Jaspers). In the field of neurology, Hughlings Jackson was initially attracted to philosophy, being persuaded to pursue medicine by Thomas Laycock and Jonathan Hutchinson.

The relationship between philosophy and neurology is obvious, but can be seen particularly acutely with regard to the question of classification of disease since this issue bears directly on epistemology. To understand some of the difficulties and complications of any classificatory scheme it is important to note the long-standing schism between two rival schools of thought, namely, rationalism and empiricism. With this in mind, the most appropriate starting point would seem to be with Plato (427–347 BC), the founder of the former, and with Hippocrates (460–377 BC) one of the first physicians to write about the subject of epilepsy.

Plato's theory of 'forms' essentially suggests that, since all things are in a state of flux and change (the Heracleitan doctrine), if knowledge is to have an object then there must be other entities which exist and persist. These 'forms' represent universals with independent existence, and are known to reason and to reason alone. Thus in the Dialogues we read:

> SOCRATES "Suppose I were to ask you about the real nature of the bee and you said that there are many and various, what would you reply if I asked you, 'Do you say that they are many and various and different one from another in respect of their being bees?' "

1

MENO ". . . There is no difference at all in respect of being bees one another."

(from Collected Dialogues)

Plato's classification of disease is given in his Timaeus. It is basically physiological, in which disease is seen to be due to lack of harmony, especially amongst the body constituents which comprise such substances as earth, fire, water and air. In the works of Hippocrates, in contrast, prognosis is given the prominent position, and no coherent classification is layed down [1]. In an analysis of the first presentation of case histories known to medicine, Temkin [2] noted how, for Hippocrates, disease was integrated into the life history of man, a parallel being drawn between this and the Aristotelian conception of tragedy. Disease was thus seen as a sequence of events, introducing into medicine, in contrast to the static conception of disease implied by Plato, an active historical element.

The rise of classificatory schemes in the seventeenth century led to reconsideration of the classification of diseases. The historical method of Hippocrates emphasised by Baglivi and Sydenham, was disregarded by those who, like Linnaeus, believe that the relationship of symptoms to disease was as clear as that between leaves and the plants from which they sprouted [3].

In the history of medicine, but in particular with reference to neurology, William Cullen (1710–1790) around this time laid a framework of classification that has had influence up to the present day. In his nosography of diseases, which he considered to be superior to those in existence at the time he was writing, four main classes were described, one of them being the neuroses. These included "all those preternatural affections of sense and motion, which are without pyrexia as part of the primary disease . . . but depend on a more general affection of the nervous system, and of those powers of the system upon which sense and motion more especially depend . . ." [4]. The classes were further subdivided into Orders and Species and, in this scheme, convulsions and epilepsy were classified under the subcategory 'spasmi', along with, for example, hysteria, hydrophobia, colic and chorea. Cullen's classification of the epilepsies was into idiopathic and sympathetic groups following Morgagni. This distinction had a long history, emanating probably from Aretaeus, who noted that epilepsy took its origin from the head, either directly, or by stimulation of nerves in sympathy with the head. Riverius dogmatically reasserted the seventeenth century position as follows ". . . in vain is that epilepsy which comes from the stomach separated from those which come by sympathy from other parts; when all ought to be called sympatheticae, or epilepsies by consent . . . Therefore we subdivide that which is by consent according to the divers parts from where these sharp and malignant vapours are sent to the Brain, for there is almost no part in the Body from which a malignant vapor cannot be sent." [5]

Idiopathic epilepsy thus found causes within the brain, while 'sympathetic' epilepsy occurred when the cause was dependant upon disease of other organs.

This distinction remained prevalent throughout the eighteenth and nineteenth centuries, although Tissot [6] introduced the term 'Essential Epilepsy' for those cases where no definite cause could be demonstrated. Pinel (1975—1826) [7] a follower of Cullen, and translater of some of his works into French, defined epilepsy as "a neurosis of cerebral function" and, according to Temkin [8], his pupil Maisonneuve in his 'Recherches et observations sur l'epilepsie' went on to distinguish ten different species of epilepsy, five idiopathic and five sympathetic. Vaporous or hypochondriacal epilepsy was one of the latter.

In the eighteenth century, the best known nosographer in neurology was Rombert (1795—1873) [9]. He set out a physiological classification emphasising two major groupings, namely the neurosis of sensibility, and the neurosis of motility. In this classification, epilepsy belonged to the latter although he sub-scribed to a divison of the disorder into central and centripetal varieties which he felt was more physiologically correct than idiopathic and sympathetic. Other terms that were introduced in this era included 'centric epilepsy' which was used in opposition to 'eccentric epilepsy', the latter which implied 'sympathetic' con-vulsions. Some authors insisted on expanding the sympathetic class to include such entities as renal epilepsy, gastric epilepsy, uterine epilepsy etc, sometimes apparently exceeding the actual number of organs that were in the body. The idiopathic group became redefined. Delasiauve (1804—1893) classified epilepsy into a) essential or idiopathic, without cerebral lesions; b) symptomatic where there was a more or less appreciable lesion; and c) sympathetic, having origin from parts of the body other than the brain [10].

In 1861, two major books on epilepsy were published wherein contemporary British ideas of classification can be seen. Radcliffe (1822—1869) [11] distin-guished 'ordinary epilepsy' from epileptiform convulsions, the latter occurring "in connection with certain diseases of the brain". Reynolds (1928—1896) said "that the qualifications of the word epilepsy had become numerous and confusing and the application of that one name to many essentially distinct affections had been productive of grave practical effects." [12] He thus reserved the term epilepsy for only "those cases in which no other disease was discoverable" — designating this idiopathic epilepsy. His own distrust of classification is expressed in the following statement: "It is not evident that any perfectly 'natural system' of classification can exist: the only natural division which is established beyond dispute is that of the individual . . ." [12, page XVI]. His own classification, based on 'organ, function and nature of morbid change' however, employed the 'eccen-tric' in opposition to the idiopathic, symptomatic epilepsy being derived from 'centric disease', either of the meninges or the nervous centres. He had a fourth category, diathetic or cachectic convulsions, which were dependant upon toxae-mia or nutritional changes of the brain. Of importance here is to note by this time the clear change from a classification based on function, introduced by Cullen and employed by others such as Romberg, to one of classification based on supposed aetiology.

Hughlings Jackson (1835–1911) is, of course, best known for his descriptions of partial epilepsy, some of which categories now bear his name [13]. With regards to the classification of epilepsy, however, he cautioned that "arrangements may be taken for classifications . . . they are only provisional groupings for more convenience." He went on to note, "there are two ways of investigating diseases, and two kinds of classification corresponding thereto, the empirical and the scientific. The former is to be illustrated by the way in which a gardener classifies plants, the latter by the way in which a botanist classifies them." [14]

Jackson is also famous for his discussion of 'dreamy states' and the description of 'the uncinate groups of fits', the latter being associated with paroxysms of smell or taste, and were related to abnormal discharging lesions in the uncinate region. Together with his delineation of dreamy states, he thus provided us with a coherent characterisation of what has become complex partial seizures.

Jackson's later attempts at classification involved the introduction of evolutionary concepts, for example, lowest level fits being 'pontobulbar', middle level fits being 'epileptiform', while highest level fits were 'epileptic'. This was based on his belief that "evolution . . . applies to the 'whole physical cosmos' . . . it would then be very marvellous if it did not apply to the whole nervous system and its diseases . . ." [15]. He was aware of the pitfalls however, emphasising ". . . because it is convenient to consider a whale as a fish for legal purposes, it would never do to consider it so in Zoology." [16]

Partial epilepsy was first clearly denoted by Prichard (1786–1848) [17] who wrote of "local convulsion or partial epilepsy." He identified examples of epilepsy without convulsions, and of a group he referred to as epileptic leipothymia in which the muscular system was relaxed, and the patient would fall to the ground "in a state of insensibility". Todd (1809–1860) [18] used the term 'epileptiform' for attacks that affected one arm, or leg or both on the same side. Jackson more fully elaborated such partial episodes, and these were designated 'Jacksonian' by Charcot. Jackson thus stated in his 'Study of Convulsions' [19] that the great majority of convulsions could be arranged into two classes: a) those in which the spasm affects both sides of the body almost contemporaneously and, b) those in which the fit begins by deliberate spasm on one side of the body, and in which parts of the body are affected one after another. The former were referred to as 'idiopathic epilepsy', although the term 'genuine' was also given to this grouping.

Gowers [20] broadly classified nervous diseases into 'organic' and 'functional' categories. With regard to epilepsy, no new system was introduced or attempted. He did, however, tackle the difficult problem of the relationship between epilepsy and hysteria, preferring the term hysteroid attacks for non-epileptic convulsions, but also recognising that attacks intermediate between epilepsy and hysteria may exist, thus acknowledging the concept of hystero-epilepsy, prevalent in the writings of contemporary French authors [21].

In this century, until the monumental work undertaken by Gastaut and colleagues [22], there has been little attempt to progress further with classification

4

in neurology generally, and epilepsy in particular. Head [23] was to write "... neurology has become frozen stiffly in the grip of pseudo metaphorical classifications which neither explain the conditions nor correspond to the clinical facts." Riese [3] was to echo a similar sentiment; he noted how nervous diseases are not grouped according to one principle, but are divided by a mixture of aetiological and pathological criteria intermingled with well known pseudonyms. His own preference was for a classification based on function, and disturbance of it, with clear recognition of the chronological element. Lesions are not diseases, a line of thought extending from Cullen to Jackson and beyond.

Aldren Turner [24] recognising that muscular spasms were not a sine qua non, and that consciousness was not always impaired, divided epilepsy into minor epilepsy, with either incomplete or complete attacks, major epilepsy with incomplete or complete attacks, and psychical epilepsy. At this time minor epilepsy was incapable of further delineation, and remained so until the 1930s and 1940s. He also used the term 'petit mal' in reference to minor epilepsy. While the Greeks, and even those before, noted cases of 'little epilepsy', for example attacks of vertigo, and 'slight epilepsy' was frequently referred to [8], it was Tissot (1728–1797) [6] who used the expressions 'grande accès' and 'petite accès', and Esquirol (1772–1840) the term 'le petit mal' in 1838 [25]. Around the same time, Calmeil (1798–1895) introduced the word 'absence' [8].

The introduction of electroencephalography however allowed classification according to observed changes in electrical activity of the brain during the disorder. Gibbs et al [26] considered that epilepsy could be classified into three main groups, namely grand mal, petit mal, and psychomotor. The latter term was introduced by this group although, as Symonds [27] pointed out, it, and the subsequent use by Lennox [28] of the term 'psychomotor triad', added little to what had been described by Hughlings Jackson, and introduction of the term temporal lobe epilepsy shortly thereafter was a reinstitution of the Jacksonian idea of the 'uncinate group of fits'.

Penfield and Jasper [29] retained the terms symptomatic and idiopathic (or essential), but from their own work derived an anatomico-clinical classification suggesting that it was important to recognise whether attacks arise from the cerebral cortex or from the subcortical region, the latter being defined as centrencephalic. These then became subdivided into several types dependant on their EEG patterns, which included petit mal, grand mal, and 'psychomotor' automotisms. Focal, or partial, epilepsies became a crucial area of investigation opened up by the EEG, and the clarification of primary and secondary generalised seizures occurred, as did clear recognition that the symptoms evoked in focal epilepsy were dependant upon the site of origin within the brain of the abnormal discharge. The state of the art was such in the late 1950s that Williams [30] could write "a classification based on the part of the brain first affected, with a statement of the clinical events, is acceptable in all countries."

In more recent times, attempts at classification of epileptic seizures have been catalysed by the development of EEG techniques, especially prolonged monitoring with video telemetry for accurate descriptions of the pattern of individual attacks and the accompanying electroencephalographic changes. The relative success of the new classification of seizures, however, has not been echoed in the classification of the epilepsies. This surely reflects the fact that seizures are not diseases, and the patients suffer from diseases, while doctors diagnose them. To quote Riese [3] ". . . nosologists did not realise with sufficient strength that a disease is a chapter of the life history and therefore by its very nature a chronological phenomenon, or a sequence of events, and the classification according to spatial criteria can do justice to symptoms, but never to the full picture of the diseases." The struggle between the empirical and the rational continues, in particular with regards to epilepsy. The dilemma was recognised over a century ago by Reynolds [10] who said' "Perhaps no disease has been treated with more perfect empiricism on the one hand or more rigid rationalism on the other, than has epilepsy. Unfortunately, both methods have often and completely failed; the former, as it must do, in a certain proportion of cases; the latter, in a still larger number because the theories upon which it has rested, have been abundantly wrong."

References

1   Adams F. *The Genuine Works of Hippocrates 1939*. Baltimore: Williams & Wilkins
2   Tempkin O *1929*, quoted by Riese *1953*
3   Riese W. *Bull History Med 1945; 18:* 465–512
4   Cullen W. *Nosology: or a systematic arrangement of diseases, by classes, orders, genera and species 1800*. Edinburgh: Creech
5   Culpeper N. *Riverius, Lazarus. The Compleat Practice of Physick 1965*. London
6   Tissot SA. *Traité de l'epilepsie 1770*. Paris
7   Pinel Ph. *Nosographie Philosophique 1813*. Paris
8   Temkin O. *The Falling Sickness, 2nd Edition 1971*. Baltimore: Johns Hopkins Press
9   Rombert MH. *A Manual of the Nervous Diseases of Man 1853*. London: The Sydenham Society
10   Delasiauve M. *Traité de l'épilepsie 1854*. Paris
11   Radcliffe CB. *Epileptic and Other Convulsive Affections of the Nervous System, 3rd Edition 1861*. London: J Churchill
12   Reynolds JR. *Epilepsy: its Symptoms, Treatment, and Relation to Other Chronic Convulsive Diseases 1861*. London: J Churchill
13   Jackson JH. In Taylor J, ed. *Selected Writings of John Hughlings Jackson 1869:* 246–250. London: Staples Press
14   Jackson JH. In Taylor J, ed. *Selected Writings of John Hughlings Jackson 1874:* 162–273. London: Staples Press
15   Jackson JH. In Taylor J, ed. *Selected Writings of John Hughlings Jackson 1888:* 365–392. London: Staples Press
16   Jackson JH. In Taylor J, ed. *Selected Writings of John Hughlings Jackson 1875:* 287–299. London: Staples Press
17   Pritchard JC. *A Treatise on Diseases of the Nervous System 1822*. London: Thomas & George Underwood
18   Todd RB. *Clinical Lectures on Paralysis, Certain Diseases of the Brain, and Other Affections of the Nervous System 1856*. London

19 Jackson JH. In Taylor J, ed. *Selected Writings of John Hughlings Jackson 1870:* 8–36. London: Staples Press
20 Gowers WR. *A Manual of Diseases of the Nervous System, 2nd Edition 1899.* London: J & A Churchill
21 Trimble MR. In Reynolds EH, Trimble MR, eds. *Epilepsy and Psychiatry 1981.* Edinburgh: Churchill Livingstone
22 Gastaut H. *Epilepsia 1969; 10:* Suppl 1–10
23 Head H. *Aphasia and Kindred Disorders 1926.* London: Cambridge University Press
24 Turner WA. *Epilepsy 1907.* London: Macmillan & Co
25 Esquirol E. *Des Maladies Mentales 1838.* Paris
26 Gibbs FA, Gibbs EL, Lennox WG. *Arch Neurol Psychiat 1938; 39:* 298–314
27 Symonds C. *Arch Neurol Psychiat 1954; 72:* 631–637
28 Lennox WG. *Neurology 1951; 1:* 357–371
29 Penfield W, Jasper H. *Epilepsy and the Functional Anatomy of the Human Brain 1954.* Boston: Little, Brown & Co
30 Williams D. *Br Med J 1958; 1:* 661–663

2

A PROPOSED COMPLETION OF THE CURRENT INTERNATIONAL CLASSIFICATION OF THE EPILEPSIES

H Gastaut

The classification of epileptic seizures has always been considered from the semiological standpoint to allow easy identification of each type of seizure. Conversely, the classification of the epilepsies has been consistently envisaged on the basis of aetiological criteria (with reference to the semiology) in order to clearly identify the prognosis of each type of epilepsy and its appropriate treatment. Accordingly, since the middle of the nineteenth century the epilepsies have been divided into two major categories: 1) epilepsies independent of an identifiable brain lesion and referred to as functional, idiopathic, essential, genuine, genetic, common, true or, with physiopathogenic connotations, as central or centrencephalic; 2) conversely, epilepsies dependent upon a brain lesion and referred to as lesional, structural, organic, symptomatic, secondary, or with physiopathogenic connotations as partial or focal.

TABLE I. Classifications of the epilepsies prior to 1969

	Functional epilepsies	Lesional epilepsies
Delasiauve, 1854 [1]	Epilepsie essentielle ou idiopathique	Epilepsie symptomatique
Russell Reynolds, 1861 [2]	True epilepsy, an idiopathic disease, a *morbus per se*	Symptomatic epilepsy with structural lesion
Gowers, 1881 [3]	Functional epilepsies*	Epilepsies resulting from recognisable brain disease
McNaughton, 1952 [4] Penfield & Jasper, 1954 [5]	Centrencephalic epilepsy (idiopathic)	Partial epilepsy (symptomatic)
Symonds, 1954 [6]	Central epilepsy (idiopathic, genetic)	Partial epilepsy (anatomical lesion present)

* "The only evidence of disease being the disordered function, they are termed functional disease" (Gowers, 1881 [3])

Remarkably, until recent years it had been generally accepted that the functional epilepsies are necessarily characterised by seizures generalised from the onset, reflecting a simultaneous discharge of both cerebral hemispheres. By contrast, the lesional epilepsies would necessarily be accompanied by partial seizures reflecting the existence of a localised cortical lesion.

TABLE II. Seizures specially related to functional and lesional epilepsies according to the older classifications

	Functional epilepsies	Lesional epilepsies
Gowers, 1881 [3]	Minor seizures characterised by brief loss of consciousness, brief muscle spasms or major seizures	Seizures either generalised or of local onset
McNaughton, 1952 [4] Penfield & Jasper, 1954 [5]	Petit mal; myoclonic petit mal; grand mal	Motor, sensory, psychical seizures reflecting a cortical focus
Symonds, 1954 [6]	Minimal lapses and jerks; major generalised seizures	Seizures with variable focal onset depending on location

It was not until the late 1950s and 1960s that full recognition was given to the existence of lesional epilepsies related to diffuse cortical disease causing seizures generalised from the onset, but distinct from the seizures of the functional generalised epilepsies. These generalised lesional epilepsies include the specific and especially the non-specific encephalopathies, the latter represented by West's and Lennox-Gastaut's syndromes. Such epileptogenic encephalopathies were referred to as the 'secondary generalised epilepsies' in the International Classification of the Epilepsies as proposed by us [7] to the Terminology Commission of the International League against Epilepsy in 1969 and presented to the General Assembly of the League by Merlis [8] in 1970 (Table III).

Finally, it was not until the last decade that full recognition was given to the existence of the 'idiopathic partial epilepsies' and the 'essential focal epilepsies' forecast by us [9] and by Masland [10] over 25 years ago, i.e. partial epilepsies lacking an identifiable brain lesion and resulting from a functional epileptogenic focus. The major form of such epilepsies is represented by 'partial epilepsy with motor symptoms and centro-midtemporal paroxysms' as identified in 1958 by Nayrac and Beaussard [11] and by Gibbs [12]. Thereafter, several other types have been described: 'partial epilepsy with affective symptoms and middle temporal spikes' [12,13]; 'partial epilepsy with sensorimotor symptoms and parietal spikes' [14]; 'partial visual epilepsy with occipital spike-waves' [15,16]. The grouping together of these epilepsies, particularly benign and proper to childhood and adolescence, has recently been considered [17,18]. We now propose that these functional partial epilepsies be included in the International Classification of the Epilepsies as shown in Table IV.

9

TABLE III. The current international classification of the epilepsies [7,8]

I. GENERALISED EPILEPSIES

A. Primary generalised epilepsies

1. Ictal semiology	typical petit mal absences and myoclonus; grand mal generalised at onset
2. Interictal semiology	usually absent
3. EEG	synchronous and symmetrical bilateral paroxysms with predominance of 3 c/s spike-waves
4. Aetiology	absence of identifiable aetiology, but family and patient history often suggestive of a constitutional predisposition to epilepsy

B. Secondary generalised epilepsies

1. Ictal semiology	atypical absences; tonic and atonic seizures
2. Interictal semiology	diffuse neurological symptoms frequent; mental retardation practically constant
3. EEG	diffuse or multifocal paroxysms with predominance of slow spike-waves and epileptic recruiting rhythm
4. Aetiology	relative rarity of an identifiable aetiology to account for the diffuse or multifocal cortical disorder causing the interictal symptoms

II. PARTIAL EPILEPSIES

1. Ictal semiology	partial seizures with elementary or complex semiology with or without secondary generalisation
2. Interictal semiology	frequent presence of neurological symptoms reflecting the existence of a focal brain lesion
3. EEG	focal paroxysms with predominance of spikes
4. Aetiology	often identified as the cause of the focal cortical lesion

The term 'primary partial epilepsies' has been chosen to designate the non lesional partial epilepsies we propose to include in the International Classification of the Epilepsies for the following two reasons: first, this term is appropriate in that it allows to distinguish these 'primary' partial epilepsies from those 'secondary' to a brain lesion; secondly and more importantly, this term is already used in the International Classification according to which the non lesional generalised epilepsies are referred to as the 'primary generalised epilepsies'. Terms such as 'functional' or 'benign' partial epilepsies could also have been chosen since they

TABLE IV. Proposed completion of the international classification of epilepsies

I. GENERALISED EPILEPSIES

A. Primary generalised epilepsies (or functional or benign) of childhood and adolescence

  1. Petit mal absence epilepsy

  2. Petit mal myoclonic epilepsy

  3. Grand mal epilepsy

  4. Combined petit mal and grand mal epilepsy

B. Secondary generalised epilepsies (or lesional or malignant) of infancy, childhood and adolescence

  1. Epilepsies secondary to specific encephalopathy

  2. Epilepsies secondary to a non-specific encephalopathy
      – West's syndrome
      – Lennox-Gastaut's syndrome
      – related syndromes

II. PARTIAL EPILEPSIES

A. Primary partial epilepsies (or functional or benign) of late childhood and adolescence

  1. Motor epilepsy with centro-midtemporal spikes

  2. Affective epilepsy with midtemporal spikes

  3. Sensorimotor epilepsy with parietal spikes

  4. Visual epilepsy with occipital spike-waves

B. Secondary partial epilepsies (or lesional or severe) occurring at all ages, but especially in adults

  1. Partial epilepsy with elementary semiology

  2. Partial epilepsy with complex semiology

are currently used in the world literature to designate the non lesional partial epilepsies [13–16,19–22], but we rejected these terms for the following two reasons: first, to avoid renaming, for the sake of symmetry, the non lesional generalised epilepsies known throughout the world as the primary generalised epilepsies; secondly, because all the primary epilepsies (generalised and partial) are neither exclusively functional nor entirely benign. These primary epilepsies

11

are indeed functional in that they are dependent upon a constitutional predisposition to epilepsy [17,18], characterised by a lower seizure threshold [23], reflecting a simple disturbance of brain function. They are not always exclusively functional since in certain cases the epileptic predisposition only plays an accessory role by unmasking the epileptogenic potential of a brain lesion that is too discrete to express itself spontaneously [15—18]. These primary epilepsies are indeed benign in that they 1) usually occur in children or adolescents with normal neuropsychiatric status; 2) display seizures easily managed by mild monotherapy without side effects, and 3) regress spontaneously prior to the end of adolescence. Nor are such epilepsies always entirely benign since in some cases a discrete brain lesion, whose epileptogenic potential was unmasked by a constitutional predisposition to epilepsy, can lead to interictal neuropsychiatric anomalies, and to seizures more resistant to treatment.

In similar fashion, the secondary epilepsies (generalised and partial) are not always exclusively lesional or necessarily severe, since an obvious brain lesion, e.g. post-traumatic scar tissue in adults or brain infarction leading to hemiplegia in neonates, may become epileptogenic only when the additional factor of epileptic predisposition is present. In such cases, the resulting seizures can often be easily controlled by medication.

Taking into account the preceding points, it is clear that the distinction between the functional and benign primary epilepsies on one hand, and the lesional and severe secondary epilepsies on the other hand, is more relative than absolute. It is on account of the relativity of this distinction that the Italian authors have suggested to individualise a variety of epilepsy, called 'intermediate' which would be classified between the 'primary' epilepsies and the 'secondary' epilepsies. Nevertheless, such a distinction remains highly useful. Accordingly, it is reasonable to preserve, with the present proposed complement, the International Classification of Epilepsies recommended by the International League against Epilepsy [7,8] accepted by the World Health Organization's Dictionary of Epilepsy [25] and since then adopted by all epileptologists who require a classification of epilepsies for their publications.

References

1   Delasiauve LJ. *Traité de l'épilepsie 1854.* Paris: Masson Co
2   Reynolds R. *Epilepsy; its symptoms, treatment and relation to other chronic convulsive diseases 1861.* London: J A Churchill
3   Gowers WR. *Epilepsy and other convulsive diseases: their causes, symptoms and treatment 1881.* London: J A Churchill
4   McNaughton FL. *Epilepsia 1952:* 7—16
5   Penfield W, Jasper H. *Epilepsy and the functional anatomy of the brain 1954.* Boston: Little Brown Co
6   Symonds C. *Arch Neurol Psychiat 1954; 72:* 631—637
7   Gastaut H. *Epilepsia 1969; 10:* Suppl 14—21
8   Merlis JK. *Epilepsia 1970; 11:* 114—119
9   Gastaut H. In *Encyclopédie Medico-Chirurgicale, Tome Systeme Nerveux.1951.* Paris: Les Epilepsies

10   Masland RL. *Epilepsia 1959–60; 1:* 512–520
11   Nayrac P, Beaussart M. *Rev Neurol 1958; 99:* 201–206
12   Gibbs F. In Baldwin M, Bailey P, eds. *Temporal Lobe Epilepsy 1958.*
       Springfield, Ill: C C Thomas
13   Dalla Bernardina B, Colamaria V. Bondavalli S et al. *Lega Italiana Contro l'epilessia.*
       Bolletino No. 29–30 1980; 131–138
14   De Marco P, Tassinari CA. *Epilepsia 1981; 22:* 569–575
15   Gastaut H. *Advances in Epileptology 1981.* New York: Raven Press 1982. In press
16   Gastaut H. L'épilepsie bénigne de l'enfant à pointes-ondes occipitales. *Bul Acad*
       Royale Med Belgique 1982. In press
17   Gastaut H. Individualisation des épilepsies dites 'bénignes' ou 'fonctionnelles' aux
       différents ages de la vie. *Rev Neurophysiol 1982.* In press
18   Gastaut H. In Broughton R, Gastaut H and the Marseilles School's Contribution to
       Neurosciences. *Electroenceph Clin Neurophysiol 1982.* Supp in press
19   Loiseau P, Beaussart M. *Epilepsia 1969; 10:* 23–31
20   Blom S, Heijbel J, Bergfors PG. *Epilepsia 1972; 13:* 609–619
21   Beaussart M. *Epilepsia 1972; 13:* 795–811
22   Aicardi J, Chevrie J. In *Compte-rendus Congrès Société Neurologie Infantile 1977*
23   Gastaut H. *EEG Clin Neurophysiol 1950; 2:* 249–261
24   Pazzaglia P, Giovanardi Rossi P, Cinignotta F et al. *Rivista di Neurologia 1977;*
       XLVII: 359–367
25   Gastaut H. *Dictionary of Epilepsy 1973.* Geneva: World Health Organization
       Distribution Service

3

INTERNATIONAL CLASSIFICATION OF EPILEPTIC SEIZURES: 1981 REVISION

R J Porter

The need for a uniform classification of epileptic seizures has become increasingly evident in the past several decades. This need is obvious to the physician who must prescribe medication according to seizure type; it is also apparent to the clinical investigator who wishes to evaluate the effectiveness of antiepileptic medications and then compare the findings with those of other evaluations. Neurologists often shun clinical classifications of disease, however, because they are usually derived from empirical data and have a highly suspect relationship to fundamental mechanisms. Fortunately, the empirical classification of epileptic seizures relates, at least in part, to these fundamental mechanisms. In humans, partial seizures and generalised toni-clonic seizures respond to drugs that affect seizure spread, whereas absence seizures respond to drugs that affect seizure threshold. The efficacy of these drugs can be quantitated in rodents by using the maximal electro-shock seizure test for the former drugs and the subcutaneous pentylenetetrazol seizure test for the latter agents. So far, all drugs clinically effective against seizures in humans are also effective in one of these two experimental models of seizures. The empirical classification of epileptic seizures is thus validated by both the clinical and experimental effects of antiepileptic drugs.

Classification of the epilepsies

The distinction between epileptic seizures and the epilepsies is important. Epileptic seizures are finite events that can be recorded on videotape with the electroencephalogram and easily compared with other similarly recorded attacks. The epilepsies, on the other hand, represent a variety of chronic disorders characterised by recurrent seizures. Merlis [1] has documented the extraordinary difficulty of defining the epilepsies, and has shown that many different but overlapping 'windows' are available. One might construct, for example, an aetiologically oriented classification (Table I). Another popular method of classifying the

14

TABLE I. Classification of the epilepsies: aetiology

Idiopathic epilepsy Primary epilepsy Genuine epilepsy Essential epilepsy Functional epilepsy Cryptogenic epilepsy Congenital (functional) epilepsy of maturation Metabolic epilepsy	Alcohol epilepsy Alcoholic epilepsy Post-traumatic epilepsy Traumatic epilepsy Pseudotraumatic epilepsy Post-surgical epilepsy Tumor epilepsy Tumoral epilepsy
Genetic epilepsy Genetic generalised epilepsy Hereditary epilepsy Familial epilepsy	Atherosclerotic epilepsy Post-encephalitic epilepsy Penicillin epilepsy
Symptomatic epilepsy Secondary epilepsy Focal symptomatic epilepsy Nonfocal symptomatic epilepsy Acquired epilepsy Organic epilepsy Residual epilepsy	Hypocalcaemic epilepsy Hypoglycaemic epilepsy Renal epilepsy Allergic epilepsy Gestation epilepsy

From Merlis [1]

TABLE II. Classification of the epilepsies: anatomico-physiological

Focal cortical epilepsy Cortical epilepsy	Cingulate epilepsy
Prefrontal lobe epilepsy	Insular epilepsy
Frontal lobe epilepsy Frontal epilepsy	Peri-insular epilepsy
	Multifocal epilepsy
Rolandic epilepsy	Diffuse epilepsy
Occipital lobe epilepsy Occipital epilepsy	Corticoreticular epilepsy
	Circuit-type epilepsy
Mesial hemispheric epilepsy	Reticular epilepsy
Temporal lobe epilepsy Temporal epilepsy Midtemporal epilepsy Hippocampal epilepsy Amygdaloid epilepsy Limbic system epilepsy	Subcortical epilepsy Centrencephalic epilepsy Diencephalic epilepsy Thalamohypothalamic epilepsy Hypothalamic epilepsy

From Merlis [1]

epilepsies is by the anatomic-physiologic systems involved in the central nervous system (Table II). Even precipitating factors are commonly referred to by clinicians (Table III). None of these approaches is mutually exclusive, although each has some utility in an individual patient. A unified classification of the epilepsies

TABLE III. Classification of the epilepsies: precipitant

Reflex epilepsy
  Sensory reflex epilepsy
  Sensory precipitation epilepsy
  Sensory evoked epilepsy
	Language induced epilepsy

	Graphogenic epilepsy
	Epilepsia arithmetices

Light induced epilepsy
  Light sensitive epilepsy
  Photosensitive epilepsy
  Photogenic epilepsy
  Photic induced epilepsy
  Optical epilepsy
	Vestibular epilepsy
	  Vestibulogenic epilepsy

	Somatosensory evoked epilepsy

	Movement induced epilepsy
	  Proprioceptive epilepsy
	  Kinaesthetic epilepsy
	  Kinetogenic epilepsy

Pattern sensitive epilepsy	Olfactory epilepsy
	  Rhinoepilepsy
	  Rhinogenic epilepsy

Television epilepsy	
Reading epilepsy	
Visual exploratory epilepsy	Laryngeal epilepsy
Startle epilepsy Acousticomotor epilepsy	Pleural epilepsy
	Water immersion epilepsy 'Hot water' epilepsy
Psophogenic epilepsy	Conditioned reflex epilepsy
Musicogenic epilepsy	Affective emotional epilepsy
Voice induced epilepsy	Self-induced epilepsy

From Merlis [1]

is the hope of a newly constituted commission of the International League Against Epilepsy (ILAE), and the subject of the preceding chapter in this volume by Professor H Gastaut.

Classification of epileptic seizures

By comparison with the classification of the epilepsies, the classification of epileptic seizures has proved more approachable. In 1970, the ILAE published a classification [2] based on the observation that most seizures have a definable localised onset and that others have no such locus; the former were termed partial seizures and the latter generalised seizures. The classification thus categorised most seizures as partial or generalised (Table IV). Six categories of information were used to determine the seizure type:

1. Clinical seizure type
2. Electroencephalographic seizure type
3. Electroencephalographic interictal expression
4. Anatomic substrate
5. Aetiology
6. Age

TABLE IV. 1970 International Classification of epileptic seizures

I PARTIAL SEIZURES (seizures beginning locally)

   A Partial seizures with elementary symptomatology (generally without impairment of consciousness)

     1. With motor symptoms [includes Jacksonian seizures]
     2. With special sensory or somatosensory symptoms
     3. With autonomic symptoms
     4. Compound forms

   B Partial seizures with complex symptomatology (generally with impairment of consciousness)

     [temporal lobe or psychomotor seizures]

     1. With impairment of consciousness only
     2. With cognitive symptomatology
     3. With affective symptomatology
     4. With 'psychosensory' symptomatology
     5. With 'psychomotor' symptomatology (automatisms)
     6. Compound forms

   C Partial seizures secondarily generalised

II GENERALISED SEIZURES (bilaterally symmetrical and without local onset)

     1. Absences [petit mal]
     2. Bilateral massive epileptic myoclonus
     3. Infantile spasms
     4. Clonic seizures
     5. Tonic seizures
     6. Tonic-clonic seizures [grand mal]
     7. Atonic seizures
     8. Akinetic seizures

III UNILATERAL SEIZURES (or predominantly)

IV UNCLASSIFIED EPILEPTIC SEIZURES (incomplete data)

Abstracted from Gastaut [2]

Partly because many epileptologists from around the world have consistently advocated its use, the classification has been successfully applied, especially with regard to the main headings. The term 'complex partial seizure', for example, has overtaken older terms such as 'psychomotor' or 'temporal lobe' as a more general term for the heterogeneous seizures of this group. Although the main categories were increasingly utilised, the subcategories were less successfully employed, especially in everyday clinical practice. Furthermore, in the early 1970s, the practice of acquiring videotape recorded data on seizures (Figure 1) allowed validation and re-evaluation of the 1970 classification. Fortunately, in 1970 the ILAE commission was "fully aware of the fact that all attempts at classification

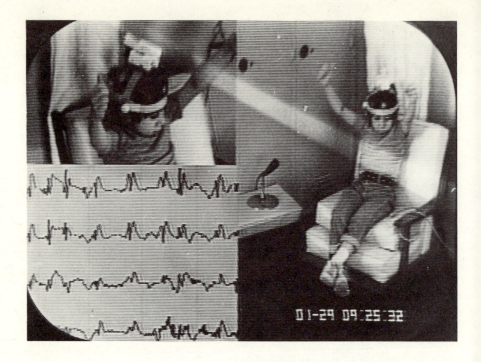

Figure 1. The split-screen video image shows a close-up view and a total-body picture of the patient having a seizure, with display of the simultaneously recorded EEG. Data from this kind of videorecording made a direct contribution to the 1981 classification

of epileptic seizures are hampered by our limited knowledge of the underlying pathological processes within the brain, and that any classification must of necessity be a tentative one and will be subject to change with every advance in the scientific understanding of epilepsy." The combination of this farsighted attitude and the availability of new scientific data allowed the evolution to the 1981 classification (Table V).

The rationale for revision of the earlier work and details of the workshops that led to the adoption of the 1981 classification have been documented [3]. The changes introduced by the 1981 classification leave the main portion of the 1970 classification intact. The changes are in fact complementary to the earlier effort and provide data to validate the majority of initial views about seizure type. The most important revisions are discussed below and summarised in Table VI.

First, the seizure classification is now based only on empirical, objective data from seizures recorded on videotape and repeatedly reviewed. The clinical seizure type, and the ictal and interictal expression on the electroencephalogram, therefore, are the only necessary criteria for classification. The 1981 classification is

18

TABLE V. 1981 International Classification of epileptic seizures

---

I   PARTIAL SEIZURES (seizures beginning locally)

    A   Simple partial seizures (consciousness not impaired)

        1. With motor signs
        2. With somatosensory or special sensory symptoms
        3. With autonomic symptoms
        4. With psychic symptoms

    B   Complex partial seizures (with impairment of consciousness)

        1. Beginning as simple partial seizures and progressing to impairment of consciousness
        2. With impairment of consciousness at onset
          (a) With impairment of consciousness only
          (b) With automatisms

    C   Partial seizures secondarily generalised

II   GENERALISED SEIZURES (bilaterally symmetrical and without local onset)

    A   1. Absence seizures
        2. Atypical absence

    B   Myoclonic seizures

    C   Clonic seizures

    D   Tonic seizures

    E   Tonic-clonic seizures

    F   Atonic seizures

III UNCLASSIFIED EPILEPTIC SEIZURES (incomplete data)

Abstracted from Commission on Classification and Terminology of the International League Against Epilepsy [3]

TABLE VI. Significant changes in the classification of epileptic seizures

---

1. Anatomic substrate, aetiology, and age are omitted as factors in determination of seizure type
2. Consciousness, operationally defined and tested, determines whether partial seizures are simple or complex
3. Seizure progression from one type to another is recognised more fully
4. Unilateral seizures are classified under partial seizures
5. Features usually observed in simple partial seizures may also occur in complex partial seizures
6. 'Compound forms', 'mixed forms', and 'akinetic' are omitted as specific seizure types

---

unabashedly a classification of the empirical event, is not dependent on anatomic substrate or aetiology, both of which are often speculative, or age. All of these factors may be important in individual diagnosis and therapy of seizures, and are appropriate considerations for classification of the epilepsies, but only empirical criteria are established for seizure classification.

Second, the differentiation between simple (elementary) and complex partial seizures is determined by the level of consciousness. The attack is considered to be simple partial when consciousness is preserved, and complex partial when consciousness is altered. Although the true meaning of consciousness remains unknown, an operational definition is quite feasible, i.e. the responsiveness or awareness of the patient. In most cases, diminished responsiveness can be documented by simple verbal questioning. In some clinical situations, such as in the presence of aphasia, the determination of consciousness may be more difficult. The use of an operational definition of consciousness is an improvement, because the critical factor (a footnote!) in the previous classification was whether the siezure involved "an organised, high-level cerebral activity" [4]. Laudable though this concept may be, this factor is not uniformly measurable and is subject to wide variations in interpretation by different observers. Alteration in consciousness usually occurs when the cerebrum is bilaterally involved. In this regard, epilepsy is just like other neurologic insults. The complex partial seizure thus implies more widespread brain involvement than does a simple partial seizure.

Third, seizure progression, especially in partial seizures, is emphasised. Many seizures are characterised by progression from one type to another, and virtually any seizure may progress to a generalised tonic-clonic seizure [5]. Partial seizures frequently progress from simple partial to complex partial to generalised tonic-clonic seizures. The possibilities for the progression of partial seizures are shown in Table VII.

TABLE VII. An overview of progression in partial seizures

(1)	SP
(2)	CP
(3)	SP → CP
(4)	SP → GTC
(5)	CP → GTC
(6)	SP → CP → GTC

SP: simple partial seizure
CP: complex partial seizure
GTC: generalised tonic-clonic seizure

Fourth, unilateral seizures are considered to be a variant of partial seizures. Even though the entity may be more frequent in young children, adults with partial seizures may also have multifocal, shifting origins of their seizures, and it was thought that unilateral seizures are not sufficiently different to warrant a separate main heading.

Fifth, features previously attributed only to simple partial seizures are also observed in complex partial seizures and are therefore permitted as criteria for their classification. For example, clonic jerking may be a common manifestation of simple partial seizures, but it can also occur during complex partial seizures. Automatisms, of course, occur only when consciousness is altered. Elementary phenomena may occur during complex partial seizures, and certain psychic phenomena, such as visual hallucinations, déjà vu, or forced thinking, may rarely occur without any measurable alteration in consciousness and, in that unusual setting, are not complex but simple partial seizures. The rationale is in the degree of spread of the discharge. The degree of localisation of visual hallucination may be no different than that of clonic jerking; if consciousness is preserved, the odds are high that the discharge has remained unilateral. Again, the 1981 classification avoids the difficulty of using 'complexity' of phenomena to determine seizure classification, and turns instead to a measurable phenomenon, the responsiveness and awareness of the patient.

Sixth, and finally, a few terms used in the earlier classification have been omitted. The concept of 'compound' or 'mixed' forms of seizures has given way to more descriptive terminology. No clinician uses these terms, and they convey nothing to the student. It is better to say that the patient had a complex partial seizure with tonic stiffening of the left side followed by automatisms and gradual return to normal responsiveness than to say that the patient had a complex partial seizure, compound form. The term 'akinetic' has also been omitted. Akinetic, meaning without motion, has been used synonymously with atonic for many years. The latter term, implying sudden loss of postural tone, has been retained. Motionlessness is clearly a feature of many types of seizures, and is not a specific seizure type.

Summary

The 1981 Classification of Epileptic Seizures more nearly approaches the seizure history taken by clinicians the world over. It is based on the clinical data from videotaped seizures. It builds on the 1970 classification and is complementary to it.

Acknowledgment

The editorial assistance of B J Hessie is gratefully acknowledged.

References

1   Merlis JK. *Acta Neurol Latinoam 1972; 18:* 42–51
2   Gastaut H. *Epilepsia 1970; 11:* 102–113
3   Commission on Classification and Terminology of the International League Against Epilepsy. *Epilepsia 1981; 22:* 489–501
4   Gastaut H. *Epilepsia 1969; 10:* 3–6
5   Porter RJ, Sato S. In Akimoto H, Kazamatsuri H, Seino M, eds. *Advances in Epileptology: XIIIth Epilepsy International Symposium 1982.* New York: Raven Press. In press

4

THE CLASSIFICATION OF EPILEPTIC SEIZURES (ILAE)

M Parsonage

Introduction

The need for an agreed classification of epileptic seizures has long been recognised and particularly so in recent years. This need has been emphasised by the continuing growth of interest in epilepsy and the corresponding growth in the volume of publications concerned with its many aspects. This growth has undoubtedly led to considerable increase in knowledge and understanding bringing with it an inevitable demand for increased precision in terminology. With its long history the study of epilepsy has, over the years, led to the introduction of a great variety of terms many of which have been in use for a very long time and some of them have outlived their usefulness. In fact, their very age and wide usage has made them household terms and ingrained them indelibly in the minds of almost everyone who has worked in the field of epilepsy. It might even be said that they have become almost hallowed to the extent that it would seem almost sacrilegious to suggest that some of them might be allowed to lapse, or at least be modified and redefined. Nevertheless, it is essential that, as far as possible, changes in terminology should keep pace with advances in knowledge and the question at issue is what changes, if any, should be made at the present time.

For many years, leading internationally known investigators have addressed themselves to the problem of the classification of seizures. They must surely have found it an arduous, even thankless, task since criticisms of their efforts have been neither lacking nor easy to refute. On the other hand, in some circles, attempts at devising classifications of this kind have often received little attention, even total disregard, but whether this be due to rejection coupled with antipathy to change, or perhaps to nothing more than mere disinterest, has never been very clear.

For my part I feel bound to applaud the efforts of those who have tried to construct systematic classifications of seizures, being in no doubt of the need.

Generally speaking, such attempts have been based on established neurophysiological principles without losing sight of the need for them to be so orientated that clinicians will find them both acceptable and useful. This is not easy to achieve since there are areas where the neurophysiological basis may not be well founded and it is here that the views of experienced clinicians can be of great value with their direct experience of epilepsy in everyday practice.

In this chapter I would like first to deal with the classification of seizures which was devised by the ILAE Commission on Terminology and Classification, under the chairmanship of Professor Gastaut, and subsequently published in Epilepsia in 1969 [1]. While accepting the impossibility of achieving perfection, I believe this classification has much to commend it and it would seem fair to say that it has achieved wide acceptance over the years. Indeed, it has survived in spite of considerable criticism from several quarters but much of this seems now to have lost its force. It is certainly not without significance that such terms as 'complex partial seizure' have successfully withstood attack and have acquired a familiarity rivalling that of some of the older terms, and they will not now be lightly discarded.

In the next part of this chapter is outlined the main features of the revised classification which the ILAE recently elected to recommend for international use, despite serious objections to some of the proposals and, finally, I shall try to give an account of the reasons why I believe this latest attempt at revision to be unsatisfactory in certain respects.

ILAE classification of epileptic seizures (1969)

An earlier ILAE scheme of classification of seizures proposed by its Commission on Terminology was first published in Epilepsia in 1964 [2]. In the following year, in response to various criticisms, it was modified by an enlarged Commission the results of whose deliberations were subsequently published in their final form in Epilepsia in 1969 [1], as stated earlier. The members of the Commission were at pains to point out at that time that any attempt at classification must be regarded as a tentative one in view of the limitation of knowledge with regard to the underlying pathological processes within the brain, and that modifications would be necessary in the future as scientific knowledge advanced.

The recommended 1969 ILAE scheme of classification is based on five main criteria, namely, clinical seizure type, electroencephalographic (EEG) seizure type, EEG interictal expression, anatomical substrate, aetiology and age. The four main groups (outlined in Table I) are as follows:

I. *Partial seizures* – or seizures beginning locally.
II. *Generalised seizures* – bilateral symmetrical seizures or seizures without local onset.
III. *Unilateral or predominantly unilateral seizures.*
IV. *Unclassified epileptic seizures.*

TABLE I. ILAE classification of epileptic seizures (1969)

I.   *PARTIAL SEIZURES OR SEIZURES BEGINNING LOCALLY*

   A.   With elementary symptomatology
   B.   With complex symptomatology
   C.   Secondarily generalised

Seen at all ages but with increasing frequency with increasing age.

II. *GENERALISED SEIZURES, BILATERAL SYMMETRICAL SEIZURES OR SEIZURES WITHOUT LOCAL ONSET*

Seen at all ages.

III. *UNILATERAL OR PREDOMINANTLY UNILATERAL SEIZURES*

Seen only in the newborn and in very young children.

IV. *UNCLASSIFIED EPILEPTIC SEIZURES*

Insufficient data to enable classification

TABLE II. ILAE classification of epileptic seizures (1969)

I.   *PARTIAL SEIZURES OR SEIZURES BEGINNING LOCALLY*

   i)   Initial clinical changes indicate activation of *an anatomical and/or functional system of neurones limited to a part of a single hemisphere.*

   ii) EEG patterns *restricted at least at their onset to one region of the scalp (the appropriate cortical area).*

   iii) *Initial neuronal discharge* usually originates *in a narrowly limited or even quite diffuse cortical part of such a system*

Partial seizures (Table II) are defined as those in which the first clinical signs indicate activation of an anatomico-functional system of neurones limited to a part of a single hemisphere. Initially the accompanying EEG discharge is localised, the underlying neuronal discharge usually originating in a narrowly limited but sometimes in a relatively diffuse cortical portion of such a system. This group is further subdivided into two sub-groups — those with elementary and those with complex symptomatology.

Partial seizures with elementary symptomatology, subsequently usually referred to as *simple partial seizures,* (Table III) are still further subdivided into those with motor, special sensory or somatosensory and autonomic symptoms with a

24

TABLE III. ILAE classification of partial seizures (1969)

A. *PARTIAL SEIZURES WITH ELEMENTARY SYMPTOMATOLOGY*
(Generally without impairment of consciousness)
1. *WITH MOTOR SYMPTOMS* – focal motor, Jacksonian, versive, postural, somatic inhibitory (?), aphasia, phonatory.
2. *WITH SPECIAL SENSORY OR SOMATO-SENSORY SYMPTOMS* – somato-sensory, visual, auditory, olfactory, gustatory, vertiginous.
3. *WITH AUTONOMIC SYMPTOMS*
4. *COMPOUND FORMS* – a joining together of elementary or (and/or) complex symptoms.

fourth group designated as compound forms. Characteristically, these seizures are regarded as consequent upon local cortical neuronal discharge arising in the appropriate area, they are generally unassociated with impairment of consciousness and are due to a variety of structural lesions in which constitutional factors may be important. These seizures are encountered at all ages, but their frequency increases as age advances.

Partial seizures with complex symptomatology, nowadays commonly termed *complex partial seizures,* comprise five primary types which are listed in Table IV. They are termed complex because they are characterised by disruptions of cognition, emotional experience, etc, and usually have a unilateral or bilateral

TABLE IV. ILAE classification of partial seizures (1969)

B. *PARTIAL SEIZURES WITH COMPLEX SYMPTOMATOLOGY*
1. *WITH IMPAIRED CONSCIOUSNESS ALONE*
2. *WITH COGNITIVE SYMPTOMATOLOGY*
    i) with *dysmnesic* disturbances (conscious amnesia, 'déjà vu', 'déjà vécu')
    ii) with ideational disturbances (including 'forced thinking', dreamy state . . .)
3. *WITH AFFECTIVE SYMPTOMATOLOGY*
4. *WITH 'PSYCHOSENSORY' SYMPTOMATOLOGY*
    i) *illusions* (e.g. macropsia, metamorphopsia . . .)
    ii) *hallucinations*
5. *WITH 'PSYCHOMOTOR' SYMPTOMATOLOGY*
    automatisms
6. *COMPOUND FORMS*

origin in temporal or fronto-temporal cortex. Related subcortical and rhinencephalic structures may also be involved and the accompanying EEG discharges are corresponding unilateral or bilateral, as well as being either focal or diffuse in the frontal and fronto-temporal regions. Their causes and age incidence are similar or identical with those of simple partial seizures.

Finally, in category C provision is made for the fact that all types of partial seizure may become *secondarily generalised,* sometimes so rapidly that their focal features may be clinically unobservable (Table V). The manifestations of such seizures may be symmetrical or asymmetrical and most commonly assume tonic-clonic form.

TABLE V. ILAE classification of partial seizures (1969)

C. *PARTIAL SEIZURES SECONDARILY GENERALISED*

all forms of partial seizure, with elementary or complex symptomatology, can develop into generalised seizures, sometimes so rapidly that the focal features may be unobservable. These generalised seizures may be symmetrical or asymmetrical, tonic or clonic, but most often tonic-clonic in type.

TABLE VI. ILAE classification (1969)

II. *GENERALISED SEIZURES, BILATERAL SYMMETRICAL SEIZURES OR SEIZURES WITHOUT LOCAL ONSET*

  i) *Clinical features do not include any sign or symptom referable to an anatomical and/or functional system localised in one hemisphere,* usually consist of initial impairment of consciousness, motor changes which are generalised or at least bilateral and more or less symmetrical and may be accompanied by autonomic discharge.

  ii) EEG patterns are from the start *bilateral,* grossly *synchronous* and *symmetrical* over the two hemispheres.

  iii) Responsible neuronal discharge is *bisynchronous* and *involves most of if not the entire central grey matter.*

The basic features of *generalised seizures* are listed in Table VI and they may have either convulsive or non-convulsive symptomatology. Their EEG accompaniment is a bilateral, essentially synchronous and symmetrical discharge from the onset but their primary anatomical substrate is unknown. Their causes are related to diffuse or multiple bilateral lesions and also to constitutional factors and toxi-metabolic disturbances in varying combinations.

The essential representatives of the *non-convulsive* group of generalised seizures

26

TABLE VII. ILAE classification of absences (1969)

1. *ABSENCES*
   (a) *SIMPLE ABSENCES* — with impairment of consciousness only
        Typical — with 3Hz spike-wave discharge
        Atypical — with fast rhythm or slow spike waves

   (b) *COMPLEX ABSENCES* — with other phenomena associated with impairment of consciousness. May be typical or atypical as in (a):
        i)   *myoclonic* — mild clonic components
        ii) *hypertonic* — increased postural tone
        iii) *atonic* — diminished or abolished postural tone
        iv) *automatic* — with automatisms
        v)   *autonomic* — with autonomic phenomena
        vi) *as mixed forms*

are the absences (Table VII). These may be either *simple* when impairment of consciousness is the only manifestation or *complex* when they are associated with other phenomena such as mild clonic components (myoclonic absences), increase or diminution of postural tone (retropulsive and atonic absences, respectively), automatisms (automatic absences) and autonomic phenomena (e.g. enuretic absences). All these associated phenomena may occur either alone or in combination. Furthermore, all types of absence may be either *typical* ('petit mal') when accompanied in the EEG by rhythmic 3Hz spike and wave discharges and *atypical* (variant of 'petit mal') when accompanied by either low voltage fast activity or by more or less rhythmic discharges of sharp and slow waves. There are also distinguishing clinical features between typical and atypical absences [3].

Generalised seizures of the *convulsive variety* are subdivided into eight types

TABLE VIII. ILAE classification of generalised convulsive epileptic seizures (1969)

2. *BILATERAL MASSIVE EPILEPTIC MYOCLONUS* — myoclonic jerks
3. *INFANTILE SPASMS*
4. *CLONIC SEIZURES*
5. *TONIC SEIZURES*
6. *TONIC-CLONIC SEIZURES* — 'grand mal' seizures
7. *ATONIC SEIZURES* — sometimes associated with myoclonic jerks (myoclonic-atonic seizures)
        (a) of very brief duration (epileptic drop attacks)
        (b) of longer duration (including atonic absences)
8. *AKINETIC SEIZURES* — loss of movement without atonia.

(Table VIII), namely bilateral myoclonic epileptic myoclonus (all ages), infantile spasms (infants only), clonic seizures (especially in children), tonic seizures (especially in children), tonic-clonic seizures (all ages except infancy), atonic seizures of either very brief or longer duration (especially in children) and, finally, akinetic seizures (especially in children).

TABLE IX. ILAE classification of epileptic seizures (1969)

III. *UNILATERAL OR PREDOMINANTLY UNILATERAL SEIZURES*

    i)   Clinical aspects are analagous to those of Group II, except that *the clinical signs are restricted principally, if not exclusively, to one side of the body.*

    ii)   EEG aspects analagous to those of Group II and *the discharges are recorded over the contralateral hemisphere.*

    iii)   Apparently depend upon *a generalised or at least very diffuse neuronal discharge which predominates in, or is restricted to, a single hemisphere* and its subcortical connections.

In the case of unilateral seizures (Table IX) the clinical and EEG aspects are analogous to those of generalised, bilaterally symmetrical convulsive seizures in Group II, except that they are expressed either predominantly or only on one side, sometimes shifting from one side to the other but usually not becoming symmetrical. Consciousness may or may not become impaired in these seizures and they are seen almost exclusively either in very young children or in the newborn. In those virtually limited to the newborn the EEG accompaniments are partial discharges which are variable both in form and in location. On the other hand, in those unilateral seizures seen almost exclusively in very young children, the accompanying EEG discharges are either partial, spreading very rapidly over only one hemisphere (contralateral seizures only), or are discharges which are generalised from the start but are markedly predominant over one hemisphere, with a tendency to change from one side to the other from one moment to another (alternating seizures). Anatomically, these seizures may be of unilateral or bilateral cortical or subcortical origin or unlocalisable. As regards aetiology they may be due to a variety of organic lesions (focal or diffuse) and to constitutional, toxic and metabolic causes operating in a setting of cerebral immaturity.

TABLE X. ILAE classification of epileptic seizures (1969)

IV. *UNCLASSIFIED EPILEPTIC SEIZURES*

    Includes all seizures which cannot be classified because of inadequate or incomplete data

---

Group IV are the *unclassified epileptic seizures* (Table X) and in the *addendum* it is pointed out that seizures may also be classified according to their frequency as follows:

(1) *Isolated epileptic seizures* which may be of any type but are usually generalised tonic-clonic seizures provoked by some accidental cause in subjects predisposed to convulsions.

(2) *Repeated epileptic seizures* occurring under a variety of circumstances: fortuitous, cyclic or provoked by non-specific factors or by sensory factors.

(3) *Prolonged repetitive seizures (status epilepticus)* — a fixed and enduring epileptic condition in which the frequently occurring seizures may be generalised, partial or unilateral.

Comment

My main criticism of this otherwise useful and comprehensive classification of seizures mainly concerns those listed under the heading of partial seizures with complex symptomatology. I would regard the first of these which is said to be characterised only by impaired consciousness as a doubtful entity since in most if not all cases it could be regarded as a component of other types of seizure, especially automatisms. In the second place, I think it would be preferable to regard seizures with 'psychomotor' symptomatology as generalised in nature rather than as manifestations of relatively localised cerebral discharge. In my later commentary I have referred to the evidence for this contention in view of its relevance to some of my objections to the 1981 revised ILAE classification.

My only other criticism of the ILAE 1969 classification is the inclusion among generalised seizures of infantile spasms (a syndrome rather than a specific type of seizure) and of akinetic seizures since there is some doubt as to whether or not it should be regarded as a separate entity.

Recommended ILAE classification of seizures (1981)

Since 1975 two further ILAE Commissions on Classification and Terminology have endeavoured to update and amend the 1969 Classification. To facilitate this task workshops were convened in Bethesda (1975) and in Berlin (1977) in order to study complex partial seizures and generalised seizures respectively. Finally, a new Commission was constituted in 1979, a further video workshop being set up to deal with variations of absence seizures, and it was assigned the task of completing the development of a revision of the 1969 ILAE Classification of Seizures based on a study of videotapes of simultaneously recorded electrical and clinical manifestations of epileptic seizures. The Commission was also charged with obtaining a majority approval of the amended classification of the active

Chapters of ILAE and also of other pertinent international societies, and of promoting its use throughout the world. The Commission was also given additional tasks which are not of immediate concern here.

The proposals of the 1975 Commission on Terminology were widely circulated for consideration and were subsequently published in Epilepsia in 1981 [4]. Finally, they were presented at the General Assembly of ILAE on the occasion of the 13th Epilepsy International Symposium held in Kyoto in September 1981. After some discussion they were accepted on the basis of a majority vote although this was opposed by representatives of five active Chapters from West Europe whose criticisms were of a fundamental nature and have not yet been met in my opinion. Indeed, I do not think that the issues raised can be lightly dismissed and it would be very desirable if some way of reconciling opposing views could be found.

The Commission has stressed that they consider their classification to be weighted clinically and that it should not be construed as 'representing the last word in the identification of the origin of the epileptic seizure, its spread through the cerebrum, or its elaboration in the mobilisation of this or that structure in its propagation'. Such stress seems hardly necessary since the incompleteness of knowledge in this sphere is so widely recognised and I am not yet satisfied that the new classification can really be regarded as a worthwhile improvement on its 1969 predecessor.

In the 1981 amended Classification of Epileptic Seizures, instead of the five basic criteria previously adopted, only clinical seizure type and ictal and interictal EEG data have been retained as criteria. The reason given for this change is the supposition that 'anatomical substrate, aetiology and age factors are largely based on historical or speculative information rather than information based on direct observation'. A fundamental new departure is the separation of partial seizures into simple and complex varieties on the basis of whether or not consciousness is disturbed. This is claimed to permit what is termed 'a longitudinal description of evolving seizure manifestations, thereby improving descriptive accuracy'. It is thereupon proposed that the term 'complex' be used in a different context, namely, to designate only those partial seizures which are associated with impairment of consciousness, irrespective of whether they commence with elementary (simple) or what has up to now always been designated complex symptomatology and arising in higher integrative (interpretive) cerebral cortex. In conjunction with this new use of the term 'complex' those seizures characterised by dysphasic, dysmnesic, cognitive and affective manifestations (grouped collectively under the term 'psychic symptoms') are now classified as 'simple partial seizures'.

The general outline of the 1981 ILAE Classification of Seizures is set out in Table XI. From this it will be seen that the group of unilateral seizures included in the 1969 scheme of classification has been omitted altogether. The sub-grouping of partial seizures is arranged in accordance with the distinction between

30

TABLE XI. ILAE classification of epileptic seizures (1981)

I.   *PARTIAL (FOCAL, LOCAL) SEIZURES*

    A. *Simple partial seizures*
       1. With motor signs
       2. With somatosensory or special sensory symptoms
       3. With autonomic symptoms or signs
       4. With psychic symptoms

    B. *Complex partial seizures*
       1. Simple partial onset followed by impairment of consciousness
       2. With impairment of consciousness at onset

    C. *Partial seizures evolving to secondarily generalised seizures*

II.   *GENERALISED SEIZURES (CONVULSIVE OR NON-CONVULSIVE)*

    A. 1. *Absence seizures*
       2. *Atypical absence*
    B. *Myoclonic*
    C. *Clonic*
    D. *Tonic*
    E. *Tonic-Clonic*
    F. *Atonic*

III.   *UNCLASSIFIED SEIZURES*
    Inadequate data or defy classification

IV.   *ADDENDUM*
    Repeated seizures occurring under a variety of circumstances

---

TABLE XII. ILAE classification of epileptic seizures (1981)

A. *SIMPLE PARTIAL SEIZURES*
   1. *With motor signs* – focal, motor, Jacksonian, versive, postural, phonatory
   2. *With autonomic symptoms or signs*
   3. *With somatosensory or special sensory symptoms (simple hallucinations, e.g. tingling, light flashes, buzzing)* – somatosensory, visual, auditory, olfactory, gustatory, vertiginous
   4. *With psychic symptoms (disturbances of higher cerebral function)* – dysphasic, dysmnesic, cognitive, affective, illusions, structured hallucinations

simple and complex seizures on the basis of whether or not consciousness is impaired, whereas the category of secondarily generalised seizures is retained although re-defined as will be seen later.

The amended classification of *simple partial seizures* is shown in Table XII and here the important point to note is that this sub-group now includes seizures having dysphasic, dysmnesic, cognitive, affective and psychosensory features, the latter including seizures characterised by illusions and 'structure hallucinations'. It will be recalled that such seizures are classified as 'complex' in the 1969 classification on the basis that they are manifestations of highly organised cortical function.

TABLE XIII. ILAE classification of epileptic seizures (1981)

B. *COMPLEX PARTIAL SEIZURES* (with impairment of consciousness; may sometimes begin with simple symptomatology)

  1. *SIMPLE PARTIAL ONSET FOLLOWED BY IMPAIRMENT OF CONSCIOUSNESS*

    (a)   With simple partial features (A1−A4) followed by impaired consciousness

    (b)   With automatisms

  2. *WITH IMPAIRMENT OF CONSCIOUSNESS AT ONSET*

    (a)   With impairment of consciousness only

    (b)   With automatisms

In Table XIII it will be seen that in the first type in the sub-group of *complex partial seizures* the onset may be characterised by any of the features listed under the heading of simple partial seizures (A1−A4), ranging from those with simple motor signs to those characterised by structured hallucinations. In the second type there is impairment of consciousness at the onset which may be either the only manifestation and both types may be associated with an automatism. It is clear therefore that impairment of consciousness is to be regarded as a feature common to all these seizures.

With regard to the *secondary generalisation of partial seizures* (Table XIV),

TABLE XIV. ILAE classification of epileptic seizures (1981)

C. *PARTIAL SEIZURES EVOLVING TO GENERALISED TONIC-CLONIC SEIZURES (GTC)*

  1. Simple partial seizures (A) evolving to GTC

  2. Complex partial seizures (B) evolving to GTC

  3. Simple partial seizures evolving to complex partial seizures evolving to GTC

    (GTC − generalised tonic-clonic seizures)

---

this is shown as becoming manifest in two main ways. Firstly, either a simple or a complex seizure may merge into a generalised tonic-clonic convulsion. Secondly, a simple partial seizure may evolve initially into a complex partial seizure, impairment of consciousness presumably resulting, and then finally into a generalised tonic-clonic seizure.

TABLE XV. ILAE classification of generalised seizures (1981)

A. 1. *Absence seizures* – with impairment of consciousness or with clonic, atonic, tonic or autonomic components or with automatisms, occurring alone or in combination
   2. *Atypical absence* – more pronounced changes of tone than in absence seizures. Onset and/or cessation not abrupt

B. *Myoclonic seizures* – (single or multiple)

C. *Clonic seizures*

D. *Tonic seizures*

E. *Tonic-clonic seizures*

F. *Atonic seizures* (Astatic)

(Combinations of the above may occur)

All varieties of *generalised seizure* are included in Group II of the 1981 Classification and are listed in Table XV. As in the 1969 ILAE Classification, they are sub-divided into non-convulsive (A) and convulsive (B–F) but it will be noted that both infantile spasms and akinetic seizures are omitted from the list.

As before, the *absence* remains as the essential representative of the non-convulsive sub-group which is further subdivided, not into simple and complex varieties as previously, but into absence and atypical absence seizures. The former may occur either with impairment of consciousness alone or in association with mild clonic, atonic, tonic and autonomic components as well as with automatisms occurring either alone or in combination. As regards the *atypical absence,* it is stated that any associated changes of tone are more pronounced than when associated with typical absence seizures and that either the onset or the cessation, or both, may be gradual. However, it is not specifically stated whether or not consciousness is impaired in these so-called atypical absence seizures.

The varieties of *convulsive seizure* are listed as myoclonic (a single or multiple myoclonic jerks), clonic, tonic, tonic-clonic and atonic (astatic). These may occur alone or in combination (Table XV).

Finally, in Group III are contained the *unclassified seizures* and in the addendum (IV) there is reference to *repeated seizures* which may be fortuitous, cyclic or provoked by non-sensory and sensory factors. Also included in the addendum are *prolonged or repetitive seizures* coming under the heading of status epilepticus

33

which is here defined as that state in which seizures occur so frequently that recovery in the intervening periods does not occur. These states may be of either the partial or generalised varieties and are no longer defined as 'fixed or enduring' as in the ILAE 1969 classifications.

Comment

The concept of epileptic seizures as 'occasional, sudden, excessive, rapid and local discharges of grey matter' which Hughlings Jackson [5] developed so extensively has more than proved its usefulness over the years. Indeed, its validity has been repeatedly confirmed by the results of modern scientific and clinical research and in this context I think that the monumental contributions made over many years in this field by Wilder Penfield and his colleagues [6] have not always been given their full due.

Although modern researches have led to some modification of older views we can still use the basic concept of the epileptic seizure as the direct consequence of abnormal neuronal discharge. This may be either generalised from its onset or have a relatively localised onset yet also possessing a natural propensity to become widely diffused as to amount to secondary generalisation. To the clinician the site of origin of relatively localised seizure discharge is particularly important in the detection of the local lesion, whereas the generalised seizure discharge, whether this be a primary or secondary phenomenon, is of less immediate importance in the sense that generalisation of discharge is a phenomenon which is at least potentially common to all seizures wherever or however they may arise.

In recent years, on the basis of his experimental studies, Gloor [7] has advanced the interesting concept of a 'first degree' of epileptogenesis in which there is a basic state of mild diffuse cortical neuronal hyperexcitability which responds abnormally to afferent thalamo-cortical volleys normally involved in the elicitation of spindles or recruiting responses. This is regarded as the neurophysiological basis of the generalised seizure of which the EEG sign is the spike-wave pattern of discharge. On the other hand Gloor conceives the focal cortical epileptogenic lesion as a 'second degree' of epileptogenesis which is the basis of the partial or focal seizure and which may in natural circumstances exist in isolation or in association with a tendency to generalised seizure discharge. Such a concept as this serves to remind us of the way in which our understanding of epileptic phenomena is gradually changing and it seems not unlikely that classifications of the future will need to move in the direction of a more unified conception of epileptic phenomena.

If the terms 'focal' and 'local' are still to be used synonymously with the term 'partial' in the classification of seizures, then it can still be maintained that its key feature is its local sign reflecting local or regional disruption of cortical function, and that its precise pattern is determined by its site of origin and by the particular function of the area of cerebral cortex involved. The terms simple and complex have long been based on the established neurophysiological principle that there is an hierarchy of cortical function ranging from the relatively simple to the highly organised. For example, so-called association or interpretive cortex subserves much more highly organised functions than is the case with primary motor and sensory cortex located in the precentral and postcentral areas. The use of the term 'complex' in relation to seizures involving intellectual function in its widest sense is therefore soundly based just as is the use of the term 'simple' in relation to seizures involving disturbances of primary motor, sensory and autonomic function.

It seems to me unwise, as in the 1981 Classification, to give the term complex an entirely different connotation, applying it solely to those partial seizures in which there is impairment of consciousness. This seems more than likely to be a source of confusion and I believe it to be a mistake to limit to one class of seizure a feature which can be associated with any kind of seizure, no matter where or how it may originate. I also find it equally difficult to accept the recommendation that seizures characterised by disturbances of language, cognition and affect, and even those giving rise to illusory and hallucinatory experiences should now be designated 'simple' partial seizures. Such functions are complex in both clinical and neurophysiological senses and could hardly be deemed otherwise.

I am also of the opinion that the whole question of the validity of distinguishing between simple and complex partial seizures on the basis of whether or not consciousness is impaired is very debatable. In this context we are handicapped by not having an adequate definition of the term 'consciousness', and we still have much to learn about its neurophysiological basis. The Commission's definition of it seems to me to be far too limited. In the appended glossary it is defined as 'the degree of awareness and/or responsiveness of the patient to externally applied stimuli', this being termed an 'operational' definition. Responsiveness is defined as 'the ability of the patient to carry out simple commands or willed movements and awareness as the patient's contact with events during the period in question'. These also seem to me to be definitions which are too restricted. Furthermore, it is hard to see how consciousness itself could be regarded as a degree of anything, although it is admittedly a phenomenon characterised by wide variations in degree. As a clinician I would prefer a much broader concept of consciousness, regarding it as a function of the brain as a whole and embodying both awareness of self and of environment as well as responsiveness, while accepting that these may all exhibit variability. Furthermore, I would regard retention of the ability to recall retrospectively experiences occurring during any episode as an indication of conscious awareness, although temporary loss of this function does not exclude consciousness during the time of the episode in question. However, the members of the Commission appear to take the view that an individual who exhibits awareness but is unresponsive (and who is presumably by definition suffering from impairment or loss of consciousness) will nevertheless be able to recount the events which occurred during a seizure. Such awareness

35

should be equated with consciousness in my view but, clearly, there is likely to be continuing debate about these issues for some time. In the meantime I would submit this as another reason for regarding it as inadvisable to differentiate seizures on the basis of whether or not consciousness is affected, given our present state of incomplete understanding of this state.

I realise, of course, that there are other ways of looking at the problem of consciousness in relation to partial seizures. For example, during the course of these seizures perceptual, hallucinatory and emotional experiences may so disturb the content of consciousness that the individual's attention may be rivetted upon them [8]. In these circumstances he may than appear to show reduced awareness of his environment as a result of his pre-occupation with his mental experiences but this might also be ascribed to reduced attentiveness to his environment. Indeed, it has frequently been my clinical experience that individuals in these circumstances can readily recall their experiences, yet at the same time maintaining awareness both of self and of environment during the episode in question. On the other hand, when there is amnesia for the events of the attack which is associated with automatic behaviour, then I believe it could be fairly claimed that the individual was unconscious during the event in the broadest sense of the term. In other words, he was unaware both of self and environment as well as being amnesic for everything that occurred during the episode. Such a state could hardly be a part of a partial seizure, so long as the seizure discharge has remained relatively localised.

There is, in fact, much which indicates that loss of awareness and automatic behaviour do not occur until seizure discharge has involved the amygdalo-hippocampal complex bilaterally with invariable spread to the mesodiencephalon and temporo-parietal cortex, often with involvement of the frontal and central areas as well [9,10]. Account must also be taken of the fact that automatisms may be initiated by discharging lesions in frontal and even parietal cortex and in cortex on the medial surface of the cerebral hemispheres [11,12] as well as in the temporal lobes, the commonest site of origin. In these circumstances the indications are that the initiating focal discharge, wherever it may be situated, spread to the anteromedial temporal lobe structures, especially the amygdala, and thereafter to the mesodiencephalon and thence widely to cerebral cortex via the diffuse projection system of the upper brain stem. It also has to be remembered that essentially similar, even identical, ictal automatisms may occur in association with either a generalised spike-wave discharge or, less commonly, with a widespread, rhythmic slow wave discharge in the fronto-temporal regions. In these circumstances the latter appears to be a primary discharge not initiated by a cortical source of discharge in the temporal regions or elsewhere [6].

There is therefore a considerable body of evidence indicating that when true impairment or loss of consciousness supervenes during the course of a seizure, the discharging process, wherever it arose, has become widely diffused by activation of antero-medial temporal lobe and upper brain stem structures and their diffuse projection systems. On the basis of such neurophysiological considerations I believe it can be maintained that those partial seizures designated as complex in category B in the 1981 ILAE scheme of classifications (Table XIV) could more properly be classified as partial seizures which have become secondarily generalised. In other words, they should be included in category C and not be regarded as a separate sub-group.

The revised classification of *generalised seizures* (Table XV) introduces no fundamental changes. The omission of infantile spasms I would regard as acceptable on the grounds that it is in reality a syndrome rather than representative of a single type of epileptic seizure. Furthermore, the so-called akinetic seizure would appear to be such a questionable entity as to justify its omission also and I believe that the point is rightly made that the various types of generalised seizure may occur in combination.

Finally, there is the question of the omission of *unilateral seizures* as a group. Those who would like the classification to be comprehensive would probably prefer to see it retained. Its omission means that there is no place for those types of seizure seen exclusively in the newborn and in very young children and my personal preference would be for the retention of this category.

Conclusion

The positive value of classifications of epileptic seizures, whatever their merits, is that they serve to stimulate thought and discussion. At the same time they underline the need for further research, both experimental and clinical, into the

TABLE XVI. Suggested classification of partial seizures

---

1. *MOTOR* - focal motor (with or without Jacksonian march), versive, postural, phonatory
2. *SENSORY* - somatic, visual, auditory, olfactory, gustatory, vertiginous
3. *AUTONOMIC* -
4. *AFFECTIVE* - fear, depression, range, elation
5. *PSYCHIC (MENTAL, PSYCHOLOGICAL)* -
       (i)   Dysphasic
       (ii)   Cognitive - dysmnesic, ideational
       (iii)   Affective
       (iv)   Psychosensory - perceptual illusions, hallucinations
6. *COMPOUND FORMS* -
7. *SECONDARILY GENERALISED* - automatisms, generalised motor manifestations
       (most commonly tonic-clonic sequences)

---

neurophysiology of seizures which remains, as ever, a fascinating and challenging field of endeavour. I have discussed this matter elsewhere [13] and, for the time being at least, there might be some merit in adopting a somewhat simplified method of classifying partial seizures, possibly along the lines set out in Table XVI. Such a scheme, admittedly much simplified, dispenses with the terms 'simple' and 'complex' and emphasises what I believe to be a fundamental feature of any seizure, namely, its site and mode of origin. For those who do not feel that ictal automatisms have sufficient claims to be regarded as generalised seizures, I would suggest that either some alternative to the term 'secondary generalisation' might be devised, or that automatisms be included in the group of seizures having 'compound form'. The latter are, in fact, the most commonly occurring types in the whole group of partial seizures.

In conclusion, many may feel that this is still not the time to make any radical changes in the 1969 ILAE Classification, despite its imperfections, and that a revised scheme should await the acquisition of new knowledge. This too has much to be said for it but, whatever happens, it is most important that the whole matter should continue to excite discussion and provide a stimulus for thought and research.

References

1   Clinical and electroencephalographic classification of epileptic seizures. *Epilepsia 1969; 10:* Suppl 2–13
2   Clinical and electroencephalographic classification of epileptic seizures. *Epilepsia 1964; 5:* 297–306
3   Gastaut H, Broughton R. *Epileptic Seizures – Clinical and Electrographic Features, Diagnosis and Treatment 1972;* 64–85. Springfield, Illinois: Charles C Thomas
4   Proposals for revised clinical and electroencephalographic classification of epileptic seizures. From the Commission on Classification and Terminology of the International League Against Epilepsy. *Epilepsia 1981; 22:* 489–501
5   Jackson JH. In Taylor J, ed. *Selected Writings of John Hughlings Jackson 1931; 1:* 90–117
6   Penfield W, Jasper H. *Epilepsy and the Functional Anatomy of the Human Brain 1954; Chapter XIII.* London: J & A Churchill
7   Gloor P. *Epilepsia 1979; 20:* 571–588
8   Gloor P, Olivier A, Ives J. In Canger R, Angeleri F, Penry JK, eds. *Advances in Epileptology: XI Epilepsy International Symposium 1980;* 349. New York: Raven Press
9   Jasper HH. *Epilepsia 1964; 5:* 1–20
10   Penfield W. In Jasper HH, Ward AA, Pope A, eds. *Brain Mechanisms of the Epilepsies 1969;* 791. London: J & A Churchill Ltd
11   Geier S, Bancaud J, Talairach J et al. *Brain 1976; 99:* 447–456
12   Fenton GW. *Irish Medical Journal 1980; 73 (No. 10):* 11–19
13   Parsonage M. *Irish Medical Journal 1980; 73 (No. 10):* 1–6

5

CLASSIFICATION OF STATUS EPILEPTICUS

H Gastaut

No classification of status epilepticus existed until the early 1960s for the simple reason that this term was applied to a single, indivisible entity, i.e. the "état de mal épileptique" as defined by Calmeil in 1824 [1] by the following features: 1) successive grand mal seizures; 2) coma and neurovegetative disturbances between seizures; 3) risk of fatal outcome. Such a definition was still accepted in the main texts on epilepsy in 1954 [2] and 1960 [3], whereas other forms of 'status epilepticus' had been considered earlier, chiefly 'petit mal status' [4] and 'temporal lobe status' [5].

The current classification, widely used across the world, was established in 1962, at the 10th Colloquium of Marseilles, based on 237 electro-clinical observations of status reported by 103 contributors. This classification was published in the Colloquium Proceedings [6], the Handbook of Neurology [7], the Handbook of EEG and Clinical Neurophysiology [8] and was adopted by the International League Against Epilepsy in an addendum to its international classification of seizures [9] and by WHO in its Dictionary of Epilepsy [10]. For an extensive review of this international classification, the reader is referred to a recent article with complete bibliography and EEG iconography [11].

EPITOME OF THE CURRENT CLASSIFICATION OF STATUS EPILEPTICUS

This classification was established after adopting a new definition of status epilepticus also adopted by the ILAE and WHO: "The term *status epilepticus* is used whenever a seizure persists for a sufficient length of time or is repeated frequently enough to produce a fixed and enduring epileptic condition". This definition implies a semiological classification including: 1) as many varieties of status as there are types of seizures; 2) grouping of these varieties in three major categories, i.e. 'generalised', 'partial' and 'unilateral' status.

I Generalised status epilepticus (SE)

A Convulsive generalised SE

1. Tonic-clonic SE or 'grand mal status' Corresponds to historical status epilepticus. Two subtypes are currently recognised:

(a) Grand mal status with seizures generalised from the onset, occurring usually in patients with known primary generalised epilepsy or, exceptionally, in non-epileptics, due to acute metabolic, toxic or infectious brain disease.

(b) Grand mal status with secondarily generalised partial seizures, occurring in patients with known partial epilepsy or, as frequently, in non-epileptics with a focal brain lesion displaying latent epileptogenic potential (referred to as 'isolated' or 'lone' status epilepticus).
  EEG recordings during status are of prime importance for differentiating between grand mal seizures with a partial or a generalised onset.

2. Tonic SE Occurring almost exclusively in children with known. secondary generalised epilepsy (usually Lennox-Gastaut syndrome), it can be easily distinguished from the preceding variety by: 1) occurrence in children rather than adults; 2) much longer duration; 3) exclusively tonic symptomatology of seizures accompanied on EEG by the typical bursts of recruiting epileptic rhythm; 4) more frequent repetition of seizures; 5) more discrete neurovegetative symptoms between seizures; 6) much better prognosis.

3. Clonic SE Occurring almost exclusively in infants and young children, it features: 1) bilateral clonic convulsions, either synchronous, symmetrical and rhythmically repeated or asynchronous, asymmetrical and arhythmically repeated; 2) EEG with bilateral synchronous slow waves mixed with epileptic recruiting rhythm yielding occasional spike-waves patterns. Prognosis depends on aetiology: benign when 'cryptogenic', i.e. occurring in apparently normal children, often during hyperthermia, severe (even fatal) when secondary to an acute brain lesion.

4. Myoclonic SE Based on aetiology, syptomatology and prognosis, two distinct types can and should be identified.

(a) Myoclonic SE arising in the course of primary generalised epilepsy. This well-defined type of status features: 1) massive bilateral myoclonus arythmically repeated, often in clusters, without impairment of consciousness; 2) bilateral synchronous multiple spike-waves on EEG; 3) benign course.

(b) Myoclonic SE arising in the course of very severe subacute or acute encephalopathies in non-epileptics (metabolic encephalopathy, especially anoxic; toxic encephalopathy, especially methylbromide; viral encephalopathy, especially Creutzfeldt-Jakob disease; degenerative encephalopathy, especially

neurolipidosis). In complete opposition to the preceding type, this SE features:
1) massive bilateral myoclonus periodically repeated, with impairment of
consciousness (often coma); 2) periodic generalised spikes or sharp waves on
EEG; usually fatal outcome.

B Non-convulsive generalised SE

1. Absence status Occurring almost exclusively in patients with, or having
presented, primary or secondary generalised epilepsy, it features: 1) more or less
profound obnubiliation, eventually accompanied by some discrete bilateral myoclonus; 2) generalised symmetrical and synchronous spike-waves (fast or slow,
continuous or intermittent) on EEG; 3) benign course.
Absence status can be divided into:

(a) Typical absence status (alias 'petit mal status' or 'spike-wave stupor'),
uncommon, related to primary generalised epilepsy and featuring solely
obnubiliation associated with rhythmic 3 c/s spike-waves, either continuous
(like a long lasting typical absence) or in bursts (like closely repeated typical
absences).

(b) Atypical absence status (alias 'minor epileptic status' or 'epilepsia minoris
continua'), much more frequent, related to secondary generalised epilepsy and
featuring: 1) obnubiliation with or without myoclonus and/or tonic seizures;
2) continuous rhythmic slow spike-wave (2 c/s) or, more often, slow dysrhythmia interspersed with fast or slow spike-waves.

2. Atonic and akinetic SE Uncommon entities occurring in infants and young
children, often in the course of fever, featuring: 1) loss of tone or loss of movement without atonia accompanied by loss of consciousness; slow dysrhythmia
interspersed with spike-waves; benign course.

II Partial status epilepticus

According to whether the symptomatology of the repeated seizures is elementary
or complex, two main types are recognised:

A Elementary partial SE

Theoretically, there are as many varieties as there are types of elementary partial
seizures, but only two varieties have been well identified:

1. Somatomotor SE On the basis of aetiology, symptomatology and prognosis,
two distinct types can and should be recognised:

41

(a) Somatomotor SE stricto-sensu, *occurring in patients with known somato-motor partial epilepsy or in non-epileptics with a focal brain lesion in the central region.* This well-defined type of status features: 1) somatomotor seizures, with or without Jacksonian march, repeated several times per hour and exceptionally associated with interictal focalised myoclonus (Kojewnikov's syndrome or epilepsia partialis continua); 2) intact state of consciousness; 3) more or less perceptible EEG ictal discharges in the controlateral central region; 4) favourable outcome.

(b) So-called somatomotor SE, arising in non-epileptics with severe brain lesion outside the central region (contusion, metastasis and especially water-shed (interterritorial) infarction). In complete opposition to the preceding type, these SE features: 1) massive myoclonus occurring periodically about one a minute, never accompanied by true somatomotor sezures; 2) severe symptomatology between seizures, often coma; 3) 'periodic lateralised epileptiform discharges' (PLEDs) in the controlateral temporo-parieto-occipital (but not central) region; 4) very severe outcome.

2. Dysphasic or aphasic SE Characterised by the repetition of aphasic seizures with EEG ictal discharges in the temporal region of the dominant hemisphere. Two subtypes have been identified according to:

(a) language disturbances occurring only during seizures, thus allowing the patient normal speech between seizures;

(b) language disturbances peristing during the interictal period.

In the latter case, the episode of aphasia is obvious and does not go overlooked by the observer, whereas in the former subtype the disturbance may be missed since aphasia lasts only 10 to 20 seconds every two or three minutes. Accordingly, aphasic status may possibly be much more frequent than currently believed.

B Complex partial SE

Occurring almost exclusively in patients with temporal lobe epilepsy it features: 1) more or less marked obnubiliation often associated with abnormal mood, hallucinations and/or automatisms; 2) more or less diffuse ictal EEG discharges predominating in temporal region. For these reasons and until recently such SE was called 'psychomotor status', 'status psychomotoricus' or 'temporal lobe status', but these terms are becoming less used as the term 'psychomotor epilepsy' is discarded and the exclusively temporal origin of complex partial seizures refuted. Accordingly, the term to be used is 'complex partial SE' with reference, when possible, to the anatomical origin of the discharge, e.g. 'temporal' or 'frontal' complex partial SE.

III Unilateral status epilepticus

A Hemiclonic SE

Peculiar to very young children it features: 1) clonic convulsions involving the entire right or left body half, but with frequency and amplitude which may vary from one segment to another; 2) progressive deterioration of consciousness; 3) slow waves mixed with epileptic recruiting rhythm yielding occasional spike-waves on the controlateral hemisphere. Prognosis depends on aetiology: benign when status is 'cryptogenic', occurring in apparently normal children, often during hyperthermia; severe (even fatal) when secondary to an acute brain lesion. But the most benign 'cryptogenic' hemiclonic SE may result in permanent hemiplegia (HH syndrome), often associated with consecutive partial epilepsy (HHE syndrome), when status is not arrested in its early stages. For these reasons unilateral SE is one of the most important neuropaediatric emergencies.

B Erratic SE

Usually discussed along with unilateral SE, this type of status should logically be considered as separate due to certain peculiar characteristics. Erratic SE is exclusive to neonates and is characterised by the repetition of seizures featuring: 1) low amplitude convulsions involving restricted parts of the body (e.g. hemifacial or only palpebral fissure, chin or tongue) and thus is often unnoticed; 2) localised ictal discharges on EEG, often changing from one part of a hemisphere to another part of the same or opposite hemisphere without a strict correspondence to the site of the convulsions. Outcome is unfavourable in most cases, especially when SE occurs during the first three days of life, consistently secondary to a severe antenatal or neonatal lesion. Conversely, erratic SE which arises after the fourth postpartum day (often 'cryptogenic' or secondary to a metabolic disturbance) has a more favourable prognosis.

ANOTHER TENTATIVE CLASSIFICATION OF STATUS EPILEPTICUS

The current classification of SE presents the advantages and disadvantages of being exclusively based on symptomatology. The obvious disadvantage is that such a classification is unstable and is interpreted differently according to one's perception of the symptoms. The advantage is that it precisely corresponds to the current international classification of epileptic seizures, a feature which is of particular usefulness to epileptologists, i.e. those who are specialists in the diagnosis and treatment of all forms of epilepsy occurring at all ages. However, aside from this small group of specialists, the present classification may be problematical for paediatricians, who are not familiar with epilepsy in adults, and for neurologists, who are unfamiliar with childhood epilepsy. Accordingly it would appear useful, as a tentative classification, to briefly present the semiological forms of SE as a function of the affected age group and prognosis.

I SE in neonates (first month of life)

1. Erratic SE, by far the most frequent. The prognosis is often very poor, especially when it occurs soon after birth.

2. Myoclonic SE with 'burst suppression'. Exceptionally observed, commonly related to hyperglycinaemia, the outcome is fatal.

II SE in infants and young children

During the first six years of life, the different types of SE are related to their component seizures. The following can be identified:

1. Clonic SE and hemiclonic SE, by far the most frequent. Prognosis is entirely different according to whether SE occurs in a) a child with an acute brain lesion or chronic encephalopathy, or b) a normal subject during the course of hyper-thermia. In the latter case, where the prognosis is much better, it should be emphasised that prolonged clonic, and chiefly hemiclonic, febrile status can leave very severe sequelae if not quickly arrested by parenteral administration of a benzodiazepine.

2. Tonic SE has a guarded prognosis because it does not necessarily respond to treatment and, in exceptional cases, can lead to death.

3. Atonic and akinetic SE, exceptional and consistently benign, since spontaneous arrest occurs within a few hours.

4. Absence SE presents a benign, short term prognosis since it yields to parenteral benzodiazepine after a few seconds or minutes. The long-term prognosis is not worse, even when absence SE is observed in secondary generalised epilepsy associated with progressive mental retardation, because the latter finding is not directly related to the presence or the degree of absence status.

III SE in older children and adolescents

Throughout these years of transition, SE progresses from the typical childhood forms to those of the adult. Accordingly:

1. Absence SE and tonic SE are still encountered, whereas

2. Clonic, hemiclonic, atonic and akinetic SE are no longer observed.

3. Myoclonic SE of primary generalised epilepsy belong to this age group as well as myoclonic SE of degenerative diseases.

4. Tonic-clonic SE with seizures generalised from the onset, occurring in patients with known generalised epilepsy is relatively frequent.

5. Partial SE, especially with elementary sumptomatology, begins to appear.

IV SE in adults and the elderly

After adolescence, SE is practically limited to the following types:

1. Tonic-clonic SE, especially with secondarily generalised seizures occurring in patients with or without chronic partial epilepsy.

2. Myoclonic SE secondary to metabolic or viral encephalopathy (especially anoxic and Creutzfeldt-Jakob disease).

3. Elementary partial SE, especially somatomotor SE *stricto-sensu* in epileptics as well as so-called somatomotor SE in non-epileptics with severe brain lesion.

4. Complex partial SE, especially temporal lobe SE.

5. Absence SE is exceptionally encountered, almost exclusively at the menopause in women who often have a personal or family history of primary generalised epilepsy.

It would be unfortunate to adopt simultaneously two different types of classification for the same series of entities so, for this reason, we suggest retaining the current semiological classification of status epilepticus, supplementing it with aetiopathogenic, prognostic and therapeutic considerations for a clearer understanding when necessary.

References

1   Calmeil L. *De l'Epilepsie, thèse Paris, 1824*
2   Penfield W, Jasper H. *Epilepsy and the Functional Anatomy of the Human Brain 1954*. Boston: Little-Brown
3   Lennox W. *Epilepsy and Related Disorders 1960*. Boston: Little-Brown and Co
4   Lennox W. *JAMA 1945; 129:* 1069–1073
5   Gastaut H, Roger J, Roger A. *Rev Neurol 1956; 94:* 298–301
6   Gastaut H, Roger J, Lob H. *Les Etats de Mal Epileptiques 1967*. Paris: Masson et Co pub
7   Roger J, Lob H, Tassinari C. In Vinken J, Bruyn GW, eds. *Handbook of Clinical Neurology Volume 15 1974*. New York: Elsevier
8   Gastaut H, Tassinari C. In *Handbook of Electroenceph·Clin Neurophysiol Volume 13 A 1975*. Amsterdam: Elsevier
9   Gastaut H. *Epilepsia 1970; 11:* 102–113
10   Gastaut H. *Dictionary of Epilepsies 1973*. Geneva: World Health Organisation
11   Gastaut H. In Delgado-Escueta A, ed. *Status Epilepticus*. New York: Raven Press. In press

6

SEIZURE DISORDER IN THE NATIONAL CHILD DEVELOPMENT STUDY

E M Ross, Catherine S Peckham

Most studies of convulsive disorders in childhood have been confined to relatively small populations [1—5], mainly hospital admissions or general practices, and the use of these two very different types of population has resulted in conflicting findings. Children with complicated convulsions are the most likely to be admitted to hospitals, so that hospital studies tend to exaggerate the severity of epilepsy, whilst general practice studies under-report the problems, especially among those hidden away in long-term institutions.

Large, cross sectional studies overcome the problems of selection and, in the last 20 years, several have been carried out in the United Kingdom [6, 7], USA [8], Iceland [9], Finland [10] and Australia [11]. These studies suggest that the prevalence of convulsive disorders in school children is in the order of 3.2 to 7.2 per 1,000 (Table I). Although these cross sectional studies demonstrate the prevalence of epilepsy at various ages and the extent of associated problems, cohort studies which start from birth are required to explore aetiology and, hopefully, prevention as well as the long-term prognosis, but there have been few such studies since they are time consuming, expensive and (in the USA) subject to legal constraints.

In the USA, Van den Berg [12] followed 19,000 births to women who were insured with the Kaiser Permenante health care scheme in the period 1960—1967 and described the patterns of seizure disorder occurring during their first six years. As part of the Collaborative project in the USA, Nelson and Ellenburg [13] reported seizure disorders occurring in the first seven years among the 54,000 children born in the period 1959—1966 to mothers delivered in 12 university centres. Cooper [14] reviewed seizures that occurred during the first 11 years of life in a subsample of 3,934 children from the 1946 perinatal study which included all births in England, Scotland and Wales in a single week in 1946. Follow-up of children from the 1958 and 1970 perinatal studies in the UK, which included all births in a single week in these two years, was also carried out, and were more

46

TABLE I. Prevalence of epilepsy in school children from cross sectional studies

Investigator	Country	Age group (years)	Population	Number with epilepsy	Rate per 1,000
Cooper (1965)	England, Scotland and Wales	11	3,934	23	7.1
Crombie et al (1960)	England and Wales	10–14	22,336	88	3.9
Gudmundsson (1966)	Iceland	10–19	32,872	143	4.3
Hauser (1975)	Rochester, USA	10–19	8,198	9	3.6
Ross (1980)	Bristol	11–16	25,165	110	4.3
Rutter et al (1970)	Isle of Wight	5–14	11,865	86	7.2
Sillanpaa (1973)	Turku, Finland	10–15	108,019	340	3.2

ambitious in scale in that details of seizures and other developmental problems were sought for all children. In this chapter we discuss some findings from the 1958 cohort study with particular reference to the natural history of convulsive disorders which first presented as febrile convulsions. Results from the 1970 cohort study are reported in the next chapter.

The National Child Development Study (NCDS) 1958 cohort [15]

During one week in March 1958, midwives in England, Scotland and Wales completed precoded questionnaires on 98 per cent of all deliveries. Extensive details were obtained on maternal health, complications of pregnancy, delivery method, and condition of the baby during the first week of life. Over 90 per cent of surviving children were traced at ages 7, 11 and 16. Children born abroad in the same week were also included.

At each follow-up the children were examined by school doctors who completed a health questionnaire after a detailed physical examination. Health visitors completed a sociological schedule which included a medical history and information about the child's family and living conditions. An educational schedule was also completed by the head or class teacher who administered some educational tests and supplied information on the child's school performance.

At each follow-up stage a series of questions were asked to ascertain whether the child had ever had any form of seizure and, if so, details of its nature and treatment. All the records of children reported to have had convulsions were scrutinised by a paediatrician who categorised them into the following groups: (i) temper tantrums, breath-holding or other non-epileptic forms of altered consciousness, (ii) febrile convulsions of a non-complicated type lasting less than 15 minutes (iii) complicated febrile seizures or non-febrile epileptic disorders. Further information was sought from general practitioners and hospital consultants for all children with more than one fit, those who had any seizures after their fifth birthday, who were on anticonvulsant medication, had electroencephalography performed, or were known to have attended or were awaiting admission to special schools.

This data included details of diagnosis, treatment, investigations, restrictions on lifestyle, possible aetiological factors and prognosis.

The prevalence of convulsive disorders

By their eleventh birthday 1,043 children (6.7 per cent) had experienced at least one episode of altered consciousness (Table II).

TABLE II. Diagnostic categories of children in the National Child Development Study with seizure disorders in their first eleven years, n = 15,496

Category	Total	Number per 1,000
'Established' epilepsy	64	4.1
Epilepsy reported by doctor but unsubstantiated	39	2.5
Febrile convulsions without later afebrile seizures	346	22.3
Febrile convulsions with later spontaneous afebrile seizures	20	1.3
Convulsions with meningitis or encephalitis	12	0.8
Breath-holding attacks, faints without convulsions, temper tantrums	280	18.1
Non-epileptic blank spells (confirmed by general practitioner or hospital)	7	0.5
Transitory afebrile convulsive episode not occurring after age five years	307	20.6
Convulsions reported by parent but not to general practitioner or hospital	12	0.8

The largest group of 606 children (58 per cent) had non-convulsive problems including transitory episodes of fainting, breath-holding attacks or temper tantrums; these children suffered no long-term disadvantages and are not discussed further in this chapter.

As many as 103 children (6.6 per 1,000) were regarded by at least one doctor as having epilepsy, but only 64 (4.1 per 1,000) of these fulfilled the study criteria of epilepsy which was 'recurrent paroxysmal disturbance of consciousness, sensation, or movement, primarily cerebral in origin, unassociated with acute febrile episodes'.

One or more seizures occurred in the course of a febrile extracranial illness in 366 children (2.4 per cent). Twenty of these children subsequently had afebrile

48

fits and are therefore also included among the 64 with epilepsy together with 24 children with fever associated fits who were regarded by their doctors as having 'epilepsy' but did not fulfil the study criteria. A further 12 children had seizures solely in the course of bacterial or viral intracranial infections.

Febrile convulsions

Febrile convulsions are now attracting a great deal of much needed research interest after years of neglect. Ellenberg and Nelson [16] reviewed seven population studies and found that the proportion with later afebrile seizures was in the narrow range 1.5 per cent to 4.6 per cent whilst 19 clinic based studies gave rates of between 2.6 per cent and 76.9 per cent. This reinforces the danger of basing clinical teaching purely on experience gained within hospital walls. Annegers et al [17] stressed that research studies have not used consistent definitions of convulsions to decide which should be regarded as febrile. Many children with fits get a concomitant rise in temperature which makes it difficult for clinicians to categorise the problem, particularly if there is no clear evidence of infectious illness. Lewis et al [18] found that 83 per cent of children with fever associated fits (compared with 40 per cent of those with enteric symptoms) harboured at least one potentially pathogenic virus which raises the possibility that some of these children may have encephalopathic conditions. The report of proceedings of a recent conference in the USA [19] discussed the nature of febrile convulsions and stressed that much confusion about their sequelae had resulted from the uncritical acceptance of non-controlled hospital studies which resulted in findings which contrasted greatly from those derived from whole population based studies. At this conference it was decided that febrile convulsions should be re-defined as 'benign, self limiting entities which in the absence of other predictors of neurologic damage do not presage epilepsy or other significant neurologic deficits'. This definition, which is a departure from the earlier more pessimistic viewpoint that had been widely held, is in line with findings from the 1958 cohort.

By the age of 11 years, 366 children (2.4 per cent) in the 1958 cohort were reported to have had at least one febrile convulsion. Over one third of this group (45 per cent boys, 35 per cent girls) had recurrent febrile convulsions and 20 (6 per cent) had at least one febrile fit followed by a non-febrile seizure. The 366 children included 205 boys (56 per cent) and 161 girls (44 per cent), but this slight excess of boys was not significant at the 5 per cent level. There was no excess of children with febrile convulsions among those from the lower socioeconomic groups. The size of family and the child's position in the family were no different in the febrile convulsion group compared with the rest of the cohort which suggests that intercurrent family infections were unlikely to be a major factor in the aetiology of fits.

Among the 322 with uncomplicated febrile convulsions there was no significant excess in the proportion with a birthweight below 2.0kg as compared with the rest of the cohort nor were the perinatal factors, such as presentation, length of the first and second stages of delivery, any more frequent.

Over a quarter of the children (93) had a history of seizures in their family. Unfortunately family history was not obtained from the whole cohort in the same detail making control data unreliable, but there is no certainty that those parents with unaffected children would know their family histories so well.

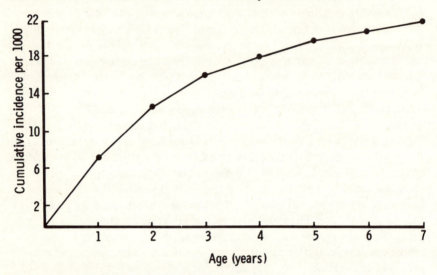

Figure 1. Cumulative incidence of febrile convulsions over the first seven years of life (NCDS 1958 cohort)

The cumulative incidence of febrile seizures is shown in Figure 1, whilst the age of onset of first fit is shown in Table III. There is no significant difference in pattern of onset between the sexes. Over half of the children had their first fit by their second birthday though in 11 per cent the first fit occurred after five years of age. Table IV shows the age of the last febrile fit among those who had multiple febrile fits; a quarter had their last fit after age seven and 7 per cent had a febrile fit after age eight.

Among the 322 with uncomplicated febrile convulsions, 12 (3.7 per cent) were receiving some form of special education by age 11, a proportion similar to the study norm. From the results of educational tests carried out at 7 and 11 to assess reading ability, mathematical attainment and general ability, the children with uncomplicated febrile convulsions did as well at school as children who had never had fits. Similarly their behaviour patterns at school as judged by their teacher was similar to that of children with febrile fits.

TABLE III. Age at first febrile convulsion

	BOYS (n = 201)					
Years	Single fit		More than one febrile fit		Total	
	Number	%	Number	%	Number	%
< 1	27	24.3	37	41.1	64	31.8
One	26	23.4	23	25.5	49	24.4
Two	18	16.2	14	15.5	32	15.9
Three	17	15.3	5	5.5	22	11.0
Four	6	5.4	5	5.5	11	5.5
Five +	17	15.3	6	6.7	23	11.4
Total with information*	111	100	90	100	201	100

	GIRLS (n = 157)					
< 1	28	27.5	19	34.6	47	29.9
One	27	26.5	15	27.3	42	26.8
Two	16	15.7	11	20.0	27	17.2
Three	8	7.8	3	5.5	11	7.0
Four	14	13.7	3	5.5	17	10.8
Five +	9	8.9	4	7.3	13	8.3
Total with information*	102	100	55	100	157	100

* Age of first fit not known in four boys and four girls of whom four had single fits and two multiple attacks

TABLE IV. Age at last febrile attack by onset age for children with multiple febrile convulsions

Age at onset (in years)	Age at last convulsions (in years)		One	Two	Three	Four	Five	Six	Seven	Eight	Nine	Ten+	Total with information
< 1	17	13	5	7	6	1	3						52
One		13	7	4	1	1	3	4	1	2			36
Two			10	7	5	2							24
Three				3	3	1							7
Four					2	3	3						8
Five +						1	6	1	1		1		10
Total with information	17	26	22	21	17	9	15	5	2	2	1		137

Note: Eight children are excluded from this table because the age of attacks is not known

TABLE V. Febrile convulsions and place of treatment

	Single fit		Multiple fit		Total	
	Number	%	Number	%	Number	%
Treated at home	131	64.9	71	35.1	202	100
Treated at hospital	86	53.1	76	46.9	162	100
TOTAL	217	59.6	147	40.4	364	100

(Fit frequency not known for two cases)

	At home		In hospital (at least once)		Total	
	Number	%	Number	%	Number	%
Boys	104	50.7	101	49.3	205	100
Girls	98	60.1	63	39.1	161	100
TOTAL	202	55.2	164	44.8	366	100

Table V shows the proportions of children treated at home and referred to hospital. Slightly more boys went to hospital than girls. Only one in 202 (0.5 per cent) children managed entirely at home by their general practitioners had later, non-febrile epilepsy by 13 years compared with 19 (12 per cent) of the 164 investigated in hospital. Continuing home and hospital treatment children gives a non-febrile recurrence rate by 13 of 5.5 per cent. These findings demonstrate that children with febrile fits who go to hospital have a more severe pattern of illness than those who remain at home and that studies based only on hospital admissions give only partial insight into the nature of the disorder.

Non-febrile epilepsy

There were 35 boys and 29 girls (4.1 per 1,000) with a history of epilepsy defined as two or more spontaneous afebrile seizures. Table VI shows their seizure pattern, which is diverse and emphasises that epilepsy in childhood should not be regarded as a single clinical entity. Table VII shows the age of onset during the first 10 years of life; information from the current 33 year follow-up on the cohort should identify the cases that have occurred subsequently.

The progress of 59 of the 64 children was followed-up to the age of 16 years. No information was available on five: two who had emigrated but had been doing well at 11 years, two were untraced but were at special schools at 11 years, and one belonged to a gypsy family, who had received little education at 11 years.

Thirty-seven of the 59 children (63 per cent) were educated in the normal

TABLE VI. Seizure patterns of the 64 children with epilepsy

	Male Number	Female Number	Total Number
Grand mal only	17	18	35
Grand and petit mal	4	5	9
Petit mal alone	1	–	1
Psychomotor/Temporal lobe seizures only	2	–	2
Changing pattern of seizure	11	6	17
Total number of children	35	29	64

TABLE VII. Age of first fit among the 64 children with epilepsy

	Years										
	<One	One	Two	Three	Four	Five	Six	Seven	Eight	Nine	Ten+
Number	15	2	6	8	8	3	8	5	5	1	3
%	23.4	3.1	9.4	12.5	12.5	4.7	12.5	7.8	7.8	1.6	4.7

educational system and results of the 16 year performance tests in this group were available for 34. Their mean reading comprehension score of 20.8 and mean mathematical attainment score of 9.9 were not significantly different from the study norms of 25.3 and 12.3 respectively. Only eight of these 37 children (22 per cent) attending normal schools had experienced a fit in their sixteenth year. In contrast, 13 of the 22 children (59 per cent) receiving special education were still having fits in their sixteenth year. These 22 children were placed in a wide variety of special schools. Fifteen were in special schools for educational backwardness (11 had been ascertained as ESN (moderate) and four as ESN (severe)). Two were in schools for physical handicap and four were in residential schools for children with epilepsy. One child was placed in a special remedial class in a normal school. The patterns of handicap among those educated in normal and special schools were very different and those who attended normal schools at 16 had a much more favourable outcome than those who required special education.

Disputed epilepsy

Although 103 children (6.6 per 1,000) were regarded by at least one doctor to have epilepsy, 39 did not fulfil the study definition. This group included 24 (14 boys and 10 girls) who presented with febrile fits and had no later afebrile seizures.

These are included among the 366 children with febrile convulsions. The average age of first fit among these 24 children was 29.4 months and the last fit 52.3 months. At 16 years, 20 were educated in ordinary schools. Of four (17 per cent) who attended special schools, two had cerebral palsy, one grossly hyperkinetic behaviour, and the other an emotional disorder. Many of these children had been prescribed anticonvulsants for many years after their last fit.

The remaining 15 children (11 boys and 4 girls) with a disputed diagnosis of epilepsy had afebrile seizures. The first fit occurred at a mean age of 38.9 months and the last fit at a mean age of 63.9 months. Nine (60 per cent) attended special schools and six normal schools. These children were not included among those with epilepsy because three had only single seizures, two recurrent breath-holding attacks, two had behavioural or hysterical problems. The remaining six had less clear cut problems including abdominal pain, seizures during acute meningitis or acute dehydrating illness. By age 16, three of these children had further seizures, one then would have fulfilled our criteria for diagnosing epilepsy. It appears that episodes of altered behaviour are more likely to be regarded as epilepsy in a retarded than a mentally normal child. This temptation should be resisted because it tends to cloud the public image of epilepsy and overstates its association with severe retardation.

Febrile convulsions and subsequent epilepsy

Ueoka et al [20] in a prospective Japanese study carried out EEGs on 255 children following a febrile convulsion. Within seven years, 12 (4.8 per cent) had developed non-febrile seizures. Their EEGs taken prior to their first non-febrile fit showed atypical 3 cps spike and wave bursts. They mainly had absence of or benign focal nocturnal seizures.

In the present study, 5.5 per cent of the children (12 boys and 8 girls) whose first fit had been associated with fever had later spontaneous seizures. Some authorities believe that febrile convulsions cause brain damage that can lead to later non-febrile fits and therefore advise long-term anticonvulsants as a preventative measure after a first convulsion. However, 14 of the 20 children had only a single febrile fit.

The mechanism by which some children first have febrile fits and later develop afebrile epilepsy remains obscure. Since one third of the 64 children with epilepsy in the NCDS initially had a febrile seizure it is important that the association be explored further through more detailed whole population studies. It is possible that some initial febrile seizures are intrinsically different from typical febrile convulsions. If this is the case then efforts should be made to distinguish the two types of child as early as possible. Nelson [13] accepted only fits lasting under 15 minutes as typical febrile convulsions but we did not have sufficiently precise records of timing to make this estimation.

The mean age of first febrile fit among our group of 20 was rather late at

TABLE VIII. The 20/64 children with epilepsy presenting with febrile fits

Age of first fit		Age of most recent fit		Type of School	Epilepsy type	Additional features
Years	Months	Years	Months			
				GIRLS		
0	< 2	9	4	N	Grand mal	Maternal bleeding < 28 weeks
0	6	8	4	N	Grand mal	–
4	6	10	4	ESN	Grand mal	Maternal fits at age 11 years
4	0	11	0	SSN	Grand mal	Microcephaly, cerebral palsy, 8th child < 2000gm
3	6	12	10	ESN	Grand mal	2nd of twins, birthweight 2–2.5kg. Intrauterine growth retardation (IUGR)
1	9	13	0	ESN	Petit mal and Grand mal	Birthweight < 2500kg
2	0	8	0	N	'Indefinite'	First fit with chicken pox
2	9	12	7	ESN	'Indefinite'	Mother had severe pre-eclampsia. Paternal fits until 25 years
				BOYS		
2	2	8	0	N	Grand mal	Maternal fits at age 11 years. Maternal bleeding 28 weeks. Gestation 34 weeks. Birthweight 1.5–2kg
2	0	10	10	ESN	Grand mal	–
2	0	12	11	Epilepsy	Grand mal	–
0	3	13	8	ESN	Grand mal	Maternal petit mal
4	1	12	0	ESN	Grand mal	Birthweight < 2500kg. 34 weeks gestation
0	11	7	9	N	Petit mal and Grand mal	Maternal fits until age 7 years
0	11	9	12	N	Petit mal and Grand mal	Fetal distress, forceps delivery –
5	9	7	2	N	Petit mal and Grand mal	Birthweight < 2500kg. IUGR
4	2	13	2	N	Petit mal and Grand mal	Otitis media, transient hemiplegia with first fit
5	0	6	0	N	'Indefinite'	First fit with measles
6	9	9	0	N	'Indefinite'	
0	9	8	0	N	'Indefinite'	First fit with gastroenteritis

32 months. Eleven had grand mal, four had a mixed form including both petit and grand mal. The remaining five had 'indefinite' forms which could not be put into a definite category. None had clear evidence of temporal lobe epilepsy. Eleven children were attending normal schools and nine were receiving special educational provision. This suggests again that the children with uncomplicated fits are different from those destined to develop epilepsy.

These findings do not suggest any easy method of predicting the one child in 750 born who will initially present with a febrile convulsion and then later have non-febrile seizures, though a wide range of perinatal problems, a family history of fits and late presentation of first fits appear to be relevant features (Table VIII).

Of the 20 who developed spontaneous epilepsy after febrile fits, nine had been started on anticonvulsants immediately after their first febrile fit and a further three after their second. Eventually the whole group were given them though one child stopped treatment against advice, after a month.

Possibilities for prevention

There is a dearth of published information on the prevention of epilepsy, which reflects the fact that this is a very difficult area to explore. Thomas in 1972, addressing a conference on the theme of prevention of epilepsy, could only find three relevant papers in the literature on the prior 25 years and a personal search of relevant literature shows that this is still a neglected field. It is often difficult to be certain whether a child's convulsive disorder did or did not follow some well remembered accident or illness. Birth injuries are often held to be the cause of epilepsy, but Illingworth [21] has suggested that most abnormalities in the new-born are due to pre-existing fetal abnormalities and not due to birth trauma. This view is supported by an analysis of the birth histories of the 64 in the NCDS with epilepsy. Of the 10 singleton infants with birthweight below 2.5kg, three had gross congenital malformations and another had a fractured skull at five months. The mean age of first fit in the non-malformed group was 42 months. This late onset suggests that low birthweight on its own was not the cause. Five children, however, had a combination of adverse perinatal factors which when considered together were regarded as possibly contributing to the child's cerebral problems and have been accepted as 'causes of epilepsy'. Of the many factors in pregnancy and delivery studied, only maternal bleeding before 28 weeks gestation was signifi- cantly more common than the study norm.

As a result of the great improvements in maternal care and wellbeing since 1958, particularly the prevention of rhesus disease, perinatal factors may now be an even less likely cause of seizure. On the other hand, many more very low birth-weight babies are now surviving and, although there is no evidence that they are particularly prone to develop epilepsy, it is important to monitor this group. Four children developed epilepsy following meningitis or encephalitis, one following a head injury and two had congenital abnormalities of a type known to be associated with epilepsy, but it is exceedingly difficult to be certain that an insult to the brain was truly the cause of a child's epilepsy, a matter of great medico-legal significance. As an illustration one child had a first fit two days after a hit on the head by a cricket bat but investigations were negative. The same difficulties apply when a child develops seizures after immunisation or other medical procedure. Immunisations are given at the very age when febrile seizures are most common. Tunstall-Pedoe and Rose [22] calculated that one in 7,500 children has a first febrile fit in any given ten day period when they are in the age range six to nine months. Although 90 per cent of children in the NCDS had pertussis immunisation, none of those known to have developed epilepsy had evidence of recent pertussis immunisation. One child had a febrile fit in the course of measles and another during chicken pox; both went on to develop later spontaneous seizures.

Despite detailed scrutiny of the considerable amount of prospectively collected data and follow-up material available we could find no definite cause for epilepsy in 49/64 cases (73 per cent) (Table IX). We regarded seven (10 per cent) children as having a cause for their epilepsy which would now be preventable. These findings are remarkably similar to those obtained in both a French study [23], where no cause could be found in 76 per cent of 3,438 children with epilepsy, and among 77 per cent of 516 patients of all ages in the Mayo clinic studies [8, 24].

TABLE IX. Possible causes of epilepsy in 64 children

Possible cause	Number
Congenital disorders:	5
tuberose sclerosis	
cerebral palsy (2)	
Down's syndrome	
multiple congenital defects	
Birth hazard:	5
maternal bleeding pre 28 weeks	
and birthweight 1500g (2)	
gestation 34 weeks	
severe rhesus disease	
severe rhesus disease and cataract	
Postnatal infection:	4
bacterial meningitis (3)	
viral meningitis	
Postnatal accident:	2
skull fracture	
subdural haemorrhage	
Clear cut role of inheritance	1
Sub total	17
No aetiological clue	47
Total	64

Findings from the NCDS demonstrate that large scale national cohort studies can throw useful light on the nature of convulsive disorder in childhood. Such studies have obvious limitations and their conclusions depend entirely on the quality of agencies which are not under the direct control of the study team. It must be remembered that our information was supplied entirely on a goodwill basis. The cohort remains under continuing study and it should be possible to review those with epilepsy through their third decade. Such information should tell much about the longer term prognosis of those who have had seizures in childhood. The study, however, has revealed largely negative information about aetiology. It is disappointing that no obvious preventable factors have been revealed in the great majority of cases. Further cohort studies should concentrate on subtler factors than we were able to study. These would include congenital virus disease, a search for mild degrees of child abuse, more detailed physical examinations, preferably undertaken by neurologically trained members of a study team, and EEGs performed under standardised conditions.

Acknowledgments

We are grateful to the National Children's Bureau for permission to publish data from the NCDS. We would also like to thank our colleagues, Professor N Butler and Dr P West, to acknowledge Mr L Fortnum for technical help and Mrs D Barnes for typing the manuscript. We were financially supported by the Epilepsy Research Fund of the British Epilepsy Association supplemented by the drug houses of Abbott, Bayer, ICI and Parke Davis.

References

1   Crombie DL, Cross KW, Fry J, et al. *Br Med J 1960; 2:* 416–422
2   Logan WPD, Cushion AA. *Morbidity Statistics from General Practice Volume 1 (General) GRO studies on medical and population subjects 1958.* London: HMSO
3   Pond DA, Bidwell BH, Stein L. *J Psychiatrica Neurologica Neurochirurgia 1960; 63:* 217–236
4   Brewis M, Poskonzi D, Rolland C, Miller H. *Acta Paediat Scand 1960; 24:* Suppl
5   Rose SW, Penry JK, Markush RE, et al. *Epilepsia (New York) 1973; 14:* 133–135
6   Rutter M, Tizard J, Whitmore K. *Education Health and Behaviour 1970.* London: Longman
7   Ross EM. In Rose FC, ed. *Clinical Neuroepidemiology 1980;* 344–350. Tunbridge Wells: Pitman Medical
8   Hauser WA, Kurland LT. *Epilepsia 1975; 16:* 1–66
9   Gudmundsson G. *Acta Neurol Scand 1966; Suppl 25*
10   Sillanpaa M. *Acta Paediat Scand 1973; 237:* Suppl
11   Rossiter EJR, Luckin J, Vile A, et al. *Med J Aust 1977; 2:* 735–740
12   Van den Berg BJ, Yerushalmy J. *Epilepsia (New York) 1973; 14:* 298–304
13   Nelson KB, Ellenberg JH. *Pediatrics 1978; 61:* 720–727
14   Cooper JE. *Br Med J 1965; 1:* 1020–1022
15   Ross EM, Peckham CS, West PB, Butler NR. *Br Med J 1980; 1:* 207–210
16   Ellenburg JH, Nelson KB. *JAMA 1980; 243:* 13: 1337–1340

17   Annegers JF, Hauser WA, Elveback LR, Kurland LT. *Neurology 1979; 29:* 297–303
18   Lewis HM, Parry JV, et al. *Arch Dis Childh 1977; 52:* 192–196
19   Nelson KB, Ellenburg JH. *Febrile Seizures 1981.* New York: Raven Press
20   Ueoka K, Mita R, Ando S, et al. *Brain and Development 1981; 3; 2:* 195
21   Illingworth RS. *Br Med J 1979; 1:* 797–801
22   Tunstall-Pedoe H, Rose G. *Frequency and outcome of febrile and non-febrile convulsions in infancy. Appendix iiiA in Whooping Cough 1981;* 50–56. Department of Health and Social Security. London: HMSO
23   Beaussart M, Beaussart-Defaye J, Delattre M. In Aicardi J, ed. *Les épilepsies de l'enfant 1981;* 339–345
24   Hauser WA, Annegers JF, Kurland LT, et al. *Am J Epidem 1977; 106:* 276

7

CONVULSIVE DISORDERS IN THE CHILD HEALTH AND EDUCATION STUDY

Jean Golding, N Butler

Introduction

As shown in the preceding chapter, study of a nationally representative sample of children over a period of time has much to offer. The Child Health and Education Study is an ongoing project designed to document social, medical, educational and biological changes in all children born in the week 5th — 11th April 1970, and resident in Great Britain. These children were studied at birth and during the first week of life [1,2]. All subsequent deaths occurring in the cohort were identified and attempts were made to trace the surviving children at five years of age. In all, 80 per cent of the original survivors were traced, their parents interviewed and detailed medical histories taken. The birth data were analysed to ascertain whether there were marked differences between the 80 per cent who were included and the 20 per cent who were not. There were no major differences in the social class or maternal age distributions, but the children born to unmarried mothers were significantly less likely to have been contacted at five years [3].

Early neonatal fits

For all babies in the birth survey, midwives filled in a proforma which included a question as to whether the child has had 'a fit or convulsion' in the first week of life. Some 72 were recorded out of 16,334 live births in England, Scotland and Wales — giving an incidence of 4.4 per 1,000 live births. Mortality was high: 16 of the 72 (22%) had died by the end of the first week and a further 5 died later — giving an overall mortality rate in this group of 292 per 1,000.

Retrospective maternal report of convulsions in the child

Convulsions are very disturbing events, especially in children. It is unlikely that any mother having seen her child having a fit will forget it. Errors might ensue in two circumstances: in cases where the child has had a fit but the mother neither saw it nor was told about it, and in instances where the mother refuses to accept or acknowledge the fact — probably because of the stigma attached to the word epilepsy. We have evidence that the first source of bias existed, because a proportion of the infants who had had convulsions in the early neonatal period were reported by their mothers as having had no such history when they were questioned at five years. It is impossible to assess the size of the second source of bias, but the fact that, as we shall show, the prevalence figures in our study are very similar to those found in other populations suggests that any such inaccuracy must either be relatively small or the same in all studies.

Prevalence

At five years, the parents were asked whether the child 'had ever had any form of convulsion, fit, seizure or other turn in which consciousness was lost or any part of the body made abnormal movements?' Information was given for 13,038 of the 13,135 children contacted at five years. Of these, 767 stated that their child had had such an episode. From the data given it was possible to classify the children into five diagnostic groups. The allocation of each case was made by a paediatrician (NRB) using relevant data from all questionnaires, including the mother's description of the attacks, and details given by her of hospital admissions, medication and investigations. As can be seen from Table I, 113 of the

TABLE I. Distribution of conditions

Medical diagnosis	Number of children	
a) *Symptomatic convulsions:*	88	(0.7%)
Non-idiopathic, but associated with underlying cerebral condition or symptomatic with other disease processes, (e.g. hypocalcaemia, meningitis)		
b) *Idiopathic epilepsy:*	36	(0.3%)
Idiopathic — no known precipitating cause. Afebrile		
c) *Febrile convulsions:*	342	(2.6%)
Associated with pyrexia		
d) *Unspecified seizures:*	188	(1.4%)
Convulsive episode but otherwise unspecified		
All with convulsive disorders	654	(5.0%)
e) *Faints and breath-holding:*	113	(0.9%)
No convulsive episode:	12,271	(94.1%)
TOTAL KNOWN	13,038	(100%)

original group had episodes that were considered to be either faints or the consequences of breath-holding. After omitting these there remained 654 children who had appeared to have had at least one convulsive attack, giving a reported prevalence of 5.0 per cent. This compares well with other population studies which have estimated that the proportion of children aged less than five years having such episodes lies between 5 and 7 per cent [4,5].

Types of convulsive episodes

Symptomatic convulsions

The 88 children who were classified as having had symptomatic convulsions comprised those who had underlying cerebral damage (e.g. 10 with cerebral palsy, and 5 with hydrocephalus), those whose fits were precipitated by other acute events such as trauma and meningitis, and infants with precipitating neonatal problems such as hypocalcaemia.

Fifty-two per cent of these children had had only one convulsive episode (Table II). These were mostly children who had suffered from a transitory abnormality such as hypocalcaemia, rather than continuing cerebral problems. In

TABLE II. Frequency of seizures by diagnosis

Medical diagnosis	No of seizures			All known
	1	2–3	4+	
Symptomatic convulsions	38 (52%)	18 (24.7%)	17 (23.3%)	73 (100%)
Idiopathic epilepsy	0 (-)	6 (18.7%)	26 (81.3%)	32 (100%)
Febrile convulsions	213 (64%)	80 (24%)	40 (12%)	333 (100%)
Unspecified seizures	110 (64.7%)	38 (22.4%)	22 (12.9%)	170 (100%)
All convulsions	361 (59.4%)	142 (23.3%)	105 (17.3%)	608 (100%)
Faints and breath-holding	35 (38%)	19 (20.7%)	38 (41.3%)	92 (100%)

contrast, most of the children who had many fits had ongoing cerebral problems, such as cerebral palsy or severe mental subnormality.

As already indicated the age of onset for symptomatic convulsions was early, 50 per cent of the children having had their first convulsion within the first year of life and 75 per cent by the age of two years (Figure 1a).

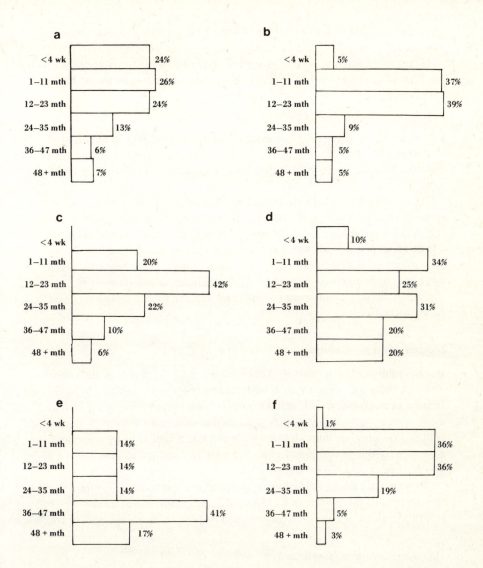

Figure 1. Age of onset of the different groups: a) Symptomatic convulsions; b) Idiopathic epilepsy; c) Febrile convulsions; d) Unspecified convulsions; e) Faints; f) Breath-holding

Idiopathic epilepsy

Thirty-six children met the criteria for epilepsy described by Gastaut [6]. By this definition, such children have more than one afebrile fit with no identifiable precipitating factor. In the event, 19 per cent of the 36 children had had two or three fits and 81 per cent had four or more fits before the age of five years (Table II).

Thus, our estimate of the prevalence of idiopathic epilepsy identifiable by five years of age is only 2.7 per 1,000.

Of the 36 children who were identified, only two had fits in the neonatal period but 75 per cent had had their first convulsion by the age of two years (Figure 1b).

Febrile convulsions

Febrile convulsions were the commonest cause of convulsions in our children, comprising 52 per cent of the whole group, with a prevalence of 26 per 1,000 children. This compares with the published data which ranges from 19 to 36 per 1,000 [7–10].

Nearly two-thirds of the children (64%) had had only one convulsion, but as many as 12 per cent had had at least four convulsions within this time period (Table II). Two children were reported to have begun their convulsions in the late neonatal period, although some investigations have suggested that febrile convulsions do not occur before the age of six months [11]. Nevertheless, in agreement with other major studies, the first febrile convulsion occurred most commonly in the second year of life (Figure 1c), the frequency of new cases falling thereafter.

Seizures of unspecified type

In 188 children (29 per cent of all convulsions and 1.4 per cent of the cohort, Table I), there was certainly an episode of lost consciousness with certain characteristics of convulsions such as jerking movements, eyes rolling, going stiff and incontinence, but we were unable to go further than classify them as 'unspecified'. A high proportion of these children were either not seen at all by a doctor or were seen by the general practitioner but were not referred to hospital so a definitive diagnosis could not be made.

There was no marked distribution in age of first occurrence (Figure 1d). Sixty-five per cent of these children had had only single convulsions, 22 per cent had had two or three, and only 13 per cent had had four or more episodes (Table II).

Faints and breath-holding attacks

Of the cohort, 113 children (0.9%) suffered from fainting or breath-holding attacks which led to brief episodes of unconsciousness. Although one-third (38%) of these children had had only one such episode, a high proportion (41%) had had four or more attacks, and many of the breath-holders had had twenty or more (Table II).

Forty per cent of children who had fainted had their first episode at age three (Figure 1e), whereas more than two-thirds of the breath-holders had had their first attack by the age of two years (Figure 1f). These two groups, though of interest in their own right, will be omitted from the rest of this chapter.

64

Demographic differences

In contrast with most causes of morbidity in our study, there were no significant differences in the prevalence of convulsions in the different regions of the country. In addition, there was no significant excess of convulsions in urban as opposed to rural areas, nor was there any increase in incidence if the home was overcrowded.

The population study from Newcastle upon Tyne [4] showed no association between convulsions and illegitimacy, but they did find an increased prevalence in the lower social classes. On further analysis they found that the association was only with those children whose convulsions were not necessarily associated with infection. The authors suggested that 'poor maternal care' was of importance in this group, but they were unable to suggest the mechanism of such an effect.

TABLE III. Proportion of children with a history of convulsions according to factors concerning the family at five years

Maternal age (at birth of child)			
Under 20	63/ 1,097	(5.7%)	
20–34	647/10,673	(6.1%)	
35+	49/ 1,075	(4.6%)	
Social Class (husband's occupation)			NS
I & II	174/ 3,223	(5.4%)	
III Nm	67/ 1,065	(6.3%)	
III M	326/ 5,690	(5.7%)	
IV & V	139/ 2,210	(6.3%)	
Parental situation at 5			NS
Child living with both natural parents	687/11,779	(5.8%)	
One natural + one step	24/351	(6.8%)	
Single mother	18/247	(7.3%)	
	38/501	(7.6%)	
Other (adopted, fostered, etc)	9/150	(6.0%)	NS
Ethnic group of parents			
Both UK	709/11,939	(5.9%)	
Both European	9/177	(5.1%)	
Both West Indian	3/171	(1.8%)	
Both Asian	11/252	(4.4%)	
Other	26/379	(6.9%)	NS
Number of older siblings			
None	289/ 4,966	(5.8%)	
One	275/ 4,515	(6.1%)	
Two	119/ 2,143	(5.6%)	
Three +	84/ 1,404	(6.0%	NS
Number of younger siblings			
None	425/ 7,225	(5.9%)	
One	293/ 4,938	(5.9%)	
Two +	49/865	(5.7%)	NS

Although we were unable to examine data on maternal care itself, we found no association with those other factors that are often associated with 'poor maternal care' (viz teenage motherhood, low social class, single-parent families, or large number of siblings, Table III). Even when subdividing our data in the way favoured by Miller and his colleagues [4], we could find no association with social class and number of siblings, which agrees with data from the previous two national cohort studies [12,13].

The child

In accord with other studies, there was an overall excess of boys with convulsions, especially in the group with febrile convulsions, but this was not statistically significant (Table IV). In addition, there were no significant differences overall in the methods of delivery of the children who later developed convulsions compared with all others in the cohort, but there were striking excesses in both the proportion of low birthweight children and those of short gestation (Figure 2).

TABLE IV. Sex distribution among children having seizures

Type of seizure	No. Males	No. Females	Sex ratio (M/F)
a) Symptomatic convulsions	48	40	1.20
b) Idiopathic epilepsy	17	19	0.89
c) Febrile convulsions	192	150	1.28
d) Unspecified seizures	100	88	1.14
All with convulsive disorders	357	297	1.20
No convulsions	6,398	5,986	1.07

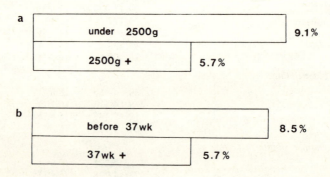

Figure 2. a) Proportion of children with history of convulsions by birthweight. b) Proportion of children with history of convulsions by gestation

These findings appeared true of all categories except the idiopathic epilepsy group, and to be most marked in the group of symptomatic convulsions (Figure 3). There was no relationship between high birthweight (over 4082gm) and any type of seizure. The association with low birthweight agrees with other studies [8,12].

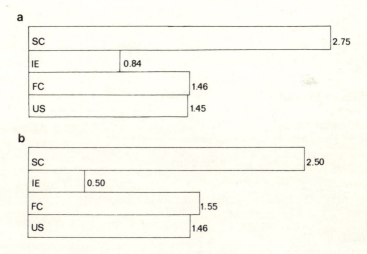

Figure 3. Relative risk of each type of convulsive disorder: a) if the infant's birthweight was under 2500g; b) if the gestation was less than 37 weeks.
SC = Symptomatic convulsions; IE = Idiopathic epilepsy; FC = febrile convulsions; US = Unspecified seizures

Behaviour patterns

Frequently during a convulsion, a child will inadvertently wet and/or soil, but the question was raised as to whether, in general, children with a history of convulsions are normally more likely to wet or soil. In the Newcastle Study, Miller and his colleagues [4] found no significant association with bed-wetting, but their numbers were very small. In our study (Figure 4) we found that there were higher proportions of children with a history of convulsions among those with frequent bed-wetting, daytime wetting and soiling problems. The associations were most marked with soiling. It is unlikely that these findings were due to the actual events occurring during seizures as very few children were having as many as one fit a week. It is, however, possible that the finding was associated with use of anticonvulsants, and this is being assessed at the moment.

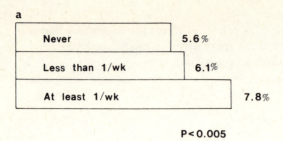

a

Never	5.6%
Less than 1/wk	6.1%
At least 1/wk	7.8%

P< 0.005

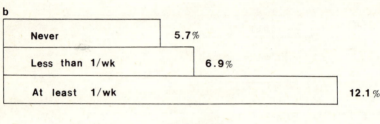

b

Never	5.7%
Less than 1/wk	6.9%
At least 1/wk	12.1%

P< 0.0001

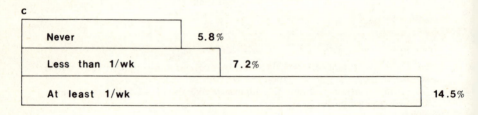

c

Never	5.8%
Less than 1/wk	7.2%
At least 1/wk	14.5%

P< 0.0001

Figure 4. See text

Accidents

Some cases of convulsions certainly occur as the result of accidents, but there is some evidence for thinking that children who have fits will also be more likely to injure themselves accidentally during seizures themselves [4]. Surprisingly, though, we found that there was no increase in the accident rate among children with convulsions.

Non-accidental injury

Of the 44 children reported by the health visitors as having non-accidental injury, as many as 13 (30%) had had convulsions whereas only 2.2 would have been expected (p <0.001). No particular category of convulsive disorder predominated. It would be wrong to ascribe all convulsions in such children to child abuse although, for example, a subdural haematoma resulting from abuse could well lead to a 'symptomatic' convulsion.

The association between child abuse and convulsions may result from medical personnel being more aware of these children and thus noticing abuse more readily. This should be true of any chronic illness, but increased incidence (i.e. reporting) of child abuse is not associated with other chronic illness (e.g. asthma).

It is possible that the characteristics of children who have had convulsions are provoking factors to a parent who is a potential batterer. It could be that lack of response consequent upon the sedative effects of anticonvulsant medication could have such an effect, or that the increased prevalence of annoying and irritating behaviour problems, such as wetting or soiling, could constitute the straw that causes the parental tolerance level to falter.

Discussion

Longitudinal studies require the assembly of information on many individuals to provide a perspective on disease which looks at a whole population rather than at what happens to each individual in it [14]. In contrast with almost all other medical conditions of early childhood, children with a history of convulsions do not appear to differ from the rest of the population in social or environmental background. The implication is that manipulation of the environment in various ways, whether by raising parental standards or improving housing conditions, is unlikely to result in any reduction in incidence of the problem. Our preliminary analyses show that a history of low birthweight and/or short gestation are of some importance. Even so, such associations account for a very small population of all children with convulsions.

The children in the cohort have just been followed-up at the age of 10, and we are currently reviewing hospital notes and questioning general practitioners as to the details surrounding the convulsions. From this we hope to derive details of the dynamics of convulsive events in the first 10 years of life: to identify children whose first episode was febrile, but then went on to have afebrile convulsions. We intend to examine factors such as the duration of the first episode, and treatment of the child, to see whether there are any associations between these and longer-term outcome. Especially exciting will be the analysis of aspects of the health and behaviour at five years of the children who subsequently have their first convulsion. Are there any factors that can distinguish them from their contemporaries that do not have convulsions? And what of the effect of the convulsion on the behaviour of the child, his growth and intellectual ability? Only a longitudinal study of a large cohort of children can possibly attempt to answer these questions.

Acknowledgments

We are extremely grateful to all the many persons involved in the design and implementation of the various facets of this cohort study. In particular, the mid-wives who filled in the questionnaires at birth, the health visitors who interviewed the mother, measured and tested the children at five. The Birth Survey was directed by Roma Chamberlain and Geoffrey Chamberlain and the five-year follow-up was designed and organised by Neville Butler, Albert Osborn, Sue Dowling and Brian Howlett. Finally we thank Penny Hicks and Yasmin Iles for typing the manuscript so well at short notice.

References

1   Chamberlain R, Chamberlain G, Howlett B, Claireaux A. *British Births 1970; Vol 1. The First Week of Life 1975.* London: Heinemann Medical Books Ltd
2   Chamberlain G, Phillipp E, Howlett B, Masters K. *British Births Vol 2: 1978 Obstetric Care.* London: Heinemann Medical Books Ltd
3   Golding J, Butler NR, Howlett B, Dowling S. *From Birth to Five;* In press. London: Spastics International Medical Publications
4   Miller FJW, Court SDM, Walton WS, Knox EG. *Growing up in Newcastle-upon-Tyne, A Continuing Study of Health and Illness in Young Children Within their Families 1960;* 164–173. London: Oxford University Press
5   Nelson KB, Ellenberg JH. *Dev Med Child Neurol 1980; 22:* 261–262
6   Gastaut H. *Epilepsia 1970; 11:* 102–113
7   Harker P. *Br med J 1977; 2:* 490–493
8   Van den Berg BJ, Yerushalmy J. *Pediat Res 1969; 3:* 298–304
9   Nelson KB, Ellenberg JH. *N Engl J Med 1976; 295:* 1029–1033
10 Oosteff H. *N Engl J Med 1965; 273:* 1410–1413
11 Livingstone S. *The Diagnosis and Treatment of Convulsive Disorders in Children 1954.* Springfield, Illinois: Charles C Thomas
12 Cooper JE. *Br med J 1965; 1:* 1020–1022
13 Ross EM, Peckham CS, West PB, Butler NR. *Br med J 1980; 1:* 207–210
14 Gruenberg EM, Le Resche L. In Mednick SA, Baert AE, Bachmann BP, eds. *Prospective Longitudinal Research: An Empirical Basis for the Primary Prevention of Psychosocial Disorders 1981;* 320–325. London: Oxford University Press

8

RECURRENCE RISKS IN EPILEPSY

M Baraitser

Introduction

The risk of having a child with a congenital malformation is 1 in 40 for anyone
in the general population. This figure is the background against which risks in
general should be assessed. Any risk greater than 1 in 10 is high but risks of 1
in 40 and lower are not too different from those that are run by the majority
of couples when planning a family. It is however true that the population is in
general unaware of the risks.

The 1 in 40 risk does not include conditions, such as epilepsy, nor does it
include the many causes of mental retardation. The risk is largely made up of
congenital malformations detectable at birth.

Genetic counselling in epilepsy is dependent on the availability of empiric
risks rather than on an understanding of Mendelian ratios. The main purpose
of counselling is to answer questions about risks to offspring or further children. The calculation of the numerical odds is made after the diagnosis has
been confirmed and a family history taken.

The general perspective is as follows:

The risk that anyone in the population will proceed to chronic epilepsy is
1 in 250 [1]. Counselling is non-directive and takes place in a setting of free
exchange between patient and counsellor. Risks should be given as odds ie,
1 in 10 and not as a risk increase over and above the risk run by the general
population. Risk increases might be disturbing, ie, the risk after a child with
generalised epilepsy is increased by a factor of 10 but the actual risk is small.
To the risk should be added the small chance of an epileptic woman on
medication having a child with a congenital abnormality. More contra-
versial is when the general risk of 1 in 40 for something completely different
and in no way related to epilepsy should be added to the equation, ie, if one
parent has grand mal seizures, the risk to offspring is about 1 in 25. There is

also the general population risk of 1 in 40 for a congenital malformation. Taken together the risk is 1 in 16. It is however best to counsel the specific risk for which the patient has asked.

It is important to have a diagnosis of the type of epilepsy under consideration before applying an appropriate figure. The pedigree information should include details about parents, sibs, cousins, uncles, aunts, nieces and nephews. Most types of epilepsy are inherited as polygenic disorders and in accordance with the postulated rules of polygenic inheritance.

Risks fall off dramatically as one progresses from first degree relatives (parents and offspring), to second degree relatives (aunts, uncles, nephews and nieces), to third degree relatives (cousins).

Grand mal

The many studies of grand mal epilepsy using different populations have shown the same tendency, that is, there are increased risks to both sibs and offspring of those with grand mal seizures, but in general these risks are seldom high ie, greater than 1 in 10. They vary from 4 to 10 in a hundred and in most situations are around the 4 per cent (1 in 25) mark [2]. The difference between 4 and 10 in a hundred is a reflection of the type of patient used in the various studies. Risks are higher when children are considered as probands, possibly because seizures tend to diminish in frequency with age [3,4]. Studies on adults especially when the survey is conducted by post or on patients in institutions, give smaller recurrence figures [5].

These risks are for clinical epilepsy. The frequency of EEG abnormalities associated with grand mal are much higher, but the risk should be calculated for clinical epilepsy and not for EEG abnormalities. Likewise, the risk would be higher if single seizures were taken into account but they do not constitute a serious burden.

It would appear as if there is a sex difference. Whereas males in the general population more frequently have epilepsy, the risk to the offspring of mothers with epilepsy is greater than the risk to the offspring of epileptic fathers.

Factors which increase the 4 per cent risk

If other first degree relatives are affected, the risk is increased on an empiric basis. No exact figures are available but using other polygenically inherited diseases such as spina bifida or cleft lip and palate as precedents, the risk factors as shown in Figure 1 are appropriate.

Temporal lobe epilepsy

The genetic contribution to temporal lobe epilepsy originates in part from the contribution of febrile convulsions. It is estimated that about one-third of those

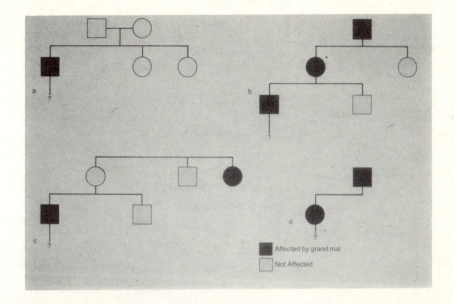

Figure 1. The following risks apply:
   a) 1 in 25
   b) 1 in 8
   c) 1 in 15
   d) 1 in 10

with mesial temporal sclerosis have had uncontrollable febrile convulsions in
early childhood [6]. The risks to sibs are 1 in 5 but only a small percentage
proceed to have temporal lobe epilepsy. The high risk is for a remediable condition and it might be possible to prevent epilepsy by adequate management of
febrile convulsions. Views about management differ but parents should at least
have the proposed management with likely outcome explained in full.

There is a separate category of mid temporal spike with seizures which start
between the ages of 1–13 years. Most patients are seizure free at 15 years. In
one study [7] 1 in 7 sibs had seizures and 1 in 5 rolandic discharges.

Petit mal

Risks to the offspring of those who have had petit mal in childhood do not differ
appreciably from the risks to offspring of those with generalised epilepsy (about
4 per cent) [8]. It is also clear that petit mal does not breed true within families
and the increased risk to first degree relatives is for either petit mal or grand mal.
The risk should be increased on an empiric basis.

When EEG evidence of 3cps spike and wave activity is present the risk is
nearer 7–8 per cent [3] (Figure 2).

73

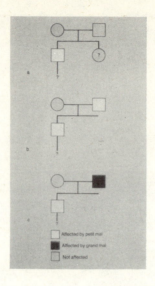

Figure 2. The following risk figures apply
  a) 1 in 25
  b) 1 in 10
  c) 1 in 10

Febrile convulsions

Risks are higher for both the sibs and offspring in this category of seizures than in any of the others. The background risk is approximately 1 in 33 — that is the risk for a child in the general population taking no account of the family history. The risk for sibs after one affected child is 1 in 5 [9].

If in addition a parent is affected, the risk should be increased to 1 in 3. There is little evidence of a genetic relationship between grand mal and febrile convulsion. Whereas a small proportion of those with febrile convulsions proceed to chronic epilepsy, those patients with epilepsy do not have a high frequency of febrile convulsions among their first degree relatives.

Hypsarrhythmia

Recurrence risks are small — about 1 in 33 for sibs. In all cases tuberose sclerosis should be excluded.

Focal epilepsy (Figure 3)

Risks are slightly increased for the offspring of those with focal epilepsy, presumably on the basis that they are more prone (on a weak genetic basis) to have seizures than others in the general population [10].

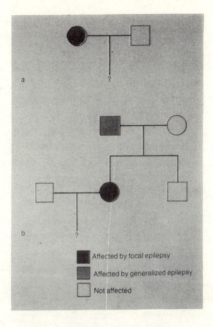

Figure 3. The following risks apply
a) 1 in 50
b) 1 in 10

Additional risks of a malformation (Background risks)

The effect of pregnancy on epilepsy

The incidence of status epilepticus in pregnancy varies from 0–10 per cent but the frequency of seizures is often altered by pregnancy. About one-third to two-thirds of epileptics have more seizures during pregnancy than they do between pregnancies. Against this background there are risks to the parent, especially to mothers who are epileptic and are on anticonvulsants, for having a child with a congenital malformation. The following drugs have been implicated:

Hydantoin Much controversy surrounds the role of anticonvulsant therapy in the observed increased incidence of congenital malformation in the offspring of epileptic mothers. The increase is 2–3 times the population risk of a malformation, i.e. 1 in 20 as opposed to 1 in 40, but there are those who doubt the role of anticonvulsants. Some studies seem to indicate that the risk of a malformation is increased irrespective of whether the epileptic mother is on anticonvulsants or not [11]. The risk is mainly for cleft lip alone or with cleft palate, congenital heart disease, microcephaly and mental retardation. None of the risks is dramatically increased and the retardation is usually mild. It has been suggested that

75

using IQ scores as a measurable scale, there is only a 5 point reduction when the group of mothers who are epileptic and on medication are compared with a control group.

A specific constellation of dysmorphic features found in the offspring of epileptic parents on epanutin is known as the fetal hydantoin syndrome. Differentiation from the fetal alcohol syndrome can be difficult. The syndrome consists of a flat, broad nasal bridge, ptosis, hypertelorism, a short upturned nose, epicanthic folds and prominent lips. The limb defects include hypoplastic nails or hypoplasia of the distal phalange. The risk for cleft lip, with or without cleft palate, in the general population is 1 in 1000. For those on antiepileptic medication it is 1 in 100. The population frequency of heart defects is 1 in 150. The increased risk for epileptics is four times this risk.

Phenobarbitone Seip [12] described two sibs who had been exposed to levels of phenobarbitone well above the usual therapeutic level, as well as to primidone. They were born with dysmorphic features which included a short nose, a low nasal bridge, hypertelorism, epicanthic folds and ptosis. One had a cleft palate and one showed retarded development. These reports are rare and difficult to evaluate, as genetic rather than environmental aetiology cannot be excluded. In the series of Lowe [13] one malformation occurred in 53 pregnancies when the mother was on phenobarbitone alone. Although not proven, it might be that phenobarbitone is less teratogenic than hydantoin.

Trimethadione This drug has been used for more than 30 years. In 1970 German et al [14] suggested a possible teratogenic effect. In seven pregnancies in a single family, 4 had congenital malformations. Cleft lip and palate, cardiac defects in 3 out of the 4, and tracheo-oesophageal anomalies were the main defects. A review of 53 pregnancies showed that 24 per cent ended in spontaneous abortions. Eighty-three per cent of the survivors had at least one major congenital anomaly — cleft lip and palate 28 per cent, low set ears 42 per cent, mental delay 50 per cent and congenital heart defect 50 per cent [15].

Sodium valproate This has been shown to be teratogenic in mice. The toxic effect in humans is as yet unproven. There have been single case reports [16] but these are exceptional.

Primidone Two sibs were reported [17], with short hirsute foreheads, epicanthic folds, upward slanting palpebral fissures, a flat nasal bridge, long philtrum and small jaw. Previously an 80 per cent risk of malformation had been noted in the offspring of women on this drug alone [18].

Management

In general patients should take the fewest number of drugs at the least possible therapeutic dosage. Those who have been seizure free for many years should consider a trial off medication before planning a pregnancy. Medication with trimethadione probably has the highest risk and the risk on phenobarbitone might be less than on hydantoin. Too little is known about carbamazepine or sodium valproate but there is little evidence to date that suggests that they are teratogenic in man. Finally, any patient who needs antiepileptic medication for adequate seizure control during pregnancy should be advised of the risks and the decision whether to plan a family be left to individual couples after full consultation and discussion with their doctors. In most instances these patients should continue with the medication.

Rare syndromes in which the inheritance might be as a single gene defect

a) There have been at least two families reported in which there is an association of neonatal hair loss with poor regrowth, epilepsy and mental retardation. In one of these the inheritance was recessive [19] whereas in the other inheritance is less certain but could be dominant [20].

b) *Benign recurrent convulsions in childhood* There have now been a number of families in which the seizures are inherited as a simple dominant. The condition is self limiting and hence benign. Risks to the offspring of those who are affected are high (1 in 2) but the condition is mild. Unfortunately a diagnosis is not possible in the absence of a family history.

References

1 Ross EM, Peckham CS, West PB, Butler NR. *Br Med J 1980; 1:* 207–210
2 Conrad K. *Z ges Neurol Psychiat 1937; 159:* 521–581
3 Metrakos K, Metrakos JD. *Neurology 1961; 2:* 470–483
4 Metrakos JD, Metrakos K. *Neurology 1960; 10:* 228–240
5 Gerken H, Dook H. *Neuropaed 1973; 4:* 88–91
6 Lindsay JMJ. *Epilepsia 1971; 12:* 47
7 Heijbel J, Blom S, Rasmuson M. *Epilepsia 1975; 16:* 285–293
8 Dalby MA. *Acta Neurol Scand* 1969; Suppl 40
9 Ounsted C. *Eugen Rev 1955; 47:* 33–49
10 Gerken H, Kiefer R, Doose H, Volske E. *Neuropaed 1977; 8:* 3–9
11 Stumpf OA, Frost M. *Am J Dis Child 1978; 132:* 746–747
12 Seip M. *Acta Pediat Scand 1976; 65:* 617–621
13 Lowe CR. *Lancet 1973; i:* 9–10
14 German J, Kowal A, Ehlers KL. *Teratology 1970; 3:* 349–361
15 Feldman GL, Weaver DD, Lovrein EW. *Am J Dis Child 1977; 131:* 1389–1392
16 Dalens B. *J Pediatric 1980; Vol 97:* 332
17 Rudd NL, Freedom RM. *J Ped 1979; 94:* 835
18 Shapiro S, Slone D, Hartz SC et al. *Lancet 1976; i:* 272
19 Perniola T, Krajewska G, Carnevale F, Lospalluti M. *J Inher Mental Dis 1980; 3:* 49–53
20 Moynahan EJ. *Proc Roy Soc Med 1962; 55:* 411–412

9

EPILEPTIC BRAIN DAMAGE

B S Meldrum, T Griffiths, M C Evans

Introduction

The term 'epileptic brain damage' is commonly used to refer to two entities. One is the chronic pathology found in patients dying (often in institutions) after suffering ill-controlled seizures for many years. The seizures are most often of the complex partial type with secondary generalisation. The pathology is usually hippocampal sclerosis and cerebellar and neocortical atrophy.

The other entity is the acute pathology (ischaemic cell change or nerve cell loss in pyramidal neurones of the hippocampus, small pyramidal neurones of lamina III of the neocortex and cerebellar Purkinje cells) found in children or adults dying a few hours or days after *status epilepticus*. These two pathological syndromes are reviewed by Corsellis and Meldrum [1]. The selective pattern of damage is broadly similar in the two cases except that neocortical damage is often relatively more severe in those dying acutely after *status epilepticus*.

Whether the chronic lesions associated with epilepsy are a cause or consequence of the seizures has been disputed for more than one hundred years [2]. In contrast the lesions after *status epilepticus* have generally been considered a consequence of physiological events associated with the seizures (e.g. impaired cerebral oxygenation or blood flow).

Over the last 12 years we have developed various experimental models of *status epilepticus* to investigate the pathogenesis of epileptic brain damage [3–8]. In baboons, sustained seizures induced by bicuculline produce ischaemic cell change in selectively vulnerable pyramidal neurones in the neocortex and hippocampus, and, provided there is no peripheral paralysis, in cerebellar Purkinje cells [3,4]. Two hours of seizure activity induced by bicuculline in paralysed ventilated rats produces similar neocortical and hippocampal lesions [6]. In this model, systemic factors do not contribute to the development of ischaemic cell change.

In April, 1980, Meldrum [9] put forward an hypothesis to account for the selective vulnerability of pyramidal neurones in the hippocampus and neocortex, and Purkinje cells. The principal elements of this are (i) that the selectively vulnerable neurones have complex dendritic trees which have high voltage-dependent calcium conductances (as shown for example by the capacity of the dendrites to develop calcium spikes), and potent excitatory inputs, which directly or indirectly open Ca^{++} channels, and the capacity to show burst firing and paroxysmal depolarising shifts, (ii) during epileptic activity the inward movement of calcium greatly exceeds the capacity of the neuronal membrane to transport calcium outwards, or exchange it for sodium, (iii) that intracellular organelles, especially the mitochondria, sequester calcium to maintain the cytoplasmic (Ca^{++}) at its normal very low level, but that if *status epilepticus* is sufficiently prolonged this mechanism becomes overloaded, leading to mitochondrial failure and a marked increase in cytoplasmic (Ca^{++}), (iv) the high intracellular (Ca^{++}) is cytotoxic and activates proteinases and phospholipases lethally injuring the cell and producing the appearance of ischaemic cell change.

Neurophysiological evidence relating to (i) and (ii) has been previously reviewed [9,10]. Substantial data relating to the movement of Ca^{++} during seizure activity, and in response to excitatory amino acids are presented by Heinemann and Lux (see this volume). We are now presenting experimental evidence to support the third component of the hypothetical sequence explaining selective vulnerability. We have used a method that permits the visualisation of Ca^{++} in electron micrographs [11] to study the intracellular accumulation of Ca^{++} in hippocampal neurones during the course of prolonged seizure activity, and have correlated this with selective pathological change. A preliminary report of some of the data has appeared [12].

Experimental methods

Rats with tracheal and femoral arterial and venous cannulae, previously implanted under halothane anaesthesia, were paralysed and maintained on mechanical respiration with nitrous oxide/oxygen. Arterial pressure and oxygenation were maintained within normal limits throughout, by adjusting ventilation and infusing donor blood. Seizures were induced with bicuculline, 3.3μmol/kg iv, or L-allylglycine, 2.4 mmol/kg iv. Seizure activity was monitored with platinum needle electrodes in the scalp, and a polygraphic EEG amplifier/recorder.

After 0.5, 1 or 2 hours of seizure activity, animals were perfusion fixed, either with 2 per cent glutaraldehyde 3 per cent paraformaldehyde solution, or with a glutaraldehyde fixative containing potassium oxalate [11]. Blocks containing the hippocampi were dissected out and processed either for standard light and electron microscopy or for the oxalate/pyroantimonate method for demonstrating calcium deposits [11–13]. Araldite embedded material was cut and stained for light and electron microscopy.

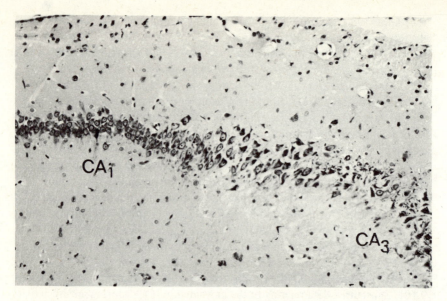

Figure 1a. Light micrograph of rat hippocampus showing lesion secondary to seizure activity induced by ipsilateral intra-amygdaloid injection of kainic acid (1mg in 0.25µl). CA_1 pyramidal neurones appear normal; CA_3 neurones are darkly staining, pyknotic, and surrounded by abnormal perineuronal spaces. Survival from seizure onset 4 hours (Cresyl fast violet; magnification x 160) (Reduced for publication)

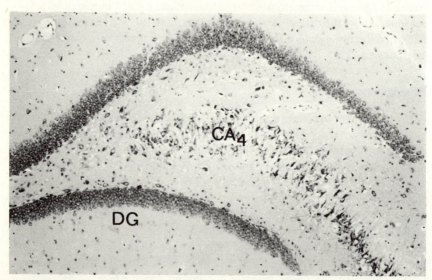

Figure 1b. Light micrograph of hippocampus from the same rat as Figure 1a to show the normal appearance of the dentate granule cells (DG) and the vacuolation, and ischaemic cell change in the endfolium (CA_4) neurones (Cresyl fast violet; magnification x 100) (Reduced for publication)

Results

Light microscopy

Marked pathological changes occur after one hour of seizure activity induced by either bicuculline or L-allylglycine. In all animals, perineuronal vacuolation due to swelling of astrocytic processes is seen in the pyramidal cell layer. In mild cases there is an element of selectivity, with most vacuolation evident in the CA_3 region, but in some severely affected animals regional selectivity is lost with vacuolation marked not only throughout the pyramidal cell layer but also at the base of the dentate granule cell layer. A proportion of selectively vulnerable pyramidal neurones show the appearance of ischaemic cell change with condensation (darkening) and shrinkage of cyto- and karyo-plasm (Figures 1a and b). Such changes are not seen in the dentate granule cells.

Electron microscopy

An electron-lucent dilatation of perineuronal and pericapillary processes of the astrocytes (Figure 2a) corresponds to the vacuolated appearance in the light microscope.

In the cell bodies of pyramidal neurones of the CA_3 and CA_4 region dilatation of intracellular organelles is identifiable after $1-2$ hours of seizure activity. The commonest such change is swelling of mitochondria, both in the soma and in the basal dendrites (stratum oriens) (Figures 2a and b). Dilatation of the Golgi apparatus and endoplasmic reticulum is also seen. In the late stage of this process (2 hours) there is often gross disorganisation of the internal cristae of the mitochondria.

After $1-2$ hours of seizure activity a condensation of the somatic cytoplasm is apparent in most cells with swollen mitochondria. In the severest form of this cellular change the cytoplasm and karyoplasm are extremely dense and intracellular structure is ill-defined.

Oxalate-pyroantimonate preparations

Control material shows calcium pyroantimonate deposits most prominent in the synaptic vesicles (Figure 3a). Some sparse deposits are also detected in mitochondria and other organelles (Figure 3b).

After seizure activity of $1-2$ hours duration, increased calcium pyroantimonate deposits are evident particularly in swollen mitochondria of pyramidal cell bodies and in swollen basal dendrites of CA_3 and CA_1 neurones (Figures 4a and b).

Discussion

The light microscopic observations of selective pyramidal neurone pathology in the hippocampus confirm our earlier observations with bicuculline-induced

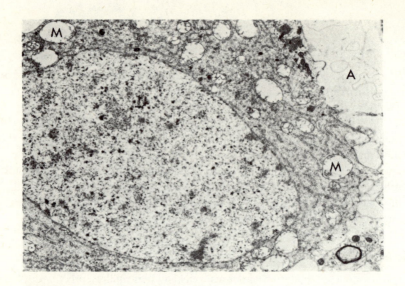

Figure 2a. Electron micrograph of early neuronal changes in a CA_4 neurone, showing micro-vacuolation (swollen mitochondria, M) and slight darkening of the cytoplasm. The cell is surrounded by enlarged, watery, astrocytic processes (A). Ventilated rat, perfused after 1 hour of continuous seizure activity induced by intravenous bicuculline (1.2mg/kg). Magnification x 8,600 (Reduced for publication)

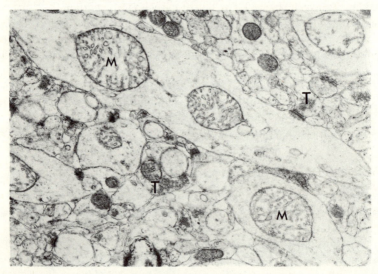

Figure 2b. Electron micrograph of neuropil in the stratum oriens from a rat perfused after 2 hours of electrographic seizure activity induced by intravenous L-allylglycine (276mg/kg). The basal dendrites of the CA_3 pyramidal neurones are enlarged and contain swollen and disrupted mitochondria (M). T = terminals contacting dendrites. Magnification x 18,200 (Reduced for publication)

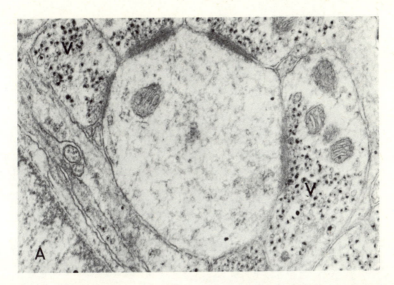

Figure 3a. Electron micrograph of control rat using oxalate-pyroantimonate method to show location of free calcium. Pyroantimonate deposits are prominent in the synaptic vesicles (V) in the terminals surrounding the dendrite of this hippocampal pyramidal neurone. Magnification x 48,000 (Reduced for publication)

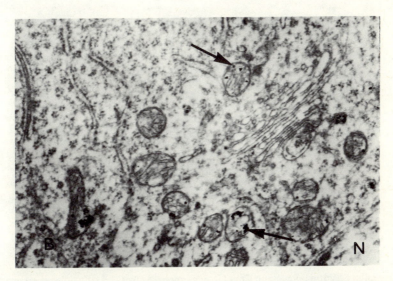

Figure 3b. Electron micrograph from hippocampus of the same control rat as Figure 3a, showing cytoplasmic structures of a pyramidal neurone. Sparse deposits of calcium pyroantimonate are visible in the mitochondria (arrows) N = nucleus. (Magnification x 34,300) (Reduced for publication)

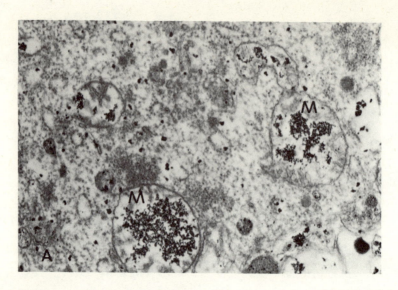

Figure 4a. Electron micrograph illustrating intracellular calcium accumulation in a pyramidal neurone following 2 hours of seizure activity, induced by intravenous L-allylglycine. Large swollen mitochondria (M) containing dense calcium pyroantimonate deposits. (Magnification x 35,500) (Reduced for publication)

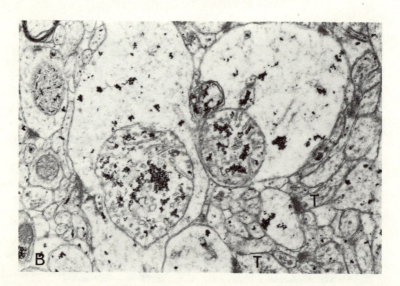

Figure 4b. Electron micrograph from the same animal as Figure 4a. Enlarged basal dendrites of CA_3 pyramidal neurones show swollen mitochondria with dense calcium pyroanti-monate deposits in both mitochondria and the surrounding dendrite cytoplasm. T = terminals. (Magnification x 23,100) (Reduced for publication)

seizures in baboons and rats [3,6], in terms of selectivity of pathology and the nature and time course of the cellular changes. We now report that L-allylglycine in the rat produces similarly selective hippocampal lesions with a comparable time course.

Our electron microscopic observations confirm our earlier tentative conclusion (based only on light microscopy) that the cellular changes induced by *status epilepticus* are indistinguishable from 'ischaemic cell change' resulting from anoxia/ischaemia as described by Brown and Brierley [14,15]. In particular, mitochondrial swelling is prominent before dense condensation of the cytoplasm. We cannot explain the failure of Söderfeldt and colleagues [16] to observe this change as a significant feature in the abnormal cortical neurones they describe during bicuculline-induced *status epilepticus* in the rat.

The use of the oxalate/pyroantimonate method to demonstrate free Ca^{++} at the fine structural level has provided a direct experimental confirmation of the third item in the hypothetical chain of events accounting for selective neuronal loss in *status epilepticus* proposed by Meldrum in April 1980 [9] and outlined above.

That mitochondria have the capacity to sequester Ca^{++} is well established [17]. They can exchange Ca^{++} for intramitochondrial H^+, or in the presence of free $PO_4^=$ can accumulate $CaPO_4$ in an osmotically active form. During drug-induced seizures in the rat, cerebral free $PO_4^=$ is dramatically increased due to hydrolysis of creatine phosphate [18]. Thus mitochondrial swelling might be a consequence of excessive calcium uptake.

The present observations provide a direct demonstration that Ca^{++} accumulates post-synaptically in mitochondria of selectively vulnerable neurones. This provides a link between (i) observations using extracellular ion sensitive electrodes showing a decrease in (Ca^{++}) during local seizure activity in the cortex or hippocampus, or in response to the iontophoretic application of glutamate or aspartate [19,20] and (ii) the concept of mitochondrial calcium overload as a step in the myopathic or ischaemic degenerative change in skeletal and smooth muscle [12,21].

We cannot say on the present evidence which are the critical steps determining irreversible destruction of the neurone. Probably failure of the metabolic role of the mitochondria and a massive increase in cytoplasmic free Ca^{++} together trigger the final phase.

Summary

Seizures have been induced by the systemic administration of bicuculline or L-allylglycine in rats whose physiological circumstances have been rigorously controlled. Perfusion fixed material has been used for a light and electron microscopic study of the genesis of hippocampal brain damage.

After 1–2 hours of seizure activity swelling of astrocytic processes gives the appearance of vacuolation around the pyramidal cell bodies. In the soma of selectively vulnerable pyramidal neurones (CA_{3-4}, CA_1), mitochondria are often distended and their cristae disrupted; dilatation is sometimes also seen in the Golgi apparatus and the endoplasmic reticulum. Condensation of the karyo- and cyto-plasm occurs in the more severely affected neurones. The appearances are those of 'ischaemic cell change'. Basal dendrites of CA_3 neurones are also dilated and contain distended mitochondria.

An abnormal accumulation of calcium in the distended mitochondria in the soma and dendrites of selectively vulnerable neurones is revealed by the oxalate/pyroantimonate method.

This provides direct evidence for the hypothesis proposed by Meldrum to account for selective neuronal vulnerability in epilepsy in terms of high calcium movements associated with burst firing and calcium cytotoxicity.

Acknowledgment

We thank the Wellcome Trust for financial support.

References

1   Corsellis JAN, Meldrum BS. In Blackwood W, Corsellis JAN, eds. *Greenfield's Neuropathology 3rd Edn 1976;* 771–795. London: Edward Arnold

2   Meldrum BS. In Williams D, ed. *Modern Trends in Neurology Vol 6 1975;* 223–239. London: Butterworths

3   Meldrum BS, Brierley JB. *Arch Neurol 1973; 28:* 10–17

4   Meldrum BS, Vigouroux RA, Brierley JB. *Arch Neurol 1973; 29:* 82–87

5   Meldrum BS, Horton RW, Brierley JB. *Brain 1974; 97:* 417–428

6   Blennow G, Brierley JB, Meldrum BS, Siesjö BK. *Brain 1978; 101:* 687–700

7   Ben-Ari Y, Tremblay E, Ottersen OP, Meldrum BS. *Brain Res 1980; 191:* 79–97

8   Menini C, Meldrum BS, Riche D et al. *Ann Neurol 1980; 8:* 501–509

9   Meldrum BS. In Rose FC, ed. *Metabolic Disorders of the Nervous System 1981;* 175–187. London: Pitman

10   Meldrum BS, In Delgado-Escueta AV, Wasterlain CG, Treiman DM, Porter RJ, eds. *Status Epilepticus: Mechanisms of Brain Damage and Treatment 1982;* 263–277. New York: Raven Press

11   Borgers M, De Brabander M, Van Reempts J et al. *Lab Invest 1977; 37:* 1–8

12   Borgers M, Thoné F, Van Neuten JM. *Acta Histochemica 1981; Suppl 24;* 327–332

13   Griffiths T, Evans MC, Meldrum BS. *Neuroscience Letters 1982; 30:* 329–334

14   Brown AW, Brierley JB. *J Neurol Sci 1972; 16:* 59–84

15   Brierley JB, Meldrum BS, Brown AW. *Arch Neurol 1973; 29:* 367–374

16   Söderfeldt B, Kalimo H, Olsson Y, Siesjö BK. *Acta Neuropathol (Berl) 1981; 54*

17   Nicholls DB, Åkerman KEO. *Phil Trans Soc Lond B 1981; 296:* 115–122

18   Chapman AG, Meldrum BS, Siesjö BK. *J Neurochem 1977; 28:* 1025–1035

19   Lux HD, Heinemann U. In Cobb WA, Van Duijn H, eds. *Contemporary Clinical Neurophysiology (EEG Suppl No 34) 1978;* 289–297. Amsterdam: Elsevier

20   Heinemann U, Pumain R. *Exp Brain Res 1980; 40:* 247–250

21   Wrogemann K, Penna SDJ. *Lancet 1976; i:* 672–674

10

IONIC CHANGES DURING EXPERIMENTALLY INDUCED EPILEPSIES

U Heinemann, H D Lux

Introduction

A number of cellular events accompany the abnormal neuronal behaviour characteristic of epilepsy (for review, see [1]). The spike, and the spike-and-wave complex of the electroencephalogram (EEG), is associated with a synchronous high frequency burst discharge of many cortical neurons. Both phenomena are caused by an abnormal paroxysmal depolarisation shift [2] of the neuronal membrane by up to 30mV, which is often but not always followed by hyperpolarisation. During the tonic phase of sustained seizure activity, neurons are continuously depolarised, but slowly repolarise during the clonic phases to eventually hyperpolarise after cessation of the ictal activity [3].

This behaviour is well known in penicillin focus epilepsy and was subsequently reported to be the characteristic feature of a number of other experimental epilepsies (for review, see Prince, [4] and [2,5–7]).

Analysis of the principal actions of a variety of epileptogenic substances has led to a survey of possible ways by which normal neurons in a given population can change their behaviour to develop paroxysmal discharge patterns [8]. These mechanisms include an accumulation in the extracellular space of excitatory dicarboxylic acids such as glutamate and aspartate [9] which, with structurally related amino acids, are known to be powerful convulsants [8,10].

Other substances, such as some amino acids [11], 4-aminopyridine [12,13], acetylcholine [14–16] and its muscarinic agonists, as well as pentetrazole [17,18] and oenanthotoxine [19], directly or indirectly interfere with K-conductances and thereby increase neuronal excitability. Often, these drugs also increase transmitter release, which could be anticipated from the interference of K-currents responsible for the termination of action potentials [12,13]. Other drugs such as picrotoxine [20], penicillin [21], pentetrazole [18,22,23], bicuculline [8] and strychnine [8], block the receptor sites for inhibitory transmitters, GABA and glycine, or prevent the activation of chloride channels which mediate the hyper-polarisation characteristic of an inhibitory synaptic potential [8].

A number of drugs also impair chloride extrusion [24–28] from neurons thereby increasing intracellular chloride concentration. This reduces the efficacy of synaptic inhibition [29], and is probably the cause of the initiation of seizure in all diseases associated with an increased ammonia concentration [27,30,31] in brain tissue.

The blocking effect of ammonia on chloride extrusion is well established (for review, see Heinemann and Lux [32] and Iles and Jack [31]). Hydrazine [33] and intracellular cobalt [34] have similar effects, and the loop diuretic, furosemide, has the same principal action [24,25] which may explain its recently reported epileptogenic action in babies.

This short list of principal convulsant drug actions, which is far from complete, reveals that very different causes can lead to the induction of epileptiform activity, but undeniable electrophysiological similarities between clinical and experimental epileptic features suggest that some common mechanisms are involved in processes such as generation, spread and termination of paroxysmal discharges. This chapter attempts to evaluate some of those mechanisms by using experimental evidence derived from electrophysiological studies of the membrane behaviour of invertebrate and vertebrate neurons, and from evaluation of the ionic conc-entration changes in the sensorimotor cortex of rats and cats, as obtained with ion selective microelectrodes. Measurements of the changes in $[Na]_o^-$, $[Cl]_o^-$, $[Ca]_o$ and $[K]_o$ take advantage of the fact that the extracellular space is small in diameter, so that ion fluxes across membranes can easily result in significant changes of ionic concentrations. Alternatively these changes can be used as moni-tors of electrogenic events at neuronal membranes. Since changes in $[K]_o$ and $[Ca]_o$ affect neuronal excitability, they contribute to the pathophysiological mechanisms underlying epileptogenesis.

Generation of paroxysmal depolarisation shifts

At present, there are three hypotheses to explain the generation of paroxysmal depolarisation shifts (PDS). The original hypothesis by Matsumo and Ajmone-Marsan [2] suggested paroxysmal depolarisation shifts (PDS) to reflect 'giant'-EPSP's that result from excessive transmitter release [3]. By overriding inhibi-tory control, recurrent excitatory pathways could be activated to the extent that epileptiform activity results. An argument in favour of this hypothesis is that the reversal potential of PDS in CA3 hippocampal pyramidal cells [35] is quite comparable with that of the EPSP [36] and of glutamate induced membrane potential changes [37]. Thus, in many neurons paroxysmal depolarisation shifts resemble the behaviour of synaptically induced potentials [38]. The two other hypotheses regard properties of single neurons suggesting that, under certain conditions, a normal cell changes into an 'epileptic' neuron [4,39–46]. These neurons should be able to produce epileptiform discharges even without synaptic context. In fact, in mollusc neurons [47], as well as in hippocampal pyramidal cells, it was demonstrated that synaptically isolated cells can produce features resembling paroxysmal depolarisation shifts. In the hippocampus, four lines of evidence strengthen this conclusion:

1 Paroxysmal depolarisation shifts can be triggered by depolarising current injection into penicillin treated cells [44,48].

2 PDS are still observable in the presence of the sodium channel blocker, terodotoxin, that prevents generation and propagation of action potentials and thus also synaptic transmission [43,49,50].

3 Spontaneous [Ca] decreases and repetitive discharges of hippocampal neurons are observed if [Ca] is lowered to a level below possible synaptic transmission (Konnerth and Heinemann, in preparation).

4 In addition, hyperpolarisation of neurons can prevent generation of paroxysmal depolarisation shifts [44,48]. This suggests that a voltage dependent inward current [51] directly or indirectly generates the PDS. Since PDS are prevented by Ca antagonists such as manganese [48] and, alternatively, since PDS generation is facilitated in the presence of barium [52—54] which enhances inward currents through Ca channels [42,55], it was suggested that a Ca inward current is the generator current for the PDS.

Considerable support for this view stems from the observation that interictal discharges are accompanied by significant reductions of $[Ca]_o$, both in neocortex [56—58] and hippocampus [18]. However, if Ca currents were the unique generators for PDS, then hyperpolarising currents should always reset the PDS because hyperpolarisation is known to rapidly close Ca-channels, but this resetting was not the case in a number of hippocampal neurons [35,44]. Moreover, the reversal potential of a directly Ca mediated PDS should be far more positive than actually observed. Therefore a third approach to this problem will be attempted using evidence from studies of the mechanisms that underlie spontaneous rhythmic burst generation in pacemaker neurons of molluscs. In these neurons, artificial injections of Ca ions into the cell [40,59], or Ca influx [55,60] during action potentials, was found to activate a non-specific current carried by cations such as Na and K with a reversal potential close to zero. This current apparently generates the depolarisation that leads to repetitive discharges. Cell firing with Ca-electrogenesis then increases intracellular [Ca] which is known to activate a potassium conductance that repolarises the neurons. Such Ca-conductances and Ca-activated K-conductance obviously occur also in motoneurons [61] and hippocampal pyramidal cells of the subfield CA1 [62—64]. Although this model would satisfactorily account for a wealth of experimental observations, it is yet unclear whether such Ca-activated non-specific membrane permeabilities also exist in cortical neurons. The condition for this mechanism is also a sufficiently intensive

Ca electrogenesis in neurons of a cortical area that is capable of generating seizures. This should also apply to neocortical neurons.

Evidence for the existence of voltage dependent Ca-conductances (see also [65–67]) in neocortical neurons was obtained by experiments in which changes in $[Ca]_o$ and $[Na]_o$ were simultaneously measured during iontophoretic application of excitatory amino acids such as glutamate, aspartate, DL-homocysteic acid, N-methyl D aspartate (NMDA) and quisqualate. All these amino acids caused dose dependent reductions in $[Ca]_o$ and $[Na]_o$. $[Ca]_o$ decreased by up to 1.1mM and $[Na]_o$ fell by up to 25mM from a baseline level of 1.2 and 147mM respectively (Figure 1). The biggest falls for $[Ca]_o$ were found in layer II of cat sensorimotor cortex [65,67] and in layer II and V of rat sensorimotor cortex. Decreases in $[Na]_o$ were much less dependent on the recording depth within the cortex. These findings could be explained by assuming that Ca leaves the extracellular space through ionophores directly controlled by the excitatory amino acids [68]. This was indeed suggested in the case of NMDA [69] activated ionophores [70–72]. In order to test this possibility we investigated the effects of iontophorectically applied Mn on $[Na]_o$ and $[Ca]_o$ changes. A typical experiment is illustrated in Figure 1, which shows a characteristic change of $[Na]_o$ and $[Ca]_o$ during iontophoretic application of aspartate. When Mn was applied the $[Ca]_o$ recovered to near normal levels whereas $[Na]_o$ remained lower. Similar observations were made with GABA, which reversed the Ca signal but did not affect the sodium decrease. This suggests that Ca and Na move through independent channels and it is likely that Ca leaves the extracellular space through a voltage dependent Ca selective ionophore.

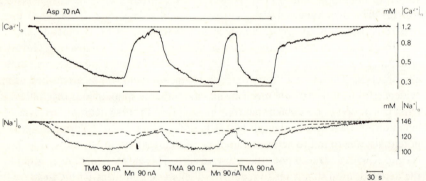

Figure 1. Simultaneous recording of $[Ca]_o$ and $[Na]_o$ with an electrode assembly consisting of a Na-selective/reference electrode, a Ca-selective/reference electrode and a multibarrelled iontophoresis electrode. The distance between tips of the ion selective electrodes was about $30\mu m$; the distance of the ion selective electrodes to the phoresis electrode was about $50\mu m$. Since Va selective electrodes are also sensitive to changes in $[Ca]_o$ by on average 8mV for a tenfold change in $[Ca]_o$, Na-signals had to be corrected according to the interference from changes in $[Ca]_o$, the dotted line represents the corrected Na-signal. Bars represent the various drug applications. Tetramethylammonium (TMA) was ejected with the same current as manganese (Mn) in order to control possible changes in transport number

Ca- and Na-changes in the in vitro hippocampal slice preparation

In the hippocampal slice preparation, stimulus induced reductions in $[Ca]_o$ are largest in the pyramidal cell layer [73–75], which suggests that Ca conductances are present in the somata of hippocampal pyramidal cells. Indeed, excitatory amino acid-induced decreases in $[Ca]_o$ were also largest in this layer. As in neocortex [66] the $[Ca]_o$ reductions were only little affected by TTX, but often completely blocked by GABA and also by Ca antagonists such as Co, Ni and Mn [75] but, in contrast to neocortex, simultaneously measured $[Na]_o$ falls were also reduced by GABA and by the Ca-antagonists. In order to test the possibility that a Ca activated non-specific conductance (Na^+ and K^+) is present in hippocampal neurons, we lowered $[Ca]_o$ to levels below 10^{-5} M. Under this condition Ca accumulation in neurons is expected to be much smaller. Indeed, $[Na]_o$ decreases were reduced to about half of control, when evoked in low Ca-solutions. When sodium in the perfusing medium was partially replaced by Tris H Cl, reductions in $[Na]_o$ and $[Ca]_o$, evoked by excitatory amino acids, were also considerably smaller. These findings raise the possibility that the Ca influx into hippocampal neurons activates, as in mollusc neurons, a depolarising inward current, which would then be the generator current for the PDS. When Ca currents serve generally to either generate or mediate membrane events underlying epileptiform discharges, it is expected that $[Ca]_o$ decreases accompany epileptiform activity, regardless of its primary cause. Therefore we compared changes in $[Ca]_o$ in normal cortex with those occurring in seizures of different aetiologies.

Changes in extracellular free Ca during epileptogenesis

In normal sensorimotor cortex, reductions in $[Ca]_o$ by up to 0.4mM could be evoked by repetitive stimulation of the cortical surface and of the thalamic ventrobasal complex [76,77]. Decreases in $[Ca]_o$ were regularly found only in depths of 100 to 700μm, with a maximum decrease in layer II. Below this depth in freshly prepared cortices, only rises in $[Ca]_o$ were observed as shown in Figure 2 A. When stimulation was repeated more than 30 times with intervals of five minutes between stimulus trains, transient reductions of $[Ca]_o$ also became apparent in depths below 700μm. This was paralleled by an increase in seizure susceptibility. The increase in $[Ca]_o$ during stimulation is probably the result of a shrinkage in extracellular space size [56]. As shown in Figure 2 B, this laminar profile of $[Ca]_o$ falls was dramatically changed by topical application of alumina cream on to the surface of the sensorimotor cortex six months to six years before the experiment. Close to the gliotic scar which develops subsequently to such manipulations, spontaneous paroxysmal activity could often be recorded. In these areas, falls in $[Ca]_o$ were up to 0.7mM and the site of maximum decrease in $[Ca]_o$ could be found in any layer of the cortex. Similar observations were made in the chronic cobalt powder focus in the sensorimotor

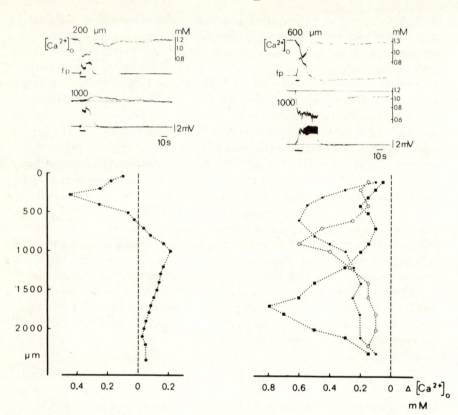

Figure 2. Stimulus induced changes in [Ca]$_o$ in normal cortex (A) and in a chronic alumina creamfocus (B). The changes in [Ca]$_o$ were evoked by repetitive cortical surface stimulation pulses of 0.1msec and in intensity of 0.8mA at 20Hz for all stimuli. Stimulus duration is indicated by bars. Numbers refer to the recording depth. Recordings in B were obtained at a distance of about 0.8mm from the border of the scar. The plots in A and B show the amplitudes of changes in [Ca]$_o$ as recording depth. Data in A are averages from the [Ca]$_o$ decreases in three different experiments. Symbols in B refer to B different experiments

cortex of rats, where we also studied the effects of excitatory amino acids on [Ca]$_o$ and found that amino acid-induced falls in [Ca]$_o$ were largest at atypical sites (Pumain and Heinemann, in preparation). The reason for this change in laminar distribution of Ca falls is as yet unclear.

Alterations of Ca-signals were also observed in acutely induced epilepsies. We studied substances which either impaired inhibitory processes, such as penicillin, pentetraxol and picrotoxin, or substances (oenanthotoxin, 4-aminopyridine, pentetrazole) which had blocking effects on repolarising K-currents. All these

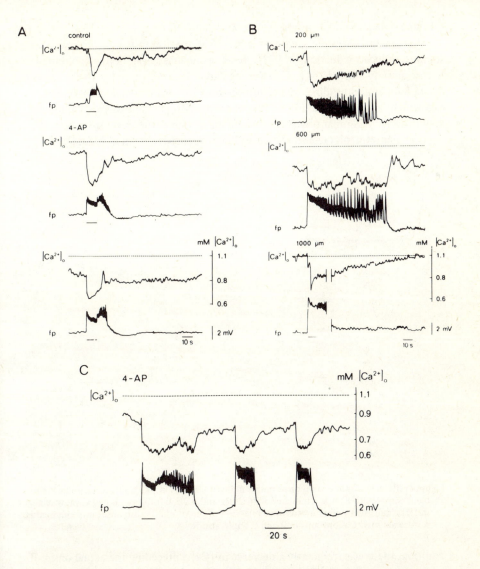

Figure 3. Effect of 4-aminopyridine (4-AP) on extracellular free calcium and field potentials (fp).

(A) Stimulus induced reduction in $[Ca]_o$ before control and after application of 4-AP. The middle recording was obtained before onset of the first spontaneous seizure; the lower recording during recovery from a spontaneous seizure. Recording depth $300\mu m$ below cortical surface. Stimulation of the ventrobasal complex with 20Hz and 0.5mA is indicated by bars.

(B) Depth profile of changes in $[Ca]_o$ during spontaneous (200 and 600 s) or stimulus induced seizures. Numbers refer to recording depth below cortical surface. Forty seconds of seizure activity are omitted in the recording.

(C) Repetitive seizure activity induced by a 20Hz CS stimulation

93

substances had a number of effects in common:

When an epileptogenic agent was topically applied on to the cortical surface, stimulus induced reductions in $[Ca]_o$ became enhanced even before spontaneous seizure activity started [56]. This was regularly observed when the focus was induced by 4-aminopyridine, by oenanthotoxin [19] or by penicillin. A typical experiment is illustrated in Figure 3 A, where 4-aminopyridine was used to induce seizure activity. Similar observations were made when drugs were systematically applied (pentetrazol, oenanthotoxin and picrotoxin) as shown in Figure 4. In

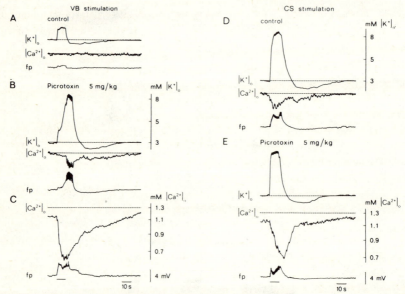

Figure 4. Effects of picrotoxin on stimulus induced changes in $[K]_o$ and $[Ca]_o$. The ventro-basal complex (VB) was stimulated with 20Hz and 0.2mA for 6 sec. B and C show changes in $[K]_o$ and $[Ca]_o$ after intravenous injection of picrotoxin before onset of spontaneous seizure activity. Calibrations in B and C apply also for A

addition, there was frequently a decrease in $[Ca]_o$ preceding the actual onset of spontaneous seizure discharges [19,57,58]. Moreover, $[Ca]_o$ could fall to much lower levels (0.5mM) than during intensive stimulation in normal cortex. After induction of a focus or of generalised seizure activity $[Ca]_o$ reductions also became apparent in more or less all cortical layers (Figure 3 B), except layer VI where only rarely were reductions in $[Ca]_o$ seen. When interictal activity was present (penicillin, oenanthotoxin), then these discharges were also accompanied by falls in $[Ca]_o$. These findings suggest that Ca-dependent mechanisms play an essential and general role in epileptogenesis.

Some caution for such a hypothesis is necessary, since cobalt application, which blocks Ca-conductances, can also induce seizure activity. We investigated this problem by analysing $[Ca]_o$ changes in an acute $CoCl_2$-focus (Konnerth and Heinemann, in preparation), which was established by application to the cortical surface of a gelform pledget soaked in a 40mM $CoCl_2$ containing Tyrode solution applied for about 20 to 40 min. This time was usually sufficient to block both amino acid- and stimulus-induced falls in $[Ca]_o$. About an hour after the end of the cobalt application, stimulus- and amino acid-evoked reductions in $[Ca]_o$ reappeared. Before the first interictal discharge appeared, stimulus- and amino acid-induced reductions in $[Ca]_o$ became even larger than in control measurements. Interictal discharges and later spontaneous seizures were accompanied by considerable reductions of $[Ca]_o$, which were present in all cortical layers but sometimes largest in the deeper layers. Thus it is likely that paroxysmal discharges first develop when the Ca blocking action of cobalt-ions has been overcome.

Changes in extracellular free Ca and their role in epileptogenesis

Reductions in extracellular free Ca increase neuronal excitability and impair synaptic transmission [78]. The increased neuronal excitability results from a reduced screening effect of negative surface charges which facilitate the activation of sodium-currents and therefore lowers the threshold for induction of action potentials [79]. On the other hand, reductions of $[Ca]_o$ decrease the efficacy of synaptic transmission due to a smaller influx of Ca into presynaptic terminals with a subsequently diminished transmitter release. It is widely accepted that generation of synaptic potentials induced by single stimuli is prevented when $[Ca]_o$ in the perfusing medium is lowered to levels of 0.5mM. In an investigation not yet published, we studied these problems further by employing Ca selective microelectrodes to measure stimulus-induced Ca changes and synaptic transfer at low Ca levels. It was found that single shock evoked synaptic potentials were largely depressed when $[Ca]_o$ was lowered to 0.3mM. When stimulus intensities of below two times threshold were used during repetitive stimulation, $[Ca]_o$ had to be lowered to 0.1mM to prevent synaptic transfer. Slight increases in stimulus frequency or intensity re-established synaptic transfer, which was paralleled by moderate variations in Ca-signals.

Stimulus induced reductions in $[Ca]_o$ were also present when no synaptic transfer was visible, as judged from simultaneously performed field potential and intracellular recordings. When stimulus intensity or frequency was slightly increased, initial $[Ca]_o$ reductions were only slightly enhanced. As soon as synaptic transfer was re-established, much larger reductions in $[Ca]_o$ became apparent. These data suggest that Ca can accumulate in presynaptic endings where Ca-concentration is very likely below 10^{-6}M. In the presence of increased intracellular Ca-levels, small Ca inward currents are probably sufficient to trigger transmitter release. Such a presynaptic Ca accumulation would in fact facilitate transmitter

95

release also under physiological conditions, and explains why epileptogenesis can be maintained even when $[Ca]_O$ falls during seizure to levels of as low as 0.5mM (Figure 2). Since spontaneous epileptiform discharges develop at low $[Ca]_O$ levels and since normal evoked responses change into burst discharges when $[Ca]_O$ is lowered in the perfusing medium (Konnerth and Heinemann, in preparation), we expect that the net effect of lowered $[Ca]_O$ is to increase neuronal excitability and to support the development of sustained seizure activity. This conclusion is supported by the finding that the frequency of spontaneous paroxysmal spikes is increased when $[Ca]_O$ is lowered in a hippocampal in vitro preparation [80].

Rises in potassium concentration during seizure activity

As shown in Figure 4, seizure activity is accompanied by increases in $[K]_O$ from a baseline level of 3mM to ceiling levels of 10 to 12mM [81–87], such increases being found in all epilepsies so far investigated [27,77,79]. Various authors have demonstrated in in vitro and in vivo experiments that elevated $[K]_O$ increases neuronal excitability in the concentration range typical for epileptiform activity [58,85,88,89].

This is mostly due to a depressant effect on repolarising K-currents due to a reduced transmembranous potassium gradient [45] which will prolong action potentials and increase evoked transmitter release. Elevated $[K]_O$ levels depolarise neuronal membranes and thus facilitate generation of action potentials [81]. In addition, spontaneous transmitter release is enhanced. Moreover, Cl will be taken into cells due to Donnan equilibration. Thus the efficacy of post-synaptic inhibition is lowered as a result of increased $[K]_O$ [27,29,90].

Potassium accumulation itself is of course the result of the intensive neuronal activity characteristic of epileptiform discharges but, since K is very likely spatially redistributed due to glial and neuronal buffering [91,92], $[K]_O$ also increases considerably in the quiescent surround of an epileptic focus, where it may support recruitment into epileptic activity [93].

Experimental evidence for such a role of K-accumulation was derived from experiments, where the effect of iontophoretically elevated $[K]_O$ levels on spreading seizure activity was investigated. When changes of $[K]_O$ are measured in sensorimotor cortex at some distance from a focal stimulating electrode pair, it is observed that $[K]_O$ rises in two phases [58,85,94]. Initially there is an elevation of $[K]_O$ from baseline to intermediate plateau levels of between 3.4 and 5mM from which develops a secondary rise in $[K]_O$, which is associated with high frequency burst discharges of increasing duration and with the development of epileptiform field potentials. When $[K]_O$ is elevated by local K-injection from an iontophoretic electrode in close proximity to the recording electrode, it is noted that the latency to the onset of the secondary rise in $[K]_O$ is shortened, and often that the amplitude of the secondary rise in $[K]_O$ is enhanced [58,83].

K-accumulation is not the sole factor supporting spread of seizure discharge;

also important is repetitive ectopic action potential generation in presynaptic endings and nerve branch points which leads to an excessive transmitter release in many locations [95–97]. Such an ectopic action potential generation has also been described in pyramidal tract neurons where it would reach not only a good number of cortical cells but also thalamic, cerebellar and other structures [96]. The mechanisms underlying ectopic action potential generation are yet unclear, but it may well be that K-accumulation and decreases in $[Ca]_O$ are important factors in generation of repetitive burst discharges in presynaptic endings.

Further, it may be possible that, at some sites in the cortex, cells are electrically coupled either by ephaptic connections or by gap junctions [98]. Such pathways may be used for synchronisation and spread of seizures.

Potassium accumulation and termination of seizure discharge

During an ictal episode, the neuronal discharge rate easily increases from average frequencies of 5 to 20/s to discharge rates of up to 200Hz. If, for the moment of seizure onset, it is assumed that none of the possible K clearing mechanisms were active, then it can be estimated that each action potential adds 0.01 to 0.03 mM to $[K]_O$. Thus $[K]_O$ could theoretically increase to levels of near 50mM if powerful K regulation mechanisms were not present. One such regulating mechanism is active K reuptake, as suggested by the observations of an increased oxygen consumption during and subsequent to seizure activity [99]. K uptake was more directly demonstrated by showing that iontophoretically induced K-signals were reduced in amplitude during stimulus induced rises and subsequent undershoots in $[K]_O$, as compared to K-signals evoked at resting levels. The iontophoretically induced K-signals were reduced by up to 50 per cent [73,84,85], so that active K-uptake appears to be an important factor in limiting the rise in $[K]_O$. It is also involved in generation of undershoots in $[K]_O$ (which follow increases in $[K]_O$), the amplitudes and durations of which are closely related to the amplitudes of preceding rises in K [83,84,100]. K-uptake is very likely linked to an electrogenic transport which is activated by intracellular Na and extracellular K accumulation and which, by excess transport of cations out of the cell, shifts the membrane potential in a hyperpolarising direction. It may well contribute to termination of seizure discharge, as evidenced by re- and hyper-polarisations of neuronal membrane potential during sustained seizure activity [5,47]. As expected, postictal depressions of neuronal discharge rate are positively correlated with the amplitude of the undershoots in $[K]_O$. This is also true for periods with depressed synaptic transfer, and for periods of reduced antidromic invasion probability for action potentials into nerve cell somata, which were generated in the synaptic endings or axonal fibres [100]. These findings suggest that activation of an electrogenic transport mechanism may be an important factor in termination of seizure activity. Indeed it was reported that seizure susceptibility is reduced during undershoots in $[K]_O$ [84,100,101].

Again this may not be the sole factor responsible for termination of seizure. Ca dependent activation of K-conductances [61,62,102] and Ca dependent uncoupling of electrotonic gap junctions in areas such as the hippocampus may be other interesting, although not as yet investigated, possibilities.

Changes in extracellular space size during seizure discharge

Reductions in iontophoretically induced K-signals can in principle also result from a widening of the extracellular space. For this reason, we performed experiments in which tetramethylammonium (TMA) or choline was iontophoretically pulsed into the extracellular space. Since TMA and choline uptake does not play an essential role for short periods of 10 to 15 sec., increases in TMA concentration are markers for the actual size of the extracellular space, whose volume fraction varies between 10 and 30 per cent and is an average of about 20 per cent [103,104]. During, and subsequent to, seizure discharge the extracellular space size decreases by 30 to 50 per cent at sites of maximum rises in $[K]_o$, which is usually layer IV of the sensorimotor cortex of cats [91,92]. This was indicated by increases in iontophoretically induced choline and TMA signals which were enhanced by up to 100 per cent. Reductions in extracellular space size in these depths are related to the amplitude and duration of a $[K]_o$ increase. This was further supported by experiments in which it was demonstrated that artificial elevation of K by local superfusion with a K enriched medium, or by local iontophoresis of K, also led to considerable reductions in extracellular space size [91,92]. We suggested an extension of the glial buffer mechanisms [105] to account for these decreases in extracellular space size.

Decreases in extracellular space size as a result of K-accumulation

Increased K not only depolarises neurons but also glial elements in sensorimotor cortex [106,107]. Since glial cells are spatially extended and/or electrically coupled [108,109], this depolarisation is electrotonically propagated to sites in which $[K]_o$ is smaller than at the sites of maximal increases in $[K]_o$, which is in about layer IV of the neocortex in most experimental epilepsies. At sites remote from maximal K-elevation, K leaves the glial compartment in order to restore the transmembranous equilibrium. Thus a current is induced which causes a compensatory current through the extracellular space, which is responsible for the slow potential shifts regularly accompanying seizure activity [1,32,109]. This spatial buffering of K very probably leads to a shrinkage of extracellular space size at sites of maximal K accumulation. Across glial membranes the current is carried only by K ions but, in the extracellular compartment, it is carried to about an equal extent by Na and Cl. Therefore, if 10 K ions leave the extracellular space at the site of maximal K elevation, only some Na ions replace them. In addition Cl ions move in the opposite direction; i.e. they leave the site of maximal K accumulation, so that extracellular osmolarity decreases and water moves into cells to restore isoosmolarity [90–92]. This hypothesis predicts that, remote from the site of maximal K elevation, widenings of the extracellular space size occur, which is indeed the case [91] and particularly impressive at border zones between normal and gliotic scar tissue. Whereas the extracellular space shrinks during seizure activity just outside a scar, it becomes wider when $[K]_o$ changes within the gliotic tissue, in spite of some remaining $[K]_o$ increases.

Na and Cl changes in epilepsy

The glial buffering of potassium also serves to prevent too large reductions in $[Na]_o$ and $[Cl]_o$ during seizure activity which is accompanied by considerable fluxes of Na and Cl into neurons. Maintenance of $[Na]_o$- and $[Cl]_o$- levels is expected, since shrinkage of extracellular space size increases the concentration of the remaining particles in the extracellular space. This was confirmed by measuring $[Na]_o$ and $[Cl]_o$ changes during stimulus [90] and penterazole induced seizures [110]. As in the case for Ca, Na increases after an initial fall by up to 7mM to levels above baselines at sites of maximal neuronal activity. Cl often does not fall at all and also increases above baseline levels.

Taking the shrinkage of extracellular space and relative volume fractions into account, it can be calculated that intracellular Na increases by up to 40mM and that $[Cl]_i$ also rises by some mM. Intracellular Cl accumulation supports development of seizure discharge by reducing efficacy of inhibitory synaptic transmission. Intracellular Na accumulation, on the other hand, as well as extracellular K accumulation, will stimulate an electrogenic pump mechanism which, by excess transport of cations out of the cell, hyperpolarises the neuronal membrane. This pump is probably the main cause for decreases of K to sub-baseline levels after the end of seizure activity (Figure 4). Apparently the Na/k-pump has a relatively long time constant, since undershoots in $[K]_o$ last for up to three minutes (Figure 4). During such decreases in $[K]_o$, seizure threshold is increased and neuronal excitability is reduced. Thus Na accumulation in cells may be one of the causes for termination of seizure activity.

In addition to decreases in intraneuronal $[K]_i$ and to increases in $[Na]_i$ and $[Cl]_i$, it is expected that intracellular calcium concentration rises. This will have many effects on the metabolism, axonal and dendritic transport and may also be responsible for cell death (see Dr Meldrum's chapter), to which alterations in cell nutrition and clearance of metabolites, due to a decreased extracellular space may contribute.

Conclusions

The effects of ionic changes in epileptogenesis may be summarised as follows:

1 Ictal activity is accompanied by increases in $[K]_o$ and $[Cl]_o$ and by reduction of $[Na]_o$, $[Ca]_o$ and of the extracellular space size.

2 Reductions in $[Ca]_o$ often precede the onset of spontaneous epileptiform activity. They are larger than in normal cortex and they can occur at atypical sites. This suggests that activation of Ca dependent mechanisms is a common feature of epileptogenesis irrespective of its primary cause.

3 Increases in $[K]_o$, decreases in $[Ca]_o$ and intracellular Cl-accumulation support the development of seizure activity.

4 Spatial redistribution of potassium supports the spread of ictal activity from a primary focus.

5 Accumulation of Na in cells, and of K in the extracellular microenvironment, will very likely stimulate electrogenic transport processes which contribute to the termination of seizure activity.

Acknowledgments

This research was supported by the DFG. Ca, Na selective resins were kindly provided by Professor Simon in Zürich.

References

1   Lux HD, Entstehung des FFG. In Simon O, ed. *Das Elektroenkephalogramm 1977;* 1–15. München, Baltimore, Wien: Urban and Schwarzenberg
2   Matsumoto H, Ajmone-Marsan C. *Exp Neurol 1964; 9:* 286–304
3   Ayala GF, Dichter M, Gumnit PJ et al. *Brain Res 1973; 52:* 1–17
4   Prince DA. *Ann Rev Neurosci 1978; 1:* 395–415
5   Oakley JC, Sypert GW, Ward AA Jr. *Exp Neurol 1972; 37:* 300–311
6   Pumain P. *Brain Res 1981;* In press
7   Pumain R. In Klee MR, Lux HD, Speckmann FJ, eds. *Physiology and Pharmacology of Epileptogenic Phenomena 1982;* 65–72. New York: Raven Press
8   Woodbury DM. In Glaser GM, Penry JK, Woodbury DM, eds. *Antiepileptic Drugs: Mechanisms of Action 1980;* 249–302. New York: Raven Press
9   Puil F. *Neurophysiol 1974; 36:* 308–310
10   Watkins JC. In McGeer FG, Olney JW, McGeer PL, eds. *Excitatory Amino Acis 1978;* 37–69. New York: Raven Press
11   Engberg I, Flatman JA, Lambert JDC. *Br J Pharmacol 1978; 64:* 384–385
12   Buckle PJ, Haas HL. *J Physiol (Lond) 1982;* In press
13   Galvan M, Grafe P, Bruggencate G. In Klee MR, Lux HD, Speckmann FJ, eds. *Pharmacology and Physiology of Epileptogenic Phenomena 1982;* 353–360. New York: Raven Press
14   Adams PR, Brown DA, Constanti A. In Klee MR, Lux HD, Speckmann FJ, eds. *Pharmacology and Physiology of Epileptogenic Phenomena 1982;* 175–187. New York: Raven Press
15   Brown DA, Adams PR. *Nature 1980; 283:* 673–676
16   Krnjevic K, Pumain R, Penaud L. *J Physiol (Lond) 1971; 215:* 247–268
17   Klee MR, Faber DS, Heiss WD. *Science 1973; 179:* 1133–1136
18   Louvel J, Heinemann U, Lux HD. *Arch Physiol 1981;* In press
19   Louvel J, Aldenhoff J, Hofmeier G, Heinemann U. In Klee MR, Lux HD, Speckman FJ, eds. *Physiology and Pharmacology of Epileptogenic Phenomena 1981;* 47–52. New York: Raven Press
20   Aickin CC, Deisz RA, Lux HD. *J Physiol (Lond) 1981; 315:* 157–173

21   Dingledine R, Gjerstad L. *Brain Res 1979; 168:* 205–209
22   MacDonald RL, Parker JL. *Nature 1977; 267:* 720–721
23   Nicoll RA, Padjen A. *Pharmacol 1976; 15:* 69–71
24   Aickin CC, Deisz RA, Lux HD. *J Physiol (Lond) 1982;* In press
25   Deisz RA, Lux HD. *Forschung/Drug Res 1978; 28:* 870–871
26   Lux HD. *Science 1971; 173:* 555–557
27   Lux HD, Heinemann U. In Cobb WA, van Duijn H, eds. *Contempory Clinical Neuro-physiology (EFG Suppl 34) 1978;* 289–297. North Holland: Elsevier, Amsterdam: Biomed Press BV
28   Lux HD, Loracher C, Neher F. *Exp Brain Res 1970; 11:* 431–447
29   Meyer H, Lux HD. *Pflueg Arch 1974; 350:* 185–195
30   Hsia JF. In Siegel GJ, Albers RW, Katzman R, Agranoff BW, eds. *Basic Neurochemistry 1976;* 500–541. Boston: Little Brown & Co
31   Iles JF, Jack JJB. *Brain Res 1980; 103:* 555–578
32   Heinemann U, Lux HD. In Speckmann FJ, Caspers H, eds. *Origin of Cerebral Field Potentials 1979;* 33–48. Stuttgart: Georg Thieme
33   Liebl L. *Exp Brain Res 1975; 23:* 125
34   Sypert GW, Bidgood WD. *Brain Res 1977; 134:* 372–376
35   Johnston D, Brown TH. *Science 1981; 211:* 294–297
36   Hablitz JJ, Langmoen IA. *J Physiol (Lond);* In press
37   Langmoen IA, Hablitz JJ. *Neurosci Lett 1981; 23:* 61–65
38   Gjerstad L, Andersen P, Langmoen IA et al. *Acta Physiol Scand 1981; 113:* 245–252
39   Crill WF. In Glaser GH, Penry JK, Woodbury DM, eds. *Antiepileptic Drugs: Mechanisms of Action 1980;* 169–183. New York: Raven Press
40   Hofmeier G, Lux HD. In Klee MR, Lux HD, Speckmann FJ, eds. *Physiology and Pharmacology of Epileptic Phenomena 1982;* 299–308. New York: Raven Press
41   Kandel ER, Spencer WA. *J Neurophysiol 1961; 24:* 243–259
42   Lux HD, Schubert P. *Advances Neurol 1975; 12:* 29–43
43   Prince DA. In Klee M, Lux HD, Speckmann FJ, eds. *Physiology and Pharmacology of Epileptogenic Phenomena 1982;* 151–162. New York: Raven Press
44   Schwartzkroin PA, Prince DA. *Brain Res 1980; 183:* 61–76
45   Schwindt P, Crill WF. *J Neurophysiol 1980; 43:* 1296–1318
46   Traub RD, Llinas R. *J Neurophysiol 1979; 42:* 476–496
47   Speckmann FJ, Casper H, Janzen RW. In Petsche H, Brazier MAB, eds. *Mechanisms of Synchronisation in Epileptic Seizures 1972.* Wein, Heidelberg: Springer
48   Wong RKS, Prince DA. *Science 1979; 204:* 1228–1231
49   Wong RKS. In Klee MR, Lux HD, Speckmann FJ, eds. *Physiology and Pharmacology of Epileptogenic Phenomena 1982;* 163–173. New York: Raven Press
50   Wong RKS, Prince DA. *Brain Res 1978; 159:* 385–390
51   Hotson JR, Prince DA, Schwartzkroin PA. *J Neurophysiol 1979; 42:* 889–895
52   Hotson JR. In Klee MR, Lux HD, Speckmann FJ, eds. *Physiology and Pharmacology of Epileptogenic Phenomena 1982;* 113–121. New York: Raven Press
53   Hotson JR, Prince DA. *Annals Neurol 1981; 10:* 11–17
54   Schwindt PC, Crill WF. *J Neurophysiol 1980; 44:* 827–846
55   Lux HD. *Nature 1974; 250:* 574–576
56   Heinemann U, Konnerth A, Louvel J et al. In Klee MR, Lux HD, Speckmann FJ, eds. *Physiology and Pharmacology of Epileptogenic Phenomena 1982;* 29–35. New York: Raven Press
57   Heinemann U, Lux HD, Gutnick MJ. *Exp Brain Res 1977; 27:* 237–243
58   Heinemann U, Lux HD, Gutnick MJ. In Chalazonitis M, Boisson M, eds. *Abnormal Neuronal Discharges 1978;* 329–345. New York: Raven Press
59   Hofmeier G, Lux HD. *Pflueg Arch 1981; 391:* 242–251
60   Lux HD, Heyer CB. In Schmitt FO, Worden FG, eds. *The Neurosciences Fourth Study Program 1979;* 601–615. Cambridge: The MIT Press
61   Krnjevic K, Lisiewicz A. *J Physiol (Lond) 1972; 225:* 363–390
62   Alger BF, Nicoll RA. *Science 1980; 210:* 1122–1124
63   Hotson JR, Prince DA. *J Neurophysiol 1980; 43:* 409–419

64   Schwartzkroin PA, Slawsky M. *Brain Res 1977; 135:* 157—161
65   Heinemann U, Pumain R. *Brain Res 1980; 40:* 247—250
66   Heinemann U, Pumain R. *Neurosci Lett 1981; 21:* 87—91
67   Heinemann U, Pumain R. *Neurosci Lett 1981; Suppl 7:* 353
68   Takeuchi N. *J Physiol (Lond) 1963; 167:* 141—155
69   Watkins JC. In DeFendis FV, Mandel P, eds. *Amino Acid Transmitters 1981;* 205—212. New York: Raven Press
70   Ault B, Evans RH, Francis AA et al. *J Physiol (Lond) 1980; 307:* 413—428
71   Davis J, Evans RH, Francis AA Watkins JC. *Adv Pharmacol Therapeut 1979; 2:* 161—170
72   McLennan H, Hicks TP, Hall JG. In DeFeudis FV, Mandel P, eds. *Amino Acid Neurotransmitters 1981;* 213—221. New York: Raven Press
73   Benninger C, Kadis J, Prince DA. *Brain Res 1980; 187:* 165—182
74   Krnjevic K, Morris ME. *Can J Physiol Pharmacol 1980; 58:* 579—583
75   Marciani MG, Louvel J, Heinemann U. *Brain Res 1982;* In press
76   Heinemann U, Konnerth A, Lux HD. *Brain Res 1981; 213:* 246—250
77   Somjen GG. *J Neurophysiol 1980; 44:* 617—632
78   Katz B, Miledi R. *J Physiol 1969; 203:* 459—487
79   Lux HD. In Glaser GH, Penry JK, Woodbury DM, eds. *Antiepileptic Drugs: Mechanisms of Action 1980;* 63—83. New York: Raven Press
80   Oliver AP, Carman JS, Hoffer RJ, Wyatt RJ. *Exp Neurol 1980; 68:* 489—499
81   Fertziger AP, Ranck JP Jr. *Exp Neurol 1970; 26:* 571—585
82   Fisher RS, Pedley TA, Moody WJ, Prince DA. *Arch Neurol 1976; 33:* 76—83
83   Gutnick MJ, Heinemann U, Lux HD. *Clin Neurophysiol 1979;* 329—344
84   Heinemann U, Lux HD. *Brain Res 1975; 93:* 63—76
85   Heinemann U, Lux HD. *Brain Res 1977; 120:* 231—249
86   Lux HD. *Epilepsia 1974; 15:* 375—393
87   Moody W, Futamachi KJ, Prince DA. *Exp Neurol 1974; 42:* 248—263
88   Hablitz JJ, Lundervold A. *Exp Neurol 1981; 71:* 410—420
89   Ogata N, Hori N, Katsuda N. *Brain Res 1976; 110:* 371—375
90   Dietzel I, Heinemann U, Hofmeier G, Lux HD. *Brain Res 1982; 181:* 1—12
91   Dietzel I, Heinemann U, Hofmeier C, Lux HD. *Exp Brain Res 1980; 40:* 432—439
92   Dietzel I, Heinemann U, Hofmeier G, Lux HD. In Klee MR, Lux HD, Speckmann FJ, eds. *Physiology and Pharmacology of Epileptogenic Phenomena 1982;* 5—12. New York: Raven Press
93   Zuckermann EC, Glaser GH. *Exp Neurol 1968; 20:* 87—110
94   Sypert GW, Ward AA Jr. *Exp Neurol 1974; 45:* 19—41
95   Gutnick MJ, Prince DA. *Science 1972; 176:* 424—426
96   Louvel J, Pumain R. *Neurosci Lett 1978; 7:* 17—22
97   Scobey RP, Cabor AJ. *J Neurophysiol 1975; 38:* 383—394
98   Schmalbruch H, Jahnsen H. *Brain Res 1981; 217:* 175—178
99   Somjen GG. In Porter E, ed. *Studies in Neurophysiology 1978;* 182—201. Cambridge: Cambridge University Press
100   Heinemann U, Gutnick MJ. *Electroenc clin Neurophysiol 1979; 47:* 345—357
101   Lux HD. In Ingvar DH, Lassen NA, eds. *Brain Work, Alfred Benzon Symp VIII 1975;* 172—181. Kopenhagen: Munksgaard
102   Nicoll RA, Alger BF. *Science 1981; 212:* 957—959
103   Nicholson C. *NRP Bulletin 1980; 18, 2:* 1—113
104   Nicholson C, Phillips JM, Gardner-Medwin AR. *Brain Res 1979; 169:* 580—584
105   Orkand RK, Nicholls JG, Kuffler SW. *J Neurophysiol 1966; 29:* 788—806
106   Futamachi KJ, Pedley TA. *Brain Res 1976; 109:* 311—322
107   Ransom BR, Goldring S. *J Neurophysiol 1973; 36:* 855—868
      Gutnick MJ, Connors BW, Ramson BR. *Brain Res 1981; 213:* 486—492
109   Somjen GG. *Ann Rev Physiol 1975; 37:* 163—190
110   Lehmenkuehler A, Zidek W, Caspers H. In Klee Mr, Lux HD, Speckmann FJ, eds. *Physiology and Pharmacology in Epileptogenic Phenomena 1982;* 37—45. New York: Raven Press

11

EEG EPILEPTIC WAVEFORMS, THEIR GENESIS AND CLINICAL CORRELATES

P B C Fenwick

Introduction

Our understanding of the mechanisms of seizure activity has advanced rapidly over the last decade. The introduction and application of micro electrode technology to the study of epilepsy has allowed individual populations of abnormal cells to be monitored closely. These new techniques applied to animal models of epilepsy have allowed deeper insights into the mechanisms underlying the generation and spread of seizure activity. Focal models of epilepsy have been studied by applying either aluminagel or penicillin directly on to the cerebral cortex of animals and then studying the generation of focal seizure activity. Generalised epilepsy in animals has been studied either by means of intravenous penicillin in cats or by the use of a flickering light to induce photoconvulsive seizures in photosensitive baboons. New evidence derived from these experiments has led to a modification of many of the previously well established concepts relating to the development and spread of seizure activity.

Abnormal neuronal discharges

There are two main groups of theories relating to the generation of abnormal activity in damaged epileptic neurones. The first group of theories relates the abnormal electrical potentials to a failure in the mechanisms of repolarisation of the cell membrane, and are adequately reviewed by Lockard [1].

The second group of theories relate the development of abnormal epileptic potentials to the mechanisms which are involved in the transmission of impulses between cells. In a normal neurone there are two types of synapses: excitatory synapses which when activated cause a depolarisation of the cell membrane, and inhibitory synapses which when activated cause a hyperpolarisation of the cell membrane. These potentials are the excitatory and inhibitory post synaptic potentials. In a damaged or epileptic neurone a third group of potentials exist and this potential is called a paroxysmal depolarisation shift, which is the hallmark of a damaged epileptic neurone. During the paroxysmal depolarisation shift potential the cell fires off rapid bursts of neuronal spikes and it is this bursting activity which leads to the identification of cells as being damaged and epileptic. The development of paroxysmal depolarisation shifts has been studied in detail by methods which use the application of penicillin to the cerebral cortex, and have been extensively and adequately reviewed [2,3].

The paroxysmal depolarisation shift after the application of topical penicillin to the cortex in a cat develops over the course of two hours. As the process continues, the cell activity becomes so disordered that repolarisation is delayed and a seizure may occur in an individual neurone. Following the seizure the neurone becomes refractory for a period of time before paroxysmal depolarisation shifts can again reappear and the procedure can be repeated. Thus in summary the paroxysmal depolarisation shift is the signature of a damaged cell that is likely to produce epileptic burst activity.

The high voltage paroxysmal burst activity developed in the centre of the focus can be measured as the electrodes are drawn away from the abnormally discharging area. It is observations such as these which lead to the conclusion that there is a close correlation between the macro EEG potential measured on the surface of the cortex and the underlying potential derived from individual abnormally firing epileptic cells.

Epileptic cells — population studies

The process by which the individual cell produces epileptic activity is now to some extent understood; as is the behaviour of populations of epileptic cells. Lockard, Ward and co-workers [4] have produced a model of the behaviour of pools of epileptic neurones in monkeys who have had alumina gel applied to the cortex. They describe two populations of neurones with different characteristics: Group 1 neurones are found at the centre of the epileptic focus. They are damaged neurones, fire only in the paroxysmal mode, and cannot be influenced by afferent activity. If much epileptic activity is present at the centre of the focus, they are liable to die but, apart from their damaged bursting mode of functioning, their importance lies with their capacity to recruit Group 2 neurones, which are found surrounding the central core of the focus. They are partially damaged, can fire in both the epileptic paroxysmal mode and in a normal mode, and can be recruited to the epileptic mode by Group 1 neurones which, in their turn, can recruit normal neurones surrounding the focus to the bursting process. The genesis of an epileptic seizure, Lockard et al suggest, is as follows: Pools of Group 1 neurones synchronise their bursting pattern and recruit the surrounding Group 2 neurones to the spread of the epileptic bursting discharge, which disrupts normal neuronal activity in the population of Group 2 neurones and it is this which constitutes the seizure discharge. The disruption of normal activity in the Group 2 pool gives rise to the symptoms of a focal seizure. Providing that the process remains within the population of Group 2 neurones, then this is a localised partial focal seizure but, if the Group 2 neurones are then able to recruit normal neurones surrounding the focus into the epileptic discharges, then the abnormal activity spreads and secondary generalisation of the seizure so as to involve the whole brain occurs.

This model therefore suggests that three processes must occur for a secondary generalised seizure to arise from an epileptic focus. Firstly, the bursting activity within the focus must be of sufficient intensity so as to be able to recruit the pool of Group 2 neurones. Secondly, the Group 2 neuronal pool must be able to fire in such a way as to recruit normal neurones to the seizure discharge and this then thirdly allows the spread of the abnormal seizure activity throughout the brain. There are thus two points at which seizure activity can be inhibited: Firstly, Group 2 neurones can be inhibited from being recruited by Group 1 neurones and secondly Group 2 neurones can be inhibited from recruiting normal neurones to the seizure process. In an elegant series of experiments, Lockard has demonstrated in her monkey model of epilepsy that attention and social anxiety inhibits the recruitment of Group 2 neurones whereas sleep enhances their recruitment and therefore the likelihood of seizure activity. Factors affecting the spread of seizure activity will be discussed further below.

The genesis and significance of EEG spikes

The grouping together of paroxysmal discharges from a pool of Group 1 neurones is seen in the cortical EEG and in the scalp EEG as a spike. The EEG definition of a spike is a wave clearly distinguished from the background activity with a duration of less than 70msecs. A sharp wave is similar except that it is slower, lasting from 70msecs to 200msecs. Both spike and sharp wave activity is therefore seen as the hallmark of paroxysmal discharges in populations of Group 1 neurones, but not all spike activity is pathological [5,6]. To quote Janine Stevens [5]: "An outstanding quality of the spike mode of transmission is the uncompromising fashion in which the spike coded message preempts access to cerebral circuitry by swamping and displacing ongoing activity." Because spike transmission occurs naturally within the nervous system, spikes may be transmitted over long distances so that the appearance of spikes on the surface of the cortex do not necessarily represent a focal lesion directly below the area where the spike appears. It is not uncommon, for example, for spikes to be generated by foci in deep cerebral lesions and be projected to the cortex at a site remote from the area of generation. Some spike foci in children are well known to migrate as the child matures. Anterior temporal spike foci in an adult may be first seen in either the posterior temporal or posterior parietal region in the child. Thus although the spike may frequently represent the paroxysmal discharge of a pool of Group 1 neurones, its appearance in the scalp electroencephalogram needs cautious interpretation.

105

The significance of a spike

Now that the mechanism of the generation of pathological cortical spikes is known, their appearance in the electroencephalogram raises important conceptual issues. If it is accepted that spikes are generated by pools of Group 1 neurones firing paroxysmally, that this activity may be transmitted over long distances within the cerebral cortex, and that the appearance of a spike in a particular cortical area distrubs the normal integrative processes of that area by swamping these processes with an imperative neuronal barrage [7], then the important question is whether or not there are specific cognitive deficits which can be related to epileptic spiking in the EEG. It is important to understand that the functioning of a system containing a spike focus contains two aspects which are frequently confused. Firstly there is the damage to the system which has led to the development of the spike focus and secondly there is the transient malfunction in that system when a spike is generated. It is not always possible to separate these two features so that this question has not as yet been satisfactorily answered although there is evidence which suggests that the appearance of spikes may not be as benign as had been previously thought.

It is also clear that the systems in which the abnormal activity arises is important. Spikes in some systems may be cognitively silent while in others such as the memory system their presence may cause a measurable interference with cognitive function. The literature from the mid 1970s has shown that the cognitive ability in children with spike foci is impaired, and has related cognitive impairment to damage within the system in which the spikes occur. It is therefore not the spike activity which has been seen as causing the cognitive impairment, but the damage to the actual system itself. Mirsky et al [8] have shown in children that spike foci occurring in the dominant temporal lobe produce an impairment of verbal memory, whereas spike foci in the non dominant temporal lobe produce a deficit in visio-spatial memory. The argument is that the memory circuits within the dominant and non dominant temporal lobes are damaged and that the presence of spikes in these areas is a reflection of the underlying damage within those systems.

It is now possible to ask the question whether or not the occurrence of spikes themselves within the brain can cause a disruption of cognition in those systems in which the spikes arise. Lockard et al [9], in their aluminagel model of epilepsy, have shown that there is a direct relationship between the numbers of spikes in the EEG and both positive and negative learning. Petersen in Copenhagen [10] has shown that children, performing a reaction time task to stimuli triggered by the occurrence of a spike, may show an increase in reaction time and occasionally miss the stimuli completely. This suggests that the occurrence of the spike in some children is not a trivial event but may impair cognition to a significant degree.

Further evidence for this view comes from a group of workers at the Epilepsy

Centre at Meer en Bosch in Holland where Binnie and co-workers [11] have shown that performance on various cognitive tests is dependent on the numbers of spikes which were occurring at the time the tests were given. Thus spike activity may directly affect the cognitive processes of patients with epilepsy and their occurrence in the EEG may not be as benign as had previously been thought. These observations raise the question as to whether the relationship between psychiatric disorder and cortical spikes in non epileptic children is as purely fortuitous as had previously been thought. Lairy and co-workers in Paris [12] have drawn attention to the occurrence of abnormal EEG activity in children with conduct disorders, and also point out that the EEGs normalise when the children's psychiatric disorder improves. It would certainly be worthwhile examining a similar group of children to see whether or not their conduct disorder is related to a change in cognition occurring at the time of the abnormal EEG activity.

The relationship between spike activity and the EEG is not absolute and it may be that only a small group of children show a direct relationship between spikes and an alteration of cognition. One report [13] compared a group of epileptic under-achieving children and normal controls, and showed that sharp waves were seen in both those children who did well, as well as those who did poorly, and that there was no difference in learning; nor was there any correlation between learning and the amount of spiking observed. Stores and Hart [14] showed in children that persistent focal discharges appear on average to be associated with impaired reading accuracy. Clearly more work is required in this area; the conflicting evidence probably relates to the different systems from which the spikes arise, some spikes being cognitively silent while others may have a profound effect on the patient's cognition.

Generalised seizures

Spike and wave activity

The traditional view reviewed by Gastaut and Fischer-Williams [15] is that spike and wave activity is initiated by the reticular system of the brain stem, and then projected to the cortex by the non-specific nuclei of the thalamus. This view sees subcortical structures as being primary in the genesis and spread of spike and wave activity. It also carries the implication that spike and wave activity will be generalised equally over both hemispheres and that each hemisphere, because of a common 'subcortical drive', will be synchronised with the other side.

In clinical practice this idealised view of spike and wave activity is rarely seen and, although most textbooks of epilepsy and manuals of neurophysiology illustrate petit mal seizures with a diagram of generalised 3 per second spike and wave activity, such activity, if it occurs, is relatively uncommon. In a major London teaching hospital, St Thomas', a review of the EEG records shows that only two to three such cases are seen during the year. It is possible that, since the introduction of ethosuximide, which is an effective anticonvulsant against three per cent spike and wave activity, many of the cases are sufficiently well controlled by their general practitioners and are therefore not referred to the major centres, or it may be that these cases are in practice very rare. Frequently spike and wave activity is not equally generalised over the scalp and focal changes are seen in different areas of the head.

Recent evidence is accumulating that it is the cortex which is of prime importance in the generation and maintenance of generalised spike and wave activity. The spikes and waves of spike and wave activity are seen to travel over the cortex at different rates and are to some extent independent of the thalamic pacemaker [16]. These observations suggested that previous hypotheses put forward by Penfield and Jasper [17] required modification. Additional evidence in man has come from observation on cortical spike and wave activity of the effect of intra-arterial metrazol. When injected into the carotid artery, which supplies mainly the cortex, this produced spike and wave activity, whereas metrazol injected into the vertebral artery failed to produce spike and wave activity, although the vertebral artery supplies the brain stem and the thalamus directly [18]. Further evidence comes from depth electrode studies, where stimulation in man showed that spike and wave activity could be elicited from the cortex, but never from deeper structures [19]. Thus both the animal evidence and the evidence in man suggest that the cortex has a prime role to play in the genesis of spike and wave activity.

The most telling and important evidence suggesting that spike and wave activity has a cortical genesis comes from animal work. The initial observation, that penicillin when applied to the cortex could generate spike and wave activity locally surrounding the focus, heralded the demise of the brain stem thalamic generator theory. Gloor and co-workers with their intramuscular penicillin model in cats have given the final blow. Musgrave and Gloor [20] have shown that, after intramuscular injection of penicillin in cats, generalised cortical spike and wave activity can be generated. They argue that this is an abnormal cortical response to 'normal' thalamic recruiting valleys. There is a suggestion that abnormal unit firing starts first in the cortex and spreads secondarily to the thalamus. If this is so, then an abnormally excitable cortex may in man be sufficient for the genesis of spike and wave activity. This excitability is thought to be coded for by a gene or group of genes with variable penetrance. Penetration begins at the age of four years and shows maximum penetrance at the age of approximately 16 years, and has ceased by the age of 40 years [21,22]. During the time that the genes are active, the cortex is excitable, and spike and wave activity rapidly generalises throughout the hemispheres.

Because the concept of the generation of spike and wave activity rested on a thalamic initiator with the cortex passively following, this type of epilepsy was called primary sub-cortical epilepsy but, as has been pointed out above, the evidence for the thalamus being the prime mover in the genesis of spike and wave activity is now no longer as secure as previously. The prime role is now given to the cortex in the genesis of spike and wave activity. If this is so, then the concept of the generation of spike and wave activity in man may need revision, and the time has now come that the idea of primary sub-cortical or centencephalic epilepsy should be abandoned.

There remains the important question as to whether or not small lesions of the cortex may be responsible in susceptible individuals, i.e. those with a high level of cortical excitability, for the genesis of spike and wave activity. It may be that this form of epilepsy, which is usually classified as idiopathic, is so classified because the lesions that cause it are small and cognitively silent. Present evidence concerning the genesis of spike and wave activity therefore raises the question as to whether or not many cases of spike wave activity actually have small discharging foci in the cortex from which the spike and wave activity arises and then rapidly generalises throughout the hemisphere. If this is so, then a more unified view of epileptic seizures becomes possible.

This view would suggest that the basic lesion in patients with epilepsy is a population of damaged neurones. Paroxysmal firing within this population can, on the one hand, trigger off a paroxysmal discharge which is seen in the EEG as a spike and which may on occasions synchronise groups of Group 2 neurones so as to produce a focal seizure. The Group 2 neurones may then of course go on to recruit normal neurones and the seizure may generalise. In the case of seizures which are generalised from the start, particularly those involving spike and wave activity, a proportion of these cases may also have focal cortical lesions. Abnormal activity arising from these lesions will then spread rapidly throughout the cortex producing generalised spike and wave, but, it is suggested that the activity arises not from a sub-cortical centre, but from a cortical focus. If this is so, then it becomes important to devise tests to show the abnormal areas from which the seizure arise.

Changes in cognition during spike and wave discharges

There is a long history of research into the cognitive changes which occur during spike and wave discharges [23], but only a few points are relevant in this chapter.

Schwab [24] was the first to demonstrate that reaction time to auditory or visual stimuli was lengthened during a spike and wave burst. Later workers used different methods to extend these observations. The overall picture which emerged is that the degree of impairment depends on the length of the burst, the degree to which the spike and wave is generalised from the start, and the degree to which it spreads over the head [25]. The extent to which the child is involved in the task is also important: passive listening produces greater impairment than active participation [26].

Tizard and Marjorison using a continual performance task produced results. The point of interest about their findings is the observation that there is a decrease in performance *before* the spike wave burst. This observation can now be explained by Gloor's experimental results in cats, if the mechanism of spike and wave generation is the same in this model as in man. If cortical synchronisation occurs before spike and wave activity is seen on the cortex, then it can be expected that cognition will also be detrimentally affected during the period of synchronisation before the spike wave burst.

Factors affecting the generation of seizures

With new evidence available on the importance of the cortex in the generation of spike wave discharges, it is possible to describe factors which are involved in the precipitation of seizures in man. If Lockard's model of epilepsy is accepted, then it follows that changes in the excitation level of groups of neurones surrounding an epileptic focus makes them either more or less easily recruited into the seizure process. Pools of cortical neurones are excited by activity in that area of the cortex which is relevant, for example, movements will excite the motor strip, sensory input will excite the sensory strip, visual activity will excite pools of neurones in the occipital cortex. It can therefore be predicted that seizure precipitation will result from cognitive activities exciting pools of neurones which are closely related to an epileptogenic focus. Wilkins et al [27] have suggested that, in photogenic epilepsy, once the levels of excitation resulting from the synchronisation has recruited a sufficiently large pool of neurones in the occipital cortex, a generalised photoconvulsive seizure will result.

Wilkins et al [28] apply this model to an interesting patient who reported that he was unable to do mental arithmetic without having a blank episode. On examination, during the blank period, this patient's EEG was found to show generalised spike and wave discharges. Wilkins measured the number of spike and wave discharges during the administration of the WAIS Intelligence Test, and noted they occurred in those sub-tests of the WAIS which required the manipulation of objects. The patient later was found to have a parietal lobe lesion. It became clear that, when this area of the brain was used in the solution of a task, a generalised spike and wave discharge would occur. These authors, therefore, link the occurrence of a generalised spike and wave discharge to a specific cortical focus.

The occurrence of spike and wave activity related to thinking had previously been reported in the literature. Cirignotta et al [29] report an increased incidence of spike and wave activity during the playing of draughts, again with the suggestion that specific stimulation of the areas of the cortex involved in this behaviour resulted in the triggering of generalised spike and wave discharges. Ingram and Ryman [30] also describe a patient whose epilepsy was triggered by calculation. There is thus evidence to confirm that activity within pools of neurones in the cortex close to an epileptic focus will precipitate a spike and wave seizure discharge. It has for some time been accepted that this is also the case for the evoked epilepsies that can be triggered by a sensory volley to an area of damaged cortex to cause a focal seizure [31]. (For a review of evoked seizures, see Merlis [32], Fenwick [33]).

So our methods of testing patients with epilepsy require refinement. It should now become routine for patients to be tested psychologically, with their EEGs being measured at the same time. This will then allow the amount of abnormal activity, either focal or spike and wave, for each cognitive task to be measured. There is then the possibility that the epileptogenic focus within the cortex may be located.

Conditioning of seizure activity

A neglected paper published by Forster and co-workers in 1969 describes Pavlovian conditioning of seizures in cats. Forster reports that, if electrodes are implanted in a normal cat's brain and the brain then stimulated via these electrodes, the cat will have a grand mal seizure. If the stimulation is then paired with an unconditioned stimulus, say, a light, then the presentation of light alone does not result in a seizure discharge. However, if the cat's brain is damaged by the production of an epileptic focus from tetanus toxin applied to the cortex, then conditioning of a seizure to a light presentation is possible. In this case, after several pairings of the light with the electrical stimulation of the brain to produce a seizure discharge, the light alone without stimulation will produce a seizure. Forster went on to show that this conditioning could be carried out across different sensory modalities so that a light could cause a focal motor seizure, or pairing with a sound could cause a visual seizure but he pointed out that conditioning of seizures was, firstly, not easy to accomplish and, secondly, was easily extinguished by a grand mal seizure. The important point is that he demonstrated in cats that conditioning of seizures was possible.

It is likely that the ability for seizures to be conditioned also exists in man. Forster and his co-workers examined the extinguishing of seizure activity in different groups of patients, and showed that they were able to extinguish photogenically-induced seizures by repeated presentation of sub-threshold flash stimuli [34,35]. They also showed that this was possible to do in the case of startle epilepsy to auditory stimuli [36]. Thus the ability to extinguish seizure activity by a process of conditioning suggests that it is also possible to condition stimuli in man. A further paper by Forster and his group showed that this indeed was possible. They were able to produce photoconvulsive responses in patients who were photosensitive by pairing the slight flash with an auditory stimulus. The auditory stimulus then could produce the abnormal activity on its own. Thus conditioning of abnormal activity in man in patients with damaged brains is possible, a finding of considerable interest because it suggests that conditioning techniques may be appropriate in the treatment of patients with epilepsy. An excellent review paper [37] describes in some detail various conditioning procedures which have been carried out in man and which are beyond the scope of this chapter but, with the new evidence suggesting that the cortex may be involved as the generator of different seizure types, conditioning of cortical activity becomes a real possibility for the treatment of epilepsy.

Psychogenic seizures

It has already been described above how activity in areas of the cortex which are damaged can precipitate seizure activity. It is therefore possible for patients to induce activation in this area of cortex voluntarily and so produce seizures themselves. Voluntary induction of seizures is possibly more widespread than is accepted at the moment. A figure of one in ten to three in seven was found in the Maudsley epileptic clinic, but the rate will depend on the sympathy of the interviewing doctor.

Classification

Primary psychogenic seizures

These are seizures which are caused by the patient deliberately activating areas of the brain which will precipitate a seizure, which can be either a simple partial seizure, partial complex seizure, or generalised seizure. The method used to precipitate a partial motor seizure is to imitate and attend to the movement which occurs at the onset of the seizure. This activates the area of the cortex which is usually involved in the seizure discharge, raises its level of excitation, and allows a seizure to be triggered in this area more easily. Partial complex seizures in patients with temporal lobe epilepsy are frequently triggered by the emotions which are part of the seizure discharge. Some patients who have auras in which feelings of sadness and anxiety arise can precipitate seizures by deliberately thinking sad and anxious thoughts. Again the process of thinking these thoughts appears to raise the activity and the excitation level in those circuits close to the epileptic focus and allows the recruitment of those cells into the seizure discharge. Generalised seizures appear to be precipitated in a less specific way. Patients with petit mal epilepsy frequently describe the mechanism by which seizures can be precipitated as a splitting of attention: a rapid shift of attention from one subject to another will frequently lead to a shower of small absences. Generalised seizures have been produced in patients of mine by making the mind blank, the pressing of consciousness into an inner void. Clearly, in these cases, the mechanisms are non-specific, and they probably alter the function of those systems which alter in a general way the activation level of the whole cortex [38].

Secondary psychogenic seizures

Seizures in this category are those which are precipitated by a specific function of mind, without a deliberate intention on the part of the patient to precipitate a seizure, and without a clear evoking peripheral stimulus. Into this category fall the thinking epilepsies of Ingram and Ryman [39], Wilkins et al [40], etc., as described above. A further group of patients that fall into this category are those where seizures are triggered by specific emotional situations. For example, a patient of mine with temporal lobe epilepsy and partial complex seizures would have a series of minor attacks if she was made to feel very guilty. It is likely that, in this patient, the feelings of guilt were associated with an increase in excitation in those neural circuits which were close to her epileptic focus; activation in this area caused by the feelings of guilt allowed their recruitment into a seizure discharge which then generalised. The significance of the occurrence of both primary and secondary psychogenic seizures is that they provide evidence for the importance of cognition in seizure generation. It is clear that a simple mechanical model of epilepsy where seizures occur randomly is no longer tenable. Seizures must now be seen as part of the dynamic interplay between the activity of the cortex and the ongoing mental life of the patient.

Summary

The paroxysmal depolarisation shift is the long lasting alteration in potential which occurs in damaged neurones and which leads to the bursting pattern of firing which is their hallmark. Pools of damaged neurones bursting together produce in the EEG the characteristic spike. Spikes can, in some patients, be responsible for a change in cognition in those systems in which they arise.

There is new evidence that spike and wave activity may mainly be due to an abnormally excitable cortex. It is suggested that cognitive activity can lead to seizure generation by changing the excitability level in pools of cortical neurones.

References

1   In Lockard JS, Ward AA, eds. *Epilepsy: A Window to Brain Mechanisms 1981*. New York: Raven Press
2   Ajmone Marsan C, Gumnit RJ. In *Handbook of Neurology. The Epilepsies 1974; 15: 30–60*
3   Russo ME. *Cornell Vet 1981; 71: 221–247*
4   Lockard JS. In Lockard JS, Ward AA, eds. *Epilepsy: A Window to Brain Mechanisms 1981*. New York: Raven Press
5   Stevens, JR. In Shagass C, Gershon S, Friedhoff AJ, eds. *Psychopathology and Brain Dysfunction 1977*. New York: Raven Press
6   Fenwick PBC. In Reynolds EH, Trimble MR, eds. *Epilepsy and Psychiatry 1981*. Edinburgh: Churchill Livingstone
7   Stevens JR. In Shagass C, Gershon S, Friedhoff AJ, eds. *Psychopathology and Brain Dysfunction 1977*. New York: Raven Press
8   Mirsky AF, Primac DW, Ajmone Marsan C et al. *Exp Neurol 1960; 2: 75–89*
9   Lockard JS. In Lockard JS, Ward AA, eds. *Epilepsy: A Window to Brain Mechanisms 1981*. New York: Raven Press
10   Petersen V. *Proceedings of the 12th International Symposium on Epilepsy 1980*. New York: Raven Press In press

11   Aarts JHP, Binnie CD, Smit A. In Kefan and Burr, eds. *Proceedings of Conference on Mobile Long-term EEG Monitoring.* In press

12   Lairy GC. *Electroenceph Clin Neurophysiol 1967; Suppl 25:* 282–298

13   Baird HW, John ER, Ahn H, Maisel E. *Electroenceph Clin Neurophysiol 1980; 48:* 283–293

14   Stores G, Hart JA. *Electroenceph Clin Neurophysiol 1976; 39(4):* 429–430

15   Gastaut H, Fischer-Williams M. *The Handbook of Physiology, Section 1: Neurophysiology 1959;* 1: 329. Washington DC: American Physiological Society

16   Petsche H, Rappelsberger P. In Brazier MAB, ed. *Epilepsy, Its Phenomena in Man 1973.* New York and London: Academic Press

17   Penfield W, Jasper HH. *Epilepsy and the Functional Anatomy of the Human Brain 1954.* Boston: Little Brown & Co

18   Cobb W. *Paper presented at the British Epilepsy Association Meeting 1975*

19   Bancaud J, Telairach J, Morel P et al.*Electroenceph Clin Neurophysiol 1974; 37:* 275–282

20   Musgrave J, Gloor P. *Epilepsia 1980; 21:* 369–378

21   Metrakos JD, Metrakos K. *Neurology (Minneap) 1961; 11:* 474–483

22   Metrakos K, Metrakos JD. In Vinken PJ, Bruyn GW, eds. *The Handbook of Neurology 1974; 15:* Chapter 24

23   Fenwick PBC. In Reynolds EH, Trimble MR, eds. *Epilepsy and Psychiatry 1981.* Edinburgh: Churchill Livingstone

24   Schwab RS. *Arch Neurol Psychiat 1939; 41:* 215–217

25   Browne TR, Penry JK, Porter RJ, Dreifuss FE. *Neurology 1974; 24:* 381–382

26   Jus A, Jus K. *Arch Gen Psychiat 1962; 6:* 71–75

27   Wilkins AJ, Binnie CD, Darby CE. In *Progress in Neurobiology 1980; 15:* 1–33. United Kingdom: Pergamon Press

28   **Wilkins AJ, Zifkin B, Anderman F, McGovern G.** *Annals of Neurology 1981.* In preparation

29   Cirignotta F, Cicogna P, Lugaresi E. *Epilepsia 1980; 21:* 137–140

30   Ingram A, Ryman H. *Neurology (Minneap) 1962; 12:* 282–287

31   Symonds C. *Brain 1959; 82(2):* 133–146

32   Merlis JK. In *Handbook of Neurology. The Epilepsies 1974; 15:* Chapter 25.

33   Fenwick PBC. In Reynolds EH, Trimble MR, eds. *Epilepsy and Psychiatry 1981.* Edinburgh: Churchill Livingstone

34   Forster FM, Campos GB. *Epilepsia 1964; 5:* 156–165

35   Forster FM, Ptacek LJ, Peterson WG. *Epilepsia 1965; 6:* 217–225

36   Booker HE, Forster FM, Klove H. *Neurology 1965; 15:* 1095–1103

37   Mostofsky DI, Balaschak BA. *Psychol Bull 1977; 84(4):* 723–759

38   Fenwick PBC. In Reynolds EH, Trimble MR, eds. *Epilepsy and Psychiatry 1981.* Edinburgh: Churchill Livingstone

39   Ingram A, Ryman H. *Neurology (Minneap) 1962; 12:* 282–287

40   **Wilkins AJ, Zifkin B, Anderman F, McGovern G.** *Annals of Neurology 1981.* In preparation

12

THE ROLE OF THE CEREBELLUM IN THE CONTROL OF EPILEPSY

I B Gartside

Why should one expect the cerebellum to have any influence on epileptiform activity? It has been suggested that, as some forms of epilepsy involve abnormal movements, then structures involved in the control of movement may play a role in the control of epilepsy.

Stimulation of the caudate nucleus in acute preparations [1–2] can temporarily suppress experimental epileptiform activity. Similarly, stimulation of the cerebellum can also suppress experimental epilepsy in unanaesthetised preparations [3–4], and in unanaesthetised monkeys [5–6]. The fact that cerebellar stimulation can suppress epilepsy does not, however, prove that the normal, unstimulated cerebellum has any influence on epileptiform activity. More direct evidence comes from experiments in which the cerebellum has been removed, and the effects of this procedure on epileptiform activity observed.

Cerebellar ablation enhances seizures from cobalt foci in unanaesthetised rats [7]. In baboons, after-discharges resulting from ventrolateral thalamic stimulation are exacerbated by cerebellar removal [8]. The duration of individual 'cortical epileptiform bursts' is increased following cerebellectomy [9]. The lifetimes of epileptiform foci produced by intra-cortical injection of benzyl penicillin are also increased by cerebellectomy [10] (Figure 1).

What could be the basis of cerebellar influence on epilepsy? There is a positive feedback loop from the motor cortex back to the motor cortex via the cerebellum. Cortical pyramidal cells project to the pontine nuclei, which in turn project to the intracerebellar nuclei. Collaterals of the pontine fibres are the mossy fibres entering the cerebellar cortex. The cells of the intracerebellar nuclei project to the ventrobasal thalamus, which projects back to the motor cortex. All the synapses in this pathway are excitatory [11]. It has been suggested that this circuit helps maintain epileptic activity [12,13], but the cerebellum damps this loop (Figure 2). The mossy fibres excite granule cells which excite Purkinje cells, and Purkinje cells inhibit the intracerebellar nuclei [14].

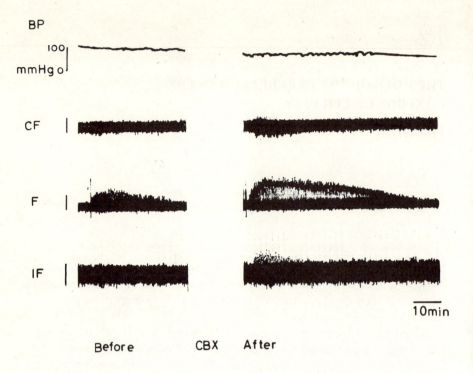

BP

100
mmHg 0

CF

F

IF

10min

Before   CBX   After

Figure 1. This shows the effects of cerebellectomy on the activity of an epileptiform focus produced by injection of 25 units of sodium penicillin into the cerebral cortex of a rat anaesthetised with urethane. The left hand group of traces were obtained before cerebellectomy and the right hand group after. Traces from top to bottom are 1) Femoral arterial pressure 2) Electrocorticogram (ECoG) recorded from the contralateral homotopic point to the focus 3) ECoG recorded from the parietal cortex ipsilateral to the focus. All amplitude calibrations are 1mv. Time bar is 10 min. Note that in this record there are increases in both duration and amplitude of the ECoG spike activity following cerebellectomy

This proposed damped positive feedback loop cannot be a correct explanation however. In experiments on the effects of cerebellectomy on focus lifetime [10], I totally removed the cerebellum, including the intracerebellar nuclei (severing the cerebellar peduncles). This action opened the loop shown in Figure 2 which on the damped positive feedback loop hypothesis, should have abbreviated the lifetime of the focus. In fact it prolonged it. I also performed experiments to study the effect of cerebellectomy on penicillin foci in the visual cortex of the rat anaesthetised with urethane. The visual cortex does not receive projections from the intracerebellar nuclei [15], and so cannot be involved in a damped positive feedback loop. Nevertheless cerebellectomy prolonged the lifetime of the visual cortical foci.

As the damped positive feedback loop hypothesis no longer holds, an alternative

116

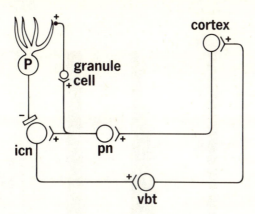

Figure 2. The positive feedback loop from the cerebral cortex and its damping by the
cerebellum. pn =pontine nucleus; N.B. The axons leaving the pontine nucleus give rise
to the mossy fibres. ICN = intracerebellar nuclei. vbt = ventro basal thalamus. P =
Purkinje cell; + = excitatory synapse; − = inhibitory synapse

hypothesis is needed. Recordings from cerebellar Purkinje cells in anaesthetised
rats with a penicillin focus in the cerebral cortex revealed that the Purkinje cells
were inhibited following an epileptiform spike [16] (Figures 4 and 6).

Inhibition of the Purkinje cells leads to disinhibition of the intracerebellar
nuclear cells, as one would predict from the work of Ito et al [14], who showed
that the Purkinje cells inhibited the cells of the intracerebellar nuclei mono-
synaptically. Thus, following an epileptiform spike in the cerebral cortex, a period
of enhanced discharge of the intracerebellar nuclear neurones is seen (Figures 5
and 6) [16,17].

This means that a burst of firing in the intracerebellar nuclear cell axons
should be projected up to the cerebral cortex. This burst of activity is very long
(up to 2 sec) compared with the epileptiform spike, which lasts for about 100
msec (see Figure 6 for perievent histograms of intracerebellar nuclear and Purkinje
cell activity around an epileptiform spike). The prolonged burst of activity, following disinhibition of the intracerebellar nuclei, can be seen in the ventrobasal
thalamus and cerebral cortex in experiments where intracerebellar nuclear disinhibition has been produced by cerebellar cortical stimulation in the urethane
anaesthetised rat (Gartside and Misson, unpublished). Also a delayed period of
increased cerebral cortical unit activity can be seen following an epileptiform
spike, and this disappears after cerebellectomy (Gartside, unpublished observations) (Figure 7).

There is a burst of enhanced cerebral cortical unit activity as a result of
activity in the cerebral cortico-cerebellar-cerebral cortical loop. At first sight,
one would expect this activity to exacerbate ongoing epileptiform activity,
(adding fuel to the fire as it were). However, this excitation is probably responsible for suppression of the epileptiform focus by the cerebellum.

117

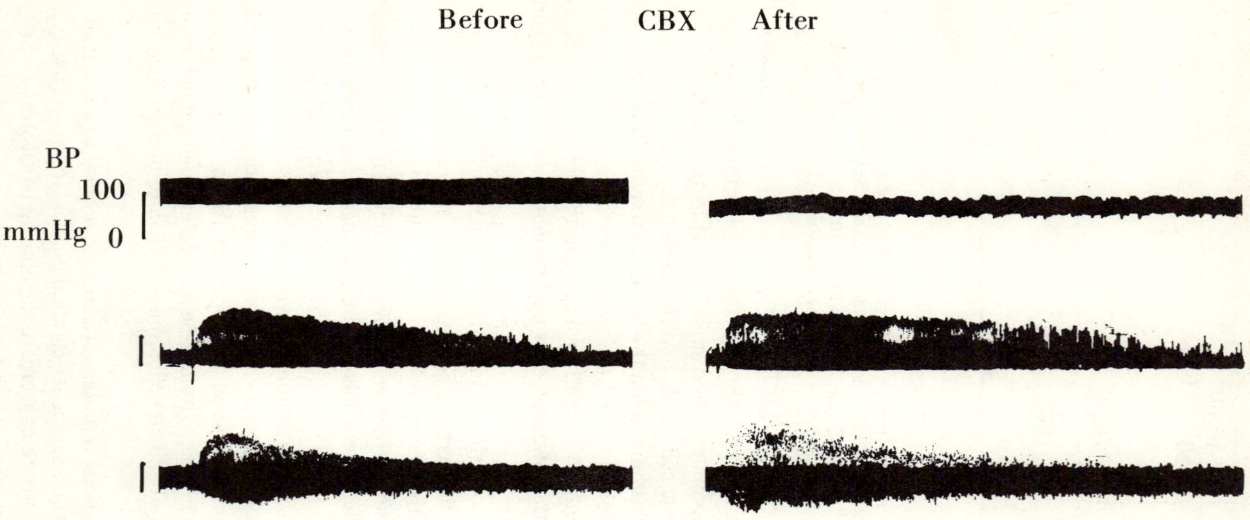

Figure 3. This shows the effects of cerebellectomy on a 25u penicillin focus in the visual cortex of the rat. The left hand set of traces were obtained before cerebellectomy, and the right hand set after. Traces from top to bottom are 1) Femoral arterial pressure; 2) ECoG recorded from the focus; and 3) ECoG recorded from the ipsilateral somato-motor cortex. Amplitude calibrations are both 1mV. Time bar = 10 min. Note the increase in duration of focal spiking following cerebellectomy

118

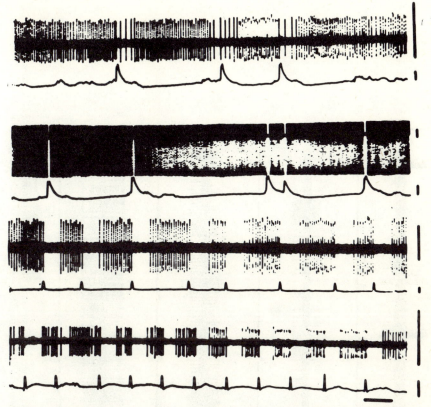

Figure 4. Showing the activity of four cerebellar Purkinje cells or inhibitory interneurones (top trace of each pair) in relation to the epileptiform spike recorded from the cerebral cortex (bottom trace of each pair).
Calibrations: All ECoG records are 1mV: all unit traces 500μV. Time calibration 1 sec

This apparently anomalous situation can be resolved if one uses the modification of Hughlings Jackson's original definition of epilepsy stated in the first chapter of the 'Basic Mechanisms of the Epilepsies' by Ward, Jasper and Pope [18], "massive discharge of many neurones in unison". The key word here is 'unison'. If the focal population of cells were unable to discharge due to refractoriness or inhibition (eg recurrent inhibition), then an epileptiform spike would be less likely to occur (assuming autogenic rhythmicity in the focal population), or would be smaller in amplitude (assuming a command from a pacemaker external to the focus).

This is illustrated by an experiment in the rat anaesthetised with urethane, where the depth of anaesthesia has been adjusted so that, although the electro-

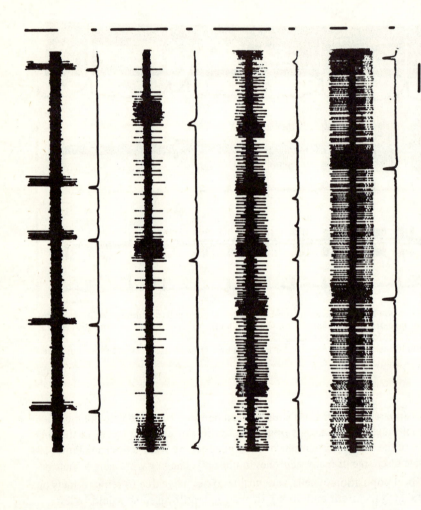

Figure 5. Showing the activity of four interpositus nuclear cells (top trace of each pair) in relation to the focal epileptiform spikes recorded from the cerebral cortex (lower traces). Note the increased discharge of each unit following the ECoG spike. Calibrations: All ECoG records are 1mV, all unit records are 500μv. Time calibration is 1 sec

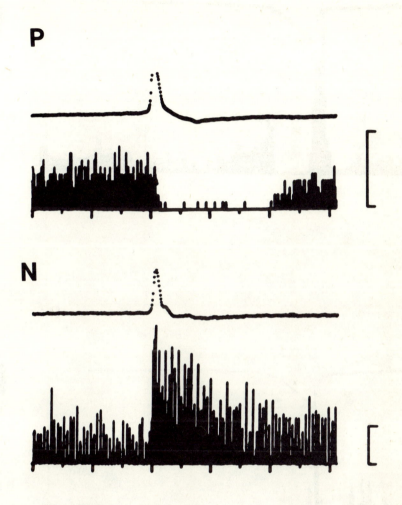

Figure 6. Averaged ECoG spikes (top trace of each pair) and perievent histograms of unit activity (lower traces). Top set of traces (P) from a Purkinje cell, bottom set of traces (N) from an interpositus nuclear cell. The calibration bars on the perievent histograms represent a probability of obtaining one spike per bin per sweep of 0.1. The sweep durations are 2.048 seconds

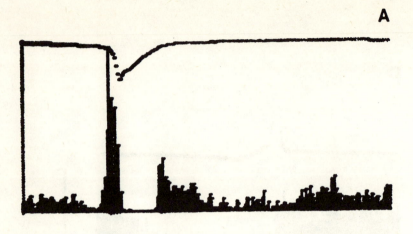

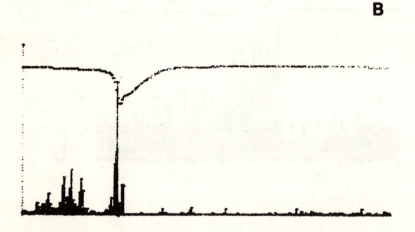

Figure 7. Averaged ECoG spikes (top trace of each pair) and perievent histograms of unit activity recorded from the cortical penicillin focus (lower traces). Top pair of traces before cerebellectomy, bottom pair after. Note the lack of the late burst of excitation after cerebellectomy. The sweep durations are 2.048 seconds

122

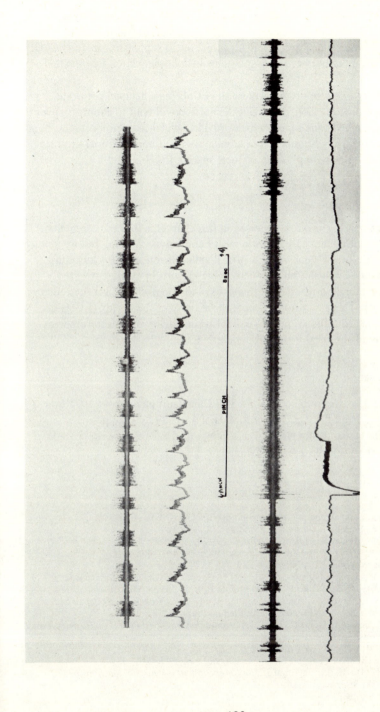

Figure 8. Two sets of traces showing cerebral cortical units (top trace of each pair) and ECoG activity (bottom traces). Note the suppression of epileptiform ECoG spiking during the application of contralateral hind paw pinches and the period of spontaneous desynchronisation

123

corticogram (ECoG) is synchronised, it can be desynchronised by peripheral stimulation. If a penicillin focus is established in this preparation, epileptiform spiking occurs when the ECoG is synchronised, but is suppressed during ECoG desynchronisation, either occurring spontaneously or stimulated by pinching a paw [19].

Thus, activity likely to desynchronise the ECoG (eg a delayed temporally-dispersed burst of excitation arriving in the cortex) will tend to suppress epileptiform activity. There is one report which provided evidence to support this hypothesis, where cerebellar stimulation in monkeys with alumina gel foci produced EEG arousal, as well as suppression of focal spiking [5].

Summary

The author's thesis in the work reviewed in this chapter is that the cerebellum does not influence epilepsy by a subtle motor control mechanism, but by a much coarser and widespread mechanism. Cortical epileptiform activity causes disinhibition of intracerebellar nuclear cells, which results in excitatory activity reaching the cerebral cortex via the thalamus, and also probably via the reticular formation [20]. This excitation disrupts the activity of the cortex (ECoG desynchronisation) and this suppresses epileptiform activity by interfering with the synchrony of the focal neuronal population.

Acknowledgments

Figures 1 and 3, are reproduced from E.E.G Clin Neurophysiol, 44 1978 and Figures 4 and 5 from E.E.G Clin Neurophysiol 46 1979 by kind permission of Elsevier/North Holland Biomedical Press. Some of this work was supported by a grant from the Medical Research Council.

References

1   Merlis JK. *Electroenceph Clin Neurophysiol 1973; 34:* 659–696
2   Mutani R, Fariello R. *Brain Res 1969; 14:* 749–753
3   Cooke PM, Snider R. *Epilepsia 1955; 4:* 19–28
4   Hutton TJ, Frost JD, Foster J. *Epilepsia 1972; 13:* 401–408
5   Lockard JS, Wyler AR. *Epilepsia 1979; 20:* 157–168
6   Cooper IS, Amin I, Gilman S, Waltz JM. In Cooper IS, Riklan M, Snider R, eds. *The Cerebellum, Epilepsy and Behaviour 1974;* 119–171. New York: Plenum Press
7   Dow RS. In Cooper IS, Riklan M, Snider R, eds. *The Cerebellum, Epilepsy and Behaviour 1974;* 57–95. New York: Plenum Press
8   Walter S, Basso A, Guiot G et al. In *Advances in Neurology 1975 Vol 10.* New York: Raven Press
9   Julien RM, Halpern LM. *Epilepsia 1972; 13:* 387–400
10 Gartside IB. *Electroenceph Clin Neurophysiol 1978; 44:* 373–379
11 Eccles JC, Ito M, Szentagothai J. *The Cerebellum as a Neuronal Machine 1967.* New York: Springer

12   Cooper IS, Snider R. In Cooper IS, Riklan M, Snider R, eds. *The Cerebellum, Epilepsy and Behaviour 1974;* 245–256. New York: Plenum Press
13   Julien RM. In Cooper IS, Riklan M, Snider R, eds. *The Cerebellum, Epilepsy and Behaviour 1974;* 97–118. New York: Plenum Press
14   Ito M, Yoshida M, Obata K et al. *Exp Brain Res 1970; 10:* 64–80
15   Evarts EV, Thach WT. *Ann Rev Physiol 1969; 31:* 451–498
16   Gartside IB. *Electroenceph Clin Neurophysiol 1979; 46:* 189–196
17   Julien RM, Laxer KD. *Electroenceph Clin Neurophysiol 1974; 37:* 123–132
18   Ward AA Jnr, Jasper HH, Pope A. In Jasper HH, Ward AA Jnr, Pope A, eds. *Basic Mechanisms of the Epilepsies 1969:* 3. Boston: Little Brown & Co
19   Gartside IB. *J Physiol 1979b; 289:* 6P
20   Bantli H, Bloedel JR, Tolbert D. *J Neurosurgery 1976; 45:* 539–554

13

DOPAMINE AND SEROTONIN IN REFLEX EPILEPSY

G M Anlezark

Introduction

Considerable experimental evidence indicates an important role for the mono-amine neurotransmitters, dopamine (DA) and 5-hydroxytryptamine (5HT, serotonin), in animal models of epilepsy, but their involvement in clinical epilepsy remains unclear.

In the hope of detecting abnormalities in brain dopaminergic and serotonin-ergic function, both before and after seizures, many authors have examined cerebro-spinal fluid (CSF) concentrations of monoamine metabolites in epileptic patients. The majority of such studies have utilised lumbar CSF, but some recent reports concerned ventricular or cisternal CSF [1]. Relationships between CSF monoamine metabolites and anticonvulsant drug treatment have also been in-vestigated, but there is little correlation between CSF concentrations of meta-bolites of 5HT and DA and type of epilepsy or drug treatment.

The principal metabolite of DA in CSF, homovanillic acid (HVA) and that of 5HT, 5-hydroxyindoleacetic acid (5HIAA) are normal, low-to-normal, or significantly reduced, in untreated or subtherapeutically treated epileptic patients [2–5]. No good correlation has been found between CSF 5HIAA and HVA concentrations and serum anticonvulsant drug concentrations [6]. A trend towards elevated 5HIAA concentrations in CSF was observed in anticonvulsant intoxicated patients [3]. In untreated epileptics, lumbar CSF 5HIAA and HVA are not different from those in non-epileptic controls [2,3,5]. In a study in which the precursors of DA or 5HT (L-dopa or L-tryptophan, respectively) plus a monoamine oxidase inhibitor were added to existing medication of drug resist-ant epileptic patients (three with generalised seizures, seven with partial seizures), no improvement in seizure frequency was observed over a 90-day period in eight out of ten patients [7].

Reflexly-induced epilepsy in man

In two reflexly-induced syndromes of human epilepsy : post-anoxic action or intention myoclonus and generalised photosensitive epilepsy (progressive myoclonus epilepsy, primary cortico-reticular epilepsy), monoaminergic drug treatment has proved effective.

The incapacitating action or intention myoclonus resulting from hypoxia or head injury [8] is abolished for 6—8 hours by treatment with the 5HT precursor, 5-hydroxytryptophan (5HTP, 2—5mg/kg, administered intravenously) and reduced following L-dopa [9,10]. Dopaminergic and serotoninergic antagonists (sulpiride, chlorpromazine, haloperidol, methysergide) increase the incidence of myoclonus. A functional cerebral 5HT deficiency in such patients is suggested by subsequent studies indicating reduced CSF 5HT concentrations, although no deficit in brain 5HT or 5HIAA was found post-mortem in two patients with post-anoxic action myoclonus (7,11,12]. In patients responsive to 5HTP there is evidence for a brain stem origin of their myoclonus, but three patients with a cortical EEG abnormality associated with myoclonus have been treated successfully with lisuride, a compound with agonist activity at 5HT and DA receptors. Severity of myoclonus is markedly reduced whereas the EEG abnormality is unaffected or increased (Marsden et al, unpublished results).

In human photosensitive epilepsy, EEG spikes induced by stroboscopic stimulation are abolished following low doses of the directly acting DA agonist apomorphine (1.25 —1.5mg, subcutaneously) [13,14]. Complete protection is short lasting (15—30 min after drug administration), but partial protection is observed for up to one hour. Visual evoked potentials are unaffected. Nausea and vomiting are seen in one-third of the patients, but these side-effects are

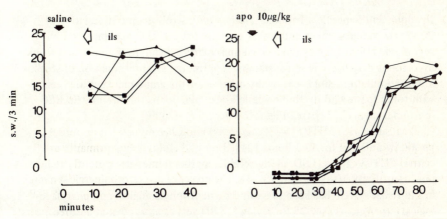

Figure 1. Photoconvulsive response in 4 patients following saline or apomorphine 10µg/kg sc. Ordinate = total number of spike and wave discharges on cortical EEG in a 3 min period of photic stimulation

transient compared with protection against photically-induced myoclonus. In another study performed by Franco Marrosu (Cagliari, Sardinia), using four patients, subcutaneous administration of apomorphine (10μg/kg) abolishes photically-induced spikes and waves for up to 40 min (Figure 1).

Thus in two stimulus-sensitive myoclonic disorders, monoaminergic drugs can reduce or abolish EEG and motor symptoms. In the case of photo-sensitive epilepsy, the development of DA agonists with a prolonged time course of action, such as the aporphines (see below), may prove a more effective treatment.

Monoamines and experimental epilepsy

In experimental epilepsy, the effects of 5HT and DA depend on the animal species and the type of seizure. Thus apomorphine raises electro-shock thresholds in rats, but not in mice [15] and exacerbates seizures induced by pentylene-tetrazol in both species [16]. Compounds which disrupt storage of brain mono-amines such as reserpine and tetrabenazine facilitate electrically- and chemically-induced seizures in rodents [17,18], but the effects of depletion of monoamines by synthesis inhibition are often equivocal and usually relatively weak [18–21]. As in the case of human myoclonus, it is in the reflexly-triggered experimental seizures that the most consistent effects of monoaminergic drugs are seen. In our laboratory, using two models of reflex epilepsy, we have established that a wide range of drugs modifying serotoninergic and dopaminergic transmission have considerable effects on seizure generation.

Photically-induced myoclonus in Senegalese baboons

In adolescent Senegalese baboons, *Papio papio,* stroboscopic stimulation at 20–25Hz induces spikes and waves on the cortical EEG accompanied by myoclonic jerks of the eyelids, facial musculature, head, neck, limbs and trunk. Myoclonus may become self-sustaining, continuing after termination of strobo-scopic stimulation, and occasionally seizures of the grand mal type are seen, with tonic spasm and rhythmic whole body myoclonus followed by an EEG 'post-ictal silence' [22] (see Figure 2 legend for grading).

Treatment with 5HTP (15–30mg/kg, iv) abolishes myoclonic responses to photic stimulation for 1–3 hours [21]. Ergot alkaloids acting primarily at central 5HT synapses (LSD, methysergide, methergoline) also potently reduce photosensitivity in this model [23,24]. The presence of a serotoninergic synapse in the visual system has been suggested by neurophysiological and pharmaco-logical experiments [see 25 for review]. LSD acts as an agonist at autoreceptors for 5HT on raphé neurones inhibiting neuronal firing, and reduction in visual evoked responses is observed following LSD in baboons [23,26]. Thus it is probable that the protective effects of serotoninergic drugs in this model are at the level of afferent transmission. Other ergot drugs which are DA agonists (as demonstrated *in vitro* and in rodent screening tests) such as ergocornine, bromocriptine and ergometrine have a protective effect [27] (Table I).

TABLE I. Effects of ergot alkaloids on photomyoclonic responses in *Papio papio* and audiogenic seizures in DBA/2 mice

	Baboons Minimal protective dose (mg/kg)	DBA/2 mice ED50 clonic phase (mg/kg)	References
LSD	0.05	9.3	23
Ergocornine	1	1.1	27, 42
Ergometrine	1	9.7	27, 42
Bromocriptine	> 4	5.0	27, 42

Seizures were graded as shown in the legends of Figures 2 and 5. Minimal protective dose = minimum dose for complete abolition of photically-induced responses. The ED50s for protection against the clonic phase of the audiogenic seizure were estimated graphically

Relatively high doses of apomorphine (0.5−1mg/kg, iv) abolish spontaneous and photically-induced cortical spikes and waves as well as myoclonus in baboons, but this effect is accompanied by behavioural and autonomic changes − agitation, vocalisation, gnawing, pupil dilation, salivation and piloerection [28]. In a subsequent study using low doses of apomorphine (10−250µg/kg, iv), a dose-dependent protective effect is seen (Figure 2). Pretreatment with the DA antagonist, domperidone (200µg/kg, iv), which does not cross the blood-brain barrier [29], abolishes the autonomic and severe behavioural changes whilst leaving protection against photically-induced myoclonus unchanged (Figure 2). Severity of behavioural changes seen following apomorphine 1.25mg/kg alone probably interfere with apomorphine's protective action. With domperidone pretreatment, a dose of apomorphine 1.25mg/kg is more effective (Figure 2). Up to 2.5mg apomorphine/kg could be administered with domperidone pretreatment without toxic side-effects.

The search for more potent DA agonists with a more prolonged action and fewer undesirable side-effects has led to the synthesis and development of apomorphine derivatives − the aporphines [30,31]. Several of the aporphines possess DA agonist activity in *in vitro* tests, but lack the excitant behavioural effects of apomorphine. These include (-) n-N-propylnorapomorphine (NPA) and (-) 2,10,11-trihydroxy-N-propylnoraporphine (TNPA) (Figure 3) which both diminish photically-induced responses over a wide dose range (0.1−2.5mg/kg, iv) whilst causing only mild sedation and yawning [32 and unpublished data]. Their anti-epileptic action is sustained, NPA lasting 1−2 hours, TNPA 3−7 hours depending on dose (Figure 4). It is likely that such compounds with or without domperidone will prove a satisfactory treatment for generalised photosensitive epilepsy in

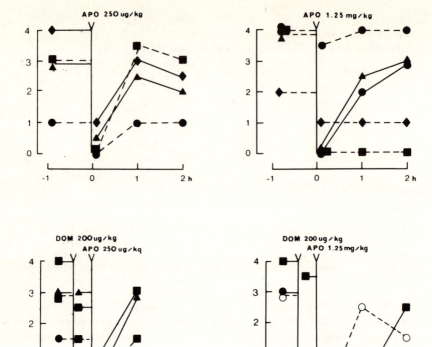

Figure 2. Reduction of myoclonic responses to photic stimulation in five baboons following apomorphine 250μg/kg and 1.25mg/kg, iv with (below), and without (above), domperidone (200μg/kg, iv) pretreatment (20 min before apomorphine). Each curve represents the responses of one animal and each different symbol represents a different animal. Myoclonic responses (ordinate) are graded as follows: 0 = no response; 1 = eyelid myoclonus; 2 = myoclonus of face, neck and upper limbs; 3 = generalised whole body myoclonus; 4 = myoclonus sustained after cessation of photic stimulation. Five minute tests with the stroboscope were carried out 5 min, 1 hr and 2 hr after apomorphine. Time in hr is shown on the abscissa

	R	R'
APOMORPHINE	CH_3	H
NPA	C_3H_7	H
TNPA	C_3H_7	OH

Figure 3. Molecular structure of DA agonist aporphines

130

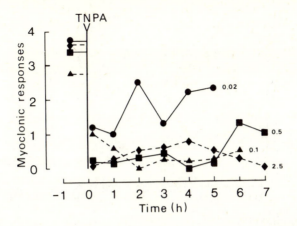

Figure 4. Effects of TNPA (0.02 –2.5mg/kg) on myoclonic responses to photic stimulation in baboons. Each point represents the mean responses of at least 3 animals. Five minute tests with stroboscopic stimulation were carried out 15 min – 7 hr following TNPA administration. Myoclonic responses were graded as described in the legend to Figure 2

man. NPA has already been used in limited trials with moderate success in Parkinsonism [33] and schizophrenia [34].

Audiogenic seizures in DBA/2 mice

Age-dependent audiogenic seizures in DBA/2 mice provide a rapid test system for pharmacological agents acting on monoaminergic transmission. On exposure to a loud sound of mixed frequency, mice aged 19–26 days exhibit a fixed sequence of seizure phenomena – 'wild running', clonic and tonic seizure with extension of the hind limbs and respiratory arrest [35] (see Figure 5 legend for grading).

5HTP and L-dopa reduce seizure susceptibility and reverse reserpine-induced enhancement of audiogenic seizures [36–40]. Apomorphine and the aporphines and DA agonist ergot alkaloids also protect mice against audiogenic seizures (Table I, Figure 5) [32,41–43]. Serotonin agonists are less effective in this test system [43].

General discussion

The site of action of monoaminergic drugs in reflex epilepsy is likely to be at the level of afferent transmission. In baboons, 5HTP and hallucinogenic ergot alkaloids which act presynaptically (LSD, psilocybin) depress visually-evoked responses [23,44] and are thought to diminish photosensitivity by blockade of visual transmission at a serotoninergic synapse in the lateral geniculate nucleus [25].

131

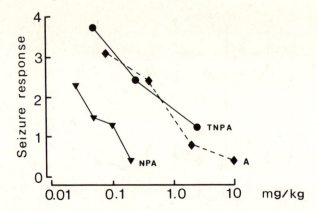

Figure 5. Comparison of effects of aporphines on audiogenic seizure response in 21—28 day old DBA/2 mice. Each point represents the mean maximum seizure response of at least 8 mice. Seizure response was graded as follows: 0 = no response; 1 = wild running; 2 = clonus; 3 = tonus; 4 = respiratory arrest; A = apomorphine; TNPA = trihydroxy n-N-propylnorapomorphine; NPA = n-N-propylnorapomorphine

Serotoninergic neurones originate in the mid-brain raphé nuclei and send ascending fibres to the neocortex, hypothalamus, thalamus, basal spinal cord and branches to the ependymal lining of the cerebral ventricles. Their diffuse projection suggests a modulatory influence over excitatory and inhibitory neurotransmission. The weaker effects of serotoninergic drugs in DBA/mice indicate a different site of action from that in baboons.

The potent effects of DA agonists in both animal models and man are likely to be mediated by dopaminergic neurones of the nigro-striatal and mesolimbic systems. In the case of photosensitive epilepsy, however, an action of DA receptors in the retina cannot be excluded, although visual evoked responses in man are not modified by apomorphine [13]. DA neurones are involved in the control of posture, movement and orientation and sensory initiation of voluntary movement. In both animal models, feedback from somatosensory afferents has a critical role in the maintenance of the seizure response [46—48]. In rats susceptible to audiogenic seizures, responses are exacerbated following caudate lesions [49] and intrastriatal injections of DA agonists in the rat block focal cortical spiking induced by cobalt [50]. The efficacy of DA agonists in reflexly evoked epileptic phenomena, compared to their lack of effect in other models, particularly chemically-induced seizures [16,27], emphasises the role of the striatum in the integration of sensory input and motor output.

Acknowledgments

I am grateful for financial support from the Medical Research Council, the Wellcome Trust and the British Epilepsy Association.

References

1   Bossi L, Zivkovic B, Scatton B et al. In Morselli PL, Lloyd KG, Löscher W et al, eds. *Neurotransmitters, Seizures and Epilepsy 1981:* 307. New York: Raven Press
2   Laxer KD, Sourkes TL, Fang TY et al. *Neurology 1979; 29:* 1157—1161
3   Chadwick D, Jenner P, Reynolds EH. *Ann Neurol 1977; 1:* 218—224
4   Garelis E, Sourkes T. *J Neurol Neurosurg Psychiat 1974; 37:* 704—710
5   Young SN, Gauthier S, Anderson GM, Purdy WC. *J Neurol Neurosurg Psychiat 1980; 43:* 438—445
6   Shaywitz BA, Cohen DJ, Bowers MB. *Neurology 1975; 25:* 72—79
7   Chadwick D, Trimble M, Jenner P et al. *Epilepsia 1978; 19:* 3—10
8   Lance JW, Adams RD. *Brain 1963; 86:* 111—136
9   Lhermitte F, Peterfalui M, Marteau R et al. *Rev Neurol (Paris) 1971; 124:* 21—31
10 Lhermitte F, Marteau R, Degos CF. *Rev Neurol (Paris) 1972; 126:* 107—114
11 Chadwick D, Hallett M, Harris R et al. *Brain 1977; 29:* 455—487
12 Van Woert MH, Sethy VH. *Neurology 1975; 25:* 135—140
13 Quesney LF, Andermann F, Lal S, Prelevic S. *Neurol (Paris) 1971; 124:* 21—31
14 Quesney LF. In Morselli PL, Lloyd KG, Loscher W et al, eds. *Neurotransmitters, Seizures and Epilepsy 1981;* 263. New York: Raven Press
15 McKenzie GM, Soroko FE. *J Pharm Pharmacol 1972; 24:* 696—701
16 Soroko FE, McKenzie GM. *Pharmacologist 1970; 12:* 294—298
17 Chen G, Ensor CR, Bohner B. *Arch Int Pharmacodyn 1968; 172:* 183—218
18 Rudzik AD, Johnson GA. In Costa E, Garattini S, eds. *International Symposium on Amphetamines and Related Compounds 1970;* 715. New York: Raven Press
19 Kilian M. Frey HH. *Neuropharmacol 1973; 12:* 681—692
20 Jobe PC, Picchioni AL, Chin L. *J Pharmacol Exp Therap 1973; 184:* 1—10
21 Wada JA, Balzano E, Meldrum BS, Naquet R. *Electroenceph Clin Neurophysiol 1972; 33:* 520—526
22 Killam KF, Killam EK, Naquet R. *Electroenceph Clin Neurophysiol 1967; 22:* 497—513
23 Walter S, Balzano E, Vuillon-Cacciuttolo G, Naquet R. *Electroenceph Clin Neurophysiol 1971; 30:* 294—305
24 Meldrum BS, Naquet R. *Electroenceph Clin Neurophysiol 1971; 31:* 563—572
25 Aghajanian G, Wang RY. In Lipton MA, Di Maseio A, Killam KF, eds. *Psychopharmacology: A Generation of Progress 1978;* 171. New York: Raven Press
26 Vuillon-Cacciuttolo G, Meldrum BS, Balzano E. *Epilepsia 1973; 14:* 213—221
27 Anlezark GM, Meldrum BS. *Psychopharmacology 1978; 57:* 57—62
28 Meldrum BS, Anlezark GM, Trimble M. *Europ J Pharmacol 1975; 32:* 203—213
29 Laduron PM, Leysen JE. *Biochem Pharmacol 1979; 28:* 2161—2165
30 Neumeyer JL, Lal S, Baldessarini RJ. In Corsini GU, Gessa GL, eds. *Apomorphine and other Dopaminomimetics, Volume 1: Basic Pharmacology 1981;* 1. New York: Raven Press
31 Neumeyer JL, Law SJ, Lamont JS. In Corsini GU, Gessa GL, eds. *Apomorphine and other Dopaminomimetics, Volume 1: Basic Pharmacology 1981;* 209. New York: Raven Press
32 Ashton C, Anlezark GM, Meldrum BS. *Europ J Pharmacol 1976; 39:* 399—401
33 Cotzias GC, Papavasilious PS, Tolosa ES et al. *N Engl J Med 1976; 294:* 567—572
34 Tamminga CA, De Fraites EG, Gotts MD, Chase TN. In Corsini GU, Gessa GL, eds. *Apomorphine and other Dopaminomimetics, Volume 2: Clinical Pharmacology 1981;* 49. New York: Raven Press
35 Collins RL. In Purpura D, Penry JK, Tower DB et al. *Experimental Models of Epilepsy 1972;* 347. New York: Raven Press
36 Boggan WO, Seiden LS. *Physiol Behav 1971; 6:* 215—217
37 Boggan WO, Seiden LS. *Physiol Behav 1973; 10:* 9—12
38 Lehmann A. *Aggressologie 1964; 5:* 311—351
39 Schlesinger K, Boggan WO, Freedman DX. *Life Sci 1968; 7:* 437—447
40 Schlesinger K, Boggan WO, Freedman DX. *Life Sci 1970; 9:* 721—729

41   Anlezark GM, Meldrum BS. *Br J Pharmacol 1975; 53:* 419—421
42   Anlezark GM, Pycock CJ, Meldrum BS. *Europ J Pharmacol 1976; 37:* 295—302
43   Anlezark GM, Horton RW, Meldrum BS. *Biochem Pharmacol 1978; 27:* 2821—2828
44   Meldrum BS, Balzano E, Wada JA, Vuillon-Cacciuttolo G. *Physiol Behav 1972; 9:*
      615—621
45   Willott JF. *Exp Neurol 1974; 43:* 359—368
46   Naquet R, Catier J, Menini C. *Adv Neurol 1975; 10:* 107—118
47   Chauvel P, Lamarche M, Pumain R. *Adv Neurol 1975; 10:* 129—132
48   Menini CH. *J Physiol (Paris) 1976; 72:* 5—44
49   Kesner RP. *Exp Neurol 1966; 15:* 192—205
50   Farjo IB, McQueen JK. *Br J Pharmacol 1979; 67:* 353—360

14

EFFECTIVENESS OF SIX ANTIEPILEPTIC DRUGS IN FOLATE-INDUCED PARTIAL EPILEPSY AND THE RELATIVE ABSENCE OF IT IN THE PENICILLIN-INDUCED FORM IN THE RAT

J Arends, O Hommes

As a part of research concerning the epileptogenic mechanism of folate, we tested the effect of six antiepileptic drugs on folate- or penicillin-induced partial epilepsy in the rat [1,2].

In our models a stereotaxic thermal lesion was made in the sensori-motor cortex followed one day later by i.v. injection of folate (0.20mmol/kg) or penicillin (0.76mmol/kg). Antiepileptic drugs were given at least 10 minutes prior to folate or penicillin by subcutaneous route.

The variables and the order of their suppressibility are shown in Table I.

TABLE I. Variables

Numerical		Not Numerical	
1 Short interval jerks	+++	1 Short interval seizures	+++
2 Medium interval jerks	++	2 Spread of long interval jerks	++
3 Long interval jerks	+	3 Medium interval seizures	+
4 Duration of epilepsy	−		

For each of six drugs the lowest dose that effectively suppressed the variable was noted; a rank order was given and added for all drugs. Short interval: <0.33 sec; medium interval: $0.33 \leqslant x \leqslant 0.80$ sec; long interval: >0.80 sec. (Compiled from [2])

From this Table, it can be seen that jerk intervals are important, two different partial seizure types exist with quite different suppressibility and that duration of epilepsy (mean: 110 minutes) is drug resistant. The results shown apply for folate- as well as penicillin-activated epilepsy.

Between the six drugs remarkable differences appeared concerning their antiepileptic profile (Tables II and III).

TABLE II. Effects of six antiepileptic drugs on folate-induced partial epilepsy. (Compiled from [2])

Drug	Duration*	Long*	Medium*	Short*	Type of action†
Clonazepam	−	+++	+++	+++	−
Carbamazepine	−	−	−	+++	−
Phenytoin	−	−	+	+++	−
Phenobarbital	−	++	++	+++	0
Valproate s.	−	+	+++	+++	+
Ethosuximide	−	+	+++	+++	0

* − no reduction $(1 < R \leqslant 2)$; + small reduction $(2 < R \leqslant 4)$; ++ intermediate reduction
   $(4 < R \leqslant 8)$; +++ strong reduction $(R > 8)$
      R = reduction factor = jerks or seconds controls/jerks or seconds drug
      Maximal effects are shown

† + disturbance of long interval rhythm precedes threshold elevation of short interval seizures
   0 disturbance of long interval rhythm at same dose as threshold elevation of short interval seizures
   − threshold elevation of short interval seizures precedes disturbance of long interval rhythm

From Table II it can be seen that:

- clonazepam has the strongest action.
- carbamazepine and phenytoin only inhibit fast components.
- in the case of valproate sodium, disturbance of long interval rhythm precedes suppression of short interval seizures. Phenobarbital and ethosuximide have an intermediate position, whereas in the three other drugs this disturbance does not occur at all or as a secondary event.

These effects were compared with those obtained after replacement of folate by penicillin injection, Table III.

TABLE III. Effects of drugs on penicillin-induced partial epilepsy

Drug	Duration*	Long*	Medium*	Short*	Type of action†
Clonazepam	−	+	+++	+++	−
Carbamazepine	−	−	+	+++	?††
Phenytoin	−	−	−	+	−
Phenobarbital	−	+	++	+++	−
Valproate s.	−	−	−	+	0 or −
Ethosuximide	−	−	−	+	−

Compiled from [2]. Legend* and † see Table II.
   †† Due to interaction of propyleneglycol with long interval rhythm no conclusion can be drawn

From Table III it can be seen that:

- all drug effects are less than after folate-induced epilepsy (due to the interaction of propyleneglycol after penicillin-induced epilepsy, the carbamazepine effect is not totally reliable).
- the types of action for all drugs except valproate sodium are alike, while no disturbance of long interval rhythm takes place. In the case of valproate sodium also, no significant reduction of seizure threshold takes place.

These findings have forced us to look for differences in epileptogenicity between folate and penicillin. Some of these can be found [1] indicating a more generalised type of epilepsy after penicillin injection [4]. In ECoG experiments multifocal activation by penicillin at electrode site was seen but not by folate [3]. Finally less interdependence between long interval jerks with the chance of short interval seizures to occur after penicillin injection was seen (to be published).

Our model of partial epilepsy can thus be regarded as unifocal (after folate injection) or unifocal with depressed threshold for generalisation (after penicillin injection).

While these rather subtle differences in epileptogenic action between folate and penicillin can explain certain unequal drug effects and therefore may be important from a clinical viewpoint, this cannot account for the fact that all drugs exhibit reduced effectiveness after penicillin-induced epilepsy (except perhaps carbamazepine, in which case propyleneglycol interfered with long interval rhythm of penicillin epilepsy). A different mechanism of action may play a role, folate interfering with monoamine metabolism [5], penicillin by also directly changing Cl$^-$-channels [6]. Apart from this it seems important to look for kinetic differences between both epileptogenic drugs and to reveal the degree of ischaemic metabolism within the focus. Experiments with regard to these questions are under way.

Acknowledgment

This study was supported by CLEO — TNO (Commission for Epilepsy research), No A-28

References

1   Arends J, Hommes O, Doesburg W et al. In Dam M, Gram L, Penry JK, eds. *Epileptology, XII Epilepsy International Symposium 1981;* 653–669. New York: Raven Press
2   Arends J, Hommes O, Schoofs M et al. *Br J Clin Pract;* In press
3   Fariello RG. *Epilepsia 1976; 17:* 217–222
4   Gloor P. *Epilepsia 1979; 20:* 571–588
5   Hommes OR. In Dam M, Gram L, Penry JK, eds. *Epileptology, XII Epilepsy International Symposium 1981;* 641–651
6   Voskuyl RA. *Experimental Epilepsy. Thesis 1978:* 16–30. Leiden: University of Leiden

15

CLINICAL ASPECTS OF MYOCLONUS EPILEPSY

J H D Millar

Myoclonus is difficult to define. It is a sudden jerk of a muscle or group of muscles, usually irregular and asymmetrical. More often than not it will cause a
movement at a joint and sometimes the movements may be violent; but at other
times it requires careful observation to detect. It must be distinguished from
fasciculation, myokymia, chorea, ballismus, spasmodic torticollis, flexor and
extensor spasms of the legs and hemifacial spasm. Myoclonus has been described
in association with most diseases of the central nervous system [1,2].

It has been classified from various viewpoints and several clinico-pathological
classifications have been published in recent years [2–4], as well as from an
electrophysiological point of view. Halliday [5] describes three types, pyramidal,
extrapyramidal and segmental, and Marsden and colleagues [2] describe two
main groups, cortical myoclonus and subcortical myoclonus.

The classification which I employ (Table I) is based on those of Swanson and
colleagues [3] and Halliday [4], but it is far from perfect. I have little experience in the neurological diseases of childhood and, like Jeavons [6], have great
difficulty in classifying the various types of myoclonus affecting children. Except
for early morning myoclonus affecting patients suffering from idiopathic epilepsy
and nocturnal jerks [7], myoclonus is a rare phenomenon in adults.

The myoclonus associated with *subacute sclerosing panencephalitis* may be
asymmetrical or even unilateral and at times has an extrapyramidal quality, an
element of 'torsion spasm'. A boy of 13 presented with chorea indistinguishable
from Sydenham's rheumatic chorea except that there was evidence of intellectual
deterioration and the EEG was generally abnormal. The antibodies to measles
virus were elevated. It was over a month before myoclonic jerks appeared and the
EEG showed the characteristic episodic discharges of subacute sclerosing pan-
encephalitis.

Creutzfeldt-Jacob disease is fortunately very rare with an incidence of less than
one patient per million of the population per year. In not all cases is it possible

TABLE I. Generalised myoclonus

Acute and Subacute

    1 Encephalitis (viral, subacute sclerosing panencephalitis, Creutzfeldt-Jacob disease)

    2 Post-hypoxia (Lance-Adams) [8]

    3 Metabolic (uraemia, cholaemia, hypoglycaemia)

    4 Non-progressive myoclonic encephalopathy (Kinsbourne – 'dancing eyes') [9]

    5 Infantile spasms [10]

    6 Subacute myoclonic spinal neuronitis (Campbell and Garland) [14]

Chronic

    1 Essential (paramyoclonus multiplex, Friedreich)

    2 Progressive familial myoclonus epilepsy (Lafora, lipidosis, degenerative type – Ramsay Hunt)

    3 Associated with idiopathic epilepsy

    4 Myoclonic astatic epilepsy (Lennox-Gastaut) [11]

    5 Nocturnal (Symonds) [7]

to find the characteristic repetitive discharges in the EEG with accompanying myoclonus. It is strange that myoclonus appears to be rare in herpes simplex encephalitis although the EEG at times shows repetitive discharges similar to Creutzfeldt-Jacob disease.

Post-anoxic myoclonus [8] in the description by Lance and Adams showed cerebellar-like features, action myoclonus, ataxia and dysarthria. The nystagmus they suggested was due to the large dose of barbiturates required to suppress the myoclonus, whilst the cerebellar-like signs appear to result from the severe myoclonus.

The myoclonus resulting from *metabolic disorders* can be rapidly reversed. I have seen severe generalised myoclonus due to hypoglycaemia disappear dramatically with intravenous glucose. In acute uraemic states the myoclonus can also be reversed but, in chronic uraemia with high blood urea and low serum calcium, treating the low calcium has little or no effect on the myoclonus. The myoclonus appears to arise in the lower brainstem reticular formation [12,13].

I include *subacute myoclonic spinal neuronitis* because it gives me an opportunity to mention a man aged 64 [15] who suffered from severe painful spasms of the legs for several months and at autopsy was found to have a demyelinating condition of the spinal cord associated with a small oat cell carcinoma of the lung without metastases to the nervous system, not unlike Case No 3 in Campbell and Garland's paper except that in their case the histology of the spinal cord was more in favour of a virus infection.

Essential myoclonus (Paramyoclonus Multiplex, Friedreich) [16] is a chronic generalised myoclonus. There is no accompanying epilepsy and no evidence of

139

intellectual deterioration. The patient may be only minimally disabled. A farmer aged 69 first noticed twitching of muscles about the age of 30. The myoclonus was generalised affecting all limbs, trunk and muscles of articulation but he was able to walk, dress and feed himself although unfit for heavy work. Seven years ago clonazepam was started with considerable improvement in the myoclonus. No other member of the family was affected but a familial form of the disease has been described [17].

A severe form of myoclonus is found in *progressive familial myoclonus epilepsy* [18]. When fully developed the myoclonus is widespread and extremely disabling. The myoclonus is increased by active and passive movements, change in posture, emotion, photic stimulation and sudden unexpected noise, but usually disappears during sleep. It is bilateral, irregular and asymmetrical. The muscles of articulation and respiration are frequently affected causing a marked dysarthria in some cases. Formal tests of co-ordination produce an intention tremor resembling that of advanced multiple sclerosis. Walking is affected by an irregular ataxia and frequent falls, and eventually in the terminal stages the patient becomes bedridden. Nystagmus is not normally seen but occasionally the extraocular muscles are affected by myoclonus. The ataxia, intention or action tremor and dysarthria resemble the findings in cerebellar disease but are related to the severity of the myoclonus. Ramsay Hunt [19] separated the cerebellar signs from the myoclonus in the condition he called *dyssynergia cerebellaris myoclonica.* He reported six cases, two of whom were twins and the other four were sporadic cases without a family history of myoclonus epilepsy. One of the twins also suffered from Friedreich's ataxia.

Major epilepsy occurs in the early stages of the disease and usually disappears in the terminal stage. The myoclonus usually increases in intensity prior to a major fit and diminshes after one.

Progressive familial myoclonus epilepsy is usually separated into three groups (1) Lafora disease (2) lipidoses (3) degenerative type which includes Ramsay Hunt's disease [20].

Lafora disease was very fully reviewed by Van Heycop ten Ham in 1974 [21]. It is a recessive autosomal disease causing curious intracellular amyloid-like deposits in brain, spinal cord, heart and liver and probably also in retina, peripheral nerves, skeletal muscles, extraocular muscles and adrenal medulla. The Lafora bodies in the brain are chiefly located in the substantia nigra and dentate nucleus. Most investigators accept an unidentified enzyme disorder as its cause. Biochemical evidence has shown that the Lafora material is essentially a glucose polymer (polyglucosan) but that the deposits in systemic organs differ in protein content. Muscle biopsy can be helpful in diagnosis [22–24].

The age of onset is usually between 12 and 17 years, the duration before death between two and ten years with an average of six. In most cases epileptic seizures preceded the myoclonus by several years. Mental changes are common; irritability, aggression, confusion and hallucinations have been described. The

140

finding of low mucopolysaccharides in the serum has not been substantiated and is possibly a secondary rather than a primary phenomenon [25,26].

The second group is caused by lipoid inclusions, a storage disease, such as *amaurotic familial idiocy* [27].

The third group, the degenerative disease, may show very little pathology in the central nervous system to account for a clinical picture just as severe as Lafora disease which shows such widespread pathological changes [28–30]. This group is frequently associated with other diseases such as Friedreich's ataxia, polyneuropathy, peroneal muscular atrophy and the cases described by Ramsay Hunt would also fall into this group [19,31].

In 1955 Harriman and I reported three families suffering from progressive familial myoclonic epilepsy [20]. In family A the onset of illness was with major epilepsy at the age of 14 years. Myoclonus appeared at 20 years and both brothers died in a mental hospital aged 24 with a duration of illness of ten years (Table II).

TABLE II. Progressive familial myoclonus epilepsy

	Epilepsy	Myoclonus	Death	Duration
Family A	14	20	24	10
	14	20	24	10
Family B	7	7	27	20
	14	14	27	13
	9	9	30	21
Family C	19	19	49	30
	20	20	61	41
	27	27	47	20

Autopsy in one showed Lafora bodies in the brain and similar material in the heart and liver which by differential staining methods was shown to be an acid mucopolysaccharide. Serum electrophoresis of mucoprotein in family B and other cases showed a very low level of the alpha 2 mucopolysaccharide component. In 1971 the third brother in family B died and an autopsy revealed no Lafora bodies but degenerative changes. In sections from the cerebral cortex there was no distinct neuronal loss although there was some gliosis of the underlying white matter. Sections from the basal ganglia did not show a distinct neuronal loss but, in sections from the brainstem, there was neuronal loss particularly in the region of the substantia nigra and pontine and medullary nuclei. In the inferior olives particularly there was cell loss with gliosis and the remaining cells showed a very marked deposition of lipofuscin. The cerebellum does not seem to have been remarked upon. In the spinal cord the anterior horn cells were relatively well preserved although there might have been a slight cell loss and some cells contained very large deposits of lipofuscin. There was no long tract degeneration. Both eyes showed degeneration of the macula region of the retina.

A younger sister (B 18) has since developed the disease. Myoclonus was first noticed in 1965 when aged 16, and major fits appeared in 1970. Electrophoresis of the serum mucoproteins in her case was normal and the evidence now suggests that the serum changes are secondary and seen only in some advanced cases and are not a primary phenomenon [25,26]. The clinical features in Family B were just as severe as in family A but more protracted, but the mental symptoms were more evident in family A.

Phenytoin in addition to other anticonvulsants was used in the patient whose autopsy has been described (B 13) when the major fits were frequent between 1957 and 1965 but not in the last seven years of his life. The recent patient (B 18) has been on sodium valproate for the past five years with some improvement in her myoclonus and major fits.

Eldridge [28] and colleagues describe 'Baltic' myoclonus epilepsy and blame the toxic effects of phenytoin for the rapid deterioration in the clinical state with improvement when phenytoin is stopped and valproic acid substituted.

Symonds distinguishes between *nocturnal jerks* which he considers to be physiological, from *nocturnal myoclonus* an 'excessive form of nocturnal jerks' and a precursor of epilepsy [7].

Focal myoclonus can arise at all levels of the nervous system:

> *Cerebral cortex* — epilepsia partialis continuans
>
> *Brainstem* — palatal myoclonus, hiccup, space occupying lesion
>
> *Spinal cord* — tumour [32], localised infection, trauma and cervical spondylitis [33]

Treatment

In recent years a number of new anticonvulsants have become available which are sometimes helpful in the treatment of myoclonus. Clonazepam, carbamazepine [34] and sodium valproate. ACTH and steroids are used in infantile spasms. Tetrabenazine has been found useful in spinal myoclonus [33].

Oral and intravenous 5-hydroxytryptophan (5HTP) in combination with carbidopa are usually successful in the treatment of post-anoxic myoclonus and possibly in other forms of myoclonus [35—37]. The combination of 1-tryptophan and a MAO inhibitor is as effective and has fewer side-effects than 5HTP.

References

1   Aigner BR, Mulder DW. *Arch Neurol 1960; 2:* 600–615
2   Marsden CD, Hall M, Fahn S. *The Nosology and Pathophysiology of Myoclonus in Movement Disorders: Modern Trends in Neurology 1982 2nd Edn.* Butterworths: In press
3   Swanson PD, Lutterell CN, Magladery JW. *Medicine 1962; 41:* 339–356
4   Halliday AM. In Williams D, ed. *Modern Trends in Neurology 1967;* 69–105. London: Butterworths
5   Halliday AM. *Brain 1967; 90:* 241–284
6   Jeavons PM. *Developmental Medicine and Child Neurology 1977; 19:* 3–8
7   Symonds CP. *Neurol Neurosurg Psychiat 1953; 16:* 166–171
8   Lance JW, Adams RD. *Brain 1963; 86:* 111–136
9   Kinsbourne M. *J Neurol Neurosurg Psychiat 1962; 25:* 271
10 Jeavons PM, Bower BD. In Vinken PJ, Bruyn GW, eds. *Handbook of Clinical Neurology 1974; 15:* 219–234. Amsterdam and New York: North Holland Publishing Co
11 Gastaut H, Broughton R, Roger J, Tassinari CA. In Vinken PJ, Bruyn GW, eds. *Handbook of Clinical Neurology 1974; 15:* 121–129. Amsterdam and New York: North Holland Publishing Co
12 Chadwick D, French AT. *J Neurol Neurosurg Psychiat 1979; 42:* 52–55
13 Zuckerman EG, Glaser GH. *Arch Neurol 1972; 27:* 14–28
14 Campbell AMG, Garland H. *J Neurol Neurosurg Psychiat 1956; 19:* 268–274
15 McCaughey WTE, Millar JHD. *Lancet 1955; ii:* 365–366
16 Friedreich N. *Virchows Archiv für Pathologie und Anatomie 1881; 86:* 421–434
17 Daube J, Peters HA. *Arch Neurol 1966; 15:* 587–594
18 Unverricht H. *Die Myclonie 1891:* 128. Leipzig and Wien: Franz Deuticke
19 Hunt JR. *Brain 1921; 44:* 490–538
20 Harriman DGF, Millar JHD. *Brain 1955; 78:* 325–349
21 Van Heycop ten Ham MW. In Vinken PJ, Bruyn GW, eds. *Handbook of Clinical Neurology 1979; 15:* 382–422. Amsterdam and New York: North Holland Publishing Co
22 Neville HE, Brooke MH, Austin JH. *Arch Neurol 1974; 30:* 466–474
23 Coleman LC, Gambetti P, Di Mauro S, Blume RE. *Arch Neurol 1974; 31:* 396–406
24 Carpenter S, Karpat G, Andermann F et al. *Neurol 1974; 24:* 531–538
25 Millar JHD, Neill DW. *Epilepsia 1959; 1:* 115–116
26 Millar JHD, Neill DW. *Quart J Med 1962; 31:* 518–519
27 Watson CW, Denny-Brown D. *Arch Neurol Psychiat 1953; 70:* 151–168
28 Eldridge R, Iivanainen M, Stern R, Korber T. *Neurol 1981; 31:* 67–68
29 Bradshaw J. *Brain 1954; 77:* 138–157
30 Matthews WB, Howell DA, Stevens DL. *J Neurol Neurosurg Psychiat 1969; 32:* 116
31 Smith NJ, Espir MLE, Matthews WB. *Brain 1978; 101:* 461–472
32 Garcin R, Rondot P, Guiot G. *Brain 1968; 91:* 75–
33 Hoehn MM, Cherington M. *Neurol 1977; 27:* 942–946
34 Hirose G, Singer P, Bass N. *JAMA 1971; 218:* 1432–1433
35 Lhermitte F, Marteau R, Degos C-F. *Rev Neurol 1972; 126:* 107–114
36 Chadwick D, Harris R, Jenner P et al. *Lancet 1975; ii:* 434–435
37 Chadwick D, Mallett M, Harris R et al. *Brain 1977; 100:* 455–487

16

EPILEPTIC DIZZINESS:
A PRESENTING FEATURE OF TEMPORAL LOBE EPILEPSY

M Swash

Dizziness and vertigo are common symptoms. Dizziness is often defined as a sudden sensation of instability, and vertigo as a similar feeling of instability accompanied by a sensation of rotation, but the separation of these two symptoms is not always clear cut. Further, there are many causes of dizziness and vertigo (Table I). Epilepsy is an important cause of transient episodes of dizziness, with or without a rotational component, but the possibility that brief episodes of dizziness may be due to epilepsy is not well known [1]. Dizziness as a manifestation of epilepsy was recognised by Hughlings Jackson more than

TABLE I. Vertigo and dizziness

Brain stem lesions	Demyelination
	Infarction and transient ischaemia
	Tumour, especially of 4th ventricle
	Drugs, e.g. Barbiturates
	Streptomycin
Cerebellar	Infarction
	Tumour
Vestibular neuronitis	(Epidemic vertigo)
Middle ear disease	Infection
	Trauma
	Ménière's disease
	Benign positional vertigo
Acoustic schwannoma	
Cortical disturbances	Temporal lobe tumour
	Temporal lobe epilepsy
Motion sickness	
Psychogenic vertigo and dizziness	
Ocular palsies	

100 years ago [2] , and was discussed by Gowers in his monograph "The Border-lands of Epilepsy" in 1907 [3] . Hughlings Jackson in 1879 recognised that in temporal lobe epilepsy dizziness is not simply an aura, but usually constitutes part of the seizure. An ill-defined complaint of episodic dizziness is a common feature of the aura preceding grand mal epilepsy, particularly in patients with idiopathic epilepsy, but this symptom is not well defined and is relatively insignificant in relation to the major seizure itself.

Since the treatment of isolated attacks of dizziness occurring as a manifestation of temporal lobe epilepsy is both simple and effective, the clinical and electro-encephalographic (EEG) features of the disorder merit more detailed description.

Patients

Thirty consecutive patients, aged 15 to 65 years (mean 35 years) were studied. Eighteen of these patients were women. Each patient had been referred for investigation of dizziness, defined as a transient sense of dysequilibrium with or without a feeling of rotation. In each of these patients investigation, and the results of treatment, indicated that dizziness was due to epilepsy rather than to any other disorder. Patients with a history of cerebral vascular disease, multiple sclerosis, or symptoms of middle ear disease were excluded as were those older than 65 years. Otological assessment, including clinical, audiometric and caloric tests, was negative in each patient. Neuroradiological investigation, by CT scan-ning of the head, was carried out in five patients, with normal results.

Clinical features

In each patient dizziness occurred in brief episodes, each lasting no more than a few seconds.

Case 1

A 40 year old housewife presented with a four year history of brief dizzy spells, often associated with a spinning feeling, occurring up to several times a day and sometimes associated with a feeling of pressure in her head. There seemed to be no particular trigger factors. Her symptoms had been attributed to anxiety, but anxiolytic drugs did not help.

Clinical and otological examinations were unremarkable, but an EEG showed a left posterior temporal sharp and slow wave focus, mainly present during hyper-ventilation.

She responded to phenytoin (300mg/day) and has remained virtually free of dizziness for over two and a half years.

A feeling of rotation was described by 14 patients (47 per cent). The symp-tom usually began abruptly as dizziness or as a feeling of instability that evolved to dizziness or rotational vertigo during a period of several seconds. In the recovery phase nausea was often experienced. Attacks were not related to postural change or to any other definite external factor. The frequency of the attacks varied both between patients and in individual patients at different times, ranging from about one a week to several episodes daily. Symptomatic dizziness had been present for from six months to 42 years (mean 10 years), but in almost two-thirds (19) of the patients it had occurred only during the previous one to five years. The mean age at onset was 25 years.

Case 2

A 45 year old woman had a long history of episodic rotatory dizziness since the age of 14. The episodes occurred in spells of several months or up to five years, alternating with similar periods when she was completely free of attacks. Sometimes the dizziness was associated with a 'swimmy feeling' in her head, a 'gassy taste' in her mouth and 'déjà vu' sensations. Treatment with Stemetil had failed to bring her any appreciable relief and she managed, over the years, to adapt herself to her symptoms. She was referred because her dizzy attacks had become increasingly frequent in the previous two years. Clinical and otological examinations were normal. A routine EEG was equivocal, but a sleep recording revealed a bitemporal theta and sharp wave abnormality.

Most of her symptoms disappeared following treatment with phenytoin 100mg bd) and she has remained well during the subsequent five years.

At the time of their first attendance seven patients (23 per cent) had also experienced generalised convulsions. In six of these patients episodic dizziness had preceded the development of generalised seizures by from 6 to 17 months. In one patient the illness began with a major seizure, itself preceded by a dizzy feeling, followed by frequent episodes of isolated vertigo. In the seven patients with generalised seizures, dizzy spells occurred both separately and immediately preceding the seizures.

Other symptoms

Other epileptic symptoms were also noted and these usually occurred separately from the episodes of dizziness (Table II). The commonest of these other components of the attacks was brief 'absences' which occurred in 15 patients. These consisted of short periods of altered consciousness without loss of posture. Sometimes the patient would retain awareness of the environment but would be momentarily unable to move or speak. Other symptoms were less common. These included generalised convulsions, depersonalisation, epigastric discomfort, nausea, headache, a sense of déjà vu', anxiety or panic, automatisms, auditory hallucinations, and gustatory hallucinations.

146

TABLE II. Other components of the attacks

Type	Number of patients
'Absences'	15 (50%)
Generalised convulsions	7 (23%)
Depersonalisation	7
Epigastric discomfort	6
Nausea	6
Headaches	5 (17%)
'Déjà vu'	2
Anxiety/panic	2
Automatisms	2
Auditory hallucinations	2
Gustatory hallucinations	1

There was evidence of an acquired cerebral lesion in only one patient who had sustained a closed head injury 13 years earlier. Two patients (7 per cent) had experienced febrile convulsions in infancy and six others (20 per cent) had a family history of epilepsy. In three of these families dizziness also occurred as a manifestation of epilepsy in the affected relatives.

EEG

An abnormal EEG was a criterion for diagnosis of epileptic dizziness in this group of patients. The EEG recordings consisted of routine waking recordings supplemented by recordings made during hyperventilation and during intermittent photic stimulation. In all but two patients the abnormality consisted of episodic temporal or bitemporal sharp or slow waves, but in some cases there were associated generalised seizure discharges (Table III). In both the patients with a generalised EEG disturbance there was a family history of epilepsy. In four patients the EEG disturbance was dubious in routine recordings, but became more definite in subsequent sleep recordings.

TABLE III. EEG features

Left posterior temporal	15
Right temporal	7
Bitemporal	6
Generalised atypical spike and wave	1
Generalised paroxysmal theta	1

147

Treatment

In this group of patients several different diagnoses had been considered before the patients had been referred for neurological opinion; these included Ménière's disease, cervical spondylosis, middle ear disease, cerebral vascular disease, and anxiety and depression. Most patients had tried various drugs, which often included phenothiazines, benzodiazepines and tricyclic antidepressants, but these treatments were usually ineffective. Two patients in whom 'absences' had been frequent had been treated with Tridione and ethosuccimide respectively without effect on their dizzy episodes.

In the 23 patients (77 per cent) in whom dizziness occurred without generalised seizures there was complete remission of symptoms in 10 (mean follow-up 18 months) and a considerable reduction in the frequency and severity of their attacks in the remainder (mean follow-up two years). Six of the seven patients who also had generalised seizures were completely free of both dizziness and other manifestations of epilepsy during one and a half to five years of follow-up. The patient with persisting seizures and dizzy episodes did not comply with treatment.

Discussion

Epileptic dizziness may often occur as part of an aura in generalised seizures but it is more specifically related to temporal lobe epilepsy, occurring as a component of temporal lobe attacks in 126 (19 per cent) of 666 patients studied by Currie et al [4]. However, in our patients dizziness was often the sole manifestation of temporal lobe epilepsy. This was indicated by the paroxysmal quality of the symptom, its close temporal relation with a generalised convulsion in some patients, and the associated electroencephalographic abnormality. The dizziness itself was often characteristic, consisting of sudden very brief episodes, lasting only a few seconds, followed by rapid recovery without sequelae. These episodes usually occurred without associated symptoms of epilepsy, but a variety of symptoms typical of temporal lobe epilepsy occurred on some occasions in this group of patients (Table I). Contrary to common belief that a subjective sensation of rotation is almost exclusively a manifestation of labyrinthine disease, rotation was experienced by nearly half our patients in their attacks. The diagnosis of epileptic dizziness could often be suspected because of the occurrence of separate symptoms of temporal lobe epilepsy, often elicited only by careful questioning. It was confirmed by the typical EEG abnormalities and by the response to treatment with appropriate anticonvulsant drugs. The 30 patients described represent an incidence of about one per cent of all new cases of epilepsy.

The underlying cause of temporal lobe epilepsy was uncertain in many cases. In some the EEG abnormalities suggested a diagnosis of idiopathic epilepsy and a family history of epilepsy of similar character was elicited in three (10 per cent) of these patients. Although this suggests the possibility of a specific genetic element the numbers are too small to allow firm conclusions to be drawn. In one patient there was evidence of an acquired cause: previous head injury.

The vestibular system projects from the brain stem to the posterior part of the superior temporal and middle temporal convolutions of the temporal lobes and thence to the supramarginal and angular gyri [5, 6]. The relatively posterior location of the vestibular representation in the temporal lobes probably accounts for the isolation of the symptom of dizziness or vertigo from other symptoms of temporal lobe epilepsy in our patients, and perhaps for the relative rarity of this isolated symptom in temporal lobe epilepsy. There have been few other reports of epileptic dizziness [7–9]. Drachman and Hart [8] found no instance in 125 patients investigated for dizziness, but Hughes and Drachman [9] noted that EEG abnormalities were more common in dizzy patients, and that dizziness was more common in epileptic patients than controls. Pedersen and Jepsen [7] recognised the concept that dizziness might occur in temporal lobe epilepsy, but they did not require EEG abnormality for diagnosis and it is therefore difficult to be certain of the accuracy of their results. However, Evistar and Evistar [10] found that epilepsy was the underlying cause in more than half of a group of 50 children with dizziness unassociated with evidence of middle ear or brain stem disease.

In previous reports a distinction has been drawn between vestibular and vestibulogenic seizures [11]. In 'vestibular seizures' the dizziness originates, as in our patients, from abnormal discharges in the cortical vestibular centres, while in 'vestibulogenic seizures' the attack is said to be initiated by labyrinthine discharges, originating in an abnormal labyrinth, which excite epileptic activity in neurones in the brain stem and temporal lobe. There was no evidence to support this concept of vestibulogenic seizures in our patients.

Dizziness is a common symptom but diagnosis is not always easy. It may result from dysfunction of the vestibular system at any point from the ear to the cerebral cortex. Dizziness due to labyrinthine disease or brain stem lesions, especially multiple sclerosis and cerebral vascular disease, is particularly common. Although in these instances dizziness may occasionally occur in isolation, the associated clinical features are usually diagnostic. Furthermore, in cerebral vascular disease the onset usually occurs later than in the patients described above, whose mean age was only 25 years. Dizziness may also occur during hyperventilation associated with anxiety or emotional distress but in such patients the EEG shows no features of epilepsy. In most of this group of 30 patients several other diagnoses had been considered for some months before a neurological opinion was sought. In most a psychogenic cause had been considered, no doubt because of the transitory nature of the attacks and the patients' perfect health between them. It is important to note, as in case 2, that despite the length of the history in many of the patients, and the development of generalised seizures in seven, anticonvulsant medication was both well tolerated and extremely effective. It is

149

thus clearly of great practical importance to consider epilepsy in the differential diagnosis of episodic dizziness or vertigo, particularly in young people.

Acknowledgment

This paper is based on data first published in the British Medical Journal [1] .

References

1   Kogeorgos J, Scott DF, Swash M. *Br Med J 1981; 282:* 687–689
2   Jackson JH. *Medical Times and Gazette 1879; 1:* 29–30
3   Gowers WR. *The Borderlands of Epilepsy 1907;* 40–75. London: Churchill
4   Currie S, Heathfield KWG, Henson RA, Scott DF. *Brain 1971; 94:* 173–190
5   Penfield W. *Ann Otol Rhinol Laryngol 1957; 66:* 691–698
6   Williams DJ. *Proc Roy Soc Med 1967; 60:* 961–964
7   Pedersen E, Jepsen O. *Acta Psychiatrica Neurologica Scandinavica 1956; (Suppl) 108:* 301–310
8   Drachman DA, Hart CW. *Neurology (Minneapolis) 1972; 22:* 323–324
9   Hughes MR, Drachman DA. *J Nerv Ment Dis 1977; 38:* 431–435
10   Evistar L, Evistar A. *Pediatrics 1977; 59:* 833–838
11   Behrman S, Wyke BD. *Brain 1958; 81:* 529–541

17

DRUG-INDUCED CONVULSIONS

D Chadwick

The study of drug-induced convulsions in animals has greatly increased our knowledge of the mechanisms involved in the production of seizures. A wide variety of natural and synthetic chemicals can induce sufficient stimulation of the central nervous system in animals to result in convulsions. Many agents have relatively non-selective effects and must be administered in high doses, and we know less of their mechanism of action than of those agents which have selective convulsant effects. The mechanism of action of convulsant drugs in animals has recently been reviewed [1], and it is helpful to consider these in order to gain some understanding of their relevance to man.

Drugs may act to enhance CNS excitation, either by direct membrane effects eg pentylenetetrazol and convulsant barbiturates, or by increasing the activity of excitory neurotransmitters eg anticholinesterases, and direct glutamate receptor agonists eg kainic acid. Alternatively, drugs may have an action in blocking inhibitory mechanisms. The GABA system is particularly important in this respect and potent convulsants, such as picrotoxin and bicuculline, all appear to act by blocking post-synaptic GABA receptors. Other convulsant agents, such as allyl-glycine and pyridoxal phosphate antagonists, produce their effects by inhibiting glutamic acid decarboxylase (GAD), and thus decreasing GABA synthesis. Strychnine appears to block the action of the inhibitory neurotransmitter glycine at its receptor [1].

In spite of this knowledge of animal experimental data, its application to the clinical situation is difficult because, in some instances, convulsants may have differing effects in different species. There may also be considerable variation in the dose of convulsant drug required to precipitate seizures in different species.

Incidence

It is difficult to obtain data on the incidence of drug-induced convulsions. The Committee on Safety of Medicines have received reports in which more than 70 different drugs were suspected of causing convulsions (personal communication). Frequently, such reports remain isolated so that, because *spontaneous* seizures are not uncommon, it is always difficult to attribute a convulsion in an individual patient (with presumed concurrent illness) to treatment with an individual drug. The fact that drug-induced convulsions are frequently reported in patients with established epilepsy adds further problems. Nevertheless, for several groups of drugs there have been a sufficient number of reports to make a causal relationship between administration of the drug and convulsions likely. It is the aim of this chapter to review the evidence in these cases, and to discuss those drugs whose ability to cause convulsions is of clinical importance or theoretical interest.

The only systematic study of the incidence of drug-induced convulsions, of which the author is aware, was undertaken by the Boston Collaborative Drug Surveillance Program [2] which reviewed the treatment of some 12,617 medical in-patients. Of these, 17 (0.13%) had convulsions associated with drug treatment; 4 with penicillins, 4 with anti-diabetic drugs (three with insulin, one with phenformin), two with lignocaine, two with phenothiazines and five others with agents as diverse as prednisone, isoniazid, vitamin K and ephedrine. Whilst there is no information on the incidence of drug-induced convulsions in out-patient populations, it appears that convulsions are relatively uncommon with drugs used in therapeutic doses, but are more common in association with accidental overdosage, and following drug abuse.

Antibiotics

The direct application of penicillin to the cerebral cortex causes focal seizures in animals [3]. More recently the parenteral administration of penicillin has been used as an experimental model for multifocal epilepsy in rats [4], and myoclonic absence seizures in cats [5]. In man, seizures occur in patients who have received high doses of penicillin intravenously, or intrathecally. Cerebrospinal fluid concentrations greater than 10 units per ml must be attained before convulsions are likely to occur [6], so that it is unwise to administer more than 10,000 units intrathecally in a single dose.

In the Boston Study [2], convulsions occurred in four patients (0.3% incidence), all of whom received intravenous penicillin, and all of whom had pre-existing renal disease. Benzylpenicillin is most frequently associated with convulsions but seizures have also been documented in patients treated with oxacillin and carbenicillin [7]. Gutnick et al [8] have suggested from animal experiments that the following drugs possess convulsant properties in a descending order of potency: benzylpenicillin, phenoxymethylpenicillin, oxacillin, methicillin, ampicillin, cephalothin, evidence that would be in keeping with the reported incidence of seizures with penicillins in man.

The convulsant action of penicillin is likely to be due to the GABA agonist properties that this drug possesses. When penicillin is applied iontophoretically

152

it reversibly blocks the inhibitory action of GABA on cortical, cuneate nucleus, and spinal neurones [9,10].

Seizures may also occur in man during treatment with antituberculous agents ie isoniazid and cycloserine [11]. It seems that both the peripheral neuropathy and seizures caused by these drugs are related to their ability to antagonise the action of pyridoxal phosphate [1]. This is a co-factor necessary for the activity of GAD, and hydrazides, such as isoniazid, whilst other carbonyl trapping agents, such as cycloserine, are able to combine with pyridoxal phosphate and thereby reduce GABA synthesis. In the case of isoniazid, genetic factors, resulting in 'slow acetylation', cause delay in inactivation of the drug, and are important in determining the susceptibility to neurological complications of this drug [12].

Hormones

Therapy with insulin was associated with tonic-clonic seizures in three (0.4%) of 763 patients in the Boston study [2]. A seizure also occurred in a patient receiving phenformin and all the diabetic drugs must be regarded as potentially convulsant, because of their ability to cause neuroglycopenia. In some patients with epilepsy, it appears that mild or moderate hypoglycaemia may precipitate typical seizures for that individual patient but, in non-epileptic patients, profound hypoglycaemia induced by insulin more usually causes myoclonus and subsequent tonic-clonic seizures [13].

Rarely, other synthetic hormonal agents may induce seizures. Prednisone was associated with a seizure in an individual patient in the Boston Study [2], possibly by causing hypocalcaemia. Oxytocin may also cause seizures when administered concurrently with a water-load resulting in a hypo-osmolar state [14].

In animals, oestrogens have been shown to be convulsant when applied to the cortex or when given systemically [15,16]; conversely, progesterone appears to protect against seizures in animals [17,18]. These findings may be relevant to cyclical exacerbations of seizures in female epileptics. Backstrom [19] found that during ovulatory cycles an increased oestrogen-progesterone ratio correlated with a higher incidence of seizures, whilst reduced seizure activity appeared in association with increased plasma progesterone levels. From this evidence it might be expected that treatment with oral contraceptive preparations could influence the occurrence of seizures in epileptic patients but this does not appear to be a major problem, although Bickerstaff [20] reported exacerbation of both partial and generalised seizures in six epileptic patients commenced on oral contraceptives. There are, however, other reports suggesting an improvement in seizure control during treatment with such preparations [21].

Local anaesthetics/anti-dysrhythmic drugs

Local anaesthetic agents with membrane stabilising properties, such as lignocaine and procaine, may provoke seizures when administered in high dosage [22]. This

153

phenomenon is of major clinical importance when such agents are used intra-venously for the control of cardiac dysrhythmia. In the Boston Study, convulsions occurred in two (0.6%) of 349 patients receiving intravenous infusions of lignocaine [2]. β-adrenoreceptor blocking drugs, propanolol and oxprenolol, have also been associated with seizures when taken in overdose [23,24]. Intravenous administration of disopyramide has been reported to cause a convulsion in one patient [25].

Cardiac glycocides inhibit active transport mechanisms for sodium and potassium, and are potent convulsants in animals when applied by intraventricular, intrathecal or intracerebral injection [26] but, because of the slow penetration of these drugs across the blood-brain barrier and very active transport mechanisms out of the CSF, encephalopathy and convulsions are rare [27]. Direct cardiac toxicity is likely to occur before cerebral concentrations of glycocide drugs reach significant levels.

Psychotropic drugs

Chlorpromazine, and to a lesser extent other anti-psychotic agents, produce an activation in the electroencephalogram, and may induce seizures in man [28]. The effect appears to be dose-related, and an increase in dosage of chlorpromazine often precedes a seizure [29]. Seizures occurred in 1.2 per cent of 859 psychiatric patients who had no previous history of epilepsy, and the risk of epilepsy increased with dosage. Patients with organic brain disease had convulsions at lower doses of chlorpromazine than those without [28].

It is tempting to speculate that the convulsant activity of antipsychotic agents may be related to their dopamine receptor antagonist properties. There is considerable evidence that monoamine systems in the brain are important in the control of threshold to reflexly-induced seizures in animals [30], and man [31], but it is more difficult to implicate monoamines in the control of threshold to spontaneous seizures [32].

Treatment with tricyclic or newer varieties of antidepressant drugs has been associated with convulsions. Myoclonus and tonic-clonic seizures were initially described in association with overdosage of imipramine or amitriptyline [33]. Tricyclic antidepressants may possess anticonvulsant properties at low doses, but have a biphasic effect on seizure threshold in animal models of epilepsy [34,35], and convulsions can occur in susceptible individuals during treatment with tricyclic antidepressants in therapeutic doses [36]. Patients with a personal or family history of seizures, those with organic brain disease and those with a previous history of electroconvulsive therapy are most at risk from these agents [37,38].

In the past, imipramine and amitriptyline have most frequently been associated with seizures, but it may prove that newer antidepressant agents such as mianserin and maprotoline may carry higher risks [39]. Viloxacine and nomifensin, along with monoamine oxidase inhibitors, may have a lesser convulsant risk and are the antidepressants of choice in epileptic patients [36].

Lithium may cause a variety of neurotoxic syndromes, including encephalopathy associated with seizures [40].

Analeptic drugs

Analeptic, or stimulant, drugs will cause seizures if administered in sufficiently large doses. Clinically the most important of these drugs is aminophylline [41], its convulsant effect being related to serum theophylline concentrations [42]. Nikethamide and older respiratory stimulants were subject to a high incidence of seizures, but the newer agent, doxapram, is safer [43] although it must still be used with caution. As most patients to whom analeptic agents are administered intravenously are in a state of respiratory or cardiac failure, the degree to which cerebral hypoxia, itself a potent cause of seizures [44], interact with these agents in the production of seizures is always difficult to ascertain.

Stimulants, such as amphetamine and its derivatives, are however less convulsant, and indeed amphetamines have been successfully used in the treatment of petit mal epilepsy [45]. The Boston Collaborative Drug Surveillance Program reported only a single patient who had a convulsion whilst being treated with ephedrine [2].

Anaesthetic agents

It is paradoxical that agents causing depression of CNS activity may also cause convulsions, particularly as anaesthesia is sometimes used in the treatment of status epilepticus. The classical descriptions of the stages of anaesthesia recognise the excitation which may occur during stages I and II of ether anaesthesia. Winters has emphasised these classical divisions and the excitatory properties of ketamine, enfluorane and γ-hydroxybuturate [46]. All these agents may produce epileptiform activity in the EEG and seizures have occurred in man associated with the use of ketamine [47], halothane [48], althesin [49], propanidid [50] and enfluorane [51]. Patients with a history of epilepsy again appear particularly at risk.

Withdrawal fits

Sudden withdrawal of any drug possessing anticonvulsant or sedative properties may result in seizures. This is particularly the case in epileptic patients, and it is likely that poor compliance with anticonvulsant therapy is one of the prime causes of admission to hospital of epileptic patients in status epilepticus. However, seizures are also seen following withdrawal of barbiturates [52], meprobamate [53], chlordiazepoxide [54], glutethemide [55] and diazepam [56]. Diazepam with-

155

drawal was one of the more important causes of drug-related seizures in a population of psychiatric in-patients [29]. Such withdrawal seizures are usually seen in patients who have a history of drug abuse.

The most studied withdrawal syndrome is that related to alcohol, and it has long been recognised that seizures are common in alcoholic patients. The careful studies of Victor [57] have demonstrated that most seizures in alcoholics occur between 12 and 24 hours after the cessation of drinking. Even short periods of drinking may result in this increased excitability [58]. Following the withdrawal of alcohol, the EEG becomes abnormal and manifests particularly photoconvulsive and photomyoclonic responses which develop at 18 to 24 hours and may persist for up to 72 hours; subsequently the EEG returns to normal. Seizures are of a tonic-clonic variety and, whilst several may occur over a number of hours, status epilepticus is rare. In patients with previous epilepsy, seizures may be precipitated by drinking, but again tend to occur in the 'sobering up' period. Small quantities of alcohol may even have a short-lasting anticonvulsant effect [59]. It is likely that the alcoholic aetiology of seizures is underestimated in the population, and large and recent studies from both Finland [58] and the USA [60] suggest that alcohol is implicated in a very high proportion of patients presenting acutely with seizures to emergency departments.

Many of the clinical features and EEG changes following sedative drug withdrawal parallel those described for alcohol [52], but the mechanisms responsible remain uncertain.

Radiographic contrast material

All aqueous iodinated contrast media are potentially epileptogenic [61], the risk being greatest when media are administered intrathecally during myelography or cisternography. Meglumine iothalamate (Conray) used for lumbar radiculo-myelography was associated with a 4—11 per cent risk of convulsions [62]; meglumine iocarmate (Dimer-x) used for similar investigations was associated with a 0.7 to 8 per cent risk. Metrizamide appears to be considerably safer; during 100,000 lumbar myelograms using metrizamide, only three convulsions were observed (0.003%) and two of these were in known epileptics [62]. The use of metrizamide for cervical myelography is associated with a higher risk (0.4%) and it is possible that cisternography using metrizamide may carry an even higher risk still. Of 22 patients with convulsions following cervical myelography only four had a predisposition to seizures, two because of idiopathic epilepsy and two because of concurrent treatment with phenothiazine medications [63].

As the risk of seizures is likely to be related to the concentration of media within the cranial cavity, patients should be nursed with the head and neck raised for at least eight hours. In patients with a previous history of epilepsy, or in patients receiving phenothiazines, it may be wise to cover any examination with anticonvulsants.

Miscellaneous agents

Baclofen was initially suspected of precipating seizures in patients with epilepsy, but further studies suggest that its use is not contraindicated, as long as adequate anticonvulsant therapy is given [64]. Baclofen is a putative GABA receptor agonist, and as such possesses anticonvulsant properties in a variety of rodent models of epilepsy [65]. However, in baboons baclofen may produce spike slow wave discharges in the EEG [66] suggesting that it may possess differing properties in primates and man, but the biochemical basis for this is uncertain.

Hyperbaric oxygen may produce seizures at pressures greater than three atmospheres [67]. It is likely that such seizures may be caused by alterations in GABA metabolism due to inactivation of the sulphahydril groups in the enzyme GAD.

Folic acid is a potent convulsant agent in animals when the blood-brain barrier is by-passed [68]. As many anticonvulsants have anti-folate activity [69], it has been suggested that folate deficiency may be important in mediating the anticonvulsant activities of some anticonvulsants. However, whilst folate therapy may occasionally exacerbate seizures in some patients, this is a relatively rare phenomenon [69].

Phenytoin possesses some excitory properties that become evident in high dosage in animals [70], and seizures have occurred following accidental overdosage in man [71]. Exacerbation of existing epilepsy may also be evident when serum levels exceed the therapeutic range for this drug [72,73]. The author has seen an individual epileptic patient who was admitted to hospital on two occasions in status epilepticus following overdosage with phenobarbitone.

Drugs which modulate cholinergic activity within the central nervous system may cause seizures. The cholinergic system appears excitory in nature, and reversible (eg physostigmine) or irreversible (eg di-isopropylfluorophosphonate) acetylcholinesterase inhibitors may cause generalised seizures in animals [74], and man [75,76].

Conclusions

The above evidence demonstrates that two factors are of major importance in drug-induced convulsions. The first of these is the concentration of the drug attained within the central nervous system, so that particular care must be exercised with drugs administered parenterally or intrathecally. Patients with renal or hepatic disease or other causes of impaired drug metabolism are particularly at risk. The second important factor is the susceptibility of the individual patient, so that patients with a previous or family history of epilepsy or pre-existing organic brain disease are more at risk of drug-induced seizures than patients in whom none of these factors applies. The presence of co-existing metabolic disturbance, eg renal failure, hepatic failure, electrolyte imbalance and blood gas disturbance, may all increase the likelihood of seizures occurring.

In common with drug-induced convulsions in animals, such seizures in man take on a relatively stereotyped form. At sub-convulsive doses of an agent, multifocal or generalised myoclonus is seen; at higher doses, generalised tonic-clonic convulsions occur. Focal seizures are rare, and their occurrence casts doubt on an aetiological relationship with a drug. They may occasionally be seen in patients with pre-existing cerebral lesions, where localised alterations in the passage of drugs across the blood-brain barrier may be important. Convulsions most commonly occur as an isolated event requiring no more than withdrawal or reduction in dosage of the offending drug. Status epilepticus is rare.

We remain ignorant of the mechanisms by which most drugs implicated in causing seizures in man have their effect, and more information on the incidence of drug-induced convulsions is required.

References

1   Woodbury DM. In Glaser GH, Penry JK, Woodbury DM, eds. *Antiepileptic Drugs: Mechanisms of Action 1980;* 249–303. New York: Raven Press
2   Boston Collaborative Drug Surveillance Program. *Lancet 1972; ii:* 677–679
3   Walker AE, Johnson HC. *Arch Surg 1945; 50:* 69–73
4   Fariello RG. *Epilepsia 1976; 17:* 217–222
5   Prince DA, Farrel D. *Neurology (Minneap) 1969; 19:* 309–310
6   Smith H, Lerner PI, Weinstein L. *Arch Int Med 1967; 120:* 47–53
7   Whelton A, Carter GG, Garth MA et al. *JAMA 1971; 218:* 1942
8   Gutnick MJ, Van Duijn H, Citri N. *Brain Res 1976; 114:* 139–143
9   Curtis DR, Game CJ, Joohnston GAR et al. *Brain Res 1972; 43:* 242–245
10 Hill RG, Simmons MA, Straughan DW. *Br J Pharmacol 1973; 49:* 37–51
11 Weinstein L. In Goodman LS, Gilman A, eds. *The Pharmacological Basis of Therapeutics 1970 4th Edn:* 1311. London: Balliere-Tindall
12 Evans DAP, Manley KA, McKusick VA. *Br Med J 1960; 2:* 485–491
13 Poire R. In Gastaut H, Jasper H, Bancaud H et al, eds. *The Pathogenesis of the Epilepsies 1969;* 75. Springfield, Illinois: Thomas
14 Leventhal J, Reid D. *Am J Obstet Gynec 1968; 102:* 310
15 Marcus EM, Watson CW, Goldman PL. *Arch Neurol 1966; 15:* 521–525
16 Marcus EM. In Purpura DP, Penry JK, Tower D et al, eds. *Experimental Models of Epilepsy 1972;* 113–146. New York: Raven Press
17 Costa PJ, Bonnycastle DD. *Arch int Physiol Biochem 1952; 91:* 330–333
18 Woolley DM, Timiras PS. *Endocrinology 1962; 70:* 196
19 Backstrom T. *Acta Neurol Scand 1976; 54:* 321–347
20 Bickerstaff ER. *Neurological Complications of Oral Contraceptives 1975;* 87–90. Oxford: Clarendon Press
21 Newmark ME, Penry JK. *Epilepsia 1980; 21:* 281–300
22 Crampton RS, Oriscello RG. *JAMA 1968; 204:* 201–204
23 Buiumsohn A, Edward SE, Jacob H et al. *Ann Int Med 1979; 91:* 860–862
24 Mattingly PC. *Br Med J 1977; 1:* 776–777
25 Johnson NM, Martin NDT, Strathdee G. *Lancet 1978; ii:* 848
26 Tower DB, In Jasper HH, Ward AA, Pope A, eds. *Basic Mechanisms of the Epilepsies 1969;* 611–638. Boston: Little, Brown
27 Hoffman BF, Biggar JJ. In Goodman LS, Gilman A, eds. *The Pharmacological Basis of Therapeutics 1980 6th Edn:* 761–792. London: Bailliere-Tindall
28 Logothetis J. *Neurology (Minneap) 1967; 17:* 869–877

29   Toone BK, Fenton GW. *Psychol Med 1977; 7:* 265–270
30   Anlezark G, Marrosu F, Meldrum BS. In Morselli PL, Lloyd KG, Loscher W, Meldrum B, Reynolds EH, eds. *Neurotransmitters, Seizures and Epilepsy 1981:* 251–263. New York: Raven Press
31   Quesney LF, Andermann F, Lal S, Prelevic S. *Neurology (Minneap) 1980; 30:* 1169–1174
32   Chadwick DW. In Sandler M, ed. *The Psychopharmacology of Anticonvulsants 1982:* in press. Oxford: Oxford University Press
33   Arneson GA. *Am J Psychiat 1961; 117:* 934–936
34   Lange SC, Julien RM, Fowler GW. *Epilepsia 1976; 17:* 183–196
35   Fromm GH, Amores CY, Thies W. *Arch Neurol 1972; 27:* 198–204
36   Trimble M. *Epilepsia 1978; 19:* 241–250
37   Betts T, Kalra P, Cooper R, Jeavons P. *Lancet 1968; i:* 390–392
38   Dallos V, Heathfield K. *Br Med J 1969; 4:* 80–82
39   Edwards JG. *Lancet 1979; ii:* 1368–1369
40   Demers R, Lukesh R, Pritchard J. *Lancet 1970; ii:* 315
41   Schwartz MS, Scott DF. *Epilepsia 1974; 15:* 501–505
42   Zwillich CW, Sutton FD, Neff TA, Cohn WM, Matthay RA, Weinberger MM. *Ann Int Med 1975; 82:* 784–787
43   Edwards G, Leszczynski SO. *Lancet 1967; ii:* 226–229
44   Meldrum B. In Davison AN, Thompson RHS, eds. *The Molecular Basis of Neuropathology 1981:* 265–301. London: Arnold
45   Livingston S. *Comprehensive Management of Epilepsy in Infancy, Childhood and Adolescence 1972:* 101. Springfield, Ill: Charles C Thomas
46   Winters WD. *Anaesthesiology 1972; 36:* 309–312
47   Thompson GE. *Anaesthesiology 1972; 37:* 662–663
48   Smith PA, Macdonald TR, Jones CS. *Anaesthesia 1966; 21:* 229–233
49   Uppington J. *Anaesthesia 1973; 28:* 546–550
50   Barron DW. *Anaesthesia 1974; 29:* 445–447
51   Virtue RW, Lund LO, Phelps M et al. *Can Anaesth Soc J 1966; 13:* 233–241
52   Wikler A, Essig CF. *Mod Probl Pharmacopsychiat 1970; 4:* 170–184
53   Haizlip TM, Ewing JA. *N Engl J Med 1958; 258:* 1181–1186
54   Hollister LE, Motzenbecker FP, Degan RO. *Psychopharmacologia 1961; 2:* 63–68
55   Essig CF. *Am J Psychiat 1963; 119:* 993
56   Hollister LE, Bennet JL, Kimbell I et al. *Dis Nerve Syst 1963; 24:* 746–750
57   Victor M. *Mod Probl Pharmacopsychiat 1970; 4:* 185–199
58   Hillbom ME. *Epilepsia 1980; 21:* 459–466
59   Mattson RH, Sturman JK, Gronowski ML, Goico H. *Neurology (Minneap) 1975; 25:* 361–362
60   Earnest MP, Yarnell PR. *Epilepsia 1976; 17:* 387–393
61   Grainger RG. In Lodge T, Steiner RE, eds. *Recent Advances in Radiology and Medical Imaging 1979; 6:* 177–194. Edinburgh: Churchill Livingstone
62   Skalpe IO. *Acta Radiol 2977; Suppl 355:* 358–370
63   Hindmarsh T, Grepe A, Widen L. *Acta Radiol Diag 1975; 15:* 497–507
64   Hattab JR. In Jukes AM, ed. *Spasticity and Cerebral Pathology 1978:* 60–67. Cambridge: Cambridge Medical Publications
65   Worms P, Lloyd KG. In Morselli PL, Lloyd KG, Loscher W, Meldrum B, Reynolds EH, eds. *Neurotransmitters, Seizures and Epilepsy 1981:* 37–46. New York: Raven Press
66   Horton RW, Collins JS, Anlezark GM, Meldrum BS. *Europ J Pharmac 1979; 59:* 75–83
67   Wood JD. In Purpura DP, Penry JK, Tower DB, Woodbury DM, Walter RD, eds. *Experimental Models of Epilepsy 1972:* 449–456. New York: Raven Press
68   Hommes OR, Obbens EAMT. *J Neurol Sci 1972; 16:* 271–281
69   Reynolds EH. *Clin Haemat 1976; 5:* 661–696
70   Woodbury DM. In Glaser GH, Penry JK, Woodbury DM, eds. *Antiepileptic Drugs: Mechanisms of Action 1980:* 447–471. New York: Raven Press
71   Schreiner GE. *Arch Int Med 1958; 102:* 896–913

72   Levy LL, Fenichel GM. *Neurology (Minneap) 1975; 15:* 716–722
73   Toupin AS, Ojemann LM. *Epilepsia 1975; 16:* 753–758
74   Maynert EW, Marczynski TJ, Browning RA. In Friedlander WJ, ed. *Adv Neurol 1975; 13:* 79–147
75   Taylor P. In Goodman LS, Gilman A, eds. *The Pharmacological Basis of Therapeutics, 6th edition 1980:* 100–116. London: Bailliere Tindall
76   Stewart GO. *Anaesth Intens Care 1979; 7:* 283

18

PROGNOSIS AND PROPHYLAXIS OF
TRAUMATIC EPILEPSY

D Janz

Introduction

The state of knowledge concerning epileptic seizures and epilepsies following brain traumas has altered during recent years in many respects. The question that has concerned us more than any other is whether prophylactic therapy is possible, necessary and how it should best be carried out. It therefore seems appropriate to deal with post-traumatic epilepsy particularly in this light, i.e. causes and course should be considered in relationship to the advantages and risks of prophylactic treatment.

Post-traumatic early seizures

On the basis of the latency period between trauma and first seizure, a distinction is made between epileptic seizures of early and late onset*. This distinction is prognostically useful, since the earlier the seizures occur the less they tend to recur, i.e. to become the first seizure of post-traumatic epilepsy; similarly, the longer this interval, the greater the probability of traumatic late epilepsy [1] (Table I). Since early seizures are definitely the expression of a direct effect of the trauma, in other words a pathological reaction, which cannot be timed accurately, there has been up to now no agreement about the maximum length of time allowed — whether one, two or even four weeks — in order to define the term 'early'.

Wesseley [1] records about the same number of seizures in each of the first two days, thereafter a gradual decrease of up to four weeks (Table I). Jennett [2] finds

---

* Many authors call this traumatic early and traumatic late epilepsy. But since the term epilepsy implies an illness with recurring epileptic seizures and since, from a prophylactic standpoint, the question is whether it is an acute reaction or a chronic process, caution in the choice of terms is necessary in order not to draw premature conclusions.

TABLE I. Time of first fit in 131 cases of traumatic early seizures within four weeks of injury (TLS = traumatic late seizures) (P Wessely 1981)

	1st day	2nd day	1st week	2nd week	4th week	Total
Without TLS	21	20	10	3	3	57
With TLS	17	15	16	12	14	74
Total	38 29%	35 26.6%	26 19.8%	15 11.4%	17 13%	131 100%

— with regard to the incidence per week — a sharp decline between the first and the following weeks, from which observation he derives the pragmatic suggestion that only those seizures occurring during the first week should be defined as early seizures (Figure 1). The fact that he, along with other authors [3—5] and

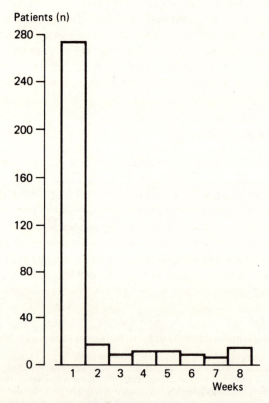

Figure 1. Time of first fit within 8 weeks of injury [2]

in contrast to Wessely [1], records early seizures most frequently in the first 24 hours, and particularly within the first hour after the trauma, suggests differences in the population under observation.

As regards the type of seizure in the case of early seizures, focal motor seizures are often encountered (Jennett [6] 41 per cent, Ketz [7] 21 of 42 cases) as well as major seizures, whereas psychomotor seizures were not observed before the second week [8]. A third of patients with early seizures have only one seizure. Status epilepticus occurs in between 3 per cent [7] and 10 per cent [2] of cases and predominantly in children under five years of age [2]; indeed, traumatic early seizures are considered to occur on the whole more frequently in children and particularly after minor head trauma [2, 4]. In a study of 35 children with mainly severe head injuries, however, Lange-Cosack et al [9] found 16 with early epileptic seizures, mainly in the form of unilateral convulsions or focal major seizures.

The following factors tend to favour the occurrence of early seizures: the length of unconsciousness or of post-traumatic amnesia. This seems to be even more important in the case of children, since seven out of eight cases of Lange-Cosack et al [9], who were unconscious for more than 24 hours had early seizures; as opposed to this, only 18 out of 154 cases of Jennett and Lewin [10] with amnesia lasting longer than one day developed early seizures (12 per cent as opposed to 2.7 per cent of those whose amnesia was of shorter duration). Moreover, early seizures also occur more frequently in the case of injuries with depressed fractures or intracranial haematomas. With the possible exception of children, in whom early seizures even after minor trauma have been observed [2, 4] (so that the interpretation as to the seizures occurring as a result of the trauma is open to question), early seizures as a rule seem to indicate the presence of severe contusion. According to Wessely [1], they should be regarded as 'alarm signs' of the presence of an intracranial complication (e.g. a space occupying haemorrhage).

Although the incidence is correlated with the severity of brain trauma, it will also vary to a great extent with the age composition and diagnostic criteria of the medical institutions to which the patients are admitted. Whilst Jennett [2] maintains that 5 per cent of all patients, who are admitted to hospital with a brain trauma, develop one or several early seizures, this is a figure more than double that reported in a very carefully conducted field study of the Mayo Clinic, i.e. 2.1 per cent [11], which approximately corresponds to the results of the investigations of Elvidge [12] (1.9 per cent) and Kollevold [5] (2.9 per cent). The greater incidence is probably due to the selection of more severe cases than those meeting only the minimal requirements of head injury with post-traumatic amnesia and to the fact that the seizures and not the brain trauma were the reason for admission [11].

Apart from the fact that early epileptic seizures can be indicative of intra-cranial bleeding or, as in the case of an early epileptic status epilepticus, may become the reason for urgent therapy, it is important to know how often and in what circumstances they persist, i.e. mark the beginning of post-traumatic epilepsy. As far as I can see, the average risk is about 25 per cent (Ketz [7] found 25.9 per cent in closed and 20 per cent in open injuries, Jennett and Lewin [10] 28.5 per cent, Jennett [2] 27 per cent in closed, 46 per cent in open injuries, Annegers et al [11] 22 per cent in severe, 13 per cent in medium, nil per cent in mild injuries). The risk of a transition from traumatic early seizures to post-traumatic epilepsy is also correlated with the severity of the trauma. It increases to 45 per cent in the case of open injuries [6, 13], lies between 13 and 27 per cent [6, 11] in the case of medium and severe closed injuries, and drops to nil per cent in the case of mild head trauma, without, however, the minimal condition of post-traumatic amnesia in all cases [11]. Considering trauma of equal severity the risk is less with children than adults [2,11]. The transition occurs mainly in the first three months after the trauma (in 63.5 per cent) and only in rare cases (26 per cent) does it still occur after six months [1].

Traumatic late seizures

When epileptic seizures occur after the acute effects of the skull and brain trauma have subsided, they are called traumatic late seizures, and when occurring repeatedly, of traumatic late epilepsy. Just as with early seizures, which tend to cease spontaneously, the prognosis of late seizures is not necessarily unfavourable so that epilepsy does not develop in all cases. Out of 51 cases in the Mayo Clinic study [11], whose course had been followed for at least six years, 19 only suffered one seizure. Of the 28 cases of Jennett and Lewin [10] with late seizures, seven cases had only one seizure, and only nine cases had had more than three seizures after a seven year follow-up investigation. The question as to whether early treatment may have had a favourable effect cannot be judged in either of these studies, but Evans [14] also showed a tendency to natural remission on the basis of a 7–11 year follow-up of 55 cases of post-traumatic epilepsy, and this has also been confirmed by other authors [1, 15, 16]. In only 18 out of 75 cases of Evans [14] did more than one major seizure still occur per year; 32 were free of seizures, 19 of whom were no longer taking antiepileptic drugs. Traumatic late epilepsies do not become chronic in approximately one quarter of cases with a variability of between 13 per cent for closed, and 45 per cent for open injuries, follow-up investigations giving the impression of a 'generally favourable course' [1]. Wessely [1] reports that 109 out of 348 cases, that is one-third, remained free from seizures for more than five years.

Looking at the latency period between trauma and seizures, it can be assumed that 2/3 of the late seizures which occur after early seizures have become manifest within the first six months. Of cases with primarily late seizures, however, only 30 to 45 per cent have become manifest within the same period of time [1, 17–20], as can be seen from the diagram of Evans [14] (Figure 2). In the

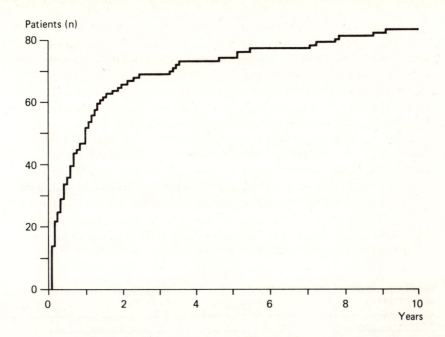

Figure 2. Time of onset of seizures expressed as a cumulative graph showing the current number of patients who had developed seizures after injury [14]

course of the first year 50 to 60 per cent have become manifest, and after two years 65 to 80 per cent [1].

The interval during which a causal relationship between seizures and preceding trauma can still be considered possible is still the subject of much discussion. Taking into account that the incidence curve clearly flattens out after about the third year, only strict criteria for a causal relationship after this period of time should be employed — such as a definite correlation between initial and paroxysmal focal signs and symptoms. The dubiety of a relationship after an interval of more than four years has been clearly demonstrated in the Mayo Clinic investigation using epidemiological methods. The authors of this study are able to show that, in comparison with the known rate of incidence for epilepsy in each age group of the population, epileptic seizures which developed later than four years after trauma did not occur for the first time statistically more frequently than would be expected in the absence of trauma [11].

The risk of traumatic epilepsy depends on the type of injury, its location, severity of trauma and complications. Thus we know from war injuries that bullet wounds, which have at least penetrated the dura, lead to traumatic epilepsies in 36 to 43 per cent of cases [15, 18, 20, 21]. The risk increases to about 70 per cent when wound infections have occurred [14] or in cases of brain abscess [22].

165

It is greater, i.e. around 42 to 44 per cent, when the injury involved the parietal and temporal region; it is less, i.e. between 17 and 24 per cent, in injuries of the frontal and occipital poles. Not only does the frequency of traumatic epilepsies apparently decrease the further away the traumatic focus is from the motor cortex, but the more distant foci require correspondingly more time to become epileptogenic, e.g. whilst it can take years for temporal lesions to lead to seizures it takes still longer with frontal and occipital foci [23].

In the case of skull and brain trauma which have not been due to bullet injuries, an increase in epilepsy risk of up to 35 per cent has been observed in the case of intracranial haematomas; of up to 17 per cent in the case of a depressed fracture [2] and, depending on the length of initial unconsciousness, of 1.7 per cent when post-traumatic amnesia was less than one hour, and up to 12 per cent when it continued for longer than seven days [10]. Annegers et al [11] demonstrated very clearly the relationship between different degrees of trauma and risks for early and late post-traumatic seizures (Table II). The risk

TABLE II. Degree of trauma severity and occurrence of post-traumatic seizures (Annegers et al [11])

Type of injury, in order of severity	All cases	Seizures, number of cases	
		Early	Late
Brain contusion, haematomas	154	30	21
Loss of consciousness for 24 hours or more	41	2	2
Depressed fracture	52	3	1
Loss of consciousness for 30 minutes to 24 hours	418	10	8
Basilar fracture	71	1	0
Linear fracture	371	2	7
Mild contusion	1,640	10	12
TOTAL	2,747	58	51

increases when several risk factors coincide and Jennett [6] has developed an empirical risk scale, whereby the statistically expected risk, which lies between 3 and 70 per cent, can be assessed in each case according to the particular combination of factors involved (Figure 3).

In the assessment of epilepsy risk the EEG strangely enough plays a surprisingly small part. In this respect, Jennett [2] is in agreement with other authors [4, 24, 25] that the "EEG (offers) little help in answering the question as to whether a late epilepsy will develop".

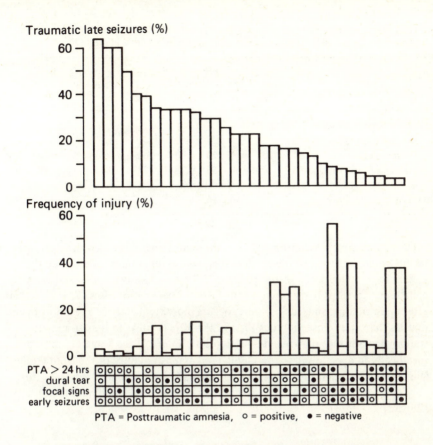

Figure 3. Risk of traumatic epilepsy according to different combinations of risk factors. The frequency with which different combinations of factors occurred is displayed below the incidence of late traumatic seizures associated with each combination [18]

Seizure type and the natural history of traumatic epilepsies differ from those of idiopathic epilepsies in that age dependent minor seizures, such as astatic seizures, absences and myoclonic seizures of the impulsive petit mal types are entirely absent; major seizures often occur spread over the day in a randomly distributed manner and less often in the form of an epilepsy on awakening which, when it does occur, more often has an evening (after work) peak [26]. With regard to the relationship between type and localisation of injuries and dependency of major seizures to the sleeping-waking cycle, little attention has been paid to the fact that traumatic sleep epilepsies often occur after trauma with unconsciousness lasting longer than 24 hours, and are related to frontal brain injuries, whereas epilepsies with a random seizure distribution often occur after parietal brain injuries [27] (Table III). It is well known that focal seizures often develop – in open injuries more often with simple, and in closed injuries more

	Localisation									
	Frontal		Parietal		Temporal		Occipital		Total	
	n	%	n	%	n	%	n	%	n	%
Grand mal predominantly										
after awakening	3	–	8	–	2	–	1	–	14	–
during sleep	21	55	9	24	4	10.5	4	10.5	28	100
random distribution	18	27	37	56	8	12	3	5	66	100
TOTAL	42	35	54	46	14	12	8	7	118	100

often with complex, symptoms [27] – the symptomatology of which corresponds to the traumatic lesion of the cortical area, whose function is reflected by the seizure in an epileptically distorted manner. Less well known is that status epilepticus develops fairly often, i.e. in 11 to 17 per cent of cases [7, 19, 28, 29] after brain trauma, and, furthermore, occurs more frequently as a result of open injuries than after closed injuries [7, 19, 28–30]. Peculiar to these traumatic status attacks is that they mainly develop after injury of the frontal brain – and specifically in open injuries after a unilateral extensive injury of the frontal lobe (Figure 4) – and that they often, either singularly or repeatedly, represent the only epileptic symptom in such cases (isolated or iterated grand mal status) [28–32].

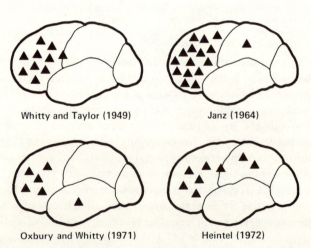

Whitty and Taylor (1949)   Janz (1964)

Oxbury and Whitty (1971)   Heintel (1972)

Figure 4. Site of lesions in cases of open head injuries and grand mal status [32]

168

Prophylactic medication

Now that we know something of the conditions whereby seizure expectancy can be assessed statistically in any given case and have an impression of the time aspects, the form and frequency of the expected seizures — in other words of their spontaneous prognosis — it is useful to consider the means and prospects of prophylactic treatment. The most favourable reports on prophylactic medication, using 160–240mg phenytoin and 30–60mg phenobarbitone daily over a period of at least three years, was carried out in a very disciplined manner in Czechoslovakia before the pharmacokinetic era of epilepsy treatment [33,35 36], and could not now be replicated. The co-workers of Servit [34], who had previously demonstrated experimentally the possibility of the medical prevention of epileptic seizures after brain trauma, have seen epileptic seizures after at least three and in most cases five years of follow-up in three out of 143 treated patients; in two of the three cases the seizures occurred only after termination of medication during the fourth and fifth year — and in six of 24 untreated patients four had already had attacks in the first year after the trauma [37]. Because the number of cases was thought to be too small, and the protocol of the investigation without placebo medication and double-blind controls unsatisfactory, a large prospective study was instigated in America using the aforementioned conditions and with the same medication and dosage [38]; the results were not published, apparently because it was concluded that a therapeutically effective serum level was generally not achieved [39] and seizures rather tended to appear more often in the treated group than in the non-treated group [40]. The results of a second study with an alteration of medication have not yet been reported. In the meantime a number of studies of prophylactic treatment have been published using a variety of drugs — carbamazepine [41], phenytoin [43, 44, 46], phenobarbitone [10], valproic acid [42, 45] in varying doses, in different forms of application — oral, i.v. and i.m. — injections, infusions — and with different treatment periods. In none of the studies could the favourable results of the Czechoslovakian authors be reproduced. Out of 24 patients who were treated for six months or longer with phenobarbitone, six developed seizures, five of them after termination of medication. Six out of 12 untreated patients with approximately equally severe trauma developed seizures [10]. Eight out of 101 patients who were treated with phenytoin after brain surgery developed seizures, as opposed to 17 out of 102 patients who were treated with placebo [46]. In a group of 84 patients in whom a therapeutic level of 10–20μg/ml was rapidly achieved by means of intravenous and intramuscular injections of phenytoin immediately after the trauma, five cases developed a seizure between the second and 52nd week, which is less frequently than would be expected on the basis of findings in the literature, but only 30 patients were still under observation after three months [44]. In a retrospective study of 50 patients who were also 'loaded' with 1,000mg phenytoin i.v. shortly after the

169

trauma and generally received 400mg daily thereafter, seizures were recorded in five cases, and out of 12 untreated patients in six cases [43]. Glötzner [41], in a methodologically satisfactory study, was recently able to show that the administration of carbamazepine beginning on the day of the trauma, whilst not being able to reduce the frequency of early seizures with certainty, led to a significant reduction in late seizures. A transition from early to late seizures occurred moreover, as in Jennett's study [6], in 28 per cent of cases. Glötzner [41] has demonstrated the effectiveness of prophylaxis in graphs of cumulative probability (Figure 5). Whereas new seizures were still appearing in the placebo-group up to

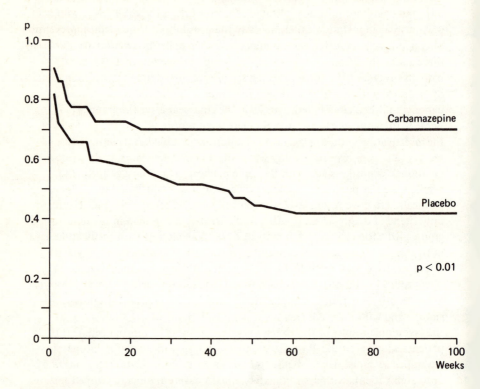

Figure 5. Effectiveness of prophylactic medication of carbamazepine in 108 patients with brain trauma. Cumulative probability (p) of remaining free of seizures until week indicated [41]

the 60th week, no new cases of post-traumatic seizures appeared after the 20th week in the treatment group, who were matched with the control group according to severity of trauma and other variables; the degree of effectiveness, with approximately 50 per cent less seizures than in the placebo group, is not very impressive.

In almost all studies the complaint is made that, whilst the level of risk can be reasonably assessed according to Jennett's [2, 6] investigations, and whilst the avoidability of post-traumatic seizures with prophylactic medication is experimentally well substantiated, the practical realisation meets with sheer insurmountable barriers. Only about 6 per cent of patients take their drugs for longer than one year [2]. Even in the case of studies which were motivated by scientific interest, therapeutic levels could still only be determined in 55 to 60 per cent of cases after six months. To what extent results prove to be much poorer when medical prophylaxis becomes routine has been seen in the Vietnam war. For the first time post-operative exhibition of prophylactic medication was made obligatory in the American group. In 75 per cent of cases it consisted of 300 to 400mg phenytoin daily, and in a further 20 per cent an additional 96mg of phenobarbitone. The incidence of traumatic epileptic seizures was somewhat greater in the case of the treated persons (177/453) than in those who had discontinued treatment or were not treated (167/577) [17].

On the basis of these reports, the following comments can be made: routine prevention of post-traumatic seizures with drugs is not indicated since the benefit bears no relationship to the effort involved. The attempt to prevent early seizures medically does not seem to be appropriate even in the case of increased risk, since such measures that need to be taken to achieve a therapeutically effective serum concentration in a very short time are only justified in status epilepticus. In all those cases with a high risk of epilepsy it is worthwhile considering conventional initiation of prophylactic medication, i.e. gradually increasing dosage. One should discuss with the patient the possibility of beginning drug treatment only after a first seizure has occurred, especially since the Czechoslovakian authors report that they were still able to prevent the recurrence of seizures, and thereby its chronicity, when treatment was started only after the first seizure [33]. Since the occurrence of one seizure after brain trauma still does not signify epilepsy, I am of the opinion that treatment should not be initiated until two seizures have occurred in a brief interval, and then given according to the usual rules. For the treatment of manifest epilepsy, the well known rules of blood level-controlled medication of the drug of choice according to type of seizure, course and expected side-effects, are valid [47].

The question as to whether the rules of treatment are also valid in the case of prophylactic medication is unclear. Phenobarbitone and valproic acid were found effective in the prevention of febrile convulsions, carbamazepine and phenytoin ineffective [47]. If the development of traumatic epilepsy were comparable with a kindling effect, then phenobarbitone would presumably be the drug of choice − to the extent that animal experiments allow conclusions − whereas phenytoin would be useless and carbamazepine and valproic acid probably effective [42, 48, 49]. On the other hand, phenytoin has proved effective in the suppression of seizures in experimentally induced cortical lesions. Apart from the choice of drug, the question as to what dosage or plasma concentration is prophylactically effective remains unanswered. Servit and Musil [37] feel that their theoretical assumption, based on practical results, that even relatively small doses, "which perhaps exert no noteworthy therapeutic effect" are prophylactically effective during the "incubation period". The unsuccessful major experiment on the treatment of brain damaged subjects of the Vietnam war with much higher doses cannot serve as an argument to the contrary, since it was hardly conducted systematically. A controlled comparison of medical regimes differing in type and dosage has so far not been done.

Last but not least there is controversy about the necessary duration of treatment. Young et al [44] — more in obeyance of necessity — pleaded for continuation for at least a number of months. Wohns and Wyler [43] have terminated medication after one year but, when specific activity was still evident in the EEG, continued medication for at least five years even in the absence of seizures. Servit and Musil [37] treated for a period of at least two years and report that even after treatment lasting three or four years, seizures occurred for the first time, though in their series, as in Jennett and Lewin's study [10], it is not clear whether they were in fact withdrawal seizures — which is moreover an additional risk of treatment. Whoever initiates treatment should have a well-founded idea of how long it should last, but the literature provides no clear guidelines for this decision.

Unless the patient himself insists, I see no necessity, either on grounds of the risk involved, or on grounds of the EEG, or of other circumstances, for prophylactic treatment. Also in the case of a first seizure there are no criteria for the likelihood that it will recur. There is not really any social complication that could be prevented by premature or early medical treatment. For example, patients with particularly risky professions — Jennett [2] mentions surgeons and pilots in this respect — will hardly remain capable of employment after brain injury involving a high risk of epilepsy that prophylactic treatment is worthy of consideration. Finally a strong motive which is repeatedly cited in favour of prophylactic medication remains the worry that the patient may lose his driving licence after a first post-traumatic seizure. The question as to whether, even with a high risk, half of all patients should receive a laborious, and in the final analysis, risky treatment is, for those who have reservations regarding prophylactic medication, [14,17,50—52] decisive.

Summary

The watershed between early and late seizures is the first week after the trauma. The development of both correlates with the severity of the trauma as does the risk of a late epilepsy after early seizures. Early seizures do not recur in 3/4 of the cases, late seizures do not recur in 1/4 of the cases, with a span between closed and open brain injuries, with and without complications. Up to 60 per cent become manifest within the first year, up to 80 per cent within the second year after the trauma. The incidence of seizures occurring more than four years after the trauma is not greater than would be expected without trauma. The risk of epileptic seizures is greatest (approximately 70 per cent) in the case of open wounds with wound infections and brain abscesses. It lies at about 30 to 40 per cent in the case of bullet wounds and about 10 to 20 per cent in the case of closed brain injuries. It is greater in the case of localised injuries of the central region than in lesions of the frontal and occipital poles. In the case of blunt skull trauma, factors which increase the risk are: depressed fracture, intracranial haematoma, long period of unconsciousness. Early and late seizures are mainly of focal type, in the case of early seizures with primarily simple, in the case of late seizures with primarily complex, symptomatology. The course of major seizures is mainly independent of the sleep-waking-cycle. Status epilepticus occurs fairly often, particularly after open frontal brain injuries. EEG investigations seem to be uninformative with regard to both prognosis and course.

The experimental, and most of the clinical, studies suggest that prophylactic antiepileptic medication reduced the incidence of traumatic late seizures. The questions as to which drug, in which dosage and plasma concentration, is sufficiently effective and reliable, and how long treatment should last, has not been answered. Even with the higher risk of epilepsy, the usefulness and risks of treatment should be weighed up with the patient and consideration should be given to the fact that, even in the case of epileptic seizures without trauma, one does not begin treatment after the first fit but only after a repetition of seizures.

References

1   Wessely P. In Remschmidt H, Rentz R, Jungmann J, eds. *Epilepsie 1980, 1981.* Stuttgart: Thieme
2   Jennett WB. In Remschmidt H, Rentz R, Jungmann J, eds. *Epilepsie 1980, 1981.* Stuttgart: Thieme
3   Stöwsand D. *Paresen und epileptische Reaktionen im Initial-Stadium des Hirntraumas 1971.* Stuttgart: Thieme
4   Ritz A, Emrich R, Jacobi G, Thorbecke R. In Remschmidt H, Rentz R, Jungmann J, eds. *Epilepsie 1980, 1981.* Stuttgart: Thieme
5   Killevold T. *J Oslo City Hosp 1976; 26:* 99–114
6   Jennett B. *Epilepsy after non-missile head injuries 1975.* London: Heinemann Medical Books
7   Ketz E. In Remschmidt H, Rentz R, Jungmann J, eds. *Epilepsie 1980, 1981.* Stuttgart: Thieme
8   Jennett B. *Lancet 1969; i:* 1023–1025
9   Lange-Cosack H, Wider B, Schlesener JH, et al. *Neuropädiatrie 1979; 10:* 105–127
10 Jennett WB, Lewin WS. *J Neurol Neurosurg Psychiat 1960; 23:* 295–301
11 Annegers JF, Grabow JD, Groover RV, et al. *Neurology (Minneap) 1980; 30:* 683–689
12 Elvidge AR. *Trans Am Neurol Assoc 1939; 65:* 125–129
13 Baum H. *Z ges Neurol Psychiat 1930; 127:* 279–311
14 Evans JH. *Neurology (Minneap) 1962; 12:* 665–674
15 Russell WR, Whitty CWM. *J Neurol Neurosurg Psychiat 1952; 15:* 93–98
16 Walker AE. *JAMA 1957; 164:* 1636–1641
17 Caveness WF, Meirowski AM, Rish BL, et al. *J Neurosurg 1979; 50:* 545–553
18 Credner L. *Z ges Neurol Psychiat 1930; 126:* 721–757
19 Prill A, Rudzki P. *Dtsch Z Nervenheilk 1969; 195:* 301–332
20 Walker AE, Jablon S. *J Neurosurg 1959; 16:* 600–610

21   Ascroft PB. *Br Med J 1941; 1:* 739—744
22   Legg NJ, Gupta PC, Scott DF. *Brain 1973; 96:* 259—268
23   Paillas JE, Paillas N, Bureau M. *Epilepsia 1970; 11:* 5—15
24   Courjon J. *Epilepsia 1970; 11:* 29—36
25   Scherzer E, Wessely P. *Eur Neurol 1978; 17:* 38—42
26   Janz D. *Dtsch Z Nervenheilk 1960; 170:* 486—513
27   Janz D. *Die Epilepsien 1969.* Stuttgart: Thieme
28   Janz D. *Dtsch Z Nervenheilk 1960; 180:* 562—594
29   Heintel H. *Der Status epilepticus 1972.* Stuttgart: Fischer
30   Oxbury JM, Whitty CWM. *Brain 1971; 94:* 733—744
31   Oxbury JM, Whitty CWM. *J Neurol Neurosurg Psychiat 1971; 34:* 182—184
32   Janz D. In Vinken PJ, Bruyn GW, eds. *Handbook of Clinical Neurology. The Epilepsies 1974: 15:* 311. Amsterdam: North Holland Publishing Co
33   Popek K, Musil F. *Cas Lek Cesk 1969; 108:* 133—147
34   Servit Z. *Nature 1960; 188:* 669—670
35   Servit Z. In Majkowski J, ed. *Posttraumatic epilepsy and pharmacological prophylaxis 1977;* 182—191. Warsaw: Polish Chapter of the ILAE
36   Servit Z, Musil F. *Epilepsia 1974; 15:* 640
37   Servit Z, Musil F. *Epilepsia 1981; 22:* 315—320
38   Rapport RL, Penry JK. *J Neurosurg 1973; 38:* 159—166
39   US-Plan:Head Injury. In *Plan For Nationwide Action on Epilepsy. US Department of Health, Education and Welfare. DHEW Publication No (NIH) 78—311 Vol II Part I 1977;* 245—255
40   Penry JK. Personal communication
41   Glötzner FL. In Remschmidt H, Rentz R, Jungmann J, eds. *Epilepsie 1980, 1981.* Stuttgart: Thieme
42   Leviel V, Naquet R. *Epilepsia 1977; 18:* 229—234
43   Wohns RNW, Wyler AR. *J Neurosurg 1979; 51:* 507—509
44   Young B, Rapp R, Brooks W, et al. *Epilepsia 1979; 20:* 671—681
45   Price DJ. In Parsonage MF, Caldwell ADS, eds. *The Place of Sodium Valproate in the Treatment of Epilepsy 1980;* 23—30. London: Academic Press
46   North JB, Ponhall RK, Hanieh A, et al. *Lancet 1980; i:* 384—386
47   Schmidt D. *Die Behandlung der Epilepsien 1981.* Stuttgart: Thieme
48   Wada JA, Osawa T, Sato M, et al. *Epilepsia 1976; 17:* 77—88
49   Wauquier A, Ashton D, Melis W. *Exp Neurol 1979; 64:* 579—586
50   Janz D. In Birkmayer W, ed. *Epileptic Seizures — Behaviour — Pain 1976;* 65—75. Bern, Stuttgart, Wien: Hans Huber Publications
51   Rish BL, Caveness WF. *J Neurosurg 1973; 38:* 155—158
52   Wolf P. In Parsonage MJ, Caldwell ADS, eds. *The Place of Sodium Valproate in the Treatment of Epilepsy 1980;* 31—32. London: Academic Press

19

PSYCHOSOMATIC ASPECTS OF EPILEPSY

Sir Desmond Pond

The term 'psychosomatic' is somewhat vague and often misunderstood, but broadly it includes the influence of psychological and social factors on the origins and course of somatic disorders, diseases or physical signs as generally understood in medicine. This chapter will thus be a general one and much of the material discussed will be more comprehensively described in other chapters.

Under this heading of 'psychosomatic' we may consider three main topics:

1(a) The triggering or precipitation of epileptic attacks by psychological states, and its converse,

(b) the stopping or reduction of attacks by psychological mechanisms.

2 The psychological content of auras.

3 The symptomatology of post-ictal states.

In addition to the study of psychological factors on clinical phenomena we can also consider the influence of psychological states on the types of discharge in the EEG which are customarily regarded as epileptic — spikes, focal or generalised spike and wave, etc.

In his recent comprehensive review, Fenwick [1] distinguishes between evoked seizures and psychogenic seizures. Under the former heading he refers to the specific stimuli (specific, that is, to the particular patient) that may cause evoked seizures. All sensory modalities have been reported as having provided appropriate stimuli. Sometimes these stimuli are very complex and concern learned perceptual activities, for example, reading. In some of these cases, as with some cases of musicogenic epilepsy, the psychological content of what is being perceived may be quite unique to the patient, and in this sense these attacks really move into what Fenwick describes as secondary psychogenic seizures.

Fenwick's primary psychogenic group refers to patients who in a variety of ways can voluntarily bring on seizures. The most famous and bizarre of such cases is, I suppose, one we looked after many years ago in the Maudsley, of the man who, by staring at open safety pins, could induce a fit which was also an orgasm [2]. The rare but well recognised cases of self-induction of seizures by photic stimulation fall into this category of primary evoked seizures [3].

It is generally assumed that the sensory input itself is normal in the sense that the stimuli reach the brain at the normal rate through normal channels, but there are also well recorded cases of patients in whom, for example, an area of peripheral nerve damage will, when stimulated, produce an epileptic attack. As far as one can tell, this is the result of a chance association of a peripheral injury whose input reaches an area of the brain which is in some sense epileptogenic. I will return later to the question of what is meant by epileptogenicity.

In addition to these various specific triggers, there are many patients who report that epileptic attacks occur more commonly in situations of psychological stress or tension, or occasionally under severe emotional states of pleasurable character. In other diseases this is almost the only aspect of psychosomatic interactions in which it is possible to conduct some research, since episodes, even in conditions like asthma, which come on in very sharp attacks, cannot usually be precipitated like epilepsy by specific sensory inputs within a matter of seconds. The unique aspect of epilepsy, of course, results from its being related to a CNS lesion or functional disorder, whereas diseases of other organs work on a different time scale. Rather surprisingly there are, as far as I know, no studies done using the life events questionnaires devised by Brown and others, but I am fairly sure from anecdotal evidence that in patients with relatively infrequent epilepsy the attacks would be found to cluster around times of stressful life events. Friis and Lund [4] found sleep deprivation the commonest 'stress' and thought there were some links between the fits thus produced and the genetic tendency to febrile convulsions.

It is possible that such relatively non-specific type of triggering operates through different mechanisms from that which is presumably involved in sensory triggering. I have the impression, for example, that stress can produce any form of epileptic attack, and one cannot hypothesise as in the case of sensory evoked seizures that the epileptogenic lesion in the brain is in the area in which the triggering stimulus is effective. The fit-precipitating effect of stress may be, as is probably the case with other diseases, mediated via metabolic or endocrine changes (steroids are currently fashionable).

As regards mechanisms, the most interesting question about triggering of stimuli is how their extraordinary specificity is acquired, i.e. learned. I deliberately use this last word as the specific nature of most of these stimuli must be selected out of the enormous and varied sensory input of any of the sensory modalities that have been involved. Once the abnormal excessive excitory process has got started in the sensitive focus, then the mechanisms of generalisation of such a discharge to other parts of the brain, if it occurs, seem to me to be just the same as with other forms of induced epilepsy. The special mystery of triggering can be probably elucidated only in relation to further studies on how cerebral function must in some way change during all learning or acquisition of new patterns of behaviour from childhood onwards (or from even earlier − in utero). The surprising thing to my mind is that, since it occurs at all, why does it not occur much more often, though, as Fenwick points out, it is probably commoner than one realises from quick and superficial questioning.

The same general points can be made about the influence of psychological states towards inhibition, and not the precipitation, of seizures. As shown in the case of triggers, a few patients discover fairly specific ways of inhibiting attacks. This applies particularly to attacks of the Jacksonian type where the movement or sensation begins in a particular limb. Patients will sometimes reduce the sensory inflow by holding the limb tight and that may abort the seizure.

A fairly common general method of seizure-stopping is by techniques self-discovered or taught designed to reduce general tension, this word being used to refer both to the somatic accompaniments of muscular tension and also to the subjective sense of ill ease. Many people have tried to use biofeedback techniques, but they have been very disappointing and seemed to have worked, if at all, largely in relation to a general improvement of the psychological state rather than the person being able to learn to block or reduce a particularly sensory input that is epileptogenic [5,6]. The effects of the reduction of stress may thus be mediated through the same general metabolic or endocrine pathways that I have suggested are used in the fit precipitating effects of stress.

The literature on the psychological content of auras is very largely anecdotal with the honorable exception of Taylor's [7] report. For a long time after Hughling Jackson's accurate description of some types of aura as a dreamy state, no-one seemed to have tried to relate the psychodynamic study of the dream, pioneered by Freud and Jung only a very few years after Jackson's original description. Several authors, for example Hill and Mitchell [8], explicity related the Freudian concepts of condensation displacement, etc, to the form and content of complex auras. A few authors [9] have described changes in the content of auras with psychotherapy, and spontaneous changes in auras over the years certainly occur, usually in the direction of simplification and general loss of detail. One may reasonably postulate that what is happening under treatment, or with the simple passage of time, is a reduction in the secondary elaboration of some quite brief and relatively simple sensory experience which alone can be directly related to the discharging epileptogenic lesion. Taylor's studies show that the type of aura varies with intelligence, more clearly in men than women. There is no relationship to the nature of the lesion and an unclear one even to sidedness. My original suggestion [10] that the frequent experience of complex auras may predispose to the development of schizophrenic-like psychoses has been disproved by subsequent studies, showing there is no clear relationship between aura experience and psychosis. The sensory modality affected by an aura is, of course, broadly related to the site of the epileptogenic lesion but, as

177

in the case of triggering mechanisms, our further understanding of the origin of nature of auras will come from studies of general brain development and change with learning, rather than with the study of epilepsy.

With regard to my last topic, the symptomatology of post-ictal states, we are here in a rather better understood field. During almost any period of recovery from loss of consciousness from whatever cause, patients may be confused, irritable, even hallucinated and deluded for variable periods of time. The post-ictal states following temporal lobe attacks may perhaps be more complex than those following grand mal attacks because the suppression of activity during the epileptic attack is focal or at least predominantly only in some parts of the cortex. There may be relative sparing of, for example, the motor region so that the subject can carry out complex activities impossible following a global disturbance of consciousness. Confusional states in epileptics can, of course, be prolonged, sometimes for days or weeks by recurrent minor focal discharges. Such minor attacks in the case of the temporal lobe variety may be relatively unnoticeable except by close and expert observation. Absence status is, of course, a different phenomenon, though it is of interest that patients in absence status are nearly always rather calm, which is in accord with their general personality characteristics that I and others have noticed over the years, though our evidence is no more than anecdotal. Post-ictal disturbances of consciousness are more often prolonged by secondary psychogenic mechanisms similar to those which produce hysterical fugues than by any mechanism that may be directly related to the original cause of the loss of consciousness. However, one or two ECT or spontaneous grand mal attacks may bring a prolonged post-ictal confusional state to an end quite dramatically.

If we turn to the question of the influence of psychological states on the various types of discharge in the EEG customarily regarded as epileptic, one finds disappointingly few observations. Several studies [11] suggest that states of heightened vigilance and attention do significantly reduce the amount of spontaneous spike and wave found in records of patients with generalised epilepsy — an observation which is, of course, in accord with the general clinical view that patients have fewer attacks when busy and occupied with interesting tasks. Certain types of epilepsy seem more related to the sleep/waking cycle than others, as Janz [12] has shown, and he relates the effects to different types of EEG discharge. The use of telemetric methods of recording EEG discharges will undoubtedly enable us to accumulate more information about the effect of patients' mental state on seizure discharges both generalised and focal. At times it will be difficult to know which comes first, for example, a focal discharge may go with an increase in irritability, and which causes which? The point particularly arises when discussing the most unknown of epileptic states, the pre-ictal period. "He's working up to a fit", has been said about many chronic epileptics by those looking after them, but we are no further on in our understanding of that situation.

Like many others, I have been excited by the spate of studies on kindling following its discovery by Goddard [13]. In Racine's recent review [14], he

178

considers there may be two mechanisms: one disinhibition, which may be related to degenerative changes in the CNS as yet undescribed; and secondly, the growth of excitatory terminals. Kindling, of course, has been so far described only as a result of the pathological excitation of a small electric current. So far no-one has been able to show that other repeated stimuli of a sensory nature can induce epileptogenesis. The induction of mirror foci suggests that epileptogenicity can be generated by the arrival of neuronal impulses, perhaps abnormal only in their quantity, intensity or some other characteristic. Such neuronal bombardment is of a different order from the electrical stimuli starting the whole thing off, and does give some hope that epileptogenicity can arise from a special combination of discharges and not only from an acquired pathological lesion.

The question of what is meant by epileptogenicity is a key issue today in our studies of this fascinating condition. There is a lot of clinical and experimental evidence that patients and animals with epileptogenic lesions show changes in mood, behaviour, vigilance and other characteristics well before overt clinical attacks begin — perhaps even before epileptic discharges are seen in routine EEGs. This is not true of patients with certain types of epilepsy, for example, children with febrile convulsions are quite normal in other ways (unless, of course, a secondary epileptogenic lesion occurs because of anoxia). I wonder whether in this condition the abnormality predisposing to febrile convulsions is not in the brain at all but simply in the body's reactions to a rapidly rising fever in organs or metabolic pathways entirely outside the brain?

Some years ago, Dr Serafitinides and I thought we would try and compare epileptogenic and non-epileptogenic temporal lobe lesions, but our study got nowhere because of the totally disparate nature of the clinical groups. We, of course, chose patients with temporal lobe epilepsy coming to operation as the first group, but the second group consisted of patients with tumours for the most part, as these are the commonest and most easily diagnosed non-epileptogenic temporal lobe lesions. The two groups turned out to be totally disparate, particularly as regards age of onset and length of time that the condition occurred. Temporal lobe tumours, primary or secondary, occur usually in middle age or later; their clinical course tends to be months, even weeks rather than years, and the secondary complications of increased intracranial pressure rapidly appear, so we regretfully had to abandon that line of investigation. It is perhaps now worth doing it again using CAT scan techniques which can pick up small temporal lobe lesions following, for example, vascular lesions or head injuries, in a much more efficient manner. I suspect that small non-epileptogenic lesions in the limbic structures, or whatever other term is appropriate for areas of greater psychiatric interest, will not have any particular psychological effects. The principles of relative equi-potentiality and vicarious function are probably valid even in these somewhat more primitive parts of the cerebrum. The ontogenetic development even of these areas may also be partly affected by learning processes — the different reactions of different people to psychological stress are not necessarily

179

entirely innate and these differences may thus profoundly affect the symptoms produced when a lesion in these areas becomes epileptogenic.

References

1   Fenwick P. In Reynolds EH, Trimble MR, eds. *Epilepsy and Psychiatry, Chapter 22 1981:* 306–321. Edinburgh: Churchill Livingstone
2   Mitchell WR, Hill D, Falconer MA. *Lancet 1954; ii:* 626–630
3   Binnie CD et al. *Epilepsia 1980; 21:* 202
4   Friis ML, Lund M. *Arch Neurol (Chicago) 1974; 31:* 155–159
5   Ray WJ, Raczynski JM, Rogers T, Kimball WH. *Evaluation of Clinical Biofeedback 1979.* New York and London: Plenum Press
6   Cabral RJ, Scott DF. *J Neurol Neurosurg Psychiat 1976; 39:* 504–509
7   Taylor DC. In Reynolds EH, Trimble MR, eds. *Epilepsy and Psychiatry, Chapter 17 1981:* 227–241. Edinburgh: Churchill Livingstone
8   Hill D, Mitchell WR. *Folia Psychiat Neerl 1953; 56:* 718
9   Epstein AW, Ervin F. *Ps-som Med 1956; 18:* 43–55
10   Pond DA. In discussion of Beard AW, Slater E. *Proc Roy Soc Med 1962; 55:* 311–316
11   Hutt SI, Fairweather H. *Brain 1971; 94:* 321–326
12   Janz D. In Vinken PJ, Bruyn GW, eds. *Handbook of Clinical Neurology. The Epilepsies 1974; 15:* 311. Amsterdam: North Holland Publishing Co
13   Goddard GV. *Nature 1967; 214:* 1020–1021
14   Racine RJ. *Neurosurgery 1978; 3:* 234–252

20

THE QUANTIFICATION OF INTERICTAL PSYCHOPATHOLOGY IN EPILEPSY

J Kogeorgos

Introduction

It is a common experience that the clinical manifestations of epilepsy include not only motor and other neurological disturbances, but also diverse changes in behaviour and subjective experience. Therefore it is not surprising that epileptic patients have been for long an important focus of attention not only for neurologists but also for psychiatrists. There are two main reasons for this. Firstly, the considerable practical problems of both diagnosis and management which may be presented by patients suffering from both epilepsy and psychiatric disturbances. Secondly, the undoubted attraction of epilepsy, as a disease model which offers the possibility of establishing meaningful links between definitive, even measurable (through the EEG), brain dysfunction and psychopathology. As a result, a great number of studies have been already carried out, aiming to identify the exact degree and type of psychopathology associated with epilepsy, but, the results particularly of earlier studies have often been at variance and caused considerable controversy. This is largely due to serious methodological deficiencies in many of them, resulting from both general methodological problems and from difficulties specific to the fields of diagnosis and classification in the absence of a definitive aetiology, although the latter have been partly resolved recently with the use of international classificatory schemes of both epilepsy [1] and psychiatric disorders [2]. Some of the main shortcomings of previous work are shown in Table I.

TABLE I. Usual methodological shortcomings of psychiatric studies of epilepsy

Very small patient samples
No control groups
Variably defined epilepsy and psychopathology
Subjective or retrospective assessment
Inadequate follow up

181

Methods and approaches in the assessment of patients with epilepsy

Increasing awareness of the inadequacies of previous research has led to considerable improvement of methodology in more recent studies, particularly in the last two decades. A most important development has been the establishment of quantitative measures of psychopathology, the use of which has been extended to studies of patients with epilepsy. These are essentially of three types:

a) Self-rated questionnaires

b) Other-rated questionnaires, and

c) Structured interviews

The validity and reliability of these instruments have usually been demonstrated by adequate research studies, but it is desirable that pilot validity studies be carried out when possible, on the particular populations where assessment is planned. Each of the above methods has advantages and disadvantages, and some of these are shown in Table II. Despite their differences, all of them share certain important characteristics: Firstly, they ensure that a predetermined range of symptoms will be covered and the corresponding information will be elicited and recorded in a uniform way. Secondly, the results are expressed in numerical scores, which are susceptible to sophisticated statistical analyses. They can also be compared with the values of other clinical or neurophysiological variables like age, length of illness, EEG abnormality, etc., and scores obtained on different occasions can provide information about the patient's clinical course. Thirdly, the psychiatric scores obtained, largely concentrate on symptoms rather than on diagnostic entities. This provides considerable flexibility in the quantification of psychopathology, irrespective of whether or not a particular diagnostic label can be assigned.

TABLE II. Basic features of standardised questionnaires and structured interviews

Self-rated questionnaire	Other-rated questionnaire	Structured interview
Relatively easy to complete	Relatively easy to complete	More time consuming
Provide less thorough assessment	Provide less thorough assessment	Provide thorough assessment
Results uninfluenced by interviewer	Results partly influenced by interviewer	Interviewer's influence reduced by procedural rules

The earliest objective tests to be used for the assessment of epileptic psychopathology, came from clinical psychology and were originally introduced for the evaluation of personality profiles. Two well known examples are the Eysenck Personality Inventory (EPI) [3], originating in this country, and the Minnesota

Multiphasic Personality Inventory (MMPI) [4], widely used in North America. The EPI is relatively easy to fill and, in its current version, ratings provide degrees of pathology along Eysenck's basic dimensions of *Extraversion/Introversion* and *Neuroticism/Psychotocism.* The MMPI, originally introduced as a screening technique for army recruits, has since been used very widely as a measure of psychopathology. The present version is rather long, consisting of 550 questions, and requires considerable time to complete, but the information derived is much more detailed and relates to several dimensions. These are in keeping with American diagnostic trends and include *hypochondriasis, depression, hysteria, psychopathy, paranoia, masculinity/femininity, psychasthenia, schizophrenia and hypomania.*

The General Health Questionnaire (GHQ) [5] and the Crown-Crisp Experimental Index (CCEI) [6,7], are two of the most well known psychiatric questionnaires in the United Kingdom, although their use with epileptic patients has been limited. The GHQ is a screening instrument, sensitive to moderate or even minor degrees of psychiatric disturbance. Scores give degrees of global psychopathology and, where they exceed a predefined threshold point, characterise an individual subject as a probable psychiatric case. The CCEI, previously known as the Middlesex Hospital Questionnaire (MHQ), has 48 items, which yield information on six main dimensions of neurotic pathology, viz *Free floating anxiety, Phobic anxiety, Obsessionality, Somatic anxiety, Depression and Hysteria.* These, in combination, can provide an overall psychiatric profile. The CCEI has extensive reliability and validity data for normal and several clinical groups and data relating CCEI scores to age, sex and social class.

Scandinavian studies have favoured the Marke-Nyman Inventory [8], which is based on Sjöbring's theory of personality structure, with its main constituent variables of *validity, solidity* and *stability.* Validity is a measure of available and effective energy; stability is a measure of control; and solidity a measure of maturity.

Other well known tests are the Hamilton [9] and Beck [10] inventories for depression, and for anxiety, the Taylor Manifest Anxiety Scale [11], the Hamilton [12] scale and the Spielberger [13] scale. The most widely used structured interviews are Spitzer's Psychiatric Status Schedule (PSS) [14] and Wing's Present State Examination (PSE) [15]. The PSS has an interview schedule based on an inventory of 321 dichotomous items; the schedule stipulates the exact words to be used, and the corresponding ratings are closely linked to the wording of the patient's reply. The PSE, containing 140 items, is less highly structured, being concerned more particularly with symptoms, especially of a psychotic nature, and the rating made represents the interviewer's final judgment on whether or not a particular symptom is present. Therefore the PSE can only be used by trained psychiatrists, while the PSS requires less training and can be also used by non-psychiatric personnel. Both interviews are equipped with decision tree computer programmes (Diagno and Catego) for the conversion of symptom patterns into diagnoses.

Similar standardised questionnaires and structured interviews have been used for the quantification of deviance in epileptic children. These rely on information about children's behaviour elicited from indirect sources, usually parents and teachers. Examples are Berg's Self-Administered Dependency Questionnaire (SADQ) [16], which measures *dependency* and is completed by the child's mother, and Conners' Teacher Rating Scale [17], measuring *conduct problems, anxiety, inattentiveness, overactivity* and *social isolation* (from other children). Other scales are those devised by Rutter and his colleagues [18], which provide scores on *neurotic disorders, conduct disorders* and *mixed disorders.* There is a trend lately for the findings by these methods to be combined with ratings based on direct observation and videotape recording of children's behaviour or of the family interaction.

Increased familiarity with these standardised techniques in recent years, led to a considerable upsurge of research in the psychopathology of patients with epilepsy. The majority of studies dealing with adults, appear to have mostly involved the use of only a small number of the available scales. This is particularly true for US studies which are based almost entirely on the MMPI. Most of the work has also concentrated upon particular research objectives, not very dissimilar to those of earlier psychiatric research. These include establishing the exact degree and pattern of psychopathology associated with epilepsy and comparing it with that of normal subjects or other non-epileptic clinical groups. Also the study of possible associations between psychopathology and type of epilepsy or laterality of the epileptic focus as detected clinically or by EEG, has often been an objective. Moreover, psychotic manifestations, especially those of schizophreniform type, have received particular attention, no doubt because of their theoretical relevance to diagnostic and theoretical conceptualisations in psychiatry. Finally, two important types of investigations have been concerned a) with the epidemiology of epileptic psychopathology in particular settings, and b) with the assessment of psychopathological changes in response to different drug regimes in clinical trials.

Psychiatric morbidity in epilepsy

The results from these investigations, show certain trends which are to some extent in line with previous more impressionistic findings.

Davies-Eysenck [19], as early as 1950, assessed 38 patients on the EPI, 18 with grand mal attacks, 7 with petit mal attacks and 13 with both types of seizures, and reported high scores on *neuroticism.*

More recently, Standage and Fenton [20], using the same instrument in combination with the PSE, also found high neuroticism scores in 37 epileptic out-patients compared, with 27 non-epileptic, matched neurological controls. These differences, however, were not significant, nor were there any significant differences between patients with primary generalised, and those with temporal lobe, epilepsy.

A number of careful American studies of different epileptic populations, using the MMPI, found no significant differences in psychopathology between patients with temporal lobe epilepsy (TLE) and others with generalised seizures [21—24]. An exception was a study by Rodin and his colleagues [25] who noted higher scores on depression and paranoia in their subgroup of patients with TLE. The scores on paranoia were particularly high in those TLE patients who also had other types of seizures. On the other hand Meier and French [26], in a study of 53 patients who were being evaluated for temporal lobe surgery, found significantly greater psychopathology in those with bilateral independent foci, especially on the MMPI scales of *depression, paranoia* and *schizophrenia.* No laterality effect was noted.

Beck and colleagues [27], using the Marke-Nyman Inventory, compared 29 patients with psychomotor epilepsy, 30 with grand mal epilepsy and 30 with juvenile myoclonic epilepsy. Those with myoclonic and psychomotor seizures scored worse on the dimension of validity, which was interpreted as indicating a psychological vulnerability to small adversities of life.

Bear and Fedio [28], using their own scale of 18 traits supposedly associated with interictal behaviour, found different characteristics between 15 patients with a right temporal lobe focus and 12 patients with a left temporal lobe focus. The former scored higher on *elation,* while the latter scored higher on *anger, paranoia* and *dependency.* Both groups showed higher scores on all traits than non-epileptic neurological, and normal control, samples but, given the very small size of their samples, the value of these findings is somewhat dubious.

The psychotic manifestations of epileptic patients have caused considerable controversy in the past, and their nature has for long been inconclusive. In a recent elegant study, Perez and Trimble [29], using the PSE, compared 23 psychotic epileptic patients, with 10 non-epileptic patients suffering from process schizophrenia. There was considerable overlap of clinical presentation between the two groups. Within the epileptic group, symptoms of affective psychosis were found to be independent of the type of epilepsy but those of schizophreniform psychosis showed significant association with temporal lobe epilepsy.

In a somewhat different approach, Kogeorgos and colleagues [30] recently assessed 66 patients with chronic epilepsy uncomplicated by other major factors, in whom interictal psychopathology and actual severity of epilepsy were both quantified and compared. Their psychopathology was measured with the GHQ and CCEI questionnaires, while their epileptic severity was quantified with reliable methods used in previous studies [31,32]. The psychiatric profiles obtained were also compared with those of 50 non-epileptic chronic neurological controls, matched for sex, socioeconomic background and length of illness. There was high correlation between scores of psychopathology and those of epileptic severity, suggesting that epileptic cerebral dysfunction has an identifiable net effect on mental functioning. This was indirectly confirmed by the overall higher psychiatric scores of the epileptics compared with those of the controls and the existing normative values. Particularly high were the scores on *phobic anxiety, somatic anxiety* and *depression.*

There are by now also a number of interesting reports on the psychiatric status of epileptic children in various settings. Rutter and his colleagues [18], in their well known study on the Isle of Wight using their own scales, identified psychiatric disorder in 28.6 per cent of 63 children with uncomplicated epilepsy, as compared with 6.6 per cent in a general population sample of over 2,000 school children. Stores [33], in a series of controlled studies, assessed children attending ordinary schools, with a combination of standardised scales including Berg's Self-Administered Dependency Questionnaire (SADQ) and Conners' Teacher Rating Scale. He found significantly greater behavioural disturbance in boys, especially those with persistent left temporal spike abnormality in the EEG. Finally, Trimble and Corbett [34], using different scales on a large population of epileptic children resident in a special school, found that phenytoin and primidone had more adverse effect than carbamazepine on mental functioning.

Conclusions

Greater care in research design and, more particularly, the use of standardised measures of psychopathology in psychiatric studies of epileptic patients have been fruitful. These studies have clarified some of the previous controversies regarding the nature of psychopathology present in these patients and its relationship to epileptic dysfunction.

It now seems clear that there is greater psychiatric morbidity among epileptic patients than the general population, and possibly than among other patients without epilepsy. This morbidity more often consists of anxiety, depression and paranoid symptomatology, and has little relation to type of epilepsy, or the lateralisation of the epileptic focus in patients with temporal lobe seizures. However, preliminary evidence suggests an association between psychopathology and clinical severity of epilepsy, as well as between behaviour disturbance and persisting left temporal lobe focus in young boys.

There is undoubtedly a great scope and need for more research in this field, with reliable means of assessment, based when possible on standardised measures. There is particularly a need to study in more detail the two major types of epileptic psychopathology, namely depression and psychosis, as well as to evaluate more accurately the relationship between mental changes and the other clinical and neurophysiological variables of the epileptic condition.

References

1   Gastaut H. *Epilepsia 1970; 2:* 102–113
2   *Mental Disorders: Glossary and guide to their classification in accordance with the Ninth Revision of the International Classification of Diseases 1974.* Geneva: WHO

3   Eysenck SBG, Eysenck HJ, *Br J Soc Clin Psychol 1969; 8:* 69–76
4   Hathaway SR, McKinley JC. *The Minnesota Multiphasic Personality Inventory Manual (Revised) 1951.* New York: Psychological Corporation
5   Goldberg D. *Manual of the General Health Questionnaire 1978.* Windsor: NFER
6   Crown S, Crisp AH. *Br J Psych 1966; 112:* 917–923
7   Crown S. In Pichot P, ed. *Psychological Measurements in Psychopharmacology 1974;* 111–124. Basel: S Karger
8   Nyman GE, Marke S. *The Differential Psychology of Sjöbring 1962.* Lund: Gleerups
9   Hamilton MA. *J Neurol Neurosurg Psychiat 1960; 23:* 56–61
10 Beck AT, Ward CH, Mendelson M et al. *Arch Gen Psychiat 1961; 4:* 561–571
11 Taylor JA. *J Abnorm Psychol 1953; 48:* 285–295
12 Hamilton M. *Br J Med Psychol 1959; 32:* 50–55
13 Spielberger CD. In Lezi L, ed. *Emotions – Their Parameters and Measurement 1975;* 713–725. New York: Raven Press
14 Spitzer RL, Endicott J, Fleiss JL, Cohen J. *Arch Gen Psychiat 1970; 23:* 41–55
15 Wing JK, Cooper JE, Sartorius N. *Instruction Manual for the Present State Examination and Catego System 1974.* Cambridge: Cambridge University Press
16 Berg I. *Br J Psychiat 1974; 124:* 1–9
17 Connors CK. *Am J Psychiat 1969; 126:* 884–888
18 Rutter M, Graham P, Yule N. *A Neuropsychiatric Study in Childhood. Clinics in Developmental Medicine Nos 35–36 1970.* London: Heinemann/SIMP
19 Davies-Eysenck M. *J Neurol Neurosurg Psychiat 1950; 13:* 237–240
20 Standage KF, Fenton GW. *Psychol Med 1975; 5:* 152–160
21 Small TG, Milstein V, Stevens JR. *Arch Neurol 1962; 7:* 330–338
22 Matthews CG, Klove H. *Epilepsia 1968; 9:* 45–53
23 Mignone RJ, Donnelly EF, Sadowsky D. *Epilepsia 1970; 11:* 345–359
24 Stevens JR. In Penry JK, Daly DD, eds. *Advances in Neurology 1975; Vol 11:* 85–107
25 Rodin EA, Katz M, Lennox K. *Epilepsia 1976; 17:* 313–320
26 Meier MJ, French LA. *J Clin Psychol 1965; 21:* 3–9
27 Beck P, Kjaersgard Pedersen K, Simonsen N, Lund M. In Penry JK, ed. *Epilepsy, the Eighth International Symposium 1977.* New York: Raven Press
28 Bear DM, Fedio P. *Arch Neurol 1977; 34:* 454–467
29 Perez MM, Trimble MR. *Br J Psychiat 1980; 137:* 245–249
30 Kogeorgos J, Fonagy P, Scott DF. *Br J Psychiat 1982; 140:* 236–243
31 Kogeorgos J, Evans S, Scott DF. In McGovern S, ed. *Perspectives on Epilepsy 1980/81.* Wokingham, Berkshire: British Epilepsy Association
32 Kogeorgos J, Scott DF, Vassilouthis J. *Materia Medica Greca 1980; 5:* 536–538
33 Stores G. *Develop Med Child Neurol 1978; 20:* 502–508
34 Trimble MR, Corbett JA. *Irish Med J 1980; Suppl; 73:* 21–28

21

EPILEPSY, PERSONALITY AND BEHAVIOUR

G W Fenton

Introduction

The behavioural manifestations of epilepsy are of special interest to the clinical disciplines of neurology and psychiatry since many such phenomena span the interface between brain and mind. The seizure itself can take the form of the classical generalised convulsion or consist of complex abnormalities of behaviour and subjective experience. Associated disorders may sometimes involve cognitive changes, personality difficulties or psychotic illnesses of various types and duration. The psychotic syndromes may be clearly 'organic' in origin, manifesting all the classical features of an organic mental state. Alternatively the psychosis can occur in clear consciousness and closely mimic one of the functional psychotic illnesses such as schizophrenia. The latter states are of particular theoretical relevance to the psychiatrist, since detailed study of such psychotic conditions is likely to throw some light in the pathophysiological basis of the functional psychotic syndromes: schizophrenic and affective psychoses. Indeed, careful investigation of the vast repertoire of behavioural and personality complications of epilepsy will undoubtedly advance our currently very limited knowledge of the brain mechanisms of behaviour.

The chronic nature of the disorder, the intermittent and unpredictable fit pattern itself, the ancient fears and prejudices surrounding epilepsy and consequent social stigma create for the person with epilepsy a series of potential psychological and social handicaps that have to be coped with. The term 'illness behaviour' was introduced by Mechanic [1] to refer to "the way in which given symptoms may be differentially perceived, evaluated and acted upon or not acted upon by different kinds of people and in different social situations". Ethnic and cultural differences as well as the person's previous life experiences and genetic endowment and the attitudes of those close to him, including the health care professionals involved, will determine the patient's reaction to the illness. Hence the range of response amongst different people to the same medical condition can be wide and variable. Epilepsy may create a special difficulty in coping because the affected individual's potential level of functioning is often normal most of the time, being only interrupted drastically and temporarily around the time of seizure occurrence. The psychological and social stresses imposed upon the person with fits and the individual's subsequent coping mechanisms make epilepsy a useful model for the demonstration and study of the impact of a chronic medical condition upon a person's social functioning. Such interaction of biological, psychological and social factors is yet another reason why epilepsy should be of special interest to psychiatrists and neurologists with an interest in brain-behaviour relationships. Clinical psychologists and medical sociologists will also find this 'medico-social' interface of particular relevance.

POTENTIAL HANDICAPS OF THE PERSON WITH EPILEPSY

The fits themselves, unpredictable in occurrence with sudden clouding of consciousness, convulsive movements or other inappropriate and often embarrassing behaviour beyond the person's control, expose the patient to the risk of injury and even death. This risk of injury to self or others places severe restrictions on choice of work. Vehicle driving may be prohibited, a prohibition with potentially serious social and vocational consequences. In severe cases there may be serious limitations of ability to leave home and travel by public transport because of the risks of having seizures crossing busy roads or while using public transport.

The occurrence of fits in public places and at work still arouses anxiety, fear and even prejudice amongst the general population. These negative feelings contribute to discrimination against the epileptic at work and may lead to difficulties in making friends outside the immediate family circle. Teasing, scape-goating and social isolation from peers can be special problems for the school child with epilepsy.

In patients with symptomatic epilepsy, cerebral dysfunction due to the underlying epileptogenic lesion, either focal or diffuse, may lead to impaired intellectual and learning abilities. The depressant action on the brain of the various drugs used in the treatment of epilepsy can also cause cognitive impairment and sometimes aggravate behaviour disorder. The effects of the underlying brain damage and/or medication may result in low intelligence, psychomotor slowing, impaired learning ability and poor educational achievement. Educational progress may be further retarded by poor concentration and attention span due to frequent minor seizures occurring in the classroom. These may be so brief as to escape the teacher's notice. Similar concentration and attention difficulties are a common finding in epileptic children with conduct disorder even in the absence of frank fits.

Parents of a child handicapped by epilepsy are concerned to protect their child from coming to harm as a result of fits. Over-protective attitudes can readily develop as a result of this parental anxiety. The inevitable but usually minor

189

restrictions as regards swimming, cycling, etc., may be exaggerated to an unnecessary degree. Usually such parental over-protective attitudes develop from natural concern for their child's well-being. Less often, more negative feelings such as anger towards and rejection of the brain damaged child may be present and are guarded against by ever increasing watchfulness. Such parental over-protectiveness may retard the natural developmental process of maturation to adult independence and result in life-long passive, dependent attitudes. An unduly restricted family and social life with limited access to peer group relationships may impede the development of social skills. Though learnt from parental and other family figures through modelling and imitation, the skills required in social interaction have to be consolidated, refined and expanded by the constant and repeated learning experiences of personal relationships with peers and adults of both sexes outside the nuclear family situation and other important authority figures such as school teachers, etc.

Self-esteem thrives on the individual's constant monitoring of his/her own performance and competence compared to that of his/her peers and will be reinforced by the latters' recognition of this competence. Self-esteem also grows as the individual demonstrates self-mastery and environmental mastery through independent action. A restricted life with limited undue dependence on parents will impair further the person's level of self-esteem already low because of the experience of being 'sick', epileptic and different.

During and after adolescence parents often find it difficult to allow their epileptic offspring to take the usual risks that growing up involves. Yet the epileptic teenager, more than others, wants to identify with peers and achieve independence without a constant overseer in the background. Hence the usual adolescent independence conflicts are often heightened in the person with epilepsy, the individual's bid for independence often clashing with his/her parents' need to maintain close supervision. Emotional difficulties and frank behaviour disorder may follow.

A discrepancy between the individual's vocational aspirations and ability to fulfill these aspirations is sometimes a problem, especially in middle class, professional or academic families. The epileptic child may acquire the aspirations and expectations prevalent in the family but may not have the intellectual equipment to carry them out, because of cortical damage due to the epileptogenic lesion and/or the depressant effects of anticonvulsant drugs. This can lead to much frustration and disappointment as well as failure to accept a work role more compatible with his/her intellectual ability. Often, parental expectations are lower than those held for their non-epileptic offspring. Long and Moore [2] found that parents were less optimistic about their epileptic child's future achievement than about that of their other children. These findings were linked with greater restrictiveness on the parents' part and the epileptic child's lower self-esteem and poorer academic achievement.

The person with epilepsy suffers from a three-fold handicap in the employment field. As well as a range of job opportunities being restricted by the liability to fits, personality and behavioural problems associated with the epilepsy may create work difficulties. In turn, such difficulties can reinforce existing psychiatric problems, when the individual finds himself unable to fulfil his work role satisfactorily. Finally there exists discrimination against the epileptic employee due to prejudice, ignorance and fear on the part of both employers and employees. Nonetheless, surveys conducted in more favourable economic times (1960s and early 1970s) have shown that three-quarters or more of all epileptics available for work have been in employment in virtually the full range of occupations. There is evidence that employers' attitudes tend to be a function of the individual employer's previous favourable experiences with epileptic persons displaying good work adjustment. Chronic unemployment or serious difficulty over holding down a job tends to be associated with IQs at the lower end of the normal range or below, organic mental changes, evidence of diffuse brain damage, the presence of temporal lobe pathology and/or personality disorder. Surprisingly enough, most studies have found that siezure frequency is less important in causing job difficulty than personality problems, psychosocial difficulty, intellectual impairment and factors related to motivation. Work problems in people with epilepsy have been reviewed by Fenton [3] and Rodin [4].

THE INFLUENCE OF TEMPORAL LOBE DYSFUNCTION

It is a common clinical experience that patients with temporal lobe epilepsy tend to show a poorer response to treatment and manifest a higher incidence of psychiatric difficulties than patients suffering from other types of epilepsy. The hypothesis presented by Gibbs [5] and other early workers that temporal lobe dysfunction specifically predisposes to behaviour, personality and psychotic disorder is still under challenge because of a number of well controlled negative studies published in the mid and late 1960s and early 1970s; reviewed by Stevens [6], Rodin [7] and Hermann et al [8]. A major methodological problem has been the study of highly selected populations with poor control of such crucial factors as duration and severity of epilepsy, fit pattern and source of referral. Nonetheless, several careful investigations of both children and adults [7, 9–12] have provided evidence in favour of the hypothesis.

The work of Rodin et al [7] is of special interest. Seventy-eight patients with temporal lobe type seizures were matched for age, sex and IQ levels with patients suffering from other seizure types. Statistically significant differences were established between the groups in regard to treatment response, causative factors and behavioural variables. Further analysis of the data showed that the behavioural problems of the temporal lobe patients were present only in that group that suffered from more than one seizure type. The temporal lobe epilepsy group having only one seizure type differed from the controls with one seizure type in regard to aetiological factors; they actually showed better performance on certain sub-scales of the WAIS as well as better employment records. Rodin et al [7] therefore conclude that the clinical impression of the temporal lobe epilepsy patient presenting more difficulties than other patients with epilepsy results from the fact that temporal lobe patients have in most cases more than one seizure type. It may be that the epileptogenic process involving the temporal-limbic structures must reach a critical threshold of severity and extent, as manifest by multiple seizure types before the individual's behaviour becomes disturbed.

Indeed, the lack of agreement in the literature about a direct link between temporal lobe dysfunction and psychopathology means that the hypothesis of Gibbs and others requires modification. It may be more appropriate to regard the temporo-limbic involvement as one of a number of aetiological agents that make people 'vulnerable' to break down when exposed to more acute stress, biological and/or psychosocial. Whether such a vulnerability factor as temporal lobe dysfunction actually leads to frank psychopathology will depend not only on the extent and severity of the temporo-limbic disorder but also upon the additive effect of other vulnerability factors (e.g. age, sex, family psychopathology, etc.) and the impact of the precipitating or provoking stress. This aetiological model will be discussed in more detail later. It is not incompatible with the views presented by Stevens and Hermann [13].

PSYCHIATRIC DISORDERS OF EPILEPSY: CLASSIFICATION AND CLINICAL FEATURES

The psychiatric disorder of epilepsy can be classified into the following three main categories: 1) Disorders due to the brain disease causing the fits; 2) Disorders related in time to seizure occurrence; and 3) Interictal disorders unrelated in time to the seizures.

Disorders due to the brain disease causing the fits

a) Mental handicap, where the seizures and intellectual impairment are both a reflection of underlying cerebral pathology; between one-fifth and a half of mentally retarded patients have epilepsy, the prevalence of fits increasing with the severity of mental handicap [14].

b) The specific epileptic syndromes of which seizures are a constant feature but are only one of a number of symptoms and signs of an organic brain syndrome e.g. West's syndrome, Unverricht-Lundberg disease, Sub-acute Sclerosing Pan-encephalitis (SSLE), the Lennox-Gastaut syndrome. These disorders are associated with global intellectual impairment, which in many cases is progressive.

c) Organic brain syndromes, in which fits may occur but are not a constant feature of the disease, e.g. Alzheimer's disease (major attacks common in the terminal phase); fits in 20 per cent of patients with arteriosclerotic dementia.

192

d) Focal brain disease especially that involving the frontal or temporal lobes. Dysfunction involving these local areas of cerebral cortex can cause organic brain syndromes with disorders of behaviour, personality and/or cognitive function; described in detail by Lishman [15].

e) Psychotic syndromes of unknown or uncertain aetiology in which recurrent fits are not an uncommon finding and appear to be a manifestation of the underlying brain dysfunction causing the psychosis: these begin before puberty and fall into the ninth International Classification of Disease (ICD-9) Category, Psychoses with Origin Specific to Childhood. This category includes infantile autism, disintegrative psychosis and atypical childhood psychosis. Such psychotic syndromes are rare in children with epilepsy apart from infantile autism in which fits occur in 29 per cent of patients.

Disorders related in time to seizure occurrence

a) Pre-ictal; prodromal irritability and dysphoria hours or days preceding the occurrence of a fit. Little is known about the prevalence of these prodromal changes nor indeed of their pathogenesis.

b) Ictal; directly due to the seizure discharge.

(i)   Complex partial seizures; mainly but not always of temporal lobe or limbic system origin; these ictal phenomena include hallucinations, perceptual illusions, ictal affect, forced thinking, illusions of memory, agnostic illusions (non-perceptive illusions during which an object is perceived normally but is poorly understood or recognised e.g. derealisation or jamais-vu experiences) and automatisms [16—19].

Automatism is perhaps the most important behavioural manifestation of complex partial seizure discharge having important forensic implications. Epileptic automatism may be defined as a state of clouding of consciousness which occurs during or immediately after a seizure and during which the individual retains control of posture and muscle tone without being aware of what is happening. It can occur either as a direct result of a seizure discharge or a post-ictal event following any type of fit, especially a generalised one.

The area most commonly involved in the initiation of an ictal automatism appears to be the periamygdaloid region. This includes the uncus, the amygdaloid nucleus, the central claustrum and the temporoinsular cortex deep in the anterior part of the sylvian fissure. Jasper [20] has pointed out that stimulation of these structures will only produce automatic behaviour in almost 50 per cent of cases. Automatism will not occur while the after discharge remains confined to the amygdala or hippocampus. There is always bilateral involvement of the amygdaloid-hippocampal structures with invariable spread to the mesial diencephalon and the temporo-parietal cortex. In many cases the frontal and central areas will be involved as well. Indeed automatic behaviour in some patients results from lesions at sites other than the mesial temporal structures, namely the frontal, orbito-frontal and parietal regions or the mesial surfaces of the hemispheres. Presumably, the discharging focus has caused secondary activation of the peri-amygdaloid-hippocampal structures. Ictal automatism can also occasionally result from prolonged generalised spike-wave discharges (petit-mal automatism) or generalised fronto-temporal or delta rhythms [20].

Behaviour during epileptic automatism varies greatly from patient to patient and in the same individual on different occasions. The person's actions have a quasi purposeful quality, but are often inappropriate to the environmental situation. There is usually impairment of awareness and lack of responsiveness to the environment. Brief attacks lasting 10 seconds or less merely cause cessation of activity. More prolonged episodes of 20 to 30 seconds' duration display stereo-typed repetitive movements e.g. chewing, swallowing, clenching fists, etc. Attacks which last several seconds are associated with more complex, variable but quasi purposeful behaviour e.g. undressing, wandering away, etc. This involves interplay with the environment and gradually merges into normal behaviour. The earlier stereotyped phenomena are a direct manifestation of the seizure discharge, while the later complex behaviour continues during the post-ictal phase of the attacks. The majority of automatisms are brief, five minutes or less in 80 per cent and never over an hour.

The inevitable clouding of consciousness associated with epileptic automatism means that well structured, goal-directed behaviour is impossible to initiate. Hence serious violence during epileptic automatism is rare. In one series of 43 patients, no aggressive conduct was observed in 36 (84%). The remaining seven tended to resist any attempt to interfere with or restrict their activities during the period of automatism. The behaviour of only one of these patients was considered dangerous [21]. This sample of 43 patients with automatism was taken from a total epileptic population of 434 outpatients.

Studies of more deviant populations have confirmed these findings. Although a survey of epileptic offenders in prisons and Borstal institutions in England and Wales had indicated that the prevalence of epilepsy in such places is significantly higher than in the general population there were only two persons out of a total of 158 whose crime was probably committed during or following a seizure: one during the post-ictal phase and the other in a possible ictal automatism. A parallel electroclinical study of the epileptic population of Broadmoor Hospital, one of the Special Hospitals in England and Wales for psychiatric offenders and patients displaying dangerously antisocial behaviour, revealed a prevalence of epilepsy similar to that of a conventional mental hospital. Of the 29 male patients who had committed offences, in only two could a definite relationship be established between their crimes and the occurrence of seizures; both behaved violently during a post-ictal confusional state [22, 23].

The International Workshop on Aggression and Epilepsy held at Bethseda, Maryland, in March 1980 [24] studied the videotape-recorded attacks of 13 patients selected because they were believed to show aggressive behaviour during seizures. These patients were selected from a total population of about 5,400 people with epilepsy from a number of different countries including USA, Canada, Germany, Italy and Japan. Seven patients were rated as exhibiting significant aggression during their seizures. The aggression varied from shouting insults and spitting to karate postures and chops and smashing of furniture. Five of the seven patients were rated as showing an angry mood during the seizure. Of the seven, four were rated as displaying violence to property only, two made threats of violence to a person (including gestures, shouting and spitting) and one was rated as displaying mild violence (the use of force against another person without inflicting serious harm e.g. pushing or shoving). This last patient, during a brief complex partial seizure, suddenly knelt on the bed and tried to scratch the face of her psychologist; she was held back by the technician. There were no ratings of serious violence. In all seven patients, the aggressive behaviour appeared suddenly, without evidence of planning and lasted an average of 29 seconds during complex partial seizures. All patients could be easily restrained. All automatic acts (e.g. kicking and boxing or attempts at grabbing an intended target and scratching his or her face) were short lived, fragmentary and unsustained.

This study confirms the clinical view that seriously aggressive behaviour is rare during epileptic seizures. Incidentally the report of the International Workshop on Aggression and Epilepsy refers to the above-mentioned work of Gunn and Fenton [23] as the only available study of prisoners whose crimes were possibly associated with epileptic automatisms. It should be drawn to the reader's attention that the summary of Gunn and Fenton's findings published in the Workshop Report is misleading. In fact, four (not two) patients were considered to have a direct relationship between criminal behaviour and the occurrence of seizures. In three, this took place during the post-ictal phase. In the fourth, it was possibly ictal.

Many of the complex seizure phenomena such as déjà-vu sensations, feelings of depersonalisation, hallucinations, etc., occur in functional psychiatric illnesses. They can be distinguished as epileptic events because of a sudden onset, transient duration lasting minutes rather than hours or days and relatively rapid resolution. The attacks are recurrent and have a stereotyped quality. Further, careful observation and enquiry will often reveal some degree of alteration of consciousness. In contrast consciousness is clear in the functional psychiatric syndromes.

(ii) Absence status; clouding of consciousness due to continuous generalised spike-wave discharge. Usually the discharge consists of spike and wave or polyspike-wave complexes more or less rhythmically and sometimes interrupted by slow rhythms of varying frequency. It may last for hours or even days. Though most common in children, absence status does occur in adults and may even present de novo in middle age.

(iii) Complex partial status; continuous temporal lobe epileptogenic discharge leads to a state of clouding of consciousness, prolonged affective disturbance (anxiety or fear), hallucinosis or frequently recurring automatism, the latter occurring without recovery of consciousness between episodes of automatic behaviour. In contrast to absence status, which is not uncommon in patients with generalised epilepsy, complex partial status is a rare event. The reasons for this are unclear, but probably result from fundamental differences in the mechanisms of generalisation and maintenance of ictal processes in absences as opposed to complex partial seizures [19, 25]. The duration of complex partial status is similar to that of absence status: hours or days.

c) Post-ictal disorders; disorders which follow one or more seizures, usually generalised convulsions. The common feature is clouding of consciousness due to post-seizure depression of cortical function leading to automatic behaviour or a post-epileptic confusional state if prolonged for hours, days or one or two weeks.

Interictal disorders unrelated in time to the seizures

Symptoms are present between attacks and often in the absence of seizures. It is assumed that the epilepsy and/or the cerebral epileptogenic lesion have played a role in the genesis of the psychiatric disorder. Though the illness is unrelated in time to seizure occurrence, the onset, intensity and course may be influenced by the fit frequency; more commonly by an exacerbation of fits; less often and more controversially by a reduction in fit frequency so that there is an inverse relation between fits and mental state [26].

Behaviour and epilepsy: general comments

There is much evidence that both children and adults have a greater prevalence of psychiatric disorder of a nature that cannot be directly related to seizure occurrence. Rutter et al [11] have demonstrated that, in children at least, this is not simply due to a reaction to the stress of coping with a chronic illness. In a survey of Isle of Wight school children, these authors found that epileptic children were five times more likely to have psychiatric disability than the general population and three times more likely than children with chronic handicaps not affecting the brain. Children with epilepsy complicated by lesions above the brainstem had the maximum prevalence (more than eight times that of the controls). This study demonstrated that multiple factors interact to cause the psychiatric disorder in people with epilepsy. Organic brain dysfunction, temporal lobe disorder as manifest by psychomotor fits and adverse familial influences were found to be predisposing factors. The symptom clusters displayed by epileptic children did not differ from those of non-epileptic patients. Antisocial and mixed neurotic/antisocial disorders were the most common.

196

However, when disturbed children with epilepsy are selected by EEG criteria, the site of origin of the epileptogenic process does influence the symptom profile. Nuffield [10] showed that children with temporal lobe spikes had high aggression and low neuroticism ratings, while those with generalised spike-wave complexes showed the reverse trend. Stores [12] has reported that boys with fits and epileptic children of either sex with left temporal lobe dysfunction are specially vulnerable to a range of behavioural difficulty.

Surveys of adult epileptics are less reliable because of sample bias. Pond and Bidwell [27] in a general practice survey reported that nearly one-third had psychological difficulties, mainly neuroses in adults and conduct disorders in children. Only four per cent showed features of the 'epileptic' personality. Seven per cent had been mental hospital patients, half of whom had temporal lobe epilepsy. In fact, temporal lobe dysfunction, low intelligence and adverse environmental factors were factors that seemed to lead to psychiatric breakdown, especially behaviour and personality disorders. As in children no specific symptom profiles could be identifed.

Indeed, the clinical features the patient develops are strongly influenced by age. Children and adolescents present with behaviour difficulties; antisocial/neurotic disorder. In contrast, adults tend to develop affective symptoms, especially those with late onset epilepsy. Suicide is five times more common amongst people with epilepsy than in the general population [28]. Personality disorder, unless a direct result of a focal brain lesion, is usually a reflection of life-long disturbance with early onset of fits and a history of maladjustment with behaviour and/or neurotic problems during childhood. The depressant effects of anticonvulsant drugs on cognitive function and emotional control also aggravate behaviour difficulties or mood disorder in both children and adults. Indeed phenobarbitone may have a paradoxical exciting effect on children with consequent increase in irritability and hyperkinetic behaviour.

Personality and epilepsy

Ever since the physiological origins of epilepsy were firmly established by Hughlings Jackson during the latter part of the nineteenth century, the thinking on the relation between the fits and mental state of epileptics has undergone a number of interesting changes [29]. Gowers in his text book about epilepsy published in 1881, in common with other writers of that period, observed that intellectual deterioration was frequently found in patients with epilepsy. The degree of deterioration or dementia varied from mild memory defects to severe mental handicap. Underlying brain disease was recognised as sometimes causing both the dementia and the epilepsy but, in most instances, the dementia was thought to be a consequence of the fits, the rate of progress of the dementia in direct proportion to the number and severity of the seizures. The earlier the onset of the seizures the greater the possibility of dementia. Frank psychosis was

197

considered rare. The contribution of prolonged medication with bromides was also recognised. The physical appearance of people with epilepsy received little attention, any changes being thought to be the result of trauma due to the seizures.

The term 'epileptic character' had occasional use throughout the latter half of the nineteenth century, being first used by the French psychiatrist, Morel. However, it was not until about 1900 that the term acquired the specific meaning it came to have. Epilepsy came to be regarded as a constitutional disorder, specific personality changes being as prominent a feature of the disorders as well as the fits. People with epilepsy were considered to be rarely, if ever, normal mentally. Profound disturbances of mood, attitudes and behaviour followed by inevitable mental deterioration were thought to be the rule. The character changes were regarded as so characteristic that a diagnosis of epilepsy could be made in the absence of fits.

Character traits specific to the epileptic personality included egocentricity, eccentricity, irritability, circumstantiality, religiosity, impulsiveness, emotional instability, hypersensitivity, paranoid attitudes. Their speech was considered to be slow and perseverative and their thought processes stereotyped and concrete. In both thought and affect, they were described as adhesive, sticky or viscous. In addition to such specific personality traits, impairment of memory, judgement and other intellectual functions, were considered common.

Both the fits and abnormal personality traits were thought to be a reflection of a genetically determined disorder with a deteriorating course. The constitutional defect causing the character changes and the seizures was also reflected in the physical characteristics of the face. Some authors described a characteristic epileptic facies; broad forehead, broad and flattened nose, prognathism, thick lips and staring eyes. In retrospect, a more plausible hypothesis is that such facial changes were acquired as the result of damage caused by falls during seizures and soft tissue hypertrophy due to chronic medication.

The concept of a specific epileptic personality evolved as the result of observations made on institutionalised patients, where bromism was common and disturbed behaviour a frequent cause for admission. Hence the epileptic personality syndrome developed as a consequence of generalisation to all people with epilepsy of clinical observations made on a minority of people with epilepsy whose disorder was so severe that they required long-term institutional care. Such selection factors have bedevilled research into the psychiatric aspects of epilepsy ever since. Surveys of patients representative of people with epilepsy living in the general population indicate that constellations of such personality change, though they do occur in occasional patients, are relatively rare in pure culture. For example in Pond and Bidwell's [27] survey of fourteeen general practices selected to be representative of the general population of England and Wales, found only 11 patients with prominent 'epileptic' personality traits out of the total of 255 epileptic patients identified (just over 4%).

Further, there is no evidence that these personality traits have a genetic basis. It is more probable that their development results from multiple handicaps: biological, social and psychological. Brain damage, diffuse and focal, specially that involving the temporal lobe, childhood deprivation, the disrupting effects of early onset epilepsy and frequent seizures on the personality development of the maturing child and adolescent, the chronic effects of medication and the psychological problems of living with severe epilepsy play a contributory role.

Indeed the assessment of personality disorder associated with epilepsy presents considerable methodological difficulties [30]. Barbara Tizard points out the biasing effects of selection factors. Observations made on patients in institutions do not generalise to patients living outside hospital. The influence of different types of epilepsy, the presence, location and extent of the brain lesion or damage causing the fits are variables that need to be controlled. She pointed out that most studies in which personality tests have been employed had not taken into consideration the intelligence of the patients nor the possible effects of medication.

More recent work carried out since Tizard's review in 1962 [30], has tended to use the Minnesota Multiphasic Personality Inventory (MMPI) as the instrument for assessing personality. There has also been much better control of such variables as age, sex, type and duration of epilepsy. Such studies have consistently shown elevated scores on most of the MMPI sub-scales. However, it is not clear to what extent these changes reflect the patient's personality (the relatively enduring or permanent traits, attitudes and patterns of behaviour which typify an individual) or a psychological response to the stresses of living with a chronic handicap such as epilepsy. Further, there is as yet no convincing evidence that such elevated scores are any more common in patients with epilepsy than in those with other types of brain disease.

An interesting recent development has been the analysis of the MMPI data using a technique that has been found to be specially sensitive in the detection of various psychopathological categories i.e. Goldberg's Rules [31]. Using this method, impaired performance on a battery of cognitive tests has been directly related to more severe degrees of psychopathology (as detected by Goldberg's Rules).

It is of interest to speculate on the reasons for the evolution of the epileptic personality concept at the turn of the century. No doubt the teachings of Kraepelin that dominated psychiatry then were highly influential. His main contribution was the description of clear cut functional psychotic syndromes such as dementia praecox (schizophrenia), a genetically determined syndrome with characteristic symptoms and signs and a deteriorating course to an inevitable end state of dementia. The epileptic personality concept fits perfectly into this model. At the same time Lombroso was applying the same biological model of disorder to criminal behaviour. The application of this particular model of mental illness to biased samples of patients living in long-term institutional care because of behaviour disorder and/or severe epilepsy and often under the adverse influences

199

of heavy bromide medication no doubt accounts for the popularity of the epileptic personality concept in the thinking of psychiatrists during the first few decades of the twentieth century.

A change in thinking about fits and mental state developed in the 1930s. Lennox in 1944 reviewed the literature about the personality of epileptics. He commented that the majority of patients he saw did not show the classical personality traits and pointed out the difficulties in unravelling the complex effects of heredity, brain damage, drug intoxication, and the reactions to the psychological and social problems the person with epilepsy has to face. Hence it became recognised that many epileptics were well adjusted people and that structural brain disease, chronic drug overdosage, frequent seizures and the psychological problems consequent upon being an epileptic all made a contribution to the genesis of psychiatric disorder in those who were mentally disturbed. As Lennox put it, much of the difficulty in assessing the mental state in epilepsy was due to the fact that 'the clear stream of essential epilepsy has been modified by symptomatic tributary'. No doubt major factors in determining this change in view were the development of more effective methods of neurological investigation and the consequent realisation that epilepsy is not a disease entity but a term used to describe a set of symptoms that can result from many different types of brain dysfunction which may cause mental changes. The change of climate in psychiatry with the development of a more psychodynamic approach also played a role in this change in attitude.

In the late 1940s and early 1950s the application of clinical electroencephalography to the study of the epilepsies and especially the work of Penfield and his colleagues in Montreal concerning the surgical treatment of focal epilepsy led to the identification of the syndrome of temporal lobe epilepsy. Surveys of large numbers of patients with epilepsy revealed an unduly high prevalence of functional psychiatric disorder in patients with temporal lobe epilepsy. Some 49 per cent of patients with anterior temporal lobe epileptogenic lesions had some type of psychiatric disorder, 32 per cent having severe personality disorder and 17 per cent being psychotic [5]. The psychiatric symptomatology was not specific in any way from a wide spectrum of personality, neurotic, psychotic and behavioural symptoms being present. In parallel with these clinical observations, the work of Papez, Maclean, and others on the physiology of the limbic system and its possible role in the control of affect, the temporal lobe ablation studies of Klüver and Bucy and the electrical stimulation studies carried out by Penfield and associates during operations for the relief of epilepsy drew attention to the relation between temporal lobe function and emotion. No doubt these experimental observations have also had a profound influence on current thinking about psychological disorder and temporal lobe dysfunction. The view that temporal lobe dysfunction predisposes the epileptic patient to a high risk of psychiatric breakdown and personality change is currently the most popular one, though it is by no means universally accepted [6].

The hypothesis by Gibbs [5] and others that behaviour and personality disorders in epilepsy can be related to the presence of long-standing seizure discharges in the mesial temporal lobe structures has led to the view that a specific temporal lobe behavioural syndrome exists [32, 33]. The syndrome includes the following features: irritability and deepened emotionality; decreased sexual interest and arousal; an excessive tendency to adhere to each thought, feeling and action (viscosity); and increased concern with philosophical, moral or religious issues, often in striking contrast to the person's education and social background.

Bear and Fedio [34] have developed a self-relating questionnaire to measure these traits. Eighteen personality traits were selected from descriptions of personality and behaviour of epileptic patients published in the literature. Each trait was sampled by five questions composed by the two investigators and judged representative of the trait in question by three additional professionals. In addition to these 90 trait derived items, ten questions were taken from the lie scale of the MMPI in order to detect any tendency of the subject to present an unduly favourable impression by the style of answers. The subsequent 100 questions about the patient's thoughts or actions are answered on a true/false basis. Two equivalent 100 item questionnaires are used: a personal inventory that the subject completes himself and a personal behaviour survey consisting of their personal versions of the same item that is completed by a close friend or relative.

At the National Institutes of Health, Bethseda, the questionnaires were given to a small series of patients with temporal lobe epilepsy and controls matched for age, sex, education, social class and place of residence. The authors found that compared to the controls which consisted of healthy members and patients with chronic neuromuscular disorders, the temporal lobe patients displayed a distinctive pattern of traits, namely humourless sobriety, dependence, circumstantiality, obsessionality, undue preoccupation with religious and philosophic concerns, emotionality and irritability.

Geschwind [35] and Bear and Fedio [34] point out that there are numerous neural connections between the primary receiving areas of the cortex and the limbic system. Their function is to give emotional significance to sensory stimuli processed by the primary receiving areas of the cortex. Destructive lesions within the temporal lobe of primates may act to disconnect the emotion mediating limbic structures, such as the amygdaloid complex and hippocampus, from the sensory association cortices of the visual and auditory system, resulting in the loss of learned emotional associations. Surgical disconnection appears to both disrupt old emotional bonds and to inhibit the formation of new stimulus-reinforcement (or sensory-limbic) linkages [36]. An extreme example of this disconnection process is the Klüver-Bucy syndrome caused by bilateral temporal lobectomy. Bear and Fedio [34] speculate that the temporal lobe epileptogenic process has a kindling effect on the medial limbic structures. A spike focus, as well as causing fits, acts as an electrode discharging from time to time into the limbic structures thus altering their reactivity. This leads to the development of new synaptic connections between the limbic system and the association cortices ('hyperconnections'). Hence, previously neutral stimuli events or concepts are given an emotional labelling. The continuous experiencing of events and objects with an unduly affective colouring will tend to engender a mystically religious view of the world. If the patient's immediate actions and thoughts are so coloured, the result will be an augmented sense of personal destiny. Sensing emotional importance in even the smallest acts lead to these being performed ritualistically and repetitively, with lengthy circumstantial speech or writing [37].

Further, Bear and Fedio [34] showed that right temporal lobe patients differed from those with left sided foci in displaying overtly emotive traits such as periods of sadness, irritability, elation, emotionality, etc. In contrast, the left temporal lobe patients had a pattern of predominantly verbal traits, for example, a ruminative intellectual tendency, religiosity, philosophical interests and an augmented sense of personal destiny. The authors tentatively interpret these results to mean that each hemisphere utilises its own characteristic style of cognitive processing in the development of limbic sensory associations. The right hemisphere uses non-verbal functions (emotive and dispositional) while the left hemisphere shows a predilection for ideational, contemplative and perhaps verbal expressions of affect. Finally, the right temporal lobe patients tended to exaggerate socially acceptable traits and deny undesirable ones. This is reminiscent of the denial of illness shown by patients with right hemisphere lesions. The left temporal patients showed the opposite pattern tending to exaggerate traits that showed them up in a bad light. The authors again speculate that such contrasting styles of self-reporting reflect specialised right and left hemisphere modes of cognitive processing.

Although the patients were drawn from five general hospital epilepsy clinics, the numbers in each sample were small (a total of 48 patients). The controls were either healthy adults or patients with neuromuscular disease. Epileptic patients without temporal lobe involvement were not studied. Hence the authors' claim that the behavioural profiles were a specific feature of temporal lobe epilepsy is open to challenge. Hermann and Riel [38] compared 14 well-matched temporal lobe epileptics and 14 patients with primary generalised seizures. There were no significant differences between the two groups with respect to chronological age, age at onset of seizures, duration of seizure disorder, sex, education and seizure control. The two groups were compared for each of the 19 trait scales and the lie scale. It was found that the temporal lobe epileptics scored significantly higher on four of the scales as follows: sense of personal destiny; dependence; paranoia and philosophical interest. None of the other 15 comparisons approached statistical significance. These results lend some support to the contention that a temporal lobe epileptogenic focus manifests itself in specific changes in behaviour and thought.

Clearly this quantitative approach to the study of behavioural profiles in

202

epilepsy is an interesting and potentially productive one. Geschwind [33] has pointed out that research on the relation between temporal lobe epilepsy and behaviour has usually asked the wrong questions e.g. "What are the behaviour disorders associated with temporal lobe epilepsy?" He suggests that the proper question is "What are the behavioural changes produced by temporal lobe epilepsy?" He feels that we should be beware of describing behavioural changes using standard nomenclature and classification of other psychiatric conditions. Such tools may be inappropriate. The behaviour change in temporal lobe epilepsy should be treated as a phenomenon in its own right.

An epidemiological approach is the only one capable of resolving the dispute over the relationship between temporal lobe epilepsy and behaviour, since it is only by total population surveys that the problem of sample bias introduced by studying hospital patients can be overcome. The Bear and Fedio questionnaire approach has the advantage that it can be readily applied to large numbers of patients identified during community prevalence surveys.

Epilepsy and sexual dysfunction

Complaints of reduced libido and impotence are known in male patients with epilepsy. As with other associations between epilepsy and behaviour, the relationships are complex. In many cases, the poor sexual skills are a reflection of poor social skills in immature, dependent persons, who have led sheltered and restricted lives with little opportunity to relate to the opposite sex because of frequent fits, parental overprotection and/or too much medication. Anticonvulsant drug-induced liver enzyme induction leads to rapid metabolism of testosterone and low serum free testosterone levels [39]. The influence of these hormone changes on sexual activity requires further evaluation. An association between sexual deviation (fetishism and transvestism) and temporal lobe epilepsy has been reported. It is tempting to speculate on a relationship between the sexual abnormalities and limbic system dysfunction but it is difficult to draw firm conclusions from such a small and highly selected group of patients. In any event temporal lobe dysfunction is rare among sexual deviants. The subject of sexual problems in epilepsy is reviewed by Scott [40].

Epilepsy and violence

Explosive aggressiveness, moodiness and irritability unrelated in time to the occurrence of fits have long been considered features of the 'epileptic personality'. During the last few decades, interictal aggressive behaviour has come to be regarded as a specific manifestation of temporal lobe epilepsy. The published studies on the relation between aggression and temporal lobe epilepsy have used a variety of definitions. Some authors have restricted their attention to outright physical assault, while others have included verbal abuse, bullying, stubbornness and assertiveness.

Kligman and Goldberg [41] have carried out a comprehensive review of the possible connections between temporal lobe epilepsy (TLE) and aggression. They critically reviewed the eight published controlled studies. All the studies were open to question because of sampling bias and only two produced definite evidence of a positive association between TLE and aggression. Only the study by Nuffield [10] on children was regarded as being methodologically sound. Though this study did offer some support for the association in children, Kligman and Goldberg feel that it will be necessary to have Nuffield's study replicated and applied to adults before a conclusion can be reached. They conclude that TLE is too heterogenous and ill-defined and human aggression too complex to allow definite interpretations of correlations between them at present.

Aggressiveness has been a not uncommon finding in those temporal lobe patients referred for anterior temporal lobectomy. About one-third of a large series of TLE patients operated on by Mr Murray Falconer were noted to have displayed overtly aggressive behaviour [42]. This behaviour was much more common in males, especially those in their teens. It tended to be associated with left-sided lesions, a pathological diagnosis of mesial temporal sclerosis and a favourable outcome in terms of successful rehabilitation after the operation and a cessation of fits.

It may well be that temporal lobe epileptic patients with drug resistant fits complicated by aggressive behaviour are more likely to be referred and selected for surgical treatment because the presence of the aggressiveness undoubtedly causes greater management and social adjustment problems. Indeed comparison of temporal lobe epileptic patients treated medically with those treated surgically indicates that the latter have an early mean age of onset and a much higher prevalence of disturbances of personality and behaviour [43]. This early age of onset within the first decade of life tends to be associated with mesial temporal sclerosis and may account for the relationship between TLE, aggression and MTS in the surgically treated patients.

As discussed previously, the occurrence of frequent fits throughout childhood may have adverse effects on parental and peer group attitudes, the processes of social learning and personality maturation. A cluster of other environmental factors that may produce a coincidental correlation between TLE and aggression by leading to a high incidence of both in the same people include low socio-economic status, parental psychopathology and child abuse. Antisocial children are more likely to have a low socio-economic background than neurotic children. The same background may expose children to poor parental and medical care with greater risks of acquiring brain damage due to poor obstetric care, head injuries due to parental neglect or abuse and infections which may provoke febrile convulsions and consequent mesial temporal lobe sclerosis. Unfortunately, little attention has been paid to controlling for socio-economic status in many of the studies on TLE and aggression.

Although epileptic automatism appears to be rare, there are more epileptic prisoners in gaols than would be expected by chance [44]: 7.2 per 1,000 prisoners in England and Wales in Gunn's survey. When a random sample of these epileptics was matched with other non-epileptic prisoners very little difference in terms of criminal behaviour could be discerned; nor was any relation between temporal lobe epilepsy and violent crime apparent. Gunn [44] has presented the following hypotheses to explain the higher prevalence of epilepsy in prisoners: (a) in some brain damage will cause both fits and behaviour disinhibition; (b) some with psychosocial problems feel stigmatised by their fits and hit back at society in an antisocial manner; (c) as already pointed out in the discussion about aggression and temporal lobe epilepsy, a deprived early environment may provide the milieu for acquiring both brain damage and learning an aggressive behavioural repertoire; and (d) finally brain damage and subsequent epilepsy may result from the person's basically disorganised impetuous life style that accompanied the criminality e.g. the juvenile thief and lorry stealer who wrecklessly smashed up an army lorry and sustained a severe head injury.

Epilepsy and psychosis

Interictal psychoses in clear consciousness do occur, though such states are rare in unselected populations of epileptic patients [45]. These psychoses are predominantly affective, schizo-affective or schizophrenia-like in presentation and are thought to have a special relationship to temporal lobe dysfunction [26].

Such interictal psychotic states in clear consciousness can be classified as follows:

1. Short-lived psychotic episodes lasting weeks or months with recovery as the usual outcome. These contrast with the epileptic and post-epileptic clouded states that last hours or days [9]. The most common clinical picture is that of classical depressive illness. For example, in his study of mental hospital admissions of epileptics in Birmingham, Betts [46] found that 31 per cent of the patients were suffering from depressive illness. Pahla et al [47] found six patients with affective psychoses out of a total of 14 psychotic patients in a sample of 80 consecutive admissions of epileptic patients at the Maudsley Hospital. A further five had schizo-affective disorders. Hence, 11 out of 14 had affective or schizo-affective psychoses. No cases of hypomania were observed. Occasionally, paranoid symptomatology is the predominant clinical feature. Toone et al [48] in a more recent study of 57 patients with epilepsy and psychosis at the same hospital found 16 with affective psychoses compared with 41 patients with schizophrenia. As well as being characterised by a primary disorder of mood, these affective and schizo-affective psychoses run a course similar to that of a typical affective illness lasting weeks or months only. Complete remission is usual but like classical depressive illness relapses and further episodes are not uncommon. In the Maudsley series

205

of Pahla and his colleagues, recovery had occurred in more than 50 per cent within three months.

In contrast to the clouded states, the onset of the psychotic state is rarely heralded by clinical seizures, but is occasionally terminated by a generalised convulsion [9]. Betts [46] in his series of 72 epileptic admissions found a significant association between a 50 per cent reduction in seizure frequency before admission in patients with depressive illness, while an increase in seizure frequency was common in those admitted with either acute behaviour disturbance or clouded states. Hence a reduction of seizure frequency may contribute to the pathogenesis of the affective psychoses of epilepsy. Reports of a direct relationship to non-dominant temporal lobe dysfunction [26] have not been replicated by more recent work [45].

2. Chronic schizophrenia-like psychoses. The mutual antagonism theory that epilepsy protected against schizophrenia led to the introduction of convulsive therapy to psychiatric practice in the 1930s. However, over subsequent years, it has become apparent that a schizophrenia-like psychosis occurs more often than can be accounted for by change in patients with epilepsy. Slater et al [49] published the first detailed study of the schizophrenia-like psychoses of epilepsy. Two-thirds had temporal lobe dysfunction, the psychoses developing on average 14 years after the onset of the fits. The most characteristic clinical presentation was of a paranoid schizophrenia-like state.

Though the symptomatology is generally similar to patients with non-epileptic schizophrenia, a number of differences were noted. Paranoid delusions were unduly common. Mystical delusional experiences were especially frequent, the patients feeling in communication with God or endowed with supernatural powers or experiencing passivity phenomena with a mystical content. Visual hallucinations were more common than in typical schizophrenia, being often experienced during dream-like states in the absence of confusion. Again, a mystical content to the hallucinations was common. The patients' affects were warmer and better retained than is usual in schizophrenia. The progress of the disorder was also more benign with less personality and social deterioration.

A more recent controlled study of the phenomenology of the schizophrenia-like psychoses of epilepsy using a structured mental state assessment technique by Toone et al [48] has partially confirmed the findings of Slater et al [49]. Toone et al [48] have found delusions of persecution and of reference to be more common in the schizophrenia-like psychoses of epilepsy and catatonic symptoms less common as compared to a control group of non-epileptic patients with schizophrenia. Abnormal premorbid personalities were less often found in the epileptic psychotic patients. Another interesting observation was that there was an excess of females in the latter group. Toone [45] and others have also reported an excess of sinistrality amongst psychotic epileptics.

There was no genetic loading for schizophrenia nor any excess of schizoid

206

premorbid personality traits amongst the patients in Slater's series. Slater and his colleagues regarded this disorder as a symptomatic schizophrenia due to the temporal lobe dysfunction. The influence of lateralisation of the epileptogenic lesion on the genesis of the schizophrenia-like psychoses remains in dispute at present. Both bilateral damage to the mesial temporal limbic structures and dominant temporal lobe dysfunction have been reported as predisposing to psychoses (reviewed by Flor-Henry[26], Fenton [50] and Toone [45]). Change in seizure frequency, either a reduction or an exacerbation, has been described as a precipitating factor, the change usually involving complex partial seizures. The increased seizure frequency may cause limbic system and/or global cortical dysfunction due to neuronal inhibition following the intense ictal activation. The phenomenon of a reduced fit frequency leading to psychosis may reflect underlying neurotransmitter changes that cause both events. Trimble [51] has presented a dopamine hypothesis that explains this phenomenon, increased dopamine activity being antiepileptic and schizophrenogenic, while diminution of such activity increases the seizure activity but has a therapeutic effect on the psychosis.

With so many varied and apparently conflicting associations between the epileptic fits, brain dysfunction and the psychotic process it is difficult to postulate a single direct causal relationship between the epilepsy and these interictal psychoses. Although global cerebral dysfunction following generalised convulsions or due to petit-mal status is almost invariably followed by clouding of consciousness, interictal psychosis in clear consciousness is a relatively rare association of temporal lobe epilepsy (2% in the series of Currie et al [43]). Therefore a direct link between temporal lobe dysfunction and interictal psychosis is unlikely. A more plausible hypothesis to account for the relatively small number of cases that occur in patients with temporal lobe epilepsy is that either the epileptogenic dysfunction localised to the dominant temporal lobe or extensive bilateral damage to the deep limbic system structures makes patients more vulnerable to psychotic breakdown. However, in any one such vulnerable individual, a florid psychosis will only develop when the person is exposed, in addition, to other pathogenic factors (biological, psychological or social). These may be either predisposing or precipitating and interact with the temporal lobe dysfunction to disrupt the person's capacity to deal with the environment. Hence the cerebral disorder caused by the epilepsy merely acts as one of a number of vulnerability or provoking factors in causing the psychosis. Indeed, such a vulnerability model can be applied to all the interictal psychiatric disorders of epilepsy.

Causation of behaviour and personality disorder

Indeed, the only aetiological model that can be plausibly applied to the interictal psychiatric disorders of epilepsy is a multifactorial one. In any one individual the disturbance of mental state or behaviour is the final manifestation of an interaction

207

of factors. Some are merely predisposing in nature, increasing the individual's vulnerability to breakdown. Others may play an important role in precipitating or provoking breakdown of the vulnerable individual. The vulnerability and precipitating factors can be biological, psychological or social, usually a complex interaction of all three, the relative importance of any one group of factors varying from one individual to another.

Vulnerability factors include genetic loading for psychiatric disorders; an early onset of epilepsy with frequent fits in the first one and a half decades of life that may adversely influence parental and peer group attitudes, educational performance, the acquisition of social skills and personality maturation; diffuse cortical damage impairing IQ and impulse control; temporal lobe dysfunction (left sided and/or bilateral involvement) with its more intractable seizure pattern and capacity to alter sensory-limbic connections and disrupt learning and memory processes; family psychopathology; the depressant effect of heavy anticonvulsant medication on cognitive function and its disinhibiting effect on behaviour; the male sex. Any combination of these factors may interact to make the individual vulnerable to breakdown.

Precipitating or provoking factors act on the vulnerable person and cause decompensation of the latter's precarious psychosocial adjustment. This is manifest by psychiatric symptoms or behaviour disorder. As discussed previously, the resulting symptoms and signs will be determined by the age of the patient, conduct disorder in the child or adolescent, anxiety or depressive symptoms in the adult with late onset epilepsy, the adult with personality disorder may present a more complex picture with difficult behaviour or paranoid symptoms. Frequently, however, such floridly disturbed behaviour represents the immature person's process of coping with an underlying mood change of depression or anxiety.

Provoking factors include crises in the person's life situation, adverse life events and social difficulties, emotional tension due to relationship problems or a role change, a marked change in seizure frequency, and drug intoxication.

References

1   Mechanic D. *Medical Sociology: A Selective View 1968*. New York: The Free Press
2   Long CG, Moore JR. *J Child Psychol Psychiatry 1979; 20:* 299–312
3   Fenton GW. *Rehabilitation 1976; 96:* 15–21
4   Rodin EA. In Laidlaw J, Richens A, eds. *Textbook of Epilepsy 2nd Edition 1982*. Edinburgh: Churchill Livingstone
5   Gibbs FA. *J Nerv Ment Dis 1951; 11:* 522–528
6   Stevens JR. In Penry JK, Daly DD, eds. *Advances in Neurology Vol II 1975*. New York: Raven Press
7   Rodin EA, Katz M, Lennox K. *Epilepsia 1976; 17:* 313–320
8   Hermann BP, Schqartz MS, Karnes WE, Vahdat P. *Epilepsia 1980; 21:* 15–23
9   Dongier S. *Epilepsia 1959; 1:* 117–142
10   Nuffield EJA. *J Ment Sci 1961; 107:* 438–458

11   Rutter M, Graham P, Yule W. *A Neuropsychiatric Study in Childhood 1970.*
      London: Heinemann
12   Stores G. *Dev Med Child Neurol 1978; 20:* 502–508
13   Stevens JR, Hermann BP. *Neurology 1981; 31:* 1127–1132
14   Corbett JA. In Reynolds EH, Trimble MR, eds. *Epilepsy and Psychiatry 1981.*
      Edinburgh: Churchill Livingstone
15   Lishman WA. *Organic Psychiatry 1978.* Oxford: Blackwell
16   Gastaut H. *Dictionary of Epilepsy 1973.* Geneva: World Health Organisation
17   Fenton GW. *Br J Hosp Med 1972; 7:* 57–64
18   Fenton GW. In *Symposium on Recent Advances in Epilepsy. Ir Med J (Suppl) 1980;*
      73: 11–19
19   Daly DD. In Laidlaw J, Richens A, eds. *A Textbook of Epilepsy 1982.* Edinburgh:
      Churchill Livingstone
20   Jasper HH. *Epilepsia 1964; 5:* 1–20
21   Knox SJ. *Med Sci Law 1968; 8:* 96–104
22   Gunn J, Fenton G. *Br Med J 1969; 4:* 326–328
23   Gunn J, Fenton G. *Lancet 1971; ii:* 1173–1176
24   Delgado-Escueta AV, Mattson RH, King L et al. *N Engl J Med 1981; 305:* 711–716
25   Daly DD. In Penry JK, Daly DD, eds. *Advances in Neurology Vol II 1975.*
      New York: Raven Press
26   Flor-Henry P. In Granville-Grossman K, ed. *Recent Advances in Clinical Psychiatry*
      1976. Edinburgh: Churchill Livingstone
27   Pond DA, Bidwell BH. *Epilepsia 1960; 1:* 285–299
28   Barraclough B. In Reynolds EH, Trimble MR, eds. *Epilepsy and Psychiatry 1981.*
      Edinburgh: Churchill Livingstone
29   Guerrant J, Anderson WW, Fischer A et al. *Personality in Epilepsy 1962.*
      Springfield, Illinois: Charles C Thomas
30   Tizard B. *Psychol Bull 1962; 59:* 196–210
31   Hermann BP. *Epilepsia 1981; 22:* 161–167
32   Waxman SG, Geschwind N. *Arch Gen Psychiatry 1975; 32:* 1580–1586
33   Geschwind N. *Psychol Med 1979; 9:* 217–219
34   Bear DM, Fedio P. *Arch Neurol 1977; 34:* 454–467
35   Geschwind N. *Brain 1965; 88:* 237–294 and 585–644
36   Jones B, Mishkin M. *Exp Neurol 1972; 36:* 362–377
37   Bear DM. *Cortex 1979; 15:* 357–384
38   Hermann BP, Riel P. *Cortex 1981; 17:* 125–128
39   Toone BK, Wheeler M, Fenwick PBC. *Clin Endocrinol 1981; 12:* 391–395
40   Scott DF. In *Epilepsy 1978.* Wokingham: British Epilepsy Association
41   Kligman D, Goldberg DA. *J Nerv Ment Dis 1975; 160:* 324–341
42   Falconer MA. *N Engl J Med 1973; 289:* 450–455
43   Currie S, Heathfield WG, Henson RA, Scott DF. *Brain 1971; 94:* 173–190
44   Gunn J. *Epileptics in Prison 1977.* New York: Academic Press
45   Toone BK. In Reynolds EH, Trimble MR, eds. *Epilepsy and Psychiatry 1981.*
      Edinburgh: Churchill Livingstone
46   Betts TA. In Harris P, Mawdsley C, eds. *Epilepsy: Proceedings of the Hans Berger*
      Centenary Symposium 1974. Edinburgh: Churchill Livingstone
47   Pahla A, Fenton GW, Driver MW, Fenwick PBC. Epilepsy and psychiatric disorder.
      In preparation
48   Toone B, Garralda E, Ron M. *Br J Psychiatry.* In press
49   Slater E, Beard AW, Glithero E. *Br J Psychiatry 1963; 109:* 95–150
50   Fenton GW. *J Ir Med Assoc 1978; 71:* 315–324
51   Trimble MR. *Biol Psychiatry 1977; 12:* 299–304

22

HYSTERICAL ATTACKS IN PATIENTS WITH EPILEPSY

Adrienne M Moffett, D F Scott

Introduction

The history of hysteria in the medical literature recently reviewed [1] contains many famous names but this chapter deals only with this condition appearing in those where a previous diagnosis of epilepsy is certain [2]. The frequency with which pseudo-seizures occur in a genuine seizure disorder is difficult to determine but they represent an important problem in terms of readmission to the neurology wards of the London Hospital.

Patients

Over the last few years we have collected 32 patients in whom it is certain that their attacks are not seizures (Table I). As expected the majority are females, they show a wide age range but tend to be clustered in the 30 to 40 range. They

TABLE I. Hysterical attacks on epileptic patients (n = 32)

Females:	30	Males:	2
Age range 16–55 years (average 35)			

TABLE II. Clues to pseudo-seizures

Very frequent
Variable in type
Neurophysiological basis difficult to 'understand'
Usually diurnal
Occur in the presence of family or consorts
EEG in attacks and soon after 'normal'

present considerable difficulty, not only in diagnosis but treatment [3]. The pseudo-seizures are very frequent (Table II), with many attacks every day They are variable in type, contrasting with genuine fits which ordinarily have a stereotyped pattern, although several types are well known in the individual patient. These attacks are almost always diurnal and occur in the presence of the family or a consort. The appearance of the pseudo-seizures is often difficult to understand on neurophysiological basis since one arm may be affected and soon after the opposite leg appears to be jerking.

The causation of these attacks (Table III) is usually related to some form of

TABLE III. Causation of attacks

Stress causing elaboration of previous attack pattern
Fear of disorder exaggerates symptoms
Previous experience of epilepsy, models behaviour
Gain by 'sick role'
Cerebral damage exaggerates previous behaviour patterns

stress and it appears that the previous experience of epilepsy models the behaviour and there may be 'gain' in this 'sick role'. In addition there is no doubt that cerebral damage, either of long standing or recent, affects these behaviour patterns.

Observation of the attacks is clearly very important (Table IV). The pattern of pseudo-seizures in contrast to fits is variable. There may be some sort of prolonged warning that an attack is about to commence, quite unlike the prodromal

TABLE IV. Features of the attack to consider

Variable pattern
Other people present
Warning of impending attack
Possible trigger factors
Micturition
Injury
Duration

or aura of the genuine seizure. Trigger factors are difficult to assess but, as Liske and Forster [4] pointed out, unusual attacks brought on by unusual triggers are suspicious in terms of their aetiology and causation. Some physicians are able by verbal means to provoke an attack.

Generally, fits have a short duration being followed by a period of confusion and sleep, but these pseudo-seizures are rather different, being often prolonged, not only in their duration but their post-ictal manifestations. It is important to bear in mind two features always regarded as cardinal [5] in distinguishing between true and pseudo-seizures, since micturition and injury both occur in pseudo-seizures.

Attack features to consider

How do we decide that the attack is in fact a pseudo-seizure when dealing with a patient with epilepsy (Table V)? In most instances the epilepsy has been of long standing. There are usually periods in which good control by drugs has

TABLE V. Factors in pseudo-seizures

Epilepsy of long standing
Previously well controlled by drugs
Sudden increase in attacks
May be very frequent even 'Status'
Family history of psychiatric disorder
Previous history of psychiatric disorder, and suicide attempts
Recent stress, related to marriage or family
Poor sexual adjustment
Drug intoxication

occurred, although it is important to appreciate that drug intoxication may lead to a sudden worsening in terms of the number of attacks [6]. They may become so frequent that they amount almost to 'status epilepticus' and two of our patients had tracheostomies with assisted ventilation at a crisis in their illness. These episodes are usually precipitated by marital and family stress, or psychiatric disorder apparently unrelated to epilepsy is often a feature, and suicidal attempts may have occurred. A family history of such disorders and poor sexual adjustment are common features [2].

These patients present great difficulty in management (Table VI). Help may be obtained from conventional EEG [2], cerebral function monitoring, telemetry or ambulatory monitor recording. Often medication has been increased markedly over the period prior to referral and rapid reduction depending on the circumstances, possibly with introduction of placebo should be contemplated. It is important to decide on anticonvulsant medication and, generally, if the patient

TABLE VI. Pointers in treatment

Rapid reduction of medication (possibly placebo 'cover')
If isolated 'genuine' fits occur maintain on a single anticonvulsant
Establish rapport and explore stress factors
Maintain a 'firm' line in relation to anticonvulsant therapy

212

does appear to have isolated fits, a single dose regime with phenytoin is suggested. It is essential, having decided on whether to continue anticonvulsant therapy, that this should be maintained at an appropriate level and not increased, otherwise the pattern of the intoxication and worsening of control will again appear. Equally important, and this may be difficult to assess and elucidate, are the stress factors. Rapport with the patient clearly has to be established and this often leads to relief from the current situation, though relapse is not infrequent.

Conclusions

Nobody would suggest that this is an easy area but two points should be emphasised. Firstly, if seizures suddenly increase in a patient with epilepsy, then consideration should be given as to whether these are pseudo-seizures. Secondly, having established that this may be the case, reduction of medication but maintenance on a standard dose of a single drug would be recommended, bearing in mind that investigation of the reason for the seizures if not established previously would be mandatory.

Acknowledgments

We are grateful to Dr R A Henson, Dr A Ridley and Dr M Swash for allowing their patients to be studied and reported, to the technicians of the EEG department for records on patients who may present difficulty and to Mrs Jean Held for indefatigable secretarial help.

References

1 Merskey H. *The analysis of hysteria 1979.* London: Bailliere Tindall
2 Roy A. *Arch Neurol 1979; 36:* 447
3 Scott DF. In Riley T, Roy A, eds. *Pseudo-seizures 1982.* Baltimore: Williams & Wilkins
4 Liske E, Forster FM. *Neurology 1964; 41:* 41–49
5 Gowers WR. *Epilepsy 1885, reprinted 1969.* New York: Dover Press
6 Niedermeyer E, Bloomer D, Holscher E, Walker BA. *Psychiat Clin 1970; 3:* 71–84

23

RELIGIOSITY, MYSTICAL EXPERIENCE AND EPILEPSY

T Sensky

Introduction

It is commonly held that temporal lobe epileptics are likely to display religiosity
and also that they are susceptible to mystical experiences [1—4]. Most of the
evidence for these associations comes from anecdotal studies involving particularly
selected patients. Almost all these studies share two basic assumptions. The first
concerns the nature and recognition of religiosity, which is seldom explicitly
defined. The second involves the putative link between religiosity and mystical
experience. Although it is possible for a mystical experience to lead to religious
conversion, such a causal relationship is contested by those who view mystical
states in general as essentially secular [5], and such an association among epileptics
thus becomes the more interesting because of its comparative rarity in the general
population.

    The prevalence of mystical states and their possible relationship to religious
inclination have been examined in a population of epileptic outpatients. The
results of this preliminary survey will be presented following a review of mystical
states and religiosity.

Mystical states

These are, almost by definition, difficult to describe, especially to someone without personal experience of them. They have a noetic quality, a form of reality
different than normal; they usually last no more than a few minutes and are
often much shorter [6]. Such states which are achieved through meditation or
other forms of active encouragement should be distinguished from similar but
subtly different experiences which arise spontaneously. The latter are likely to
be the more interesting, if not also the more important, among epileptics. All such
states characteristically also have an intensely emotional quality.

It is noteworthy that the same features can be recognised in many temporal lobe fits, but mystical states have an additional feature, a feeling of proximity to some supernatural force. This has been variously described as "an awareness of, or influence from, a presence or power different from everyday life" [7] ; "closeness to a powerful force that seems to lift one out of oneself" [8] ; "being in touch with the Universal" etc. Conspicuous omissions in all these statements are explicit references to God or religion. As already noted, some would go so far as to argue that mystical states are secular experiences given a religious interpretation [5].

Mystical experiences in the general population

The nature of mystical states makes assessment of their frequency difficult. Using lengthy semi-structured interviews, Hay found that up to two people in every three will report having had a mystical experience [9,10].

A simpler but less thorough approach involves incorporating one or more of the descriptive phrases already mentioned regarding the experience of proximity to some supernatural force as a question in an interview or questionnaire. Regardless of which of the forms of the question is used, this produces an overall response rate of around 30 per cent [8]. Females are more likely to report such experiences than males, and the response rate rises with age, higher socio-economic status and education. Positive responders tend towards higher ratings on scales of global 'psychological wellbeing' [8,10].

The link between religious background and reported mystical experience is particularly interesting. Twenty-three per cent of a group of postgraduate students reporting personal experience of a mystical state affirmed that this experience was not of a religious nature [9]. Although there is a positive correlation between reported mystical states and religious inclination, the same kinds of experiences are also reported by atheists and agnostics. The frequencies of such reported experiences are very similar in Britain and the United States, despite the much larger percentage of churchgoers in the population of the latter country. This supports the separation of religious inclination into 'ritualistic' and 'experiential' dimensions; it is argued that church attendance is a manifestation of the former, while mystical experience may be more firmly linked with the latter. A similar distinction may be relevant to the religiosity accorded to some epileptics and the link between this and mystical experience.

Mystical states in epilepsy

Interest in this was generated particularly by the work of Beard and his colleagues [1,2]. Their original study [1] suggested that "mystical delusional experiences" were a common feature of the schizophrenia-like psychoses of epilepsy. It must be stressed that all their patients were selected as psychotic as well as epileptic, and it is far from clear what relationships these mystical experiences might have to the psychoses, or to mystical states in general.

Twenty-six of Slater et al's [1] 69 patients (38%) showed what was described as 'religiosity'. Six of these religiose patients had sudden religious conversions, and it is this group from the 1963 study which was described in more detail in Dewhurst and Beard's subsequent paper [2]. One distinction between these six and the religiose group as a whole was that, whereas few of the latter (8 of 26) displayed any religious interest before the onset of their illnesses, five of the six patients who experienced sudden religious conversions had a background of religious interest, either personally or within their family (Table I). As has been

TABLE I. Details of the family and personal religious backgrounds of the cases reported by Dewhurst and Beard [2], together with the sites of their focal epileptic discharges (L = left temporal lobe, R = right temporal lobe)

| Case | RELIGIOUS BACKGROUND | | Focus |
	Family	Personal	
1	?	+	L + R
2	+	+	L
3	+	+	R
4	+	?	L
5	?	+	R + L
6	–	–	L + R

argued for mystical states in general, it is possible that these five invested the experiences described as mystical with religious significance because of their backgrounds. Admittedly, similar arguments do not apply to the anecdotal accounts of sudden religious conversions in epileptics reported in other studies [11–13], although the information reported might be incomplete.

There is no suggestion from Dewhurst and Beard's study, as Table I shows, that mystical experiences are associated exclusively or even predominantly with foci in one or other temporal lobe. The preponderance of right temporal foci found in other studies where sudden religious conversions are recorded as incidental findings may have been due to bias introduced by specific selection criteria [11–13].

Religiosity and epilepsy

Although Slater et al [1] did not explicitly define what they meant by religiosity, the case histories they quoted suggest that they took it to mean religious interest of an excessive and possibly idiosyncratic kind. As in the case of their "mystical

216

delusional experiences", it is impossible from their study to distinguish how religiosity might relate on the one hand to epilepsy and on the other to the psychoses which accompanied it. Would, for example, a schizophrenic who asserted that he was God qualify as religiose in the same way as someone whose life had apparently been changed by a sudden religious conversion experience?

Other studies have also failed to define the limits of religiosity [3,14,15]. Bear and Fedio [3] looked at this as one of the possible interictal characteristics of temporal lobe epilepsy but the limited information available from their paper suggests that they may have been considering 'religious inclination' rather than 'religiosity'. Their results as a whole are in any case of limited value because of inadequate information on the cerebral dominance of their patients (epileptic foci were referred to as 'left' or 'right' with no indication of the handedness of their patients) and also the absence from their study of a control group of patients with generalised epilepsy. Their results could apply just as easily to all epileptics as to temporal lobe epileptics specifically; their conclusions could even apply to patients with other forms of brain damage. Hermann and Riel [15] made an attempt to resolve this question by comparing patients with temporal lobe epilepsy with another group who had generalised epilepsy, but they had no control group of non-epileptics. As they used the same protocol as Bear and Fedio, they too may not have examined religiosity as such.

There may even be problems in assuming that religious inclination is a necessary prerequisite for religiosity [10], although this assumption seems very reasonable. However, because of the difficulties already mentioned in defining religiosity and to allow comparison with previous studies, the present survey, of a group of outpatients attending the Maudsley Hospital Epilepsy Clinic, has concerned itself with religious inclination of its subjects rather than their possible religiosity.

The Maudsley Epilepsy Clinic study

Details of the survey, together with results relating to paranormal states other than mystical, are reported elsewhere [16]. In brief, questions asked in a self-administered questionnaire incorporating 51 items included: "Do you consider yourself a religious person? (Yes/No)"; "Did your faith come gradually, or was there a point at which you 'suddenly saw the light'? (Gradual/Sudden/Combination of both)" and "Have you ever felt at one with the Universe, or in touch with the Universal? (Never/Once/Sometimes/Often)". Subjects were asked specifically how these experiences related to their fits, and were encouraged to elaborate on their answers where possible. After initial blind rating of the responses, further information was sought from the medical case notes.

The results are summarised in Table II. In no case was a reported mystical experience related directly by a respondent to a fit, nor was there any association apparent between such experiences and fit frequency or past psychiatric history. In particular, patients were excluded who were, according to their medical records,

TABLE II. Reported religious inclination and mystical experiences among epileptics and the general population

| | Per cent respondents | | |
	TLE (N = 30)	Generalised epilepsy (N = 16)	Controls* (N = 1865)
Religious	56	72	78
Experienced sudden coming of faith	40	62	
"In touch with the Universal"	12	33	36

* Data from Hay and Morisy [8], based on a stratified sample of the UK population

clearly psychotic either at the time of the reported mystical experience or when answering the questionnaire.

Among those who professed to be non-religious, only one of 20 subjects reported having experienced a mystical state, compared with seven of 27 'religious' respondents. This trend towards an association between being religious and reporting experience of a mystical state failed to reach significance ($p = 0.13$, χ^2 test). Although the figures involved are small, it is interesting that this result mirrors Hay's findings among non-epileptics [9]. The small numbers of cases involved also prevented adequate comparisons between epileptics with foci in one or other temporal lobe but, such as they are, our data reveal no differences in this respect between dominant and non-dominant temporal lobe foci.

Discussion

Our patients with temporal lobe epilepsy are not only less likely than other subjects to have experienced mystical states (or at least to report having done so), but are also less likely to profess to being religious. By contrast, patients with generalised epilepsy appear no different in their religious inclination and reports of mystical experience than the UK population as a whole. This same trend holds true for belief in and experience of other paranormal phenomena [16]. As already mentioned, Hay and Morisy [8] identified a strongly positive association between mystical experience and increasing age, and the difference between our two groups is the more striking because the mean age of the temporal lobe epileptics (44.5 years) was 10.5 years greater than that of the other group. Neither of the two patient groups differed from the control population with respect to other significant variables such as sex and mean IQ or education.

If the assumption has any validity that religiosity should be demonstrable primarily in those who consider themselves religious, our results suggest that religiosity is unlikely to be a quantitatively important characteristic of epileptics. From the evidence of previous studies, it is only possible to say that some epileptics are religiose and some experience mystical states. These are unlikely to be associated exclusively with temporal lobe epileptics, as the present evidence implies; available studies are largely biased in their selection of patients [17]. In fact, Gastaut [18] has argued that perhaps the best known of all recorded mystical states associated with epilepsy, those of Dostoevsky, were not associated with temporal lobe epilepsy as has commonly been supposed.

Furthermore, as in the case of non-epileptics, evidence has yet to be found to firmly establish a link between mystical states and religiosity in epileptics. Even if such an association is ultimately verified, its nature may turn out to be complex. Some of the shortcomings of studies on the interictal characteristics of epileptics have already been mentioned. However, one might speculate that many of the suggested attributes, such as obsessionality, viscosity and even interest in personal destiny, may be seen as responses to a need to bring maximal order into life. The development of religiosity in this context could thus be a different or additional response to the same need. As such, it would appear to represent religion at its ritualistic extreme, relatively distant from mystical experience. Alternatively, religiosity may represent the response, particularly of a 'rigid' individual, to the chaotic effects of a seizure-related mystical experience. Although this idea would seem to have been favoured in the past, it leads to the expectation (assuming that mystical states in epilepsy are in general ictal) that the interictal characteristics of epileptics should be tied more closely to the nature of their ictal experiences.

One further consideration deserves mention, namely the possible relationships of religiosity and mystical experience to psychiatric history in general and psychosis in particular. Although people reporting mystical states tend to be "happier and more optimistic about life than other people" [10], depression and despair are common antecedents of mystical experiences [7] and the role played by psychiatric illness awaits further clarification. This is relevant to the results of the survey described above, which was conducted on patients attending a psychiatric hospital and needs to be replicated in the setting of a neurological clinic.

There are reports of epileptics free of psychosis experiencing either mystical states [4], religiosity (e.g. possibly case 5 of Waxman and Geshwind [11]) or both (e.g. case 3 of Roberts, Robertson and Trimble [13]), but most such reports in the literature involve patients who were psychotic as well as epileptic [2] and whose behaviour cannot be assumed to be that of epileptics in general. Schizophrenics who do not have fits can also experience mystical states [19] and their families tend to be more religious than others [20], thus there may be greater involvement of psychosis than has previously been assumed in the development of religiosity and experience of mystical states among epileptics.

Models are currently available which aim to explain the neuropsychology [21] and neurophysiology [22,23] of mystical experience. Research into the behavioural and other correlates of epilepsy will undoubtedly have a part to play in testing such models, but only after the thorough reappraisal of existing information and the rigorous collection of further data.

References

1   Slater E, Beard AW. *Br J Psychiat 1963; 109:* 95–150
2   Dewhurst K, Beard AW. *Br J Psychiat 1970; 117:* 497–507
3   Bear DM, Fedio P. *Arch Neurol 1977; 34:* 454–467
4   Cirignotta F, Todesco CV, Lugaresi E. *Epilepsia 1980; 21:* 705–710
5   Laski M. *Everyday Ecstasy 1980.* London: Thames & Hudson
6   James W. *The Varieties of Religious Experience 1902.* London: Longmans,Green & Co
7   Hardy A. *The Spiritual Nature of Man 1979.* Oxford: Oxford University Press
8   Hay D, Morisy A. *J Scientific Study of Religion 1978; 17:* 255–268
9   Hay D. *J Scientific Study of Religion 1979; 18:* 164–182
10   Hay D. *Exploring Inner Space: Is God Still Possible in the Twentieth Century? 1982.* Harmondsworth: Penguin Books
11   Waxman SG, Geshwind N. *Neurology 1974; 24:* 629–636
12   Waxman SG, Geshwind N. *Arch Gen Psychiatry 1975; 32:* 1580–1586
13   Roberts JKA, Robertson M, Trimble MR. *J Neurol Neurosurg Psychiat 1982:* in press
14   Small JG, Small IF, Hayden MP. *Am J Psychiat 1966; 123:* 303–310
15   Hermann BP, Riel P. *Cortex 1981; 17:* 125–128
16   Sensky T, Fenwick PBC. *Br J Clin Prac 1982:* in press
17   Stevens JR. *Arch Gen Psychiat 1966; 14:* 461–471
18   Gastaut H. *Epilepsia 1978; 19:* 185–201
19   Jaspers K. *General Psychopathology 1963.* Manchester: Manchester University Press
20   Heston LL. *Br J Psychiat 1966; 112:* 819–825
21   Deikman AJ. In Ornstein RE, ed. *The Nature of Human Consciousness 1973:* 216–233. San Francisco: WH Freeman & Co
22   Sargant W. *Br J Psychiat 1969; 115:* 505–518
23   Fenwick PBC. *The Neurophysiology of the Brain: its Relationship to Altered States of Consciousness 1980 (Wrekin Trust Lecture).* Little Birch, Hereford: The Wrekin Trust

24

BEHAVIOURAL ASPECTS OF CHILDHOOD EPILEPSY

G Stores

Introduction

The problems of learning and behaviour in children with epilepsy have been discussed by Stores [1]. The approach to the topic is all important, since generalisations and impressionistic accounts have been the source of much confusion in the past. For effective clinical practice, and for research in this area, distinctions need to be made between the many different disorders and circumstances that are collected under the term 'epilepsy'. A similar degree of precision is required in the definition of operative terms such as 'learning problems', 'education underachievement', or 'behavioural problems'. Glib, uncritical formulations are unhelpful and even harmful to patients.

Extent of behavioural problems

The true rate of learning and behaviour problems in children with epilepsy is unknown. Surveys have been carried out in various countries but comparisons are difficult because of differences in criteria and methods of assessment. However, the general picture suggests that although many children with epilepsy behave normally at school, proportionally more of them have learning and behaviour problems than their non-epileptic counterparts, i.e. children with epilepsy can be considered a high risk group for the development of such problems. A recent survey of children admitted to a special epilepsy centre [2] suggests that such behavioural problems are often overlooked because of a preoccupation with the neurological aspects of each case. The same appears to be true of family problems in this series, which were frequently identified during hospital assessment although rarely mentioned on referral.

Associated factors

Although the determinants of such problems are far from being fully understood, certain factors can be identified which might underlie an individual child's difficulties. Such factors often operate in combination.

Biological determinants include severity and type of seizure disorder, antiepileptic drug treatment and the child's sex.

Seizure disorders caused by gross cerebral lesions are likely to seriously affect intellectual capacity and behaviour and, in the case of focal lesions, may produce specific syndromes. Frequent, prolonged or frightening seizures can be a source of further damage or distress. Severity can also be judged in terms of early onset which may well carry a poor prognosis for intellectual and social development.

Drugs are an important part of treatment but, because of their incautious use, some children with epilepsy suffer avoidable adverse physical or behavioural effects [3]. Behaviour may improve strikingly when treatment is reduced or changed. Barbiturates are a particular source of behavioural problems and phenytoin has a disfiguring effect on personal appearance in some patients. Adverse effects of drugs may produce a different clinical picture in children compared with adults, even in the case of intoxication.

Broad, ambiguous categories such as 'grand mal' or 'petit mal' ought to be abandoned in favour of the more precise, clinically descriptive terms as indicated in the International Classification of Seizures [4]. This should allow anticipation of the more specific learning and behavioural problems that are associated with certain types of seizure [1]. Traditional views such as that conerning a relationship between seizures of temporal lobe origin and antisocial behaviour have recently been subjected to critical review [5].

In keeping with the findings in certain non-epileptic conditions that boys are more vulnerable than girls to physical or psychological trauma, there are indications that boys with epilepsy are especially subject to various learning and emotional problems. The biological and social factors that underlie these difficulties are not clear.

Important though the above biological factors may be in individual cases, they may account for very little of the total amount of behavioural disturbance in children with epilepsy. In contrast, psychosocial problems often appear to have direct bearing on the child's difficulties.

The still common public miconceptions about the nature of epilepsy and its consequences make it a particularly socially disadvantageous condition. Parents' reactions are often inappropriate and unhelpful to the child who may be rejected or overprotected. The same often applies at school where encouragement to succeed may be withheld and initiative stifled. Predictably, children with epilepsy (perhaps especially the more intellectually competent) become bored or frustrated in such circumstances and develop lack of confidence or self esteem. Very often an unhealthy emotional climate develops within the family as a whole. This requires close and sustained attention in its own right to allow the epileptic child to realise his potential in life.

Conclusions

Combined medical, psychological and social assessment is required to deal effectively with the complicated disorder and predicament shown by many children with epilepsy. There can be no short cuts. Basic requirements include accurate diagnosis of the type, cause and severity of the child's seizure disorder. Treatment effects (both good and bad) need to be documented accurately. Children with epilepsy should be considered at special risk of developing educational and emotional problems. The family situation and attitudes need to be ascertained as well as the emotional state of the parents and that of any sibs. Teachers' attitudes and expectations often need to be explored and the child's academic and social progress at school monitored carefully avoiding intrusiveness or overconcern. If problems arise, referral (where possible) to a special epilepsy clinic for children is highly desirable for a comprehensive reassessment to be carried out. Piecemeal and poorly integrated care of children with epilepsy can be both ineffective and a source of confusion to all concerned.

Adolescence may be a particularly difficult time and yet it is a period of life which has been very little studied from the epilepsy point of view. Although some seizures may improve with age, others may intensify at puberty and drug treatment may need adjustment because of metabolic changes. The social consequences of epilepsy can, of course, be felt more acutely by the adolescent patient who may be especially sensitive about his condition or resentful about the limitations that it imposes on his activities such as finding a job or driving.

The many and diverse problems that can be associated with childhood epilepsy exemplify the need for a multidisciplinary approach by well-informed professionals whose efforts are likely to be required over long periods of time for both the patient and his family.

References

1 Stores G. In Reynolds EH, Trimble MR, eds. *Epilepsy and Psychiatry 1981;* 33. London: Churchill Livingstone
2 Stores G. In *Proceedings of Annual Meeting of German Chapter of International League Against Epilepsy. Marburg, West Germany, October 1981;* In press
3 Stores G. In Werry JS, ed. *Pediatric Psychopharmacology. The use of behaviour modifying drugs in children 1978;* 274. New York: Brunner/Mazel
4 Gastaut H. *Epilepsia 1970; 11:* 102–113
5 Hermann BP, Stevens J. In Hermann BP, ed. *A Multidisciplinary Handbook of Epilepsy 1980;* 272. Springfield, Illinois: Thomas

25

NON-EPILEPTIC ATTACKS IN CHILDHOOD

P M Jeavons

I have previously reported [1, 2] that 20 per cent of patients referred to my epilepsy clinics did not, in my opinion, have epilepsy. In a recent survey the figure had risen to 25 per cent. If an incorrect label of epilepsy is applied to a child or adult it can have profound and regrettable consequences because of the prejudice of society, and can influence schooling, social life, and employment. Furthermore, the patient may suffer side effects from unnecessary medication. It is because epilepsy continues to be misdiagnosed that I have spent some time on diagnosis, whilst realising that much of the information will be familiar, if not naive. The most frequent misdiagnoses are shown in Table I, the commonest conditions to be mistaken for epilepsy being syncopal or vaso-vagal attacks.

TABLE I. Non-epileptic attacks

Diagnosis	Children	Adults
Syncope	87 (44%)	71 (43%)
Psychiatric	39 (20%)	62 (38%)
Migraine	12 (6%)	15 (9%)
Daydreams	9 (5%)	
Breath holding	21 (11%)	
Night terrors	11 (6%)	
Other	21 (11%)	18 (10%)
TOTALS	200	166
	366	

There are five main reasons for the misdiagnosis of epilepsy: an inadequate history, the occurrence of clonic movements, jactitation or incontinence, a family history of epilepsy, a past history of febrile convulsions, and an abnormal

224

EEG. To these must be added an inadequate knowledge of the nature of epilepsy. Epileptic attacks are brief, usually lasting seconds or minutes, they are stereotyped and repeated, often with a tendency to cluster. Although seizures may occur in relation to drowsiness, waking from sleep, anxiety, or in the premenstrual or menstrual phases, immediate precipitants are rare, apart from photosensitive epilepsy, whilst precipitating factors are almost invariable in syncopal, vaso-vagal and breath holding attacks, and in psychiatric disorders. One advantage of a special epilepsy clinic is the time available for taking a detailed history. It is absolutely essential to obtain a description of an attack from an observer, and to avoid jumping to conclusions. I have previously commented on the phrase 'known epileptic' so commonly encountered in patients' notes. This phrase can be translated 'someone has already diagnosed epilepsy so I do not need to take a history'. It is quite common, in children around puberty whose tonic-clonic seizures have been controlled by medication since early childhood, to present with an attack of loss of consciousness which is syncopal, and it may then be assumed that they have relapsed, unless an accurate description of the recent attack is obtained. One should always ask for details of any recent attack which occurs in a patient of any age who has previously been controlled by the medication. Furthermore, if a patient with primary generalised tonic-clonic seizures is not rendered free from seizures by an appropriate antiepileptic drug given in adequate dosage, one should suspect that the attacks are not epileptic. This does not apply to patients with partial seizures or secondary generalised tonic-clonic seizures.

In 1967 Lombroso and Lerman [3] described two types of breath holding spells, cyanotic and pallid, calling the latter pallid infantile syncope. Stephenson [4] called white breath holding attacks reflex anoxic seizures. The cyanotic breath holding attacks are well known and it is usually easy to obtain a history that the infant has been hurt or frustrated or frightened. The upward deviation of the eyes, stiffness of limbs, occasional incontinence and twitching or jerking movements may lead to the diagnosis of epilepsy. In pallid infantile syncope the precipitant may be less obvious, but bathing, learning to walk, new experiences, slight blows on the head, may all be precipitants.

Case history 1

Joanne's first pallid breath holding attack occurred at the age of one, after a bath. Cyanotic breath holding attacks, usually in response to frustration, started at three years and were followed by syncopal attacks precipitated by knocks or falls up to the age of 11 years. The original EEG was normal. Phenobarbitone had been prescribed up to the age of 12 and when this was withdrawn the girl became more alert and her schooling improved.

225

Case history 2

At the age of 15 months Emma had pertussis. During the third week she inspired deeply, became cyanosed and rigid, with upward deviation of her eyes, and held her breath until she went limp. Recovery was rapid. Further attacks occurred after coughing, episodes of temper, and minor pain. Presumably because of a family history of epilepsy in two aunts and of febrile convulsions in a cousin, phenobarbitone 15mg tds was prescribed, and this 'pepped her up no end'. When seen in the clinic aged 17 months she was overactive and irritable, and improved on withdrawal of phenobarbitone.

Case history 3

Christina, aged 3½ had characteristic breath holding attacks since the age of one year, precipitated by falls or frustration. She was referred because her epilepsy had not responded to medication with phenytoin 120mg daily. Her EEG had been normal. Her father had tonic-clonic seizures from the age of 8 years, treated with phenytoin. Her brother had simple absences, treated with ethosuximide. The girl had slight hyperplasia of her gums and there were considerable behavioural problems. These disappeared after withdrawal of the phenytoin, as did the breath holding attacks.

A very rare form of non-epileptic attack is benign vertigo which appears between one and three years. In the attack the child holds on to something for support, or may sit or lie down. The attack lasts less than a minute. Diagnosis usually depends on the description from the child [5, 6] of a sensation of rotation or falling. Consciousness is not lost.

Three relatively rare causes of misdiagnosis of epilepsy are daydreams, night terrors, and migraine. Daydreams may be mistaken for absences though the differentiation is usually easy. Waving a hand in front of the child's eyes will usually elicit a response in a child who is daydreaming, but not in one who has an absence. Children who daydream may smile or frown or screw up their eyes, but these responses are most unlikely in absences even if complex. Absences in an untreated child can be induced by hyperventilation. Daydreams may increase or decrease in relation to circumstances such as a change in house, or school, or friends.

Night terrors may be diagnosed as complex partial seizures because of the profound change in level of awareness and the apparent automatic behaviour and emotional disturbance, and because it is usually extremely difficult to 'get through' to a child who has a night terror. In fact, complex partial seizures occurring during sleep in children are extremely rare.

226

Case history 4

Robert was diagnosed by a paediatrician as having complex partial seizures because of having unpleasant sensations, fear, visual and auditory hallucinations and being in a semi-conscious state. The history revealed that he had had a single attack on waking from sleep, and he was white and shaking and afraid and said that noises were twice as loud as usual. His original EEG had shown slight slow activity but the second was normal. He was the youngest of three children, with a very anxious mother.

Attacks of migraine may be mistaken for epilepsy if the symptoms are focal — hemiplegic, hemianopic or sensory.

Case history 5

Moira, age 14, was referred by her family doctor with a diagnosis of focal fits. In her attacks she had a left sided headache with hemianopia and tunnel vision, and paraesthesia in the left hand. Clinical examination, EEG and neuroradiological examination were all normal. Her mother had had similar attacks of migraine in adolescence.

Since epileptic attacks are by definition episodic, episodic psychiatric symptoms may be regarded as being epileptic and evidence of psychiatric disorder was present in 20 per cent of the 200 children with non-epileptic attacks. The most common psychiatric disorders were anxiety, depression or behavioural disorder. In general the differential diagnosis depended on obtaining a psychiatric history, and an accurate account of the duration of the symptoms during the attack. Attacks which last hours are most unlikely to be epileptic (apart from status). Palpitations and 'butterflies' in the stomach may be regarded as temporal lobe phenomena. Déjà vu (not uncommon in childhood) is very brief in epilepsy, but may last for minutes or hours when it is of psychological origin. Episodic disturbances of behaviour, including aggression, especially if occurring under precipitating circumstances, are unlikely to be epilepsy.

Case history 6

Nelson, aged 5, was referred from Casualty with a diagnosis of grand mal or temporal lobe epilepsy, probably post-traumatic. He had been knocked down by a car four months previously and had been unconscious. His behaviour had altered since the accident and he had become aggressive, frequently lost his temper, screamed and kicked, but never lost consciousness. He would not go to bed until 3 am and cried in his sleep.

Hyperventilation, often following precipitating circumstances, is a common cause of non-epileptic disturbances of consciousness or behaviour. Simulation of seizures is very rare in paediatric out-patients. A number of normal physiological or psychological experiences may be regarded as abnormal and misinterpreted as indicating epilepsy. 'Funny feelings' which the child often finds impossible to describe, may be due to emotional upset. Hypnogogic hallucinations and single myoclonic jerks on falling asleep are commonly mistaken for an epileptic phenomenon. Premenstrual symptoms, mild feelings of depersonalisation or derealisation may be regarded as epileptic phenomena because they are brief, peculiar, and episodic. It is not only adults who experience such symptoms and one cannot stress too highly the importance of obtaining (and not ignoring) a history from a child, however young.

The most common misdiagnosis of epilepsy is made in children with syncopal or vaso-vagal attacks, and the most common reason for misdiagnosis appears to be a belief that jerking or incontinence indicate an epileptic fit. Jactitation is quite common, although sustained clonic movements are rare — incontinence is common. It is possible to cut the tongue when falling, though true tongue biting does not occur. Severe injury, including fracture of vertebrae, may occur in adults.

The diagnosis depends on what happened before the loss of consciousness, and what happened afterwards. In syncopal attacks there is a precipitant, and a warning sensation before consciousness is lost. Afterwards, recovery is rapid, without confusion, sleep or headache, unless the head was hit in falling, resulting in mild concussion.

Posture is commonly a factor in syncopal attacks, especially in association with prolonged standing, hot atmosphere, and sudden change in posture. Fainting is common in school assembly, whilst fits are very rare. Jactitation may often be misinterpreted by the teacher.

Other common precipitants include pain, injections, the sight of needles or syringes, the sight of blood, the sight or description of something unpleasant — TV films on accidents, operations, etc.

In girls, fainting may occur when the hair is being combed or brushed, and faints occur on getting out of the bath or going to the toilet.

Loss of consciousness is almost always preceded by some subjective sensation, often described as a funny feeling in the head, dizziness, blurring, darkening or clouding of vision, legs feeling weak, or things going 'far away'. This warning feeling may be misinterpreted as an epileptic aura. Apart from the subjective sensations, one usually obtains a history of extreme pallor and of perspiration. The pulse is slow or imperceptible in syncopal and vaso-vagal attacks, fast in a seizure.

Case history 7

Debra, age 10, was referred because of tonic-clonic seizures. At age 9 she lost consciousness whilst having her hair combed before going to school. A month later, again whilst her mother was combing her hair she said she felt funny, sat in a chair, arched backwards, shook a little, fell and cut the tip of her tongue, and was incontinent. She was not confused nor did she have a headache after the attacks, and recovery was rapid. Physical examination was normal, as was her EEG.

Case history 8

Kerry, age 6, was referred because of major fits. She had had six attacks, in all of which she had become very pale, her lips slightly cyanosed, she had stiffened and shaken a little, with a brief loss of consciousness. Recovery was always rapid. The precipitants of the attacks were: bathing of a finger abscess, witnessing her younger brother fall and cut his mouth, seeing her cousin's ears being pierced, bending her thumb back, cutting her hand, and falling and grazing her knee.

Case history 9

Elaine, aged 15, had five blackouts, the first at 11 years after she cut her finger. In all she slid to the ground, made some thrashing movements of her arms, her head jerked slightly, and she then recovered rapidly. Attacks were all precipitated by injury or the sight of her own blood, and one attack occurred with a painful period. She would go grey if her blood was taken, but was not affected by injections, or the sight of other peoples' blood. She worked in a butcher's shop. She had not improved with phenytoin which was withdrawn.

Case history 10

Stephen, age 13, was referred because his epilepsy had not responded to phenytoin and later to carbamazepine, despite apparently satisfactory serum levels. His first attack followed a severe reprimand from his mother. He went pale, fell, made mouthing movements and salivated. There were some limb movements but these (on direct questioning) were not clonic. A further attack occurred when he was severely reprimanded at school, and this frightened the teacher. He had an attack whilst watching a film on road accidents. He had four attacks, on each occasion of an EEG examination, stick-on electrodes being used. His mother commented that he disliked having his head touched in any way. All his attacks were preceded by a feeling of dizziness.

Finally, the effect of misdiagnosis on a child's future is indicated by the following case history.

Case history 11

Stephen, age 16, had been under the care of a neurologist who stated that there was no doubt about the diagnosis of epilepsy. He had originally been treated with phenobarbitone and later with phenytoin. There was a history of behaviour problems and he had been treated at a child guidance clinic. He had recently been working on a farm and been very happy and wished to take up farming as a career, but had been refused because he could not apply in due course for a driving licence, because of his continuing epilepsy. He had had five attacks, one when standing in church, one when watching a film on industrial accidents, one in a hot classroom, one when watching a demonstration. The account of the latter was obtained from the lecturer. He collapsed, was slightly stiff and there was a slight twitch in his left arm. His face was ashen. He was not confused on recovery. At the time of his EEG when the electrode jelly was being applied, using a syringe and blunt needle, he had a severe syncopal attack. The label of epilepsy was removed and medication withdrawn permitting the possibility of obtaining a driving licence and thus entering on a chosen career.

References

1   Jeavons PM. *Update 1975; 10:* 269–280
2   Jeavons PM. In Mani KS, Walker AE, Tandon PN, eds. *Proceedings of the National Seminar on Epilepsy 1976;* 85. Bangalore: Indian Epilepsy Association
3   Lombroso CT, Lerman P. *Paediatrics 1967; 39:* 563–581
4   Stephenson JBP. *Arch Dis Childh 1978; 53:* 193–200
5   Bower BD. *Br J Hosp Med 1974; 12:* 527–534
6   Chutorian AM. *Dev Med Child Neurol 1972; 14:* 513–515

26

THE BENIGN EPILEPSIES OF CHILDHOOD

J Aicardi

The term 'benign epilepsy', as used in this chapter, refers to the chronic convulsive disorders of childhood whose natural course is predictably towards a prolonged, and apparently definitive, remission in at least 90–95 per cent of the cases before the patients reach adulthood. The epilepsies which produce severe seizures, capable of leaving residua are not included, even though remission is obtained. Febrile or other occasional epileptic seizures are also not considered.

Although a number of epilepsies of childhood often run a fairly benign course (e.g. petit mal, many cases of idiopathic grand mal, some myoclonic epilepsies), they cannot be termed 'benign' according to the above definition, since their remission rate is unpredictable and usually of the order of 70–80 per cent at most [1–5]. The benign epilepsies of childhood at this moment are represented mainly by the syndrome of Benign Epilepsy of Childhood with Rolandic Spikes (BECRS) [5–7], but other benign epileptic syndromes have been reported, even though their delineation is not yet complete or generally accepted. These various syndromes will be reviewed successively.

Benign Epilepsy of Childhood with Rolandic Spikes (BECRS) or benign partial epilepsy of childhood

BECRS is defined by four main criteria:

1. An onset between 2 and 14 years of age, mostly between 6 and 10 years.

2. The occurrence of partial seizures in 80 per cent of the patients, electively involving the face and mouth, and related to sleep in 75 per cent of the cases.

3. The presence in the EEG of a focus of sharp waves or spikes, typically recorded on the lowermost Rolandic area, appearing on a normal background record.

231

4. Neurological and intellectual normality.

These criteria may be present simultaneously or in succession and some of them may be missing at any one examination, but the diagnosis is easy in most patients as the fits and the EEG are fairly characteristic.

The seizures may be generalised (often secondarily and especially during deep, middle of the night, sleep), unilateral or partial, the latter being most common [5,6]. Seizures involving the face are of two types [8], simple and complex. Simple seizures occur mainly when the patient is awake and consist only of a conscious tonic or clonic contraction of one side of the face, of very brief duration, at times accompanied by paraesthesiae in the same territory or inside the mouth; occasionally paraesthesiae may be the only manifestation of a seizure [5]. Complex seizures occur most commonly during sleep, especially during the first hour after falling asleep or during the two hours that precede awakening. They are marked by a tonic contraction of the jaw and/or pharynx, by rhythmical jaw motions, sialorrhoea (30 per cent of the cases) or inability to speak ('aphemia') in spite of the preservation of language mechanisms and comprehension (40 per cent of the cases). These seizures are often noticed because of the chuckling and

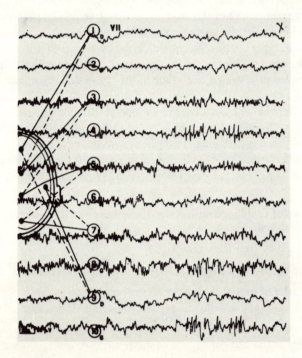

Figure 1. Benign epilepsy with Rolandic spikes. Repetitive spikes at 4Hz over the left temporo-central area

232

gurgling noises produced, which awaken the parents, but the child is entirely conscious and recalls the attack.

The EEG shows a unilateral spike or sharp wave focus in 70 per cent of the patients [6]. The spikes often occur in repetitive trains and have a characteristic shape (Figure 1), although many variants are possible. The foci are bilateral and asynchronous in 30 per cent of the cases. Their location may vary from one record to the next, although an anterior temporal location is not observed. The foci may shift from one hemisphere to the other, and they are apt to disappear and reappear suddenly, their shape, rhythm and voltage being quite variable in any given patient. These modifications bear no relation to the clinical course so that the EEG should not be used as a guide to therapy [5]. In a few patients

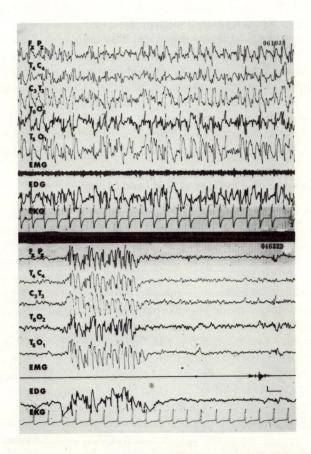

Figure 2. Partial epilepsy with Rolandic focus. Intense and diffuse paroxysmal activity during slow wave sleep (upper trace). Diffuse paroxysmal bursts during REM sleep

233

paroxysms consistently cannot be obtained in awake records, which is a definite indication for a sleep tracing, as it is not possible to accept a diagnosis of BECRS without EEG evidence. In fact, the rate of discharges is considerably increased during sleep, even during REM sleep [5,9,10]. The spikes may increase only in frequency or also in amplitude and diffusion. In occasional patients, extremely intense and diffuse paroxysmal activity may be seen (Figure 2).

The outcome of BECRS is almost constantly favourable, the epilepsy remitting by 12 years in 92 per cent of patients, and in 99 per cent by 17 years [6]. The rare patient may develop a second epileptic syndrome, in my experience primary generalised epilepsy. Treatment with carbamazepine or other drugs is very effective in 60 per cent of the patients. Considering the benign course and character of the symptoms, therapeutic escalation should be avoided, even in those patients who respond poorly or not at all to monotherapy [6], as they do not differ from the others in their ultimate outcome.

Despite the sharply localised seizures and EEG paroxysms, BECRS is not a lesional epilepsy and CT scan or other neuroradiological investigations are not indicated when there is a typical electroclinical picture. Genetic factors play a central role in its aetiology. According to Heijbel et al, BECRS is transmitted as a dominant trait which, however, is often expressed only in the EEG [11], and is manifested during only a limited period of life (3–15 years). BECRS is very common, the incidence being 15 to 25 per cent of all the epilepsies in school age children [2,7], an incidence vastly in excess of that of petit mal epilepsy.

Atypical Benign Partial Epilepsy of Childhood (ABPEC)

Since 1974, several workers [13–18] have reported cases that shared some of the features of BECRS but that also displayed unusual clinical and EEG phenomena, especially absence seizures [13,14], an intense paroxysmal EEG activity during sleep [14,15,18], and bursts of spike-wave complexes at various rhythms while awake [14,19]. Some of the authors who studied this problem were mainly interested in the relationship that, they thought, existed between BECRS and primary generalised epilepsy, a relationship illustrated by the co-existence of typical partial seizures and EEG spikes with absences of the petit mal type associated with generalised 3Hz spike-wave bursts during wakefulness or sleep [13]. Other authors [14,15,18] emphasised the EEG abnormalities seen in some children who, initially, presented as typical cases of BECRS, and related them to the condition earlier described by Patry et al [20] as "Electrical Status Epilepticus during Sleep", a clinical syndrome of absences and intellectual and behavioural deterioration, associated with the EEG changes. Still others drew attention to the resemblance of these unusual cases with the Lennox-Gastaut syndrome and warned of the dangers of misdiagnosis [17].

These reported cases are probably heterogeneous from the clinical, EEG and aetiological viewpoints. In particular, the paroxysmal EEG activity during slow

234

wave sleep is said to be uninterrupted and to occur every night for years in some reports [14,18], whilst it seems to be less consistent, or has been less extensively studied in others [13,19]. This activity is probably not specific for any one type of epilepsy: Morikawa et al [10] have shown that similar tracings can be recorded in various types of partial epilepsy in children, including epilepsies with partial complex seizures. From the point of view of aetiology, this electro-clinical picture can be observed both with lesional and nonlesional epileptic foci. Dalla Bernardina et al [14] reported it in association with infantile hemiplegia and Marikawa et al reported briefly on six children with "combined sylvian and absence seizures", most of them displaying "psychomotor retardation and positive findings on their CT scans" [16].

We believe [19] that, among this group of patients, there exists an uncommon, but relatively well defined, epileptic syndrome that is important to recognise, as it resembles the Lennox-Gastaut syndrome or other severe myoclonic epilepsies for which it is regularly mistaken. This syndrome is characterised by the following features:

1. Its onset is between two and six years of age.

2. Affected children have developed normally before the onset of the seizures, have no neurological deficits, and continue to be normal in spite of frequently repeated fits.

3. They all have two or more types of seizures. These include partial motor seizures during sleep, reminiscent of those in BECRS, absences, generalised tonic-clonic fits and, especially, myoclonic and/or atonic seizures, which may be repeated many times daily and often supervene in clusters separated by free periods lasting several months.

4. The EEGs during sleep, and even in the drowsy state, record an intense, bilateral, if not always symmetrical, slow spike-wave activity which persists throughout the stages of slow wave sleep, even though it is not necessarily continuous. This activity is recorded during the periods when seizure activity is also intense.

5. The awake EEG tracings are much less abnormal (although in two children a continuous spike-wave activity was present with the eyes closed and disappeared on eye opening) (Figure 3). During active periods, bursts of 3Hz spike-waves are often seen. Spike foci, often with contralateral diffusion, are recorded in at least part of the waking records.

Although the repeated falls and the continuous, high voltage, slow spike-wave activity are reminiscent of the Lennox-Gastaut syndrome, certain features can suggest the correct diagnosis: the persistence of a normal mental and neurological functioning in the face of repeated fits; the frequent occurrence, especially at onset, of nocturnal partial motor seizures; the absence of tonic fits; the gross contrast between the waking and sleep EEGs; the presence of focal spikes in a

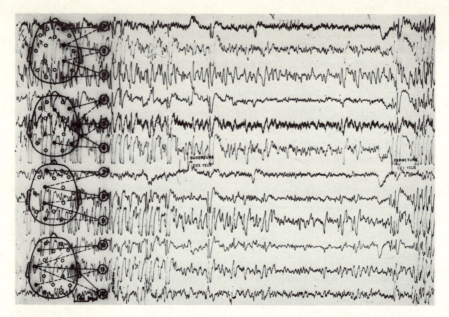

Figure 3. A typical partial benign epilepsy. High amplitude, diffuse slow spike-waves with eyes closed. Suppression of paroxysmal activity while the eyes are open

Rolandic or parietal location in at least some records.

The course seems to be a self-limited one: seven of our nine patients were apparently cured before eight years of age, although a longer follow up is necessary. Bad periods, that last weeks or months, alternate with relatively fit-free periods. No mental deterioration or severe behaviour disorder is ever observed. Antiepileptic drugs seem to be of no avail against fits or EEG abnormalities during the bad periods, so that polytherapy and dosage escalation are useless and dangerous.

This syndrome might represent a very atypical form of BECRS but its mechanism is unknown, and its exact limits remain to be determined.

Benign Affective Epilepsy of Childhood (BAEC)

Under this heading, Dalla Bernardina et al [21] have reported on 20 children with an epileptic syndrome which displayed the following features:

1. The onset is between three and ten years of age.

2. The mental and neurological development is normal both before and after onset of the fits.

3. The seizures are only of one type: partial complex seizures remarkable for the predominance of affective components, i.e. expression of terror, screaming

236

etc. Motor signs and symptoms are limited to a few chewing or swallowing automatisms, occasionally with unilateral facial twitching. Consciousness is preserved. The seizures are often reported several times daily and occur in the same form during night and day.

4. The EEG may show interictal, central spikes or occasional bilateral spike-waves, similar to the tracings in BECRS or it may be normal. Ictal EEGs record typical partial seizures (Figure 4).

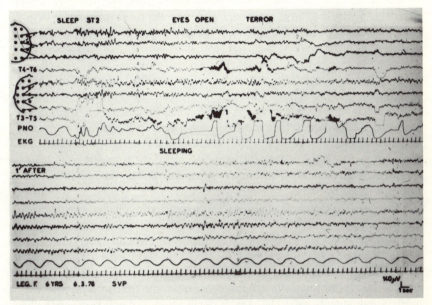

Figure 4. Ictal discharge in a 5-year old boy with 'benign affective epilepsy'. Left sided temporo-central rhythmic activity concomitant with a brief nocturnal seizure with fear. PNO = respiration

The course is said to be consistently favourable. Treatment is rapidly effective and eventual complete remission can be expected before 15–16 years.

The report by Dalla Bernardina et al draws attention to the often overlooked fact that 'psychomotor' (partial complex) seizures, usually regarded as particularly resistant to treatment, are capable of remitting completely before adulthood is reached. The same conclusion has been reached by Lindsay et al [22] who showed that one-third of their children with 'temporal lobe epilepsy' had achieved complete remission after a 25-year follow-up.

The retrospective character of the study, as well as the lack of precision on the total series from which the reported patients were drawn and on the criteria upon which they were selected, makes it difficult to determine whether the syndrome of BAEC can be recognised as such early enough for its categorisation to be meaningful. The answer to this essential question must await further studies.

237

Other benign epileptic syndromes of infancy and childhood

Benign Partial Epilepsy with Occipital Spike Waves has been described by Gastaut [23].

Benign Sensory-Motor Epilepsy with Parietal Spikes is considered by De Marco and Tassinari to be distinct from BECRS [24,25]. It is characterised by the occurrence of giant evoked somatosensory potentials, produced over the parietal area by tapping the heel, contralaterally to the stimulus or bilaterally. The evoked parietal spikes often precede the seizures by several years and probably remain isolated in a large majority. Later on, a parietal spike focus may appear during sleep, then during wakefulness. Clinical seizures may then develop, which are usually of an adversive type and tend to supervene with a low frequency. They remit spontaneously within one year in almost all patients.

Although the benign epileptic syndromes so described belong to the partial epilepsies, some syndromes featuring generalised seizures may also be tentatively considered as benign. This may apply to petit mal (or absence epilepsy) or at least to one type of petit mal: that which begins between four and eight years of age, responds rapidly to treatment, features only typical absences to the exclusion of any other seizure type, and remits before the age of ten to twelve years. The existence of such a benign type, however, is based only on clinical impression and further data are obviously necessary.

Dravet et al have described cases of early myoclonic epilepsy, responding very rapidly to drugs (valproate or ethosuximide) and remitting after only a few years of treatment [26]. The myoclonias were mainly of the axial type, brief, accompanied by short bursts of irregular fast (3Hz) spike-waves on a basically normal record. They represented the only type of seizures and their onset was before one year of age. Although benign forms of myoclonic epilepsy with such characteristics undoubtedly exist [1], it is, at the moment, difficult to separate them early from the more severe types. The condition is distinct from the 'Benign myoclonus of early infancy' described by Lombroso and Fejerman [27] which presents like infantile spasms occurring in series more than brief myoclonias. The jerks, in this condition, are unaccompanied by any EEG abnormality and are not of an epileptic nature.

It seems possible that other benign epileptic syndromes will be recognised in the future. In the present stage of knowledge however, it is probably wise to accept only the well-established and easily recognisable syndromes (e.g. BECRS) regularly associated with a very high remission rate, if the concept of benign epilepsy is to maintain its usefulness. More information on the other syndromes is highly desirable since their recognition may avoid tragic diagnostic mistakes, with their serious consequences on prognosis and management. Every effort should be made to recognise the benign epilepsies that should not be made 'malignant' by improper counselling or therapy.

238

References

1   Aicardi J, Chevrie JJ. *Neuropaediatrie 1971; 3:* 177–190
2   Emerson R, D'Souza BJ, Vining EP et al. *N Engl J Med 1981; 304:* 1125–1129
3   Holowach J, Thurston DL, O'Leary J. *N Engl J Med 1972; 286:* 169–174
4   Juul-Jensen P. *Epilepsia 1964; 5:* 4, 352–363
5   O'Donohoe NV. *Epilepsies of Childhood 1979.* London: Butterworth
6   Beaussart M, Loiseau P. In Lugaresi E, Pazzaglia P, Tassinari CA, eds. *Evolution and Prognosis of Epilepsies 1973.* Bologna: Aulo Gaggi
7   Heijbel J, Blom S, Bergfors PG. *Epilepsia 1975; 16:* 657
8   Loiseau P, Beaussart M. *Epilepsia 1973; 14:* 381–389
9   Dalla Bernardina B, Beghini V. *Epilepsia 1976; 17:* 161–167
10   Morikawa T, Osawa T, Ishara O, Seino M. *Brain Develop 1979; 1:* 257–265
11   Heijbel J, Blom S, Rasmusson M. *Epilepsia 1975; 16:* 285–293
12   Cavazzuti GB. *Epilepsia 1980; 21:* 57–62
13   Beaumanoir A, Ballis T, Varfis G, Ansari K. *Epilepsia 1974; 15:* 301–315
14   Dalla Bernardina B, Tassinari CA, Dravet C et al. *Rev EEG Neurophysiol 1978; 8:* 350–353
15   Laurette G, Arfel G. *Rev EEG Neurophysiol 1976; 6:* 137–139
16   Morikawa T, Osawa T, Seino M. *Brain Develop 1980; 2:* 262
17   Rucquoy-Ponsar M, Mechler M, Sorel L. *Compte-rendu des Journées de la Société Belge de Pédiatrie, Bruxelles 1975*
18   Tassinari CA, Terzano G, Capocchi G et al. In Penry JK, ed. *Epilepsy, the 8th International Symposium 1977:* 345–354. New York: Raven Press
19   Aicardi J, Chevrie JJ. *Develop Med Child Neurol 1982:* in press
20   Patry G, Lyagoubi S, Tassinari CA. *Arch Neurol 1971; 24:* 242–252
21   Dalla Bernardina B, Bureau M, Dravet C et al. *Rev EEG Neurophysiol 1980; 10:* 8–18
22   Lindsay J, Ounsted C, Richards P. *Develop Med Child Neurol 1979; 21:* 285–298
23   Gastaut H. A new type of epilepsy: Benign partial epilepsy of childhood with occipital spike-wave. *Clinical EEG 1982; 13:* 13–22
24   De Marco P. *Arch Neurol 1980; 37:* 291–292
25   De Marco P, Tassinari CA. *Epilepsia 1981; 22:* 569–575
26   Dravet C. *Rev EEG Neurophysiol 1981:* in press
27   Lombroso CT, Fejerman N. *Ann Neurol 1977; 1:* 138–143

27

BENIGN FOCAL EPILEPSY OF CHILDHOOD

N V O'Donohoe

In a recent historical review of epilepsy, Sir Denis Hill [1] commented on the surprising fact that, only 20 years ago, epilepsy alone or epilepsy 'per se', as it was called (that is, epilepsy unassociated with mental abnormality or psychosis) was still regarded by many internationally known physicians and psychiatrists as having a uniformly poor prognosis. The concept of the epileptic personality, with its implication of a constitutionally hereditary psychopathic make-up, was still flourishing and played a major role in causing the enormous stigma which attached to the individual with epilepsy, making him a person apart and one doomed to inevitable failure in life and to intellectual, moral and social deterioration.

Fortunately, the great advances in the understanding and diagnosis of epilepsy in this century and the increasing awareness of the many epileptic syndromes which may occur have led to improvements in these attitudes. It is now realised that, especially in childhood, a number of the epilepsies pursue a natural history to full recovery in a majority of cases. This is especially true of those epilepsies characterised by normal intellect and by the lack of any demonstrable brain damage or neurological deficit. These include primary generalised epilepsy of the petit mal type, primary generalised tonic-clonic seizures (grand mal) and photo-sensitive epilepsy. In all of these disorders, genetic factors are important in the aetiology. These epilepsies are generalised but there is also a well-recognised partial epilepsy occurring in childhood with an excellent prognosis.

The International Classification of Epileptic Seizures [2] recognised a sub-division of partial seizures into those of simple and complex symptomatology. In the former, the clinical phenomena are determined by the part and side of the brain involved by the epileptogenic focus and mixtures of motor and sensory symptoms occur. Nayrac and Beaussart [3] described what is now recognised as the most frequently occurring partial epilepsy in childhood and it has been variously called benign focal or benign centro-temporal epilepsy of childhood, Sylvian or Rolandic epilepsy (because of the situation of the EEG abnormality), and the lingual syndrome. This epilepsy has an incidence of 16 per cent among children affected by epilepsy [4] which is four times the incidence of true petit mal. A ready response to therapy and an excellent prognosis for permanent clinical remission soon after puberty or by the middle teens are the general experience, but the EEG may take longer to revert to normal.

Benign focal epilepsy occurs in both sexes, usually presents between seven and ten years of age, and its most characteristic feature is the relationship of the attacks, in over three-quarters of the patients, with sleep. Nocturnal attacks may occur at any time of night and usually commence as partial seizures which become rapidly generalised. They may first be observed by parents when the child falls asleep during a long car journey as, for example, when the family is going on holiday. Diurnal attacks, which may occur in about 20 per cent of affected patients, are characteristically partial and are associated with hemifacial twitching and with oropharyngeal motor and sensory phenomena consisting of salivation, drooling, gurgling, contractions of the jaw, peculiar tongue sensations, feelings of suffocation, and an inability to speak without impairment of hearing or comprehension of speech. The bilateral oropharyngeal motor and sensory changes have been explained on the basis of bilateral cortical representation of mouth, tongue and throat.

A personal series of 66 children with the clinical features of this variety of epilepsy was studied retrospectively [5]. As in other reported series, boys outnumbered girls (37 to 29). Birth history and development were normal in all and the mean age of onset was eight and a half years. The usual time of onset is between seven and ten years of age; it rarely begins before three years, is uncommon before seven and rarely starts after the age of 12 [6].

Familial predisposition to seizure disorders was evident in a number of cases. There were three children who had siblings with a similar epilepsy and parents of two of the children had been affected in childhood in the same way. Furthermore, six children had siblings who had experienced febrile convulsions and, in one case, both parents had had febrile seizures.

The convulsions were described as generalised in 34 cases, partial in 16 cases, and of both types in 16 cases. Occasional attacks were recorded in 41 children, moderately frequent attacks in 12, and frequent seizures occurred in six. Of the remaining seven children, six had a single convulsion and one had only two attacks. This relative infrequency of seizures accords with the observation [7] that three-quarters of the children have less than five seizures ever and only 8 to 10 per cent have numerous attacks.

The seizures were experienced at night by 39 children, were nocturnal and diurnal in 19, and were exclusively diurnal in eight patients. In 16 children, numbness of lips, tongue and mouth was complained of, usually associated with an inability to speak. Hemifacial twitching was noted in eight, paraesthesiae of the limbs were experienced in five, and twitching of an arm or leg or weakness of a limb occurred in 10 children.

The characteristic EEG pattern is one of a normal background activity combined with spike discharges in the inferior Rolandic area. Unilateral discharges of this nature were observed in all but five cases in this series and the remaining cases had bilateral discharges. It is important to note that similar discharges may be found in normal children of school age who do not have epilepsy but may have learning difficulties [8].

After a mean follow-up of four and a half years, complete remission occurred in 52 patients and another 12 had infrequent seizures. Only two children continued to have frequent attacks, and, in such circumstances, the validity of the 'benign' diagnosis should be questioned. Various drugs were employed, usually phenobarbitone in the 1960s and carbamazepine in the 1970s. Dosage was usually modest in amount. Carbamazepine is the drug of choice for this epilepsy and often controls it in apparently sub-therapeutic dosage and even in a single dose at bedtime. It is possible that many cases would do well without any drug therapy but, nevertheless, the effective use of carbamazepine promotes confidence and trust among parents and should be employed when recurrent attacks are a feature.

Genetic factors seem to play an important part in causing this epilepsy and Heijbel et al [9] favour an autosomal dominant inheritance with an age-dependent penetrance which reaches its maximum between 5 and 15 years of age. The presumed functional disturbance in the brain causing the epilepsy gradually disappears as maturation into puberty and adolescence proceeds. Epileptic propensities of this nature, however, usually result in generalised rather than partial epilepsies and perhaps there is some other local factor in the brain combining with genetic influences to produce a focal disturbance. There may, for example, be an element of minimal brain damage or other local abnormality which combines with the constitutional or inherited epileptic tendency to produce a clinical partial epilepsy at a particular age.

The clear definition of this epilepsy has been an important advance. Advances in epileptology concern concept and terminology as much as therapy and the recognition of the benign or functional epilepsies has been beneficial for parents and patients. It has enabled the paediatrician to give exact information to parents about the natural history and prognosis, thereby allaying unnecessary anguish and concern about the diagnosis and avoiding reactive emotional disturbance in the child.

References

1   Hill D. In Reynolds EG, Trimble MR, eds. *Epilepsy and Psychiatry 1981;* 1—11. Edinburgh, London, Melbourne, New York: Churchill Livingstone
2   Gastaut H. *Epilepsia 1969; 10:* Suppl 2—21
3   Nayrac P, Beaussart M. *Rev Neurol (Paris) 1958; 99:* 201—206
4   Heijbel J, Blom S, Bergfors PG. *Epilepsia 1975; 16:* 657—664
5   O'Donohoe NV. *Irish Med J 1980; 73:* Suppl 62—65

6   Beaussart M, Loiseau P. In Lugaresi E, Pazzaglia P, Tassinari CA, eds. *Evolution and Prognosis of Epilepsies 1973;* 215. Bologna: Italseber

7   Aicardi J. *Brain and Development 1979; 1:* 71–73

8   Eeg-Olofsson O, Petersen I, Sellden U. *Neuropädiatrie 1971; 2:* 375–404

9   Heijbel J, Blom S, Rasmuson M. *Epilepsia 1975; 16:* 285–293

28

FEBRILE CONVULSIONS AND REFLEX ANOXIC SEIZURES

J B P Stephenson

The term 'febrile convulsion' is commonly applied to any seizure accompanying fever, whether convulsive or not. The difficulties encountered in this definition are discussed elsewhere [1]. In this chapter I develop the hypothesis that several distinct genetic and non-genetic mechanisms are implicated, and in particular to delineate the non-epileptic 'anoxic' mechanism.

The theoretical framework is displayed in Table I. The *anoxic* mechanism implies that the seizure is in effect febrile syncope [2]. This aspect will be elaborated later in the chapter, but here it should be noted that this concept has recently been extended to the pathogenesis of 'cot death' [3]. If true, there should be an excess of cot deaths in siblings of children with (anoxic) febrile seizures, and vice versa: evidence on this point is not yet available.

TABLE I. Febrile convulsion interactions – theoretical

Anoxic	Epileptic
Convulsive syncope	Generalised
Simple Syncope	Partial – temporal lobe epilepsy
(? cot death)	– benign focal epilepsy of childhood
	– extreme somatosensory evoked potentials
Anoxic-Epileptic	
Cerebral pathology	
chronic } { overt	
acute } { subtle	
absent	

244

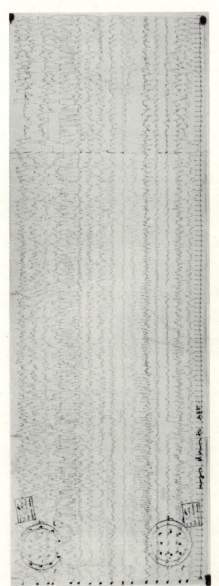

Figure 1. Onset of brief febrile seizure in otherwise normal 1½ year old girl. Spikes begin in left anterior temporal region. Transient right-sided weakness followed

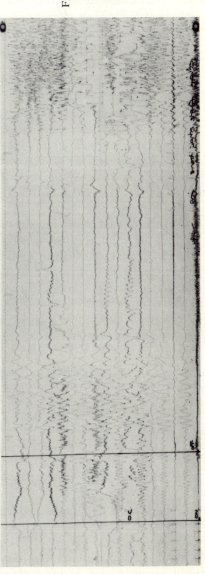

Figure 2. An experimental 'anoxic-epileptic' seizure induced by ocular compression: EEG and ECG channels (montage not important). See text

245

Epileptic mechanisms for febrile seizures are best known but the genetic subdivisions are only now being clarified. A generalised epileptic mechanism is most widely recognised [4], but genetic links to temporal lobe epilepsy (TLE) [5], benign focal epilepsy of childhood (BFEC) [6, 7], and somatomotor seizures with extreme somatosensory evoked potentials (ESEP) [8] have been described. In general it is clear that, when epilepsies evolve after febrile seizures with an uncomplicated epileptic mechanism, then the epilepsies are likely to be benign, and in any case an epileptic outcome is improbable [9]. Direct recordings of brief febrile seizures of any of these types are very rare. One of generalised spike-wave manifestation was reproduced by the injection of sulphur oil in a susceptible child [10]; the EEG onset of a febrile seizure from the left anterior temporal region is illustrated in Figure 1.

The title *anoxic-epileptic* in Table I refers to a hypothetical interaction whereby an anoxic seizure would itself induce an epileptic seizure. The experimental induction of such a seizure is illustrated in Figure 2, in which ocular compression induced cardiac asystole after which the resultant EEG flattening was followed not by the usual recovery delta activity but by generalised spiking and then spike and wave with clonic jerking. In this example the induced seizure exactly reproduced the child's spontaneous attacks which in fact followed noxious stimuli rather than fever.

Population studies, in particular that of Nelson and Ellenberger [9, 11], have clarified the role of *cerebral pathology* of *chronic* type in the genesis of febrile seizures. In the terminology of Table I, *overt* refers to a child definitely abnormal before the first fit, and *subtle* to a child with suspect neuro-developmental status. Most authors exclude these with *acute* cerebral pathology from the definition of febrile seizures, but it makes more sense to make no such exclusion [1].

In a recent unpublished study of pyogenic meningitis I have found that 27 per cent of children who presented with generalised seizures solely before admission

TABLE II. Pyogenic meningitis in children (253 attacks)

Seizures solely before admission		Febrile convulsion predisposition
Generalised	26	7 (27%)
Hemi-(unilateral)	10	0

to hospital had a predisposition to febrile seizures (Table II). By predisposition is meant a history of febrile seizures before the attack of meningitis, or at a later date, and/or a family history of febrile seizures in siblings. No such predisposition was evident when the presenting seizures were hemi-clonic and it is likely that here acute cerebral pathology was the more important factor [12].

246

I would now like to turn to personal studies of the *anoxic* mechanism, which followed the earlier work of McGreal [13, 14] and Gastaut [15]. The diagnostic tool in these studies was the vagal-mediated oculocardiac reflex which has been shown to be especially sensitive, with the induction of asystole and consequent anoxic seizures, in 'white' breath holding attacks and reflex anoxic seizures [16–18]. Gastaut showed that anoxic seizures could be induced by this method in a substantial percentage of children with febrile convulsions [15], and I extended this by looking at the response to ocular compression in 100 children with different subtypes of febrile seizures [2].

Between 1977 and 1978, a total of 630 consecutive children aged seven years or less presenting for EEG after one or more febrile seizures were studied by ocular compression, as previously described [17, 18]. The children were divided entirely on clinical grounds, into four groups, 'anoxic', 'hemi', 'cerebral pathology', and 'others' (Figure 3). 'Anoxic' indicates that the febrile seizure resembled an ordinary pain-induced reflex anoxic seizure, being predominantly tonic. 'Hemi'

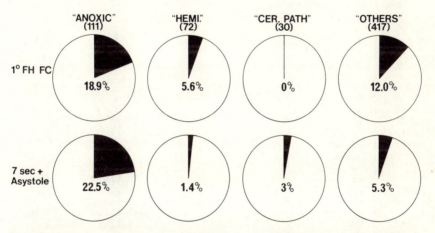

Figure 3. Ocular compression study of 630 children with febrile seizures, in four clinical groupings (see text). Top row shows percentage with first degree relative with febrile seizures. Bottom row shows percentage with grossly prolonged asystole

refers to lateralised, commonly hemi-clonic seizures. Those under the heading 'Cerebral pathology' had overt evidence of acute or chronic cerebral pathology preceding the febrile seizure, for example pyogenic meningitis, herpes simplex encephalitis, hydrocephalus, spastic tetraplegia. Those who could not be classified into these three groups were called 'others'. It is evident that those whose febrile seizures were on clinical grounds 'anoxic' frequently had very long asystole on ocular compression and had a first degree relative affected by febrile seizures, while the unclassified 'others' were intermediate between the 'anoxic' and the

247

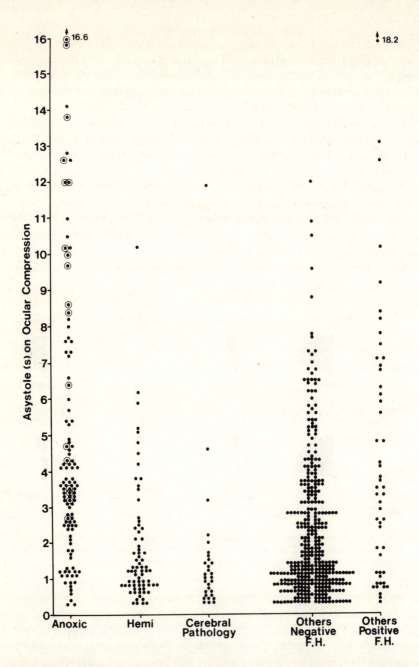

Figure 4. Individual ocular compression asystole values in 630 children with febrile seizures. The circled dots are 18 children who had reflex anoxic seizures from other stimuli as well as febrile convulsions. The 'others' are divided into those with and without a positive family history of febrile seizures in first degree relatives

248

'hemi' and 'cerebral pathology' groups. The individual asystole values are displayed in Figure 4. The 'others' are divided into those with and without a positive family history of febrile seizures in first degree relatives, and those of the 'anoxic' group who also had ordinary reflex anoxic seizures (from pain, emotion, etc.) are separately identified. It is apparent that (1) the children with seizures triggered both by fever and by unpleasant stimuli all have prolonged asystole, mostly of gross degree and (2) a positive family history for febrile seizures delineates a sub-population of the unclassified 'others' with a pattern of ocular compression response similar to those of the 'anoxic' group who had seizures solely with fever.

The observation that seizures can be triggered by both fever and other noxious stimuli such as pain in the same child suggests a common mechanism. The best defined non-febrile trigger for reflex anoxic seizures is a pain or bump [16, 19]. The combination of fever and pain as triggers has been noted by Lennox-Buchthal [20] "the child with febrile convulsions (an estimated 5 to 10 per cent) may have an occasional afebrile convulsion, usually one or two, and often under certain circumstances such as after a *slight blow to the head* or during violent struggling or crying" (my italics). Similar observations were made in the unpublished study of fits in young persons [21]. I therefore compared a group of children who had seizures exclusively triggered by blows to the head (Table III) and another group who had the combination of fever and pain (mainly head bumps) as triggers (Table IV). It is clear from these tables that the two groups are identical in their grossly exaggerated ocular compression response. Further, there was a close concordance between the type of febrile seizure described in any given child and the

TABLE III. Motor anoxic seizures (convulsive syncope) exclusively after bumps to the head

Number of children examined	29
aged three years or over at test	20 (range 17 months to 7½ years)
7+ seconds asystole on ocular compression	18 (62%)
EEG spikes	1 (left occipital)

TABLE IV. Febrile convulsions and pain-induced seizures in the same child

Number of children examined	28
aged three years or over at test	20 (ragne 10 months to 14 years)
head bump a trigger	13
7+ seconds asystole on ocular compression	18 (64%)
EEG spikes	0
Fever/pain seizure type concordance	21 (75%)

TABLE V. Seizure type concordance – fever and pain triggers

			PAIN or BUMP			
		Tonic	Jerks	Limp	?	Total
FEVER	Tonic	11	1	–	–	12
	Jerks	2	8	–	–	10
	Limp	–	–	2	–	2
	?	2	–	1	1	4
	Total	15	9	3	1	28

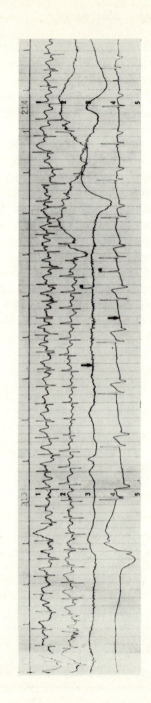

Figure 5. Effect of a bump to the head in a two year old: four sequential 16 second epochs from the ECG channel of an ambulatory ECG/EEG monitor. There was 22 seconds asystole and a pure anoxic motor seizure. The arrows mark the beginning and the end of the anoxic flattening seen on the simultaneous EEG trace; x indicates transcription artefact

seizure induced by the head bump or other painful stimulus (Table V). Since we now know that seizures induced by head bumps are anoxic seizures (convulsive syncope) mediated by reflex cardiac asystole (Figure 5), it follows that the concordant febrile seizures should have the same anoxic mechanism. Doubtless such febrile syncopes, convulsive or otherwise, continue into adolescence and even adulthood.

The relationship of oculocardiac sensitivity to febrile seizure hereditability, as suggested by the data in Figure 4, is more speculative. I have previously suggested [2] that prolonged asystole on ocular compression implies an anoxic mechanism such as must be the case in children who have *both* fever and pain triggered seizures. An alternative explanation for the others might be that cardiac sensitivity to ocular compression parallels the 'epileptic' convulsive threshold. It is now known that the cell bodies of the vagal neurones which inhibit the heart lie in the nucleus ambiguus [22]. Injection of bicuculline into the nucleus ambiguus leads to sinus arrest [23] reversed by the GABA-agonist muscinol, and further experiments have shown that GABA inhibition is powerful in physiological control at this site [24], that is, a state of reduced GABAergic inhibition would be associated with increased vagal activity and presumably a greater sensitivity of the oculocardiac reflex. If GABA activity in nucleus ambiguus neurones parallels the level of anti-convulsive (anti-epileptic) GABAergic inhibition, then the sensitivity of the oculo-cardiac reflex might be a genetic marker reflecting the epileptic convulsive threshold.

Evidence to support such a speculation would have bearing on treatment or prophylaxis of febrile seizures. In a single study [25] GABA was found to be reduced in the CSF of children with febrile convulsions, and the use of GABA agonists deserves further study. In cases where a purely anoxic mechanism, vagally mediated, is presumed, then atropine sulphate would, I think, be contraindicated because of its ability to reverse the central cholinergic mechanisms [26] of temperature regulation. By contrast, atropine methonitrate [27], although it also inhibits sweating, will not slow heat loss if the ambient temperature is kept low, and merits a controlled trial.

Conclusion

Febrile seizures — predominantly convulsive — depend on the interplay of pyrogenic infections with (1) syncopal (anoxic) mechanisms, (2) genetic (benign) epilepsies and (3) cerebral pathology, acute or chronic. One or more of these three factors may co-exist. Febrile convulsive syncope, not confined to young children, is a non-epileptic condition characterised by an exquisitely sensitive oculovagal reflex. Even when a genetic epileptic mechanism is operating, it is possible that the oculocardiac reflex mirrors a GABA-dependent convulsive threshold. Further studies in febrile seizures should have no exclusions (such as 'cerebral infection'), and yet critically specify the interacting factors involved.

References

1 Stephenson JBP, Ounsted C. In Milton AS, ed. *Pyretics and Antipyretics, Handbook of Experimental Pharmacology Volume 60 1982;* In press. Heidelberg: Springer-Verlag
2 Stephenson JBP. *Br Med J 1978; 2:* 726–728
3 Sunderland R, Emery JL. *Lancet 1981; ii:* 176–178
4 Tsuboi T, Endo SH. *Neuropädiatrie 1977; 8:* 209–223
5 Lindsay J, Ounsted C, Richards P. *Develop Med Child Neurol 1980; 22:* 429–439
6 Morikawa T, Osawa T, Ishihara O, Seino M. *Brain and Development 1979; 4:* 257–265
7 Kajitani T, Ueoka K, Nakamura M, Kumanomidou Y. *Brain and Development 1981; 3:* 351–359
8 De Marco P, Tassinari CA. *Epilepsia 1981; 22:* 569–575
9 Nelson KB, Ellenberg JH. *Pediatrics 1978; 61:* 720–727
10 Gastaut H, Tassinari CA. *Epilepsia 1966; 7:* 85–138
11 Nelson KB, Ellenberg JH. *N Engl J Med 1976; 295:* 1029–1033
12 Ounsted C. *Lancet 1951; i:* 1245–1248
13 McGreal DA. *Am J Dis Child 1956; 92:* 504–505
14 McGreal DA. *Convulsions in childhood. A clinical and electroencephalographic study of 500 cases in children under the age of seven.* MD Thesis, University of St Andrews 1957
15 Gastaut H, Gastaut Y. *Rev Neurol (Paris) 1957; 96:* 158–163
16 Lombroso CT, Lerman P. *Pediatrics 1967; 39:* 563–581
17 Stephenson JBP. *Arch Dis Childh 1978; 53:* 193–200
18 Stephenson JBP. *Develop Med Child Neurol 1980; 22:* 380–386
19 Mausby R, Kellaway P. In Kellaway P, Petersen I, eds. *Neurological and Electroencephalographic Correlative Studies in Infancy 1964:* 349–360. New York Grune and Stratton
20 Lennox-Buchthal MA. In Brazier MAB, Coceani F, eds. *Brain Dysfunction in Infantile Febrile Convulsions 1976;* 327–351. New York: Raven Press
21 Hope-Simpson RE, Laidlaw W, Morrison SL, Ounsted C, Watts CHH. *Fits in young persons. Study by the MRC Committee for research in general practice.* Unpublished
22 Chen HI, Chai CY. *Am J Physiol 1976; 231:* 454–461
23 Di Micco JA, Gale K, Hamilton B, Gillis RA. *Science 1979; 204:* 1106–1109
24 Williford DJ, Hamilton BL, Gillis RA. *Brain Research 1980; 193:* 584–588
25 Löscher W, Rating D, Siemes H. *Epilepsia 1981; 22:* 697–702
26 Tangri KK, Misra N, Bhargava KP. In Brazier MAB, Coceani F, eds. *Brain Dysfunction in Infantile Febrile Convulsions 1976;* 89–106. New York: Raven Press
27 Stephenson JBP. *Lancet 1979; ii:* 955

29

GROWTH IN CHILDREN WITH EPILEPSY

Marian E L McGowan

Introduction

There is a relative paucity of information about the physical growth of children with epilepsy, although clinicians often have the impression that children with severe epilepsy tend to be short. It has been suggested that antiepileptic drugs may affect growth [1]. There is also evidence that the administration of certain antiepileptic drugs during pregnancy results in a reduction in fetal growth [2] and in fetal head circumference [3].

In a recent study carried out among pupils with epilepsy at a residential school [4], it was found that these children had similar growth and development patterns to normal adolescents but, as a population, were of less than average height and often failed to reach their predicted final height. These findings seemed to be due to an early growth spurt and lower than normal growth velocity. In addition these children displayed advanced skeletal maturation, which would tend to be associated with earlier puberty, early closure of the epiphyses and a reduction in final stature. Among the girls menarche was reached earlier than average.

Factors which might affect growth in children with epilepsy would include seizure activity per se, and the action of antiepileptic drugs but, in addition, some children with severe epilepsy have brain damage, which is commonly associated with short stature. Finally, children resident in institutions may display adverse effects on growth related to emotional deprivation [5].

This chapter presents firstly the results of a retrospective study of final adult height attained in patients with epilepsy, and secondly some preliminary results from a prospective, longitudinal study of children followed from the time of diagnosis of epilepsy.

RETROSPECTIVE STUDY

The aim of this study was to determine the final adult heights attained by patients with epilepsy. Subjects included people who had taken antiepileptic drugs contin-

253

uously from childhood and people who had begun taking antiepileptic medication only in adult life. Any reduction in stature related to drug effects should have been apparent in the first group but not the second. However, in case factors related to epilepsy per se had played any part in determining the height of these subjects and had been present in the second group even before they began taking antiepileptic medication, the data for both groups were compared with established data for the general population of the United Kingdom [6].

Method

The standing heights of 39 men over age 18 and 49 pre-menopausal women over age 16 attending neurological outpatient clinics were measured by one observer. All subjects were Caucasian and had no other condition associated with abnormal growth (e.g. chromosome disorders, organic brain disease). All were taking antiepileptic medication, and none had been resident in institutions.

TABLE I. Composition of the study population

	Males	Females
Antiepileptic therapy started before age 10	12	14
Antiepileptic therapy started between 10 and 18	10	15
Antiepileptic therapy started in adult life	17	20
TOTAL	39	49

The patients were divided into the following three groups (see Table I):

1. Those who had begun therapy before age 10 years, i.e. before the prepubertal growth spurt.

2. Those who had begun therapy between age 10 years and the completion of growth.

3. Those who had begun antiepileptic therapy after completing their growth.

Results

a) Overall

The mean heights for patients in each group are shown in Table II. There was no significant difference between the mean heights of any of the groups, nor did any group's mean height differ from the known mean for the general population [6]. However, women who had begun therapy before age 10 showed a tendency to be shorter than both the other women in the study and the national average.

254

TABLE II. Mean adult heights of patients starting antiepileptic therapy at different ages

	MALES		FEMALES	
	Mean height (cms)	Standard deviation	Mean height (cms)	Standard deviation
United Kingdom population	174.7	6.65	162.2	6.00
Antiepileptic therapy before age 10	173.46	5.24	159.79	5.97
Antiepileptic therapy between ages 10 and 18/16	174.15	8.02	161.87	5.94
Antiepileptic therapy in adult life	173.09	8.02	161.77	5.48

b) Heights observed in relation to different seizure types

From the population of the study a number of patients were identified who had begun having seizures before completing their growth, and who had only one type of seizure, either grand mal (10 men and 18 women) or partial seizures (6 men and 9 women). The mean heights of these subjects were calculated separately (Table III) — the height distribution is illustrated in Figures 1 and 2. The mean height of men with partial seizures was significantly less than that of men with grand mal (0.01 > p > 0.001) and than that of the normal male population (0.02 > p > 0.01), but women with different seizure types displayed no such difference.

TABLE III. Mean adult height in patients with different seizure types beginning before completion of growth

	MALES			FEMALES		
	Number of patients	Mean height (cms)	Standard deviation	Number of patients	Mean height (cms)	Standard deviation
Grand mal	10	176.55	4.66	18	160.28	5.69
Partial	6	166.92*	5.14	9	160.06	6.08

* Significantly different from mean value for general UK population

c) Heights observed in relation to different antiepileptic drugs

The subjects measured had taken a wide range of antiepileptic drugs, singly or in combination but, among patients who had begun therapy in childhood or ado-

255

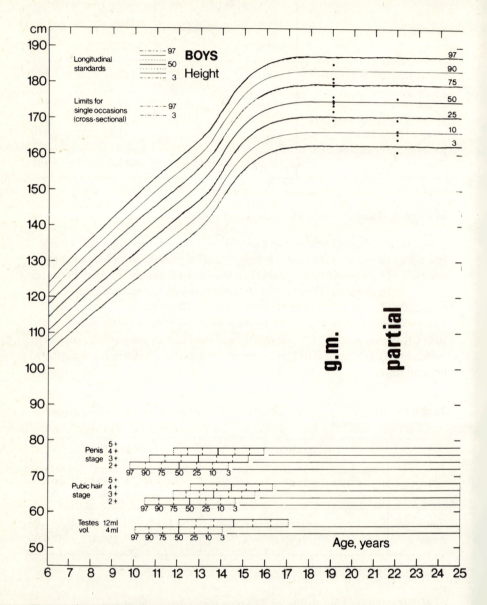

Figure 1. Distribution of observed heights in men with partial or grand mal seizures

256

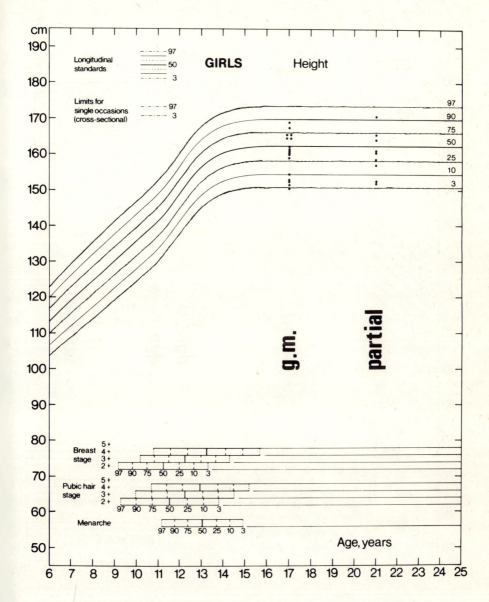

Figure 2. Distribution of observed heights in women with partial or grand mal seizures

257

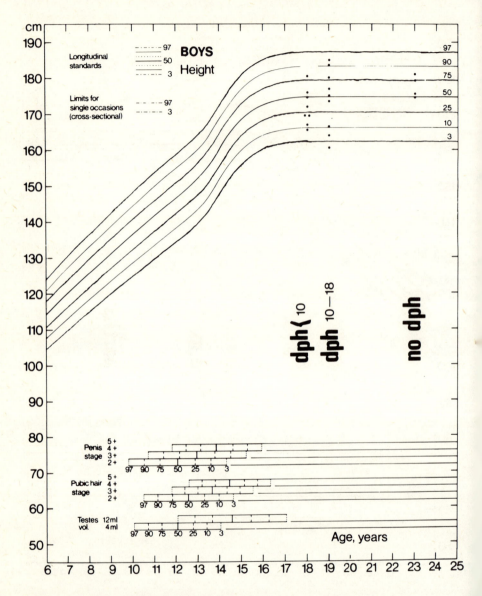

Figure 3. Distribution of observed heights in men in relation to phenytoin therapy

258

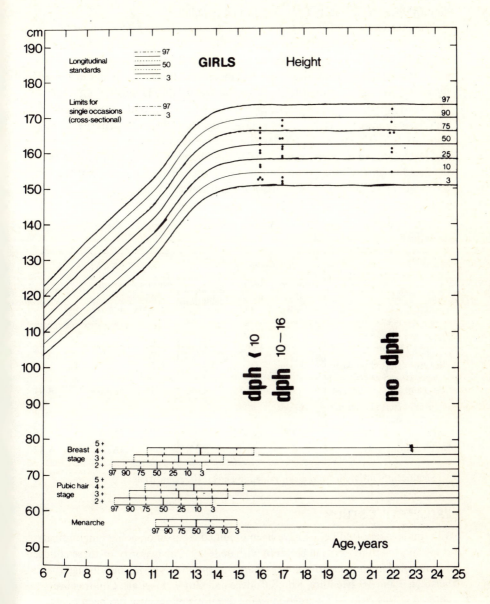

Figure 4. Distribution of observed heights in women in relation to phenytoin therapy

259

lescence, exposure to phenytoin and phenobarbitone was particularly common. The heights of those who had taken phenobarbitone before completion of growth did not differ significantly from the normal population.

The mean heights of the 17 men and 22 women who had taken phenytoin before reaching adulthood were calculated (Table IV) — the distributions are illustrated in Figures 3 and 4. Men who had received the drug before the age of 18 were no different from the norm, but there was a tendency for those among them who had been exposed to it before the age of 10 to be shorter, although this trend did not reach statistical significance. Women who had received phenytoin before the age of 16 had a mean height significantly lower than the normal population ($0.05 > p > 0.02$). When this group was sub-divided into those who had been exposed to phenytoin before 10, and between the ages of 10 and 16, the mean heights of each group were less than the population mean, but the differences just failed to reach statistical significance.

TABLE IV. Mean adult height in patients who had taken phenytoin at different periods during their growth

	MALES			FEMALES		
	Number of patients	Mean height (cms)	Standard deviation	Number of patients	Mean height (cms)	Standard deviation
Phenytoin started before age 10 (group 1)	8	171.81	4.98	11	159.05	5.28
Phenytoin started between ages 10 and 18/16 (group 2)	9	173.89	8.63	11	160.09	6.01
Phenytoin started anytime before age 18/16 (group 1 + group 2)	17	172.91	7.02	22	159.57*	5.55
No Phenytoin	4	177.50	3.03	7	163.86	5.82

* Significantly different from mean value for general UK population

PROSPECTIVE STUDY

The findings reported below have been obtained from an on-going longitudinal study of growth patterns in children with epilepsy. The majority of these children are included in a prospective study of antiepileptic therapy in children aged between 3 and 16 attending King's College and Guy's Hospitals. Children are entered in this latter study as soon as the diagnosis of epilepsy has been made, and only if they have not previously received antiepileptic medication. This enables initial data concerning growth to be collected before antiepileptic therapy is instituted.

Method

When the diagnosis of epilepsy has been established, and before treatment is prescribed, the child's standing height, weight and head circumference are measured by one observer who also records the stage of sexual maturity attained in accordance with Tanner's criteria [7]. For girls the age of menarche is recorded, if this has already occurred. The children are then reviewed at three-monthly intervals, and the same data recorded by the same observer. The child's bone age is determined at the start of the study and is repeated at yearly intervals.

Results

a) Heights

As yet, only a small amount of preliminary data is available from this study. The distribution of standing height in 11 girls and 13 boys, recorded before the inception of antiepileptic therapy is shown in Figures 5 and 6. None of the children has brain damage and all are Caucasian. The group includes four girls and two boys with grand mal epilepsy, two girls and seven boys with partial seizures, two girls and one boy with petit mal absences and three girls and three boys with mixed seizure types.

The heights recorded before treatment are normally distributed, and do not vary significantly from standard for normal children of the same age suggesting that, at the time a diagnosis of epilepsy is made, children with this disorder do not yet show any disturbance in growth.

As yet, no girls in the study have been followed up for six months, but Figure 7 illustrates the growth patterns of nine boys who have been measured six months after starting treatment – the antiepileptic drugs having been allocated randomly. Three boys were receiving carbamazepine, three sodium valproate, two phenobarbitone and one phenytoin. The heights recorded after six months' treatment do not vary significantly from the population mean, indicating that overall these boys do not differ from normal children. However, when one considers the individual growth patterns of the nine subjects over six months, it can be seen from Figure 7 that three boys are displaying a slightly slower than normal growth and have not maintained their position on their original centile line. These three boys have all responded relatively badly to antiepileptic therapy and have continued to have seizures, whereas of the six boys who are growing normally, only one has continued to have frequent seizures. It is too early, and the data are too limited, to draw any meaningful conclusions from this finding but it does suggest that the possibility should be explored, at a later stage, that a disturbance of growth may be related to continuing seizure activity, rather than to the effects of drugs.

261

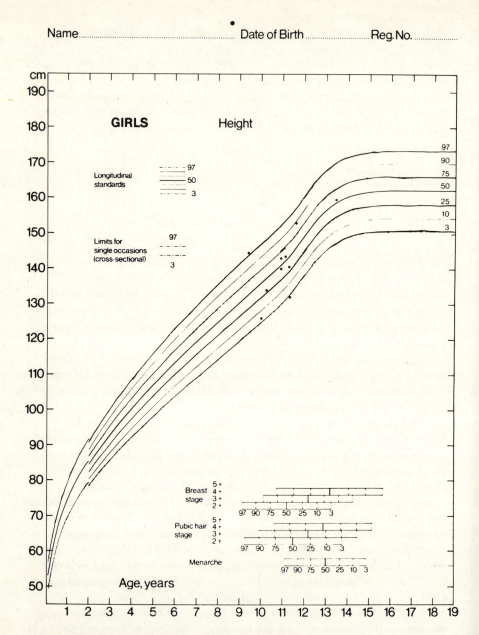

Name.. • Date of Birth.......................... Reg. No. ....

Figure 5. Heights of girls at the start of antiepileptic therapy

262

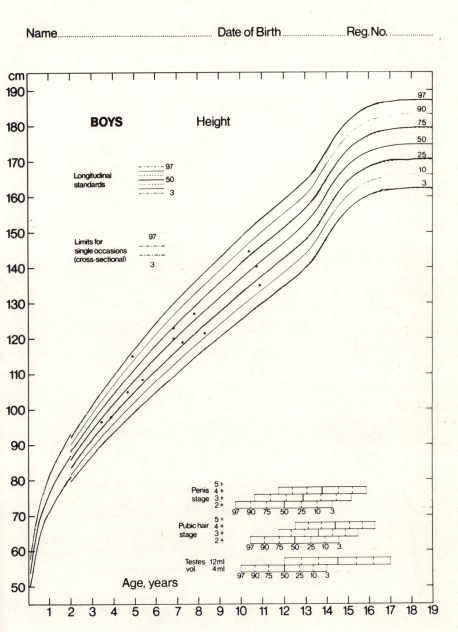

Figure 6. Heights of boys at the start of antiepileptic therapy

263

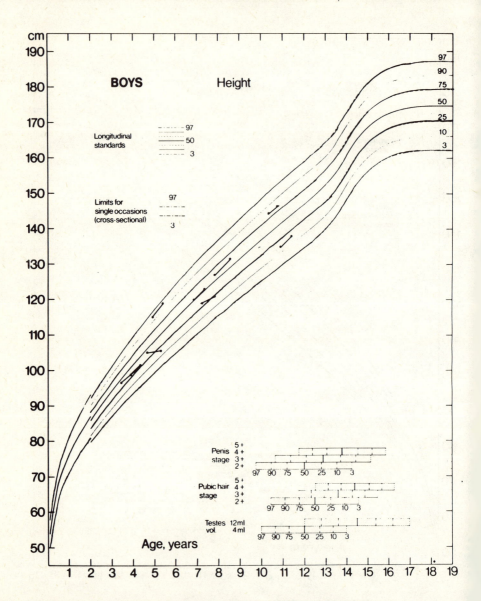

Figure 7. Growth of boys during first six months of antiepileptic therapy

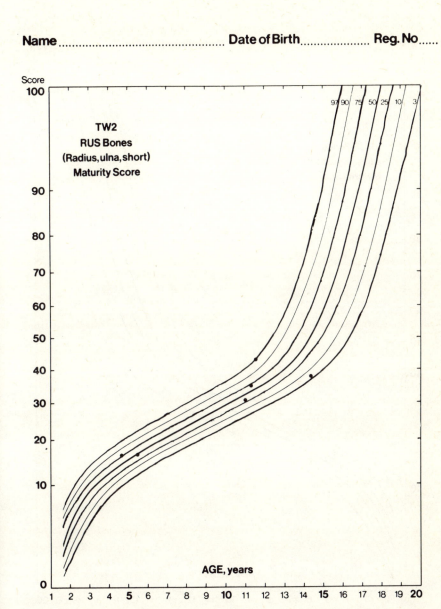

Figure 8. Skeletal maturity scores (*RUS system*) in children at the start of antiepileptic therapy

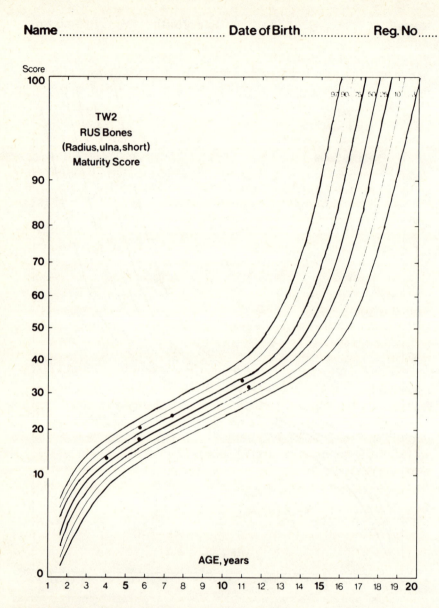

Figure 9. Skeletal maturity scores (*RUS system*) in children after six to twelve months' antiepileptic therapy

b) Skeletal maturity

The distribution of skeletal maturity scores derived from standard hand and wrist X-rays of six children entering the study are shown in Figure 8. These do not differ significantly from values seen in normal children, suggesting that at the time epilepsy is diagnosed there is no evidence of advanced skeletal maturation.

Unfortunately none of the children in this study has been followed for long enough to enable a bone age score determined after treatment with antiepileptic drugs to be available for comparison with the initial one. However, Figure 9 shows the distribution of skeletal maturity scores observed in six children on antiepileptic therapy for between 6 and 12 months, who are already attending a hospital epilepsy clinic. Again these show no difference, as a population, from normal children but it is unfortunate that data for skeletal maturity before treatment is not available in these children to enable an assessment of the rate of skeletal maturation in individuals during treatment.

Conclusions

From the retrospective study, no overall differences in final adult height emerged between patients who had begun antiepileptic treatment in childhood, patients who had begun treatment in adult life and the normal population. This lends support to the view that previous findings [4] may reflect the adverse effects of institutionalisation on growth. However, this study has revealed the existence of two groups of patients whose height is significantly less than that of the general population — namely men with partial seizures of early onset and women who have taken phenytoin before adulthood. Concerning the first group one might argue that they might be more likely to have a greater degree of brain damage than patients with generalised epilepsy, despite attempts to exclude such cases from the study, but this would not explain why the phenomenon was not observed in women. A similar difficulty arises in explaining why only women are sensitive to the apparent effect of phenytoin, but it should be noted that men, who had taken this drug before puberty, did tend to be shorter and that fewer men than women were involved in the study. Had more men been measured it is conceivable that a more significant difference might have emerged. It is also interesting to note that in Round's study [4] of institutionalised children with apparent slowing of growth, the majority of patients (43 out of 49) were taking phenytoin.

Unfortunately it is impossible, in this type of retrospective study, to collect meaningful information about growth patterns or the degree of seizure control during childhood and adolescence, as this depends in most cases on the patients' recollections. One can, of course, assume that the patients who had begun therapy in childhood probably had relatively severe epilepsy since treatment had continued into adult life.

For the limited information available as yet from the prospective study, it seems that children presenting with epilepsy are not different from normal children in respect of height and skeletal maturation. The results of follow-up at six months do suggest that uncontrolled epilepsy may play a part in adversely influencing growth, and clearly further information will need to be collected throughout the study on the relationship between seizure control and growth patterns. As the study continues information will become available about the age of onset of puberty and the rate of skeletal maturation following the institution of drug therapy, as well as about growth patterns, and it will be possible to compare the effects, if any, of individual anti-epileptic drugs on these parameters.

Summary

There have been suggestions that physical growth is impaired in children with epilepsy, but data are lacking. Such impairment could be related to multiple factors. In a retrospective study, measurements of standing height in 88 adult patients with epilepsy revealed no overall difference between these subjects and the general population of the United Kingdom, whatever the age of starting anti-epileptic therapy. Within the sample, however, men with partial seizures beginning before the age of 18 were shorter than non-epileptic males, or men with grand mal seizures; women who had taken phenytoin before the age of 16 years were significantly shorter than the normal female population; and, although the difference was not statistically significant, men who had taken phenytoin before the age of 10 showed a similar tendency.

In a prospective longitudinal study of growth in children with epilepsy, 24 subjects aged between 3 and 16 have been measured at the time of diagnosis, and show no difference in respect to height from the normal population. Six children who have had bone age estimation show no difference in skeletal maturation at the time epilepsy is diagnosed. Nine boys who have been followed for six months from the time of starting antiepileptic therapy have normal growth patterns, except in those cases where seizure control has not been achieved.

Acknowledgments

I should like to thank Dr E H Reynolds and Dr B G R Neville for permission to study patients under their care.

References

1   Landon MJ. *Lancet 1974; ii:* 1327
2   Montouris GD, Fenichie GM, McLain LW Jn. *Arch Neurol 1979; 36:* 601–603
3   Hulesmaa VK, Terama K, Granström ML, Bardy AH. *Lancet 1981; ii:* 165–167
4   Round JM. In Dam, M, Gram L, Penny JK, eds. *Advances in Epileptology: XIIth Epilepsy International Symposium 1981.* New York: Raven Press
5   Tanner JM. In *Foetus into Man 1978;* 206–219. London: Open Books Publishing Ltd
6   Tanner JM, Whitehouse R, Takaishi M. *Arch Dis Childh 1966; 41:* 454
7   Tanner JM. *Growth at Adolescence, 2nd edition 1962.* Oxford: Blackwell Scientific Publications

30

AMBULATORY EEG MONITORING

R E Cull

Over the past seven years advances in the electronics industry have allowed the development of miniature tape recorders for monitoring EEG in ambulant patients [1–3]. The system described in this chapter was developed by Quy et al [3] at the Institute of Neurology, National Hospital, Queen Square, London, in conjunction with Oxford Medical Systems. I shall describe experience with, and applications of, this system at the National Hospital.

The recording system is based on the Oxford Medical Systems Medilog 4-24 cassette tape recorder which permits registration of up to four channels of data in combinations of EEG, ECG, body movement or digital time code. In clinical practice, it has been useful to have available two such recorders: the first set up for recording four channels of EEG alone for the investigation of problems known to be purely epileptic, and the second set up for two channels of EEG, one channel ECG and one channel receiving a digital time code, for the investigation of patients with disorders of loss of consciousness of uncertain pathogenesis.

Preamplification of the EEG signals is carried out by small scalp-mounting amplifiers [4] which are glued to the scalp with collodion. Use of these preamplifiers permits the length of electrode wires to be kept very short, greatly reducing cable movement artefacts and interference from external fields. It is often preferable to site electrodes well away from the frontalis and temporalis muscles to avoid muscle artefact, but the position of the electrodes will depend on the type of clinical problem. With anterior or mid-temporal montages, muscle artefact is very difficult to avoid. ECG is recorded using conventional stick-on chest electrodes and, where applicable, body movement can be registered by a small head-mounted accelerometer. The use of a digital time code generator in place of one recording channel greatly improves the accuracy with which recorded events can be placed in time.

The signals are recorded in analogue form onto a standard C 120 magnetic tape cassette which provides 24 hours' continuous recording time. Event marks can be superimposed on to either the time code channel or one of the EEG channels, and can be detected on playback for checking timing and searching for events. The recording system is compact and lightweight; with preamplifiers and electrodes hidden under hair, and cables concealed beneath clothing, it can be worn inconspicuously and without impediment by most patients.

Playback of recordings is carried out using the Oxford Medical Systems page-mode display unit (PMD-12) which allows review of recordings to be made at 20 or 60 times real time. The system presents on a television screen sequential 8 or 16 second 'pages' of recording, each 'page' remaining on the screen for a brief time, unless the tape is stopped by the operator, thus enabling a single 'page' to be held in view. An audio signal can be taken from any channel and transferred to a loudspeaker; abnormalities in the EEG or ECG are often readily detected by ear in this way. The playback system can be linked to a standard EEG machine for production of hard copies of portions of the record, and the signals can be transferred to a computer for automated analysis (see below).

Interpretation of the data recorded and displayed in this way takes some practice. As with all forms of EEG, artefacts arise frequently and must be recognised. Eye movements and blinks, chewing and swallowing and body movement all interfere with interpretation. Thus, although it is possible theoretically to allow patients home or to work during the recording, these benefits must be weighed against the improved quality of recording obtained when the subject is confined to a relatively sedentary day in the hospital ward. This latter situation also permits electrodes to be checked and re-jellied during the recording period which also tends to produce better results.

Where the EEG shows repeated runs of characteristic abnormality, such as in petit mal epilepsy, rapid automatic analysis is very useful. An analogue detection system for spike and wave devised by Quy et al [5] can be set up to detect and log bursts of 2−4/sec rhythmical spike and wave activity, and will produce numerical and graphical representation of this for the 24 hours of recorded time. Comparison of different records from the same patient can be used to assess the efficacy of drug treatment. Variations in the amount of spike and wave activity at different times of day can also be detected. Figure 1 shows the amount of spike and wave activity detected automatically over sequential 15 minute epochs in six ambulant patients with petit mal who were recorded over 24-hour periods [6]. Rhythmical spike and wave is seen to decrease during overnight sleep (horizontal bars) but to rise to a maximum during the first two hours after wakening in the morning. It is important to consider the duration of epileptic activity which is required to trigger such automatic detection systems. At least one second of well formed rhythmical spike and wave activity is required to register on the system described above [5]; but since, during slow wave sleep, spike and wave paroxysms become brief and ill-formed [7], despite their increased frequency of appearance, these altered bursts of epileptic activity are not detected by the automated system. It can be argued that, since spike and wave paroxysms

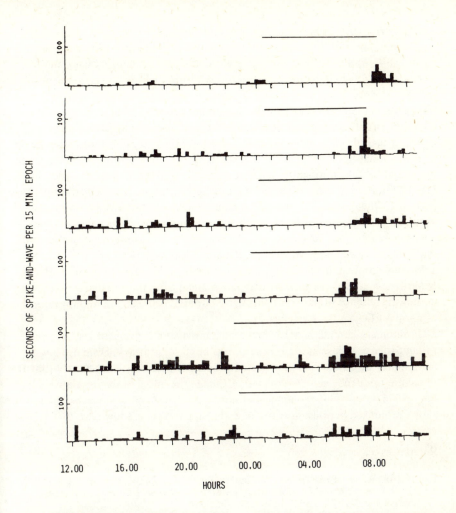

Figure 1. Bar charts showing amount of spike and wave activity in consecutive 15 minute epochs throughout a 24-hour period in each of six patients with petit mal. Horizontal bars above each chart indicate overnight sleep. Note the reduction in epileptic activity during sleep and the increased amount on morning wakening

of less than 5 seconds duration are unlikely to cause clinical symptoms, a system which ignores bursts of epileptic activity lasting less than one second is very adequate for clinical purposes.

It is probable that other automatic detection systems will be developed in the future. Detection of single spike or sharp wave discharges poses a greater problem than that of rhythmical spike and wave, because, although these transients are readily detected on the basis of frequency and amplitude, they are less easily

271

separated from artefacts due to eye blinks or muscle activity.

The suitability of different kinds of patient for ambulatory EEG monitoring needs to be considered, and depends both on the type of clinical attack and the frequency with which they occur. Patients with petit mal epilepsy are the most suitable because of the usually high frequency of attacks, and the highly characteristic generalised EEG changes which accompany each attack. Patients with complex partial seizures may be suitable if attacks are sufficiently frequent (0.5–1 attack/day is preferable), and it is helpful if some prior information about EEG abnormalities is obtained from a routine record to aid appropriate electrode placement. EEG abnormalities during complex partial seizures are variable; they may be localised or generalised and are usually less easy to detect than those of petit mal. When attacks of loss of consciousness are of unknown pathogenesis, simultaneous EEG and ECG monitoring is warranted, since many such patients are not epileptic [8]. As before, attacks need to be sufficiently frequent for prolonged monitoring to be worthwhile. Patients with 'hysterical' seizures present a difficult problem, particularly in the absence of a video record of their attacks. Nevertheless, useful information may be obtained from the ambulatory recording in showing absence of paroxysmal activity during the attack and prompt return of normal EEG rhythms afterwards.

In summary, ambulatory EEG recording provides a convenient way of monitoring patients with seizures or other forms of episodic attack. Diagnostic information may be obtained and, in petit mal epilepsy particularly, accurate estimates of seizure frequency can be provided. Although the initial outlay is relatively high, the system described is economical of both physicians' and technicians' time, and allows prolonged periods of recording to be undertaken at a low cost.

References

1   Ives JR, Woods JF. *Electroenceph Clin Neurophysiol 1975; 39:* 88–92
2   SRI Intermin Report. *Development of a wearable 4-channel EEG cassette recording system March 1975.* Standford Research Institute
3   Quy RJ, Willison RG, Fitch P, Gilliatt RW. In Stott FD, Raftery EB, Sleight P, Gouding L, eds. *Proceedings of the Third International Symposium on Ambulatory Monitoring 1980;* 393–398. London: Academic Press
4   Quy RJ. *J Physiol (Lond) 1978; 234:* 23–24P
5   Quy RJ, Fitch P, Willison RG. *Electroenceph Clin Neurophysiol 1980; 49:* 187–189
6   Cull RE, Fitch P, Gilliatt RW. *Diurnal variations in spike-and-wave activity in petit mal epilepsy.* In preparation
7   Sato S, Dreifuss FE, Penry JK. *Neurology 1973; 23:* 1335–1345
8   Schott GD, McLeod AA, Jewitt DE. *Br Med J 1977; 1:* 1454–1457

31

RECENT APPLICATIONS OF AMBULATORY EEG MONITORING IN CHILDREN

G Stores

Introduction

Increasingly, ambulatory EEG monitoring is becoming part of the range of techniques available in modern electroencephalography. Compared with more traditional EEG procedures, it has the advantage of permitting long-term recordings (for days or weeks if necessary) and allowing patients to be investigated in their everyday environment without it being apparent that the investigation is in progress. It is a relatively inexpensive procedure available to any EEG department.

The clinical use of ambulatory monitoring has been described in three centres in particular: Montreal [1], London [2] and Oxford [3]. Publications from these centres give the details of the Medilog System used there, the three main components of which are (1) a small cassette recorder which provides four channels of data (EEG, ECG or other physiological variables), (2) on-head preamplifiers which greatly reduce movement artefacts, and (3) a replay and visual display unit which allows rapid presentation of data in familiar form. The system has been used on a wide variety of patients of different ages and intellectual level.

Diagnosis

The main clinical application of the system has been the differential diagnosis of attacks of uncertain origin, where the range of diagnostic possiblities is wide [4].

Several series of patients have been recently described [5]. For example, Forrest and Crawford [6] describe the use of ambulatory monitoring in 76 children between the ages of 4½ and 17½ years with undiagnosed attacks of disturbed behaviour. The intellectual level of these children ranged from severely subnormal to above average. The behaviours in diagnostic doubt included falls, lapses of concentration, visual hallucinations, abnormal movements and flushing and sweating attacks. Recordings (mainly EEG alone) were carried out, usually for 24 hours, during general activities in hospital or at home. In 20 of these children the findings confirmed that the attacks were a form of epileptic seizure. In 18 the absence of seizure discharge at the time of the attacks provided additional evidence of a psychological disturbance. The investigation was inconclusive in 38 children who had no attack and no EEG or ECG abnormality during the recording period.

Certain important points arise from this and other reports. Ambulatory monitoring is not a substitute for careful clinical assessment which in most cases allows an accurate diagnosis of attacks to be made. Where the diagnosis remains in doubt after such clinical inquiry, and where more traditional forms of EEG investigation have been unhelpful, ambulatory monitoring is useful. It is also of value where simultaneous video monitoring of the patient's clinical state and EEG is either unavailable or where no attacks have occurred during its use.

Sometimes the diagnostic value of ambulatory monitoring has been limited by restricting the recording period to 24 hours. It is generally more appropriate to choose patients whose attack frequency is at least once or twice a week, and to continue recording until an attack occurs, but interictal abnormalities may be diagnostically helpful, even when no attack occurs during the recording period.

In only a minority of reported cases has combined EEG and ECG monitoring been carried out. Perhaps especially in infants and middle aged to elderly patients, this combination is advisable in order to explore the possibility that attacks (even of a convulsive type) are the result primarily of cardiac arrhythmia. This is well illustrated in the report by Eyre and Crawford [7] who have used prolonged EEG recording in babies on a neonatal intensive care unit.

A common question concerns the detection of seizure discharge of focal origin by means of a four channel system. Such a system is not an appropriate way of localising discharges, and EEG recordings of preferably sixteen channels are required for this purpose. Unfortunately, conventional brief recordings often do not contain spontaneous seizures. Whilst the Medilog System is not suitable for precise localisation of seizures, it may be useful in the less ambitious role of lateralisation of the seizure source. Support for this limited use is provided by Stores [8], Forrest and Crawford [6], Docherty [9], and especially Ives and Woods [10] who report the use of the system in 100 patients with focal seizures.

When a patient's attacks are not accompanied by EEG or other physiological abnormalities during ambulatory monitoring, interpretation requires careful consideration. Clearly, negative findings in scalp recorded EEGs at the time of the attack do not exclude the possibility of epileptic seizures at those times. Such findings do, however, increase the likelihood that these attacks are not epileptic in type and may be seen as adding significantly to all other information available about the patient. Such patients need to be followed up carefully and the diagnosis reviewed in the light of subsequent events.

Patterns of occurrence of seizure activity

There is a need for a means whereby patterns of occurrence of seizures can be accurately documented and preferably quantified in relation to possible precipitating or inhibiting factors. Ordinary clinical assessment for this purpose can be difficult especially in the case of frequently occurring, subtle, non-convulsive seizures. There are indications that ambulatory monitoring can meet this need in certain types of patient. Stores and Lwin [11] carried out 24-hour Medilog recordings on 28 children between the ages of 6 and 16 years each suffering from absence seizures accompanied by generalised spike and wave EEG activity. The recordings were carried out either in hospital, at home or at school. The cassette tapes were replayed and the time and amount of seizure discharge measured by hand. Charts compiled to show the distribution of epileptic activity over the 24-hour period showed individual differences in many of these children. Differences were seen in the relative amounts of epileptic activity in the awake and asleep periods, and in five children the peak occurrence of seizure discharge was associated with psychological or physiological factors as recorded by observers who had kept a diary of the child's activities over the same 24-hour period. These preliminary results suggest that ambulatory monitoring can provide important insights into patterns of occurrence which might not be obvious by other means of assessment. Before acting on these findings it would, of course, be necessary to demonstrate that the pattern of occurrence was consistent from one period to another.

Drug evaluation

Several groups have used ambulatory monitoring in an attempt to achieve a more objective evaluation of response to antiepileptic drug treatment than is usually possible by clinical means or more traditional forms of EEG recording.

Ives et al [12] have used the technique to assess patients' response to ethosuximide. Milligan and Richens [13] report similar studies and discuss the advantages and limitations of such procedures. Serial monitoring of this type can be of particular value in children with subtle, generalised seizures and either mental handicap or slowness which makes the recognition of such seizures especially difficult [1].

Sleep recordings

Traditionally sleep studies are carried out in special laboratories and the lengthy polygraphic records are analysed by hand into classical sleep stages. The need for these special facilities has limited clinical studies of sleep disorders especially in disturbed patients or children. For the study of many common sleep problems, it seems that useful clinical information can be obtained by monitoring sleep states in an elementary way by means of a cassette recorder worn by the patient while sleeping in his own bed. Kayed et al [14] have developed a technique using the Medilog recorder by which eye movements, EMG and body movements are monitored. The overnight recording is replayed at high speed and written out on an ink jet recorder running at low paper speed to provide a highly compressed complete night's recording in which the awake state, REM and non-REM periods can be distinguished. This type of analysis is being extended [15] by adding a single EEG channel with the overall aim of producing a simple recording procedure which will be acceptable to patients, including children, and where results are presented in an easily reviewed form.

Automated analysis

Hand scoring of prolonged recordings is a time consuming and tedious process, but Bailey [16] has reported an evaluation study of an automated three per second spike and wave processor designed to overcome this problem. The study involved the use of a Medilog replay and display system, an analogue spike and wave detector, a micro-computer and a printer. Twenty-four hour recordings were selected to represent different types of spike and wave activity ranging from 'classical' three per second activity with normal background rhythms to irregular spike and wave bursts with abnormal background rhythms. Comparison of automated analysis with hand scoring showed good overall agreement except when the regular morphology of daytime seizure discharge was degraded during sleep.

Conclusions

In patients of all ages, including quite young children, ambulatory monitoring is proving to be of value in the investigation of clinical problems for which more conventional EEG procedures have been of little help. This is particularly so in the differential diagnosis of attacks of an uncertain nature and it seems likely that the more recent developments may also find a place in a wide variety of clinical circumstances.

References

1   Ives JR, Woods JF. *Electroenceph Clin Neurophysiol 1975; 39:* 88–92
2   Quy RJ, Fitch P, Willison RG, Gilliatt RW. In Wada JA, Penry JK, eds. *Advances in Epileptology. The 10th Epilepsy International Symposium 1980; 69*. New York: Raven Press
3   Stores G, Brankin P. In *Proceedings of Meeting of British, Dutch and Danish branches of International League Against Epilepsy. Heeze, Netherlands, October 1981*. In press
4   Stores G. In Dam M, Gram L, Penry JK, eds. *Advances in Epileptology. The 12th Epilepsy International Symposium 1981; 259*. New York: Raven Press
5   Stott FD, Raftery EB, Clement DL, Wright SL, eds. *ISAM 1981. Proceedings of the 4th International Symposium on Ambulatory Monitoring. Gent, Netherlands*. In press. London: Academic Press

6   Forrest GC, Crawford C. In Stott FD, ed. *ISAM 1981. Proceedings of the 4th International Symposium on Ambulatory Monitoring. Gent, Netherlands.* In press. London: Academic Press

7   Eyre J, Crawford C. In Stott FD, ed. *ISAM 1981. Proceedings of the 4th International Symposium on Ambulatory Monitoring. Gent, Netherlands.* In press. London: Academic Press

8   Stores G. In Parsonage MG, ed. *Aspects of Epilepsy. Res and Clin Forums 1980; 2:* 141–148

9   Docherty TB. *J Electrophysiol Technol 1981; 7:* 141–158

10 Ives JR, Woods JF. In Stott FD, Raftery EB, Goulding L, eds. *ISAM 1979. Proceedings of the 3rd International Symposium on Ambulatory Monitoring 1980;* 383. London: Academic Press

11 Stores G, Lwin R. In Dam M, Gram L, Penry JK, eds. *Advances in Epileptology. The 12th Epilepsy International Symposium 1981;* 421–422. New York: Raven Press

12 Woods JF, Gloor P. *Electroenceph Clin Neurophysiol 1975; 39:* 295

13 Milligan N, Richens A. *Br J Clin Pharmacol 1981; 11:* 443–456

14 Kayed K, Hesla PE, Rosjo O. *Sleep 1979; 2:* 253–260

15 Brankin P. *Proceedings of Annual Meeting of the American Medical EEG Association. Lake Tahoe, Nevada, June 1981.* In press

16 Bailey C. In Stott FD, ed. *ISAM 1981. Proceedings of the 4th International Symposium on Ambulatory Monitoring 1981. Gent, Netherlands.* In press. London: Academic Press

32

STATUS EPILEPTICUS: EEG MONITORING DURING THERAPEUTIC TRIALS OF ANTICONVULSANTS

G Pampiglione

The term 'status epilepticus' includes a variety of clinical manifestations which may occur in both adults and children. Seizures, prolonged seizures, and status epilepticus tend to merge in a continuum of time and the exact duration of a seizure for classification as 'status epilepticus' does not appear to be specified in any of the many dictionaries. Even Gastaut [1] had to use several lines to conclude that status epilepticus is 'a condition characterised by an epileptic state . . . to produce an unvarying and enduring epileptic condition'! Various authors have added further adjectives in order to specify variants such as 'major epileptic status', 'minor epileptic status', 'partial epileptic state', 'uncontrolled seizure activity', 'twilight state', 'unilateral status epilepticus' and so on.

Status epilepticus with whatever manifestations is a medical emergency requiring urgent treatment. A great variety of drugs have been employed to interrupt status epilepticus since the introduction of bromides in 1851, chloral hydrate in 1872 and paraldehyde in 1882, just a century ago. More recently thiopentone and particularly diazepam have been used with considerable success. However, in the recommended doses these drugs have a marked soporific effect which makes it impossible to assess clinically whether the patient remains unrousable because of the effect of the drug or because the cerebral condition continues to interfere with the return of consciousness.

In a previous paper [2], it has been shown that small doses of some anticonvulsant drugs if injected rapidly as a bolus may have a very prompt beneficial effect interrupting prolonged seizures without soporific effect. However, continuous clinical and EEG monitoring is essential to assess whether or not brain function has improved. The present EEG study of 101 babies and children shows that either a short acting barbiturate (methohexitone) or a benzodiazepine (diazepam) *in very small doses* interrupt status epilepticus within half a minute or less provided the drug is injected intravenously as a bolus. However, different patients with apparently similar clinical manifestations may respond quite differently to one or the other group of drugs, a fact which remains incomprehensible at present.

Over the last 15 years (1967–1981), 101 children were referred for neurophysiological investigations at Great Ormond Street, during an episode of status epilepticus (75 boys and 26 girls, 38 below one year, 42 between one and six years and 21 between six and 15 years). One or more attempts to control status epilepticus were made with clinical and EEG monitoring at the patient's bedside. Of these 101 cases, 84 were studied during a single episode of status epilepticus, and the remaining 17 during two and three episodes. A total of 288 injections of either methohexitone or diazepam was given, in small doses, to these 101 children during status epilepticus.

The EEGs were taken with a uniform technique using silver/silver chloride electrodes stuck to the scalp with collodion according to measurements from bony landmarks [3]. On occasions 2–4 channels were used for poly EMG (surface recording EMG) (as well as a lead one electrocardiogram) with techniques previously described [4]. The apparatus was either an Offner/Beckman eight channel type T or a Grass 8–10 type. The time constant usually employed was 0.3 or 0.4 seconds, though sometimes increased to one second. The high frequency response was linear within 10 per cent up to 70Hz and the sensitivity was usually of 10 microvolts per one millimetre/pen deflection, though often decreased appropriately when the amplitude of the spontaneous activity was very high. The contact resistance of the electrodes to the skin was of the order of 5K Ohms. The EEG was taken as soon as possible in the ward or in the intensive care units. Depending on both clinical and EEG features during status epilepticus, as well as on the drugs already given prior to admission to our hospital, either methohexitone or diazepam was selected and rapidly injected intravenously as a bolus (about three seconds). Whenever possible an anaesthetist was present but in any case an appropriate resuscitation trolley was kept at hand. No undesirable side-effects (depressed respiration or hypotension) occurred with the small doses employed. The dose of methohexitone was between 3 and 10mg from a solution of 10mg/ml made up in distilled water (Brictol sodium, Eli Lilly) while diazepam was injected in doses of 0.5 to 2mg using a solution of 5mg/ml concentration (valium supplied by Roche). With diazepam a 1ml syringe was used, loaded with two or three times the selected dose so that the injection could be repeated if desired without removing the syringe. With methohexitone, a 2ml syringe was used for the same reasons. It is important to inject the bolus very rapidly (within three seconds) preferably directly into a vein. When it was necessary to inject through an intravenous line, the effect was less satisfactory because of the slower rate of administration and because of the dilution of the drugs.

Close clinical observation as well as EEG monitoring continued before, during and after the injection: particular note was taken of the events some 15–40 seconds after the injection because the more dramatic clinical and EEG changes are to be expected during this phase. A second dose of the same drug was given

1–5 minutes after the first if clinical and/or EEG changes were difficult to evaluate. The effect of methohexitone in such small doses usually lasts about three minutes while diazepam may have an effect for five or more minutes. In those cases where methohexitone had failed to control seizures, diazepam was administered five or more minutes later. Follow-up EEGs were taken a few hours later or the next day. It became apparent over the years that it was an advantage to begin with methohexitone particularly in patients who had not received large doses of barbiturates prior to arrival at our hospital, because its effect disappears in such a short time and there is minimal accumulation when a second dose is injected. The timing of events was pencilled on the EEG paper (type and amount of drugs, duration of the rapid injection, clinical and EEG changes). The patients were studied at the bedside after ascertaining that no respiratory or cardio-circulatory troubles were present and that resuscitation equipment was promptly available. Of course, if there was a disappearance of the seizures and of the discharges in the EEG the patient continued to be observed without injections.

Results

There was a great deal of variability in the clinical manifestations as well as in the EEG features before the therapeutic trial (Table I).

The clinical features in the first year of life were more variable than in older children with seizures lasting many minutes or hours. During a single prolonged episode there were also considerable variations in amplitude and morphology of the EEG phenomena even if the clinical phenomena remained apparently constant.

TABLE I. Total of 141 episodes of status epilepticus in 101 children

Main clinical features	Main EEG features	Number
Stupor or coma ('non-convulsive')	Continuous mostly spike or spike and wave discharges	6
Generalised tonic/clonic seizures	Either generalised or multifocal discharges	6
Unilateral or focal tonic and/or clonic phenomena (with or without hemiparesis)	Either contralateral or generalised discharges	20
Mixed/variable manifestations	Variable types of discharges usually with multifocal distribution	24
Ataxia, grogginess, minor twitching, often loss of contact	Variety of discharges but often spike and wave complexes 2–4 per second	38
Continuous myoclonic phenomena often with variable distribution and some preservation of contact	Multiple spikes with variable distribution mixed with slow waves and occasional complexes	47

The rapid injection of methohexitone usually interrupted the clinical phenomena within half a minute but the discharges in the EEG took 2–5 seconds more to disappear. However, in eight patients such effects on the EEG occurred much more slowly, being delayed at least for 1–2 minutes, while the clinical seizures returned after a few minutes. In these cases the drug probably did not reach the areas of the brain responsible for the clinical seizures because of impairment of cerebral circulation, as when multiple emboli are blocking small cerebral vessels. In three of these cases who died within a few hours, the presence of such small emboli were verified at post-mortem. A delay therefore in the EEG effect of the drug given as a bolus, in spite of cessation of convulsions, is important in the evaluation of differential diagnostic problems.

Both clinical and EEG effects of the drug were much less obvious and often indefinite when the intravenous injections could not be administered as rapidly as desirable for various reasons. In such cases a repetition of the injection at a faster rate, some minutes later, did in some cases interrupt both the clinical manifestations and also the discharges in the EEG. In 42 of the children, a transitory arrest of the motor pheomena occurred within half a minute without any EEG improvement and in all these patients the clinical manifestations reappeared some 3–5 minutes later. Rapid amelioration of the EEG features without a parallel clinical improvement was never seen.

An increase in the EEG discharges *without* change in the clinical manifestations of the status epilepticus (whatever its features) occurred in some 10 per cent of children who had received methohexitone. Such increase in EEG spikes lasted only 2–3 minutes and was probably due to an idiosyncratic sensitivity of some individuals to this drug. This phenomenon has also been reported in the literature in relation to thiopentone. It was interesting to note that a child who showed an increase in EEG discharges following methohexitone (with no clinical deterioration) could respond to a bolus of diazepam injected a few minutes later with the opposite effect i.e. a disappearance of the clinical manifestations and the discharges in the EEG.

There was another group of patients who did not respond to diazepam but in whom methohexitone reduced or suppressed the discharges in the EEG together with a rapid clinical improvement. Although there were 40 children who did not benefit from either drug 61 responded favourably to one or other or both drugs. In 12 children further therapy was not necessary as clinical and EEG improvement occurred within half a minute following the injection. In these cases there was no reappearance of either EEG discharges or seizures for days or months and the bolus of drug given disrupted a vicious circle of seizures.

The following cases illustrate some of the advantages and limitations of a present approach to the control of status epilepticus in particular circumstances.

Case 1 This boy of five years was referred for an EEG on 4 May 1970 (Figure 1A) with a provisional diagnosis of 'minor status, myoclonic seizures, major epilepsy'.

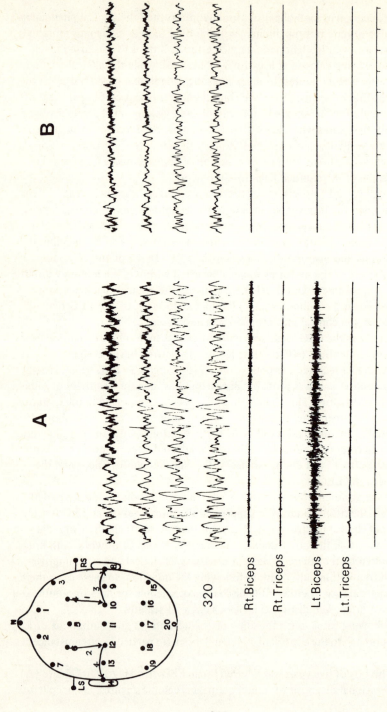

Figure 1. Five year old boy (Case 1). Top 4 channel EEG and lower 4 channels surface EMG. Paper speed at 1.5 cm a second.
A) Note sensitivity at 320 microvolts/10 millimetre-pen-deflection. Diazepam 1 mg injected rapidly intravenously during a status.
B) Forty seconds later disappearance of muscle activity and of EEG discharges. Sensitivity now of 100 microvolts/10 millimetres

He had been admitted to this hospital under the care of Dr John Wilson and was receiving mysoline, epanutin, phenobarbitone and valium. At the time of this test there were nearly continuous fast twitching movements involving the fingers, sometimes the thumb and less frequently the legs with variable lateralised preponderance. There were also small twitching movements of the muscles of the face mostly of the eyelids. There were also more violent jerks affecting trunk and limbs, but he was able to close and open his eyes to command, though very slowly, and was able to try hyperventilation to command.

The EEG on 4 May 1970 showed a severe generalised abnormality with practically continuous discharges accompanied by myoclonic phenomena of variable severity. Intravenous valium 1mg was given as a bolus and in less than half a minute there was a marked diminution of the discharges in the EEG while there was a disappearance of the muscle activities of the right and left biceps and triceps (Figure 1B).

In less than seven minutes the myoclonic phenomena returned. This boy was then treated with a variety of other drugs with reasonably good results. After removal of the polypharmacy and treatment with ACTH the major seizures and the status myoclonicus disappeared though he occasionally fell at school.

In 1973 he had no more fits and was attending an ESN school. The EEG showed a marked improvement while there was a residual excess of slow components particularly over the anterior half of the two hemispheres and an asymmetry in the posterior temporal regions suggesting that the underlying pathological process was in a quiescent phase.

Case 2 This 18 month old girl was a patient of Dr Philip Evans who referred her for EEG investigations. She had been 'off colour' for two weeks and on that day (14 December 1967) had a prolonged generalised convulsion which was terminated with 1.75ml of paraldehyde after three-quarters of an hour. She remained semi-comatose and two hours later the seizures reappeared with clonic movements involving the right arm and fast twitching of the right side of the face. She was given 1ml of paraldehyde at 11a.m. without effect and the jerking continued with similar distribution. In the EEG there was large amplitude slow activity (500 to over 1000 microvolts) at about 1–2 per second, maximal in the posterior half of the left hemisphere mixed with small sharp waves and spikes. The activity on the right side was of slightly lower amplitude particularly in the posterior third of the hemisphere. Methohexitone was given intravenously as a bolus (6mg) and in about 20 seconds there was complete relaxation of face and limbs and disappearance of the discharges in the EEG (Figure 2A) with disappearance of the grouping of muscle activities which were superimposed upon the electrocardiogram. In the EEG fast activity elicited by the Brietal was present over a wide area of the right hemisphere but not over the left and irregular very slow activity was seen on the left side suggesting a fairly large involvement of the left hemisphere (Figure 2B). No more seizures occurred although the patient remained

Figure 2. 18 month old girl (Case 2)

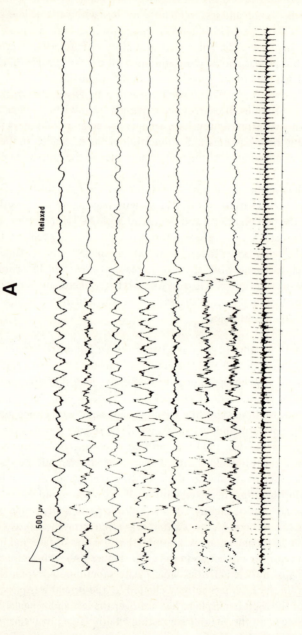

Relaxed

500 μv

A

A) In status with preponderant right sided convulsions. Paper speed 1.5cm/sec. EEG sensitivity 500 microvolts/10 millimetres. Only 6mg of methohexitone given intravenously as a bolus. In less than 20 seconds the large discharges and the muscle activity (superimposed on the electrocardiogram) disappeared. The asymmetry between the two hemispheres was just visible with such a low sensitivity

284

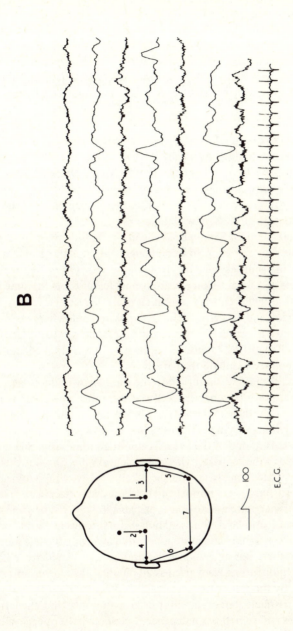

B

285

B) Two minutes after methohexitone bolus. Paper speed 3cm/sec. Child relaxed, awake. EEG sensitivity 100 microvolts/10 millimetres. Gross asymmetry between the activities of the two hemispheres with large very slow activity on the left. The fast activity on right side indicates a normal effect of methohexitone. On the left side, the absence of fast activity response to the drug is due to the extensive cortical damage

rather drowsy for several hours, probably due to the administration of the paraldehyde. No further seizures occurred in subsequent days and further EEGs showed a rapid improvement. It emerged that this girl had sustained a left parietal fracture and a lumbar air encephalogram showed only slightly widened sulci without real brain atrophy. Further follow-ups showed a moderate EEG abnormality with patchy distribution over the two hemispheres maximal in the left temporo-occipital region and to some extent also in the right temporal area with small multifocal discharges in 1974 (probably sequelae to the head injury mentioned above) but no further seizures had occurred and the patient was on no drugs.

Case 3 This girl had congenital heart disease with transposition of the great arteries and pulmonary stenosis. As a baby she was seen at the local hospital and then transferred to The Cardio Thoracic Unit at Great Ormond Street on 27 November 1961 where the diagnosis was made and the child was followed up as an outpatient for several years, was re-admitted on 27 September 1966 for further investigations, breathless on walking.

The first EEG taken on 28 September 1966 at the bedside prior to angio-cardiography showed an excess of slow components in the waking state for a child of five years and some asymmetry between the activities of the two hemi-spheres but no signs of a focal lesion or paroxysmal features. At the time we were doing a survey of children with congenital heart disease before, during and after angiocardiograms and no definite changes appeared following two injections of contrast media into the cardiac ventricles under gas/oxygen/halothane anaesthesia between 16.30 and 17.22 hours when the wound was stitched and the anaesthetist was about to extubate the patient.

However, when the child was returned to the ward a few minutes later it was noticed that she was not breathing very well and there was generalised twitching more marked on the right than on the left side. In the subsequent two hours there was an increase in jerking varying in intensity and involving the legs more than the arms with upwards rolling of the eyeballs almost continuously. She was intubated and connected to the ventilator via a nasotracheal tube. She was then given intravenous thiopentone 25mg twice and she became behaviourally in deep sleep or in semi-coma. Her fundi were normal and her limbs were flaccid at first but at about 21.30 hours her pulse was no longer palpable in the wrist or groin though still recognisable at carotid level. Resuscitation procedures were carried out and soon after midnight generalised convulsions occurred involving the left more than the right limbs and there was no response to intramuscular paraldehyde (2ml). Ten milligrams of thiopentone were given as a bolus and the convulsions stopped for three minutes. By the following morning 29 September 1966 the patient was still in coma with frequent stereotype short lived spasms involving the left more than the right limbs and sometimes independent periodic jerks of each side of the face.

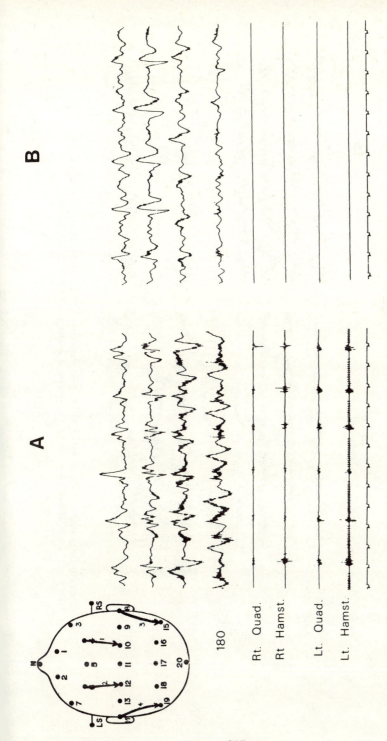

Figure 3. Five year old girl (Case 3). In coma with continuing jerks of right and left limbs with variable lateralised preponderance.
A) Somewhat periodic complex bursts in the EEG, during repetitive but variable muscular contractions. Two milligrams diazepam injected as a bolus.
B) Two minutes later patient was relaxed and the EMG was silent but in the EEG the repetitive complexes persisted, in keeping with extensive bilateral inadequate cerebral perfusion

287

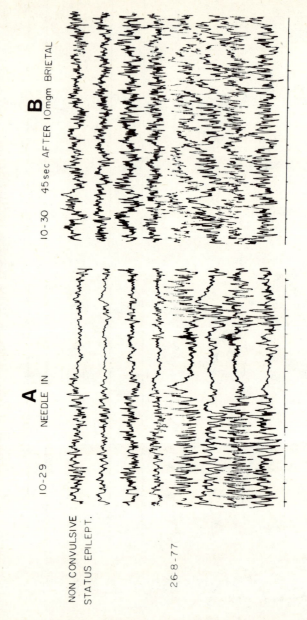

Figure 4. Four year old boy (Case 4). In 'non-convulsive status epilepticus'

A) Fluctuating very frequent spikes. Paper speed 1.5cm. Sensitivity 200 microvolts/10 millivolts. No jerks

B) After 10mg of methohexitone there was an increase in discharges but no clinical changes

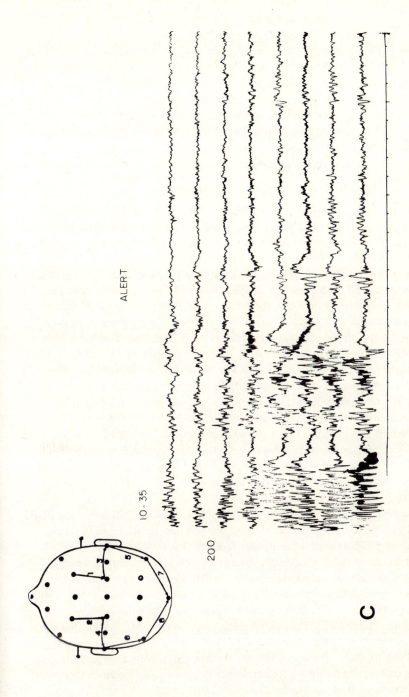

C) Five minutes after B, 1mg of diazepam was injected as a bolus and there was a prompt (20 seconds)
   disappearance of EEG discharges and the boy became fully alert and cheerful

289

In the EEG there were large amplitude slow waves with small sharp elements with variable lateralised preponderance reaching well over half a millivolt while in the poly EMG (surface EMG electrodes) there were groupings of muscle activity during the contractions every 2–3 records (Figure 3A). Intravenous valium was given as a bolus (2mg) and two minutes later there was a complete disappearance of the movements and general clinical relaxation but in the EEG the large amplitude repetitive complex slow waves persisted (Figure 3B). In the afternoon the patient went into ventricular fibrillation with failure to respond to resuscitation procedures and the child died.

Post-mortem showed embolic injury of gut and kidneys but the brain was not investigated.

Case 4 This case was referred by Dr Brett at the age of four years because of 'lots of petit mal and myoclonic episodes and ? in minor motor status or ? effect of drugs'. The patient at the time was treated with dexamphetamine, zarontin, diamox and epilim. There was a strong family history of seizures.

The first EEGs showed a large amount of very frequent discharges (spikes, sharp waves and 2–4 per second complex waves and spikes, much more prominent over the posterior than over the anterior half of the two hemispheres). These discharges were practically continuous and increased during passive eye closure and also during photic stimulation at high rates of flickering. This boy's history was complex and he had started having seizures at the age of 11 months and had been treated with many drugs without any benefit in various hospitals. There were transient periods of blankness and blinking of the eyelids as well as sudden jerking of one or more limbs; there were also periods of generalised rigidity for up to a minute without loss of consciousness. At 20 months the jerking became more violent and treatment with clonazepam apparently stopped the seizures for two months. Later, however, he was seen at various hospitals and each doctor gave his or her preferred combination of drugs. He was transferred to Great Ormond Street with a view to 'either ketogenic diet or ACTH for his intractable epilepsy'.

A second EEG on 7 April 1977 showed similar features to those of the first record and further combination of drugs was not beneficial. An EEG taken on 26 August 1977 showed again similar features (Figure 4A). After 10mg of Brietal intravenously as a bolus the discharges increased without however any change in the patient's clinical state (Figure 4B). However, five minutes later valium 1mg was given intravenously and in less than 20 seconds this boy turned promptly around to look at people and became aware of what was going on around him (Figure 4C). The complex discharges in the EEG disappeared for about two minutes and then reappeared together with the return of his grogginess and twitching state. Therapy with many other drugs, including prednisolone, ACTH, epilim, phenytoin and tegretol were not beneficial. However there was some benefit with ketogenic diet for a limited period.

In 1978 he gradually improved with decrease of phenytoin and removal of prednisolone. A CT scan in December 1978 showed no evidence of any focal abnormality. Further increase in tegretol was not beneficial and another course of ACTH made him miserable.

Conclusions

In conclusion the most important aim in an emergency situation such as that of status epilepticus is to make sure that the patient's respiratory and cardiovascular functions are cared for. In a well equipped hospital with good experience of the intensive care situation, the patient's risks are relatively small. It is therefore possible in selected circumstances to study patients in status epilepticus both clinically and with EEG monitoring while attempting to control the condition, particularly in infants and children. Since the work of Naquet et al [5] diazepam has been considered very useful: the recommended doses in the literature vary from 5mg to over 100mg as a slow infusion over a period of many minutes, hours or days. The main disadvantage of this method is that the patient remains asleep, sometimes very deeply for long periods. Even if the motor phenomena disappear over a period of minutes or hours, the patient may remain out of touch or in coma for long periods and without the EEG monitoring it is impossible to appreciate fully whether cerebral function has substantially improved or not.

The small dose of diazepam given as a bolus, instead, may be sufficient to control the clinical status and may stop the discharges in the EEG as well, with the advantage of being able to document the possible reversibility of the cerebral condition. A slight increase of fast activity in the EEG (due to the small dose of diazepam) helps further in assessing the extent of cortical involvement. With such small doses no complications occurred in the 288 injections and in particular there was no hypotension, respiratory depression, cardiac arrest or the tonic status epilepticus met by Prior et al [6].

The use of methohexitone in small doses, injected intravenously as a bolus achieved the same results. The advantage of methohexitone in small doses is that it has very little soporific effect and that one or two injections at intervals of two or three minutes do not have cumulative effect in contrast with diazepam. The disadvantage of methohexitone, however, seems to be only an increase in EEG spikes in about 10 per cent of patients: this usually indicates that a beneficial effect was unlikely to be achieved. No clinically detectable seizures were triggered with such small doses in spite of the increase of spikes in the EEG.

It is difficult at present to understand why some patients respond to one or the other drug or even to both. If one or the other drug is given in small amounts as a bolus and status epilepticus is not interrupted within half a minute, two possibilities remain: either there is a partial vascular occlusion in some areas which prevents the bolus being promptly distributed in the brain; or there has been some saturation effect due to the amount and type of drugs already given in the previous day or so.

We must remember, however, that if instead of a fast bolus injection (2–3 seconds) the drug is administered slowly (intravenous, intramuscular, oral or rectal) the results will be poor as the pharmacokinetic properties are considerably distorted.

References

1   Gastaut H. *Dictionary of Epilepsy 1973;* 72. Geneva: World Health Organisation
2   Pampiglione G, Da Costa AA. *J Neurol Neurosurg Psychiatry 1975; 38:* (4) 371–377
3   Pampiglione G. *Proceedings of the Electrophysiological Technologists Association (EPTA) 1956; 7:* 20–30
4   Pampiglione G. *Electroencephalogr Clin Neurophysiol 1965; 19:* 314
5   Naquet R, Soulayrol R, Dolce G, et al. *Electroencephalogr Clin Neurophysiol 1965; 18:* 427
6   Prior PF, MacLaine GN, Scott DF, Laurance BM. *Epilepsia (Amst) 1972; 13:* 467–472

33

COMPUTERISED TOMOGRAPHY IN POST-TRAUMATIC EPILEPSY

I F Moseley, J Silie Ruiz

Late epileptic seizures are not a common complication of head injury. Annegers et al [1] found a maximum incidence of 11.5 per cent in five years following severe trauma (brain contusion, intracranial haematoma or 24 hours of unconsciousness or amnesia). In many cases, where the aetiology is clear, investigation is rather limited. Computerised tomography (CT) has the great advantage of being a non-invasive imaging modality which can show changes within the cerebral parenchyma.

An earlier study of 500 patients with epileptic seizures of different types included 35 patients with a known head injury antedating the first seizure. They showed a higher incidence of hydrocephalus than the remaining patients, but the results were otherwise almost identical in the two groups [2]. This chapter is concerned with a larger group of patients thought to have post-traumatic epilepsy.

Material and Methods

One hundred consecutive patients undergoing CT examinations as part of the investigation of presumed post-traumatic epilepsy were reviewed. There were 63 males and 37 females.

Criteria for inclusion in the study were:

(i)   normal development, without seizures, up to the time of head injury;

(ii) a documented closed head injury of at least moderate severity;

(iii) well documented seizures extending beyond the early post-traumatic period (in effect, at least one year);

(iv) no other established cause of epilepsy;

(v)   CT study performed at the National Hospital, Queen Square.

The following data were recorded: age at time of head injury; duration of loss of consciousness; post-traumatic amnesia and hospitalisation; presence of a skull fracture; cranial surgery; interval to onset of seizures; type and frequency of attacks; presence of physical signs; type and site of EEG abnormalities; CT findings: ventricular size and any focal or generalised abnormality.

Results

Age at time of trauma Approximately one quarter of the patients suffered head injuries in each of the first three decades, and the remainder when more than 30 years of age. Three patients had had at least two severe head injuries.

Duration of loss of consciousness, etc. Since the injuries had in many cases occurred in childhood, many of these details were imprecise e.g. data on length of the period of unconsciousness were available for only 69 patients. Of these, 11 (14%) claimed not to have lost consciousness, while nine (11%) had been unconscious for more than one week, and two (2.5%) for more than a month. There were 16 patients (20%) who had lost consciousness for less than one hour; of the remainder 12 (15%) had been unconscious for less than a day and 30 (37.5%) for less than one week.

Post-traumatic amnesia Data were available for 65 patients. Of these, 20 (21%) had had no amnesia, but an amnesic period of more than one day was reported by 36 per cent.

Hospital admission Only 50 patients gave presumably accurate information, of whom 15 (30%) had not been admitted, while 14 patients (28%) had spent more than one month in hospital.

Skull fractures at the time of injury were reported in 33 cases; five were depressed. Sixteen patients had undergone cranial operations, of whom four had been known to have subdural haematomas.

Interval to onset of seizures This was known in 88 patients. Seizures commenced within one year in 43 per cent of patients but there were 10 (11%) in whom seizures did not supervene for at least 10 years and 13 (15%) in whom delay was greater than 20 years. In both of these groups, no other cause of epilepsy was revealed.

Seizures occurred at least one per month in 68 per cent of patients, and less than twice per year in only 8 per cent. They were classified as: generalised, focal, temporal lobe and psychomotor; 28 patients had attacks of more than one type. Using the most specific type as the basis of classification, seizures were generalised in 42 per cent, focal motor or sensory in 24 per cent and temporal lobe and/or psychomotor in 34 per cent.

Physical signs No abnormal signs were present in 56 patients; 27 showed evidence of focal cerebral damage, six had cranial nerve palsies and in 11 cases there were non-focal signs of cerebral damage, six had cranial nerve palsies and in 11 cases there were non-focal signs of cerebral disease — dementia, retardation, etc.

The EEG was classified as normal, diffusely abnormal, or showing a localised abnormality. In five cases the data were insufficient, but of the remainder 28 patients (29%) had normal records, 15 (16%) showed a diffuse abnormality, and more focal changes were present in 52.

CT The studies were classified as normal: 31 cases; non-focal atrophy (enlargement of the cerebrospinal fluid spaces): 18 cases; hydrocephalus (ventricular enlargement only): 5 cases; focal lesion(s): 41 cases; and miscellaneous: 5 cases. The most frequent focal abnormality was low attenuation in the inferior frontal white matter on one or both sides, sometimes extending to the overlying cortex and associated with focal atrophy (9 cases).
   CT findings were correlated with duration of post-traumatic amnesia, and of loss of consciousness, delay to onset of seizures, their type, EEG findings and physical signs.

CT and post-traumatic amnesia (Table I)

In the 45 patients who had reported post-traumatic amnesia, lasting from several minutes to two years, focal CT findings increased with its duration. Thus, those in whom amnesia lasted less than one day had normal CT studies in 78 per cent; with a duration of 1–7 days this fell to 44 per cent, whereas 39 per cent showed focal abnormalities, and of the patients in whom the period of amnesia exceeded

TABLE I. Post-traumatic amnesia and CT findings

| | CT | | | | |
	Normal	Atrophy	Hydrocephalus	Focal lesion	Other
Duration of post-traumatic amnesia					
< 1 week (27)	16 (60)	2 (7)	2 (7)	7 (26)	–
< 1 month (13)	2 (15)	3 (23)	–	8 (62)	–
> 1 month (5)	–	–	1 (20)	3 (60)	1 (20)

one week, 60 per cent showed focal lesions and only 11 per cent were normal. Of the eight patients with an amnesic period of less than one month, four showed frontal lesions at CT, as did three in whom amnesia lasted for more than one month.

CT and duration of unconsciousness (Table II)

A similar pattern was seen here; 62 per cent of those patients who had been unconscious for one hour or less had normal CT studies, compared with 25 per cent when consciousness had been regained within one week, and 12.5 per cent (one patient) when it was more long-lasting. Conversely, the proportion of patients with focal lesions was 15 per cent, 47 per cent and 75 per cent respectively in the three groups.

TABLE II. Loss of consciousness and CT findings

Duration of loss of consciousness	CT				
	Normal	Atrophy	Hydrocephalus	Focal lesion	Other
< 1 hour (13)	8 (62)	3 (23)	–	2 (15)	–
< 1 week (35)	8 (25)	5 (16)	3 (9)	15 (47)	1 (3)
> 1 week (8)	1 (12.5)	1 (12.5)	–	6 (75)	–

CT and time of onset of seizures (Table III)

There was no evidence that seizures commenced sooner in patients with focal cerebral damage as demonstrated by CT; indeed, the onset appeared more rapid in patients with normal CT studies, and in those with generalised atrophic changes. Onset was relatively rapid in the small group of patients with hydrocephalus.

TABLE III

CT finding		% of patients having seizures by this time after trauma			
		1 yr	5 yr	10 yr	20 yr
Normal	(42)	66	83	88	100
Non-focal atrophy	(18)	72	83	100	-
Hydrocephalus	(5)	60	100	-	-
Focal lesion	(31)	43	52	67	100
Other	(4)	100	-	-	-
TOTAL		60	72	81	100

CT and type of epilepsy (Table IV)

Of 42 patients with *generalised* seizures only, almost half had normal or atrophic CT studies, or showed other abnormalities which were probably irrelevant; four of the five patients in whom CT revealed hydrocephalus had generalised attacks. Focal CT abnormalities were slightly more common in those with focal motor seizures, and in those with temporal lobe attacks. Patients with temporal lobe epilepsy also showed the highest proportion (41%) of normal scans.

TABLE IV. CT findings and seizure type

Seizure type	CT				
	Normal	Non focal atrophy	Hydrocephalus	Focal lesion	Other
Generalised	10 (24)	9 (21)	4 (9.5)	15 (36)	4 (9.5)
Focal motor	7 (29)	5 (21)	1 (4)	11 (46)	–
Temporal lobe and/or psychomotor	14 (41)	4 (12)	–	15 (44)	1 (3)

CT and the EEG (Table V)

There was a good correlation between focal CT findings and localised abnormalities in the EEG. However, focal EEG changes were also common in patients with hydrocephalus and in those with normal CT studies. Closer inspection of the group with focal lesions revealed a close correlation between the *site* of the EEG and CT abnormalities (Table VI). Thus, 31 of 50 patients with focal lesions on the EEG had focal abnormalities on CT, of which 20 were in the same quadrant.

TABLE V. CT and EEG findings

EEG	CT				
	Normal	Non focal atrophy	Hydrocephalus	Focal lesion	Other
Normal	15 (38)	4 (29)	–	6 (19)	–
Diffuse	5 (12)	4 (29)	–	3 (10)	–
Localised	20 (50)	6 (42)	5 (100)	22 (71)	–

TABLE VI. 50 patients with focal EEG abnormalities

CT:	normal	15 (30)
	non focal atrophy	4 (8)
	hydrocephalus	2 (4)
	focal lesion	29 (58)

same quadrant	12
same side, different quadrant	4
bilateral, same quadrant	6
bilateral, different quadrant	1
EEG bilateral, same quadrant	2
no agreement	4

CT and physical signs (Table VII)

There was a broad correlation between the presence of focal signs and focal anomalies on the CT scan.

TABLE VII. CT findings and physical signs

Physical signs	CT					Total
	Normal	Non focal atrophy	Hydrocephalus	Focal lesion	Other	
Focal	10 (37)	5 (19)	1 (4)	11 (40)	–	27
Other cerebral	6 (35)	4 (24)	1 (6)	5 (29)	1 (6)	17
None	26 (47)	9 (16)	3 (5)	15 (27)	3 (5)	56

Other radiological investigations

Radionuclide scans were carried out in 13 cases, 10 were normal, two showed abnormalities probably related to old craniotomies and one was wrongly interpreted as indicating a subdural haematoma. Intrathecal radioisotope cisternography gave a normal result in one case of suspected hydrocephalus.

Five carotid angiograms were performed, two preceding temporal lobectomy. None showed a structural abnormality confirmed at CT.

Three of six pneumoencephalograms showed atrophy; one was normal, one demonstrated a porencephalic cyst, while in the last no ventricular filling occurred.

Effects on management

Two patients with normal CT studies underwent temporal lobectomy; two in whom CT had revealed hydrocephalus had ventricular shunting procedures. No active therapy resulted from the CT findings in any other case.

Discussion

A very large number of publications have dealt with CT findings in various types of epilepsy, but few have specifically concerned that of traumatic origin.

However, Moseley and Bull [2], dealing with a very heterogenous group, noted that hydrocephalus and tumours, which they found in 13 per cent and 9 per cent of patients with a history of head injury, were respectively less and more common in the group as a whole – 5 per cent and 16 per cent. They also noted that changes indicating 'atrophy' – enlargement of the sulci, fissures and ventricles – were extremely common, particularly in the elderly and in chronic epileptics. Thus, atrophic changes were present in 39 per cent of patients aged more than 40 at onset of epilepsy and in 40 per cent of those who had had seizures for 20 years or more. The discovery of non focal atrophy in patients with post-traumatic epilepsy is therefore of questionable significance. The correlation of CT atrophy with cerebral deficit is also rather poor [3].

A systemic study of post-traumatic epilepsy was carried out by Yoshii et al [4]. They identified 41 patients among an assiduously followed group of 262 cases of head injury. However, although they followed criteria similar to those in the present series (no seizures prior to the trauma, no evidence of cerebral or systemic disease other than the seizures, and 'purely epileptic' seizures), patients were admitted who had spike and wave EEG abnormalities, even if they never suffered clinical seizures. Moreover, the proportion of clinical and electro-encephalographic 'seizures' was not stated; they were classified as generalised (63.6%), partial (15.2%) or of other types (21.2%). In the 83 patients who attended for at least six months with post-traumatic sequelae, the Japanese workers found seizures or EEG abnormalities in 49 per cent. CT findings of normal appearances, generalised atrophy, asymmetrical ventricular dilatation or possible subdural effusions were not associated with an increased incidence (41–54.5%) of epilepsy, but parenchymal low density lesions into which category the frontal lesions noted in the present series fall, were associated with a 72.7 per cent incidence, and in cases with lesions of this type in which there was a known skull fracture, the incidence increased to 87.5 per cent.

The widespread rather poor correlation between CT and EEG findings in the present series is not surprising; the former shows only morphological abnormalities, whereas the EEG is essentially a functional investigation. A similarly high proportion of normal CT findings in temporal lobe epilepsy has been noted previously; it is due in part to a high rate of positive EEG studies in this condition, and to technical difficulties in obtaining diagnostic CT images of the contents of the middle cranial fossa [2]. Oakley et al [5] suggested that comparison of pre- and post-contrast CT images could assist in lateralisation of temporal lobe epileptogenic foci, but their conclusions are highly debatable; in the large majority of cases, the EEG is much more reliable.

299

The clear relationship between post-traumatic amnesia and the presence of focal lesions, especially frontal, is in agreement with the known significance of amnesia as a predictor of epilepsy after head injury [6].

No reason is apparent for the later appearance of epilepsy in patients with focal lesions than in those without. It is possible that in some cases the focal lesions revealed by CT were the result of, for example, a subsequent vascular accident.

Yoshii et al [4] concluded that the 'CT scan appears to be indispensable in the diagnosis of post-traumatic epilepsy'. While the findings at CT may be of extreme interest, they rarely affect management, as shown by the present study. The chief value of CT lies in the exclusion of a superimposed lesion.

References

1   Annegers JF, Grabow JD, Groover RV et al. *Neurology 1980; 30:* 683–689
2   Moseley IF, Bull JWD. *Epilepsia 1976; 17:* 327
3   Claveria LE, Moseley IF, Stevenson JF. In Du Boulay GH, Moseley IF, eds. *The First European Seminar on Computerised axial tomography in Clinical Practice 1977;* 213–217. Berlin: Springer
4   Yoshii N, Samejima H, Sakiyama R, Mizokami T. *Neuroradiology 1978; 16:* 311–313
5   Oakley J, Ojemann GA, Ojemann LM, Cromwell L. *Arch Neurol 1979; 36:* 669–671
6   Jennett WB, Lewin W. *J Neurol Neurosurg Psychiat 1960; 23:* 295–301

34

FUNCTIONAL IMAGING OF THE EPILEPTIC BRAIN WITH POSITRON COMPUTED TOMOGRAPHY

J Engel, D E Kuhl, M E Phelps

The clinical diagnosis of specific epileptic disorders and research into the basic mechanisms of human epileptogenesis depend largely upon techniques which reveal abnormalities of neuronal function, as opposed to structure. For this reason, the recent advances in radiological imaging of structure have not been as important to epilepsy as to many other neurological conditions, and diagnoses of seizure disorders continue to depend largely on electrophysiological measurements. However, while the EEG is sensitive to epileptic disturbances of cerebral function, it is severely limited with respect to anatomical localisation. The EEG records activity only from regions of neocortex directly underlying scalp electrodes and, even with stereotaxically implanted depth electrodes (SEEG), the number of anatomical sites that can be sampled is relatively small. Consequently, a complete picture of the spatial distribution of functional abnormalities is impossible to obtain by this method. Furthermore, both interictal and ictal epileptiform electrical events propagate, and a falsely localising focus is not uncommonly observed [1–3].

In most clinical situations the information obtained from epileptic patients by electrophysiological testing is adequate but, when accurate localisation is required, additional evaluation techniques are necessary. This is particularly true when surgical therapy is considered, but is also important in other situations, not the least of which is research into the anatomical substrates of human epileptic behaviour and other epilepsy related phenomena.

Other methods for localising abnormalities of cerebral function in man are available, such as the xenon-133 method for measuring regional cerebral blood flow, a technique capable of revealing focal disturbances in epileptic patients [4–8], but results have been inconsistent and investigation is still limited to relatively large superficial cerebral structures accessible to scalp monitoring. More recent advances in nuclear medicine have applied techniques of computerised imaging to radionuclide scanning, which provides alternative methods for measuring local cerebral function in man with improved spatial resolution. Computerised imaging of biologically active radiopharmaceuticals beginning with single-photon emission computed tomography [9,10], and more recently involving positron computed tomography (PCT) [11,12], now provides a noninvasive means of visualising patterns of local function for the entire human brain.

In PCT, positron emitters such as ^{18}F, ^{13}N, ^{15}O and ^{11}C are incorporated into a wide variety of radiopharmaceuticals and metabolic precursors which are taken up by the brain. The annihilation radiation that occurs when a positron collides with an electron consists of two photons emitted in opposite directions (Figure 1). The path of this emission can be determined when both photons are simultaneously identified (coincidence detection) at opposite sides of the head. Using a circumferential array of sodium iodide or bismuth germinate radiation detectors (Figure 2), sufficient coincidence data are collected to mathematically reconstruct the cross sectional tissue concentration distribution of positron activity in the brain [11–14]. The mathematical image reconstruction used with PCT is the same as that used with the x-ray CT scanners. PCT of ^{18}F labelled 2-fluorodeoxyglucose (FDG) [14–16] is used to measure local cerebral metabolism for glucose (LCMRGlc) in a manner analogous to the ^{14}C-2-deoxyglucose (2DG) autoradiographic technique of Sokoloff [17]. Metabolic rate for glucose is calculated for specific brain structures using an extension of Sokoloff's operational

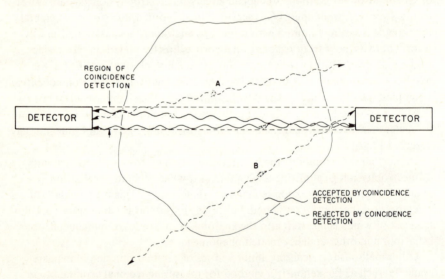

Figure 1. Illustrates the principle of annihilation coincidence detection employed in positron computed tomography. In the radioactive decay process of positron emission, two 511-keV photons are emitted 180 degrees apart. The photons are simultaneously recorded (ie, in coincidence) in opposing detectors to assure the radioactivity originated in a well-defined region between the two opposing detectors (solid lines). If an event strikes one detector but misses the opposing one, then it is rejected since it lies outside the region between the two opposing detectors (dashed lines) [12]

302

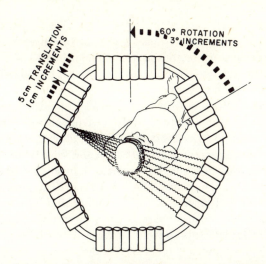

Figure 2. Schematic illustration of a circumferential arrangement of radiation detectors employed in a PCT system. The fan beam set of lines illustrates that the coincidence technique cannot only record events from a pair of directly opposing detectors, but also from all combinations of opposing detectors. Thus a circumferential array of detectors in a PCT system can simultaneously collect data from many different angles around the head. These sets of data are then used to mathematically reconstruct the cross section of tomographic distribution of the tissue concentration of the positron emitting radionuclide [58]

equation [14,16]. $^{13}NH_3$ has been used to demonstrate patterns of local cerebral blood flow [18,19]; ^{15}O labelled CO_2 or H_2O have also been used for blood flow measurements and, in conjunction with ^{15}O labelled O_2, measure metabolic rate for oxygen [20,21], while ^{11}CO labelled haemoglobin demonstrates the distribution of cerebral blood volume [22]. Other compounds labelled with positron emitters are presently being developed that may allow, among other things, demonstration of patterns of protein synthesis, amino acid metabolism, myelin, water and localisation of receptor sites for specific neurotransmitters.

At UCLA, patients with epilepsy have been studied with PCT of $^{13}NH_3$ and FDG [2,23–31]. In general, changes in blood flow have followed changes in metabolic rate, although the latter measurement is the more sensitive [30]. Consequently, most of the PCT studies of epilepsy to date have used FDG and only these will be discussed.

Methods

FDG is a competitive substrate with glucose for facilitated membrane transport sites and for hexokinase, the end product being FDG-6-PO_4, which is trapped essentially in the cells because it is not a substrate for the subsequent glycolytic reactions or the formation of glycogen [14–17]. It has a low membrane perme-

303

ability, and is only slowly dephosphorylated by phosphatase [14–17]. The rate of FDG phosphorylation is proportional to the rate of exogenous glucose utilisation. An operational equation for the calculation of LCMRGlc in man, which takes the dephosphorylation reaction into account, has been developed by Phelps and Huang [14,16] as an extension of the Sokoloff model [17].

Because of the relatively slow fixation rate (ie, tissue FDG turnover rate of $t^{1/2} = 4$ min), the calculated value of LCMRGlc represents an average value of the glucose metabolic rate over the period of the study but, since the plasma FDG concentration decreases rapidly with time, this value is heavily weighted to the earlier times after injection. For example, normally 55, 70 and 85 per cent of the LCMRGlc is determined within 5, 10 and 20 minutes after the injection, when scans are performed at about 40 minutes after injection [16]. If short duration changes in glucose metabolism occur, such as in ictal studies, then the calculated LCMRGlc represents a weighted average of the ictal and nonictal states. This weighting depends primarily upon the time the events occurred after injection and the duration of these events. The detailed effects of these transient changes in glucose metabolism have been analytically examined by Huang et al [16].

For the present studies, FDG with a specific activity of 10–20 mCi/mg was synthesised using the method developed by Ido et al [32] and modified by Barrio et al [33]. The radiochemical purity, as determined by thin layer and high pressure chromatography, was greater than 95 per cent. Following intravenous injection of approximately 10 mCi of FDG, 'arterialised' venous blood samples [14] were drawn from a hand heated in a water bath. These samples were used to measure the plasma FDG and glucose concentrations. Approximately 40 minutes were allowed for a near steady state condition to be reached before PCT scanning was initiated. Scanning of the full extent of the brain required another 40–60 minutes. Studies were carried out in an ambient environment without attempts to limit sensory input.

PCT studies have been performed at UCLA with the ECAT positron computed tomograph [13] (EG&G/ORTEC, Inc, Oakridge, TN), which has a resolution of 16mm in the plane of section. This scanner consists of a hexagonal ring of 66 sodium iodide detectors circumferentially located around the patient. A more sensitive and higher resolution instrument, the Neuro ECAT, has just begun operation at UCLA and is designed especially for the brain [34]. This scanner has three octagonal rings containing a total of 264 bismuth germinate detectors and a smaller opening, which places the detectors closer to the head. Three to five planes can be scanned simultaneously and resolution can be selected at 8 or 11mm in the image plane.

Results

The details of specific results have been published elsewhere and a summary of the important findings follow. These can be conveniently divided into interictal and ictal studies carried out in partial and generalised seizure disorders.

Over 100 patients with partial seizure disorders have been studied with PCT of FDG with concurrent EEG and/or SEEG monitoring. Detailed analyses were made for the first 50 patients for whom ictal as well as interictal EEG data were available [27,28]. Only two of these patients had x-ray CT scan abnormalities at the site of the presumed epileptogenic lesion. Approximately 70 per cent of these patients demonstrated one or more zones of hypometabolism, which correlated in most cases with the site of the epileptic focus as ultimately determined by combined interictal and ictal EEG and SEEG data [28] (Figure 3). However, there was no correlation between quantitative measures of LCMRGlc within the zone of hypometabolism and the frequency of SEEG recorded interictal epileptiform events [27]. Only one patient in this series demonstrated a zone of hypermetabolism in the interictal state, and this was within a larger zone of decreased metabolic activity [27].

Complete disagreement between positive electrophysiological and metabolic localisation of the epileptogenic lesion was observed for only three patients (6%) in this series [28]. In one, there was reason to believe the zone of hypometabolism, which subsequently disappeared, represented focal edematous changes due to irritation from depth electrodes and not the epileptic focus. In the second, retrospective analysis suggested the electrophysiological localisation may have been incorrect. The third patient was found to have multiple and diffuse lesions, some of which coincided with EEG abnormalities while others coincided with hypometabolism seen on PCT.

Pathological studies were carried out on anterior temporal lobes resected from 25 patients who had previously undergone PCT with FDG [23]. Twenty-two of these scans demonstrated a zone of hypometabolism and, in 19, this zone coincided with a pathological abnormality identified in the resected surgical specimens. Two of the remaining three FDG abnormalities were felt to be induced by depth electrodes while the third may have indicated a lesion posterior to the resection. The 19 lesions, which were not suspected by presurgical radiological studies, included mesial temporal sclerosis, one glial tumour, one fibrous meningioma, one heteratopia, and an angioma of the temporal pole. None of the three patients with normal FDG scans demonstrated structural lesions in their resected temporal lobe specimens.

In most patients with lesions, the extent of the hypometabolic zone was much greater than the extent of the pathological changes observed with light microscopy, and it could be demonstrated that this discrepancy was not a partial volume effect. It is not known whether the more extensive metabolic abnormalities represent structural disruption of synaptic organisation not seen with routine pathological evaluation, such as decreases in dendritic domains and absence of dendritic spines [35], or whether this could represent some epilepsy related suppression of neuronal function [36,37].

305

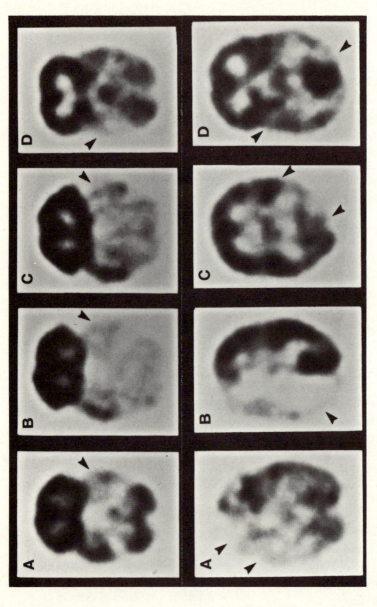

Figure 3. Examples of FDG scans from patients with partial seizure disorders. Top row, A–D: Representative temporal lobe hypometabolism (arrows). X-ray CT scans in these patients failed to demonstrate focal abnormalities. Bottom row, A–D: Representative FDG scan sections from patients with multiple or diffuse zones of hypometabolism, A) shows left frontal and temporal hypometabolism. The left frontal area appeared atrophic on x-ray CT scan, but the left temporal lobe was the site of ictal onset. B) shows hypometabolism of the entire left hemisphere in a patient with hemiatrophy. There was a left parietal focus on EEG (arrow). C) demonstrates right occipital and posterior temporal hypometabolism in a patient with a small cystic astrocytoma in the occipital lobe and seizures originating from this site. D) shows left temporal and right occipital hypometabolism in a patient with a normal x-ray CT scan. The left temporal lobe was demonstrated to be the site of the epileptogenic lesion

Interictal studies in generalised epilepsy

To date, no abnormal patterns of metabolic activity have been observed on interictal FDG scans of patients with absence seizures who were diagnosed as having petit mal epilepsy [30].

Ictal studies in partial epilepsy

PCT studies with FDG, as with 2DG autoradiography, require steady state conditions of glycolysis before absolute LCMRGlc can be accurately calculated, but these techniques can provide useful anatomical information in the nonsteady state conditions that characterise transient ictal events. For example, the technique can be used to examine the patterns of involvement of cerebral structures during various epileptic behaviours. We have previously used 2DG autoradiography for this purpose to study kindled seizures in rats [38]. Others have investigated epileptic spread from neocortical penicillin foci in rats [39–42] and monkeys [43–45], and limbic seizures in rats induced by penicillin [46] and kainic acid [47]. Analogous ictal FDG studies have now been carried out in a series of patients with partial seizures [24–26, 31]. Because ^{18}F has such a short half-life, these studies were possible only on patients whose seizures were sufficiently frequent to assure the occurrence of ictal events during FDG uptake, or on others in whom seizures could be easily activated.

Most patients studied during partial seizures have demonstrated a marked increase in metabolic activity at the site of the EEG ictal onset (Figure 4), but the anatomical pattern of hypermetabolism was different for each patients and, in some, included a variety of ipsilateral structures in addition to the primary focus. In one patient with hemiatrophy and a parietal ictal onset, the entire hemisphere was hypermetabolic with the highest degree of hypermetabolism occurring in the frontal lobe [31]. Another patient had a zone of relative hypometabolism surrounding a hypermetabolic temporal lobe [31] while, in two others, the entire brain beyond the zone or zones of hypermetabolism was markedly hypometabolic compared to control studies. A scan from a patient who had a brief focal seizure induced by electrical stimulation of one hippocampus showed relative hypometabolism of the ipsilateral temporal lobe, excluding the hippocampus. In general, when hypermetabolism was present, there was no quantitative correlation between the degree of increase in LCMRGlc and either the duration or frequency of ictal events.

These studies clearly show that the anatomical patterns of metabolic activity reflect both spread of ictal discharge and the site of ictal onset. In addition, these patterns appear to be unique for each individual patient rather than stereotyped, as in animal models [39–47]. Because of the temporal limitations of the metabolic measurements, it is not possible to determine whether the hypometabolism observed on ictal scans represents ictal mechanisms leading to metabolic suppression,

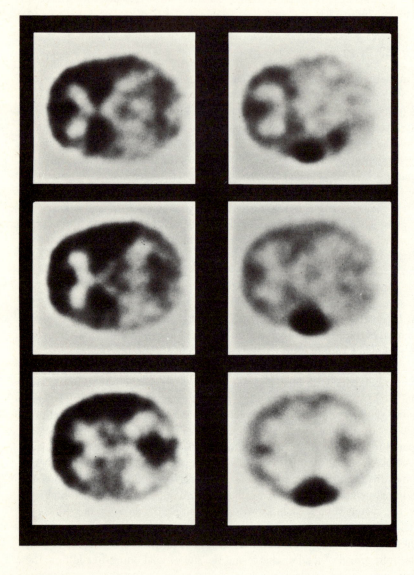

Figure 4. Three representative interictal (top row) and ictal (bottom row) FDG scan sections from a patient with partial seizures originating in the left sylvian area. The ictal hypermetabolism involves the left temporal lobe and suprasylvian structures, and is within the area of interictal hypometabolism

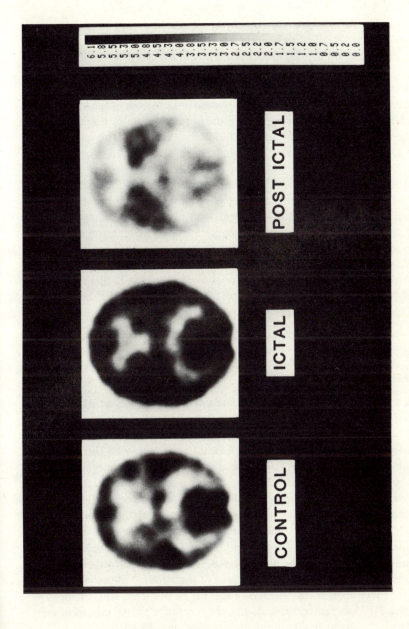

Figure 5. Sections from control, ictal and postictal FDG scans of a patient undergoing a series of electroconvulsive shock treatments for behavioural depression. Note the diffuse increase in metabolic activity ictally, and the decrease postictally, which does not appear to involve the basal ganglia. Scale at right indicates estimated LCMRGlc in mg glucose/min/100g tissue

or whether this can be explained entirely on the basis of postictal depression [24,25].

Ictal studies, generalised seizures

In order to investigate the metabolic correlates of postictal depression more specifically, FDG scans were carried out on a patient undergoing a series of electroconvulsive shock treatments [24,25]. FDG injected at the time of electroshock was associated with a diffuse increase in estimated LCMRGlc, while FDG injected at the end of the seizure and beginning of the postictal depression was associated with a generalised decrease in estimated LCMRGlc (Figure 5). This indicates that at least some of the hypometabolism seen during ictal FDG studies of partial seizures may be attributed to postictal phenomena.

Ictal scans performed on patients during petit mal seizures induced by 10 minutes of hyperventilation were compared to control scans performed after successful treatment with ethosuximide or valproic acid [30]. Control scans were also carried out during 10 minutes of hyperventilation when no absences occurred. Ictal episodes consisting of brief lapses of consciousness associated with generalised 3/second spike and wave EEG discharges produced a diffuse increase in LCMRGlc and the number or duration of ictal episodes during hyperventilation. The patterns of LCMRGlc observed on ictal and control scans were identical for each patient and no specific anatomical generator of petit mal absences could be identified.

Discussion

Significance for basic research

Chronic partial epilepsy in man, as in animals, is usually associated with focal structural changes in the brain and resultant loss of energy requiring elements [48–50]. Cell loss, however, cannot adequately account for the interictal metabolic patterns seen in the majority of FDG scans of patients with chronic partial seizure disorders, not only because the zones of hypometabolism appeared to extend beyond the pathological changes noted in resected temporal lobe specimens, but also because the hypometabolic zones became markedly hypermetabolic during seizures. The functional significance of these findings is, as yet, unknown. Although enhanced inhibitory phenomena have been well described in the experimental epileptic focus [49,50], recent experimental evidence indicates that active inhibition, at least in the hippocampus, results in an increase in glucose metabolism [51]. The neuronal mechanisms of the transient hypometabolism observed on ictal FDG scans, which may actually be postictal, also remain to be elucidated. 2DG autoradiographic studies of appropriate animal models of epilepsy are in progress in an attempt to answer these questions.

Ictal FDG scans appear to demonstrate sites of propagation as well as sites

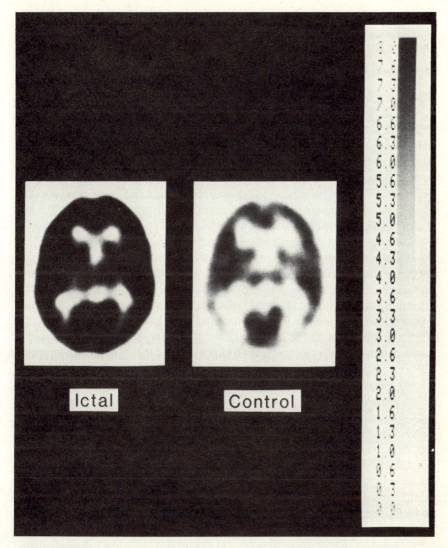

Figure 6. Two FDG scans performed on a child with petit mal seizures during 10 minutes of hyperventilation. For the ictal scan, hyperventilation produced frequent recurrent absences. The control scan was performed after successful treatment and hyperventilation failed to produce either behavioural or EEG abnormalities. Scale at the right indicates estimated LCMRGlc as in Figure 5

of seizure origin, and should improve our understanding of the anatomical substrates of specific epileptic behaviours. Comparison of ictal FDG scans obtained during spontaneous seizures in man with 2DG autoradiographic studies of experimental animal models of epilepsy may also help to determine which of these

311

experimental conditions actually do resemble human disorders and, thereby, improve the clinical relevance of animal research on basic mechanisms of epilepsy.

Significance for clinical diagnosis

The most useful aspect of PCT for the clinician appears to be enhanced spatial resolution of functional disturbances. The only proven diagnostic application of PCT to date has been its use for improving localisation of lesions in epileptic patients considered for resective surgical therapy [1,2]. PCT of FDG can help to determine whether an EEG spike focus is associated with an epileptogenic lesion or is propagated from a distance. On the other hand, many types of lesions can appear on FDG scans as a zone of hypometabolism and EEG studies are always necessary to determine whether this abnormality is epileptogenic.

At UCLA, PCT of FDG has become an important confirmatory test in the evaluation of epileptic patients who are candidates for surgical resection [1,2]. As discussed by Crandall et al elsewhere in this volume [52], the UCLA presurgical protocol includes tests to localise cerebral areas of epileptic excitability and also areas of focal dysfunction. Scalp and depth electrode EEG telemetry is used to identify sites of interictal spike discharges and spontaneous ictal onsets. Confirmatory tests include EEG and neuropsychological measures of focal dysfunction, and PCT with FDG. Although the UCLA approach initially required implantation of depth electrodes in all patients in order to confidently localise the epileptogenic lesion most responsible for the patient's habitual seizures [2,53], reliable localisation of abnormal tissue with PCT with FDG led to a change in the protocol in 1977 [1]. Since 1977, patients with well defined focal ictal onsets recorded with scalp and sphenoidal EEG telemetry have undergone surgical resection without depth electrode evaluation when the EEG determined epileptic focus also appeared hypometabolic on the interictal FDG scan, and one additional test of dysfunction confirmed the presence of a lesion in the same location [1]. In several patients with consistently focal ictal EEG onsets but no confirmatory focal dysfunction, the ictal EEG localisation was later determined to be incorrect [2]. However, all patients meeting the above criteria so far have revealed structural abnormalities in their resected tissue and benefited from surgery. Over 80 per cent are seizure free. At the present time approximately one-third of all patients who undergo anterior temporal lobectomy at UCLA do so without depth electrode evaluation, as a result of the addition of PCT to the presurgical protocol.

Ictal FDG scans do not appear to be useful for localisation of the epileptic focus since hypermetabolism is also seen in areas of propagation, but these scans may be helpful in the future as an aid to classification of epileptic disorders, if specific patterns are eventually identified. For instance, ictal and interictal scans may help to differentiate relatively benign disorders such as true petit mal and Sylvian epilepsy [54] from more malignant focal and generalised epileptic conditions.

312

PCT studies of FDG, as well as other newly developed biologically active compounds, have great potential for expanding our knowledge of epileptic conditions in man. Although it is too early to know to what extent PCT, or any of the other recently developed approaches to functional imaging of the brain such as single-photon emission computed tomography [9,10] and nuclear magnetic resonance [55], will have practical applications in routine clinical diagnosis, they will certainly become significant tools in neuroscience research [56,57]. None of these techniques, however, appears to rival the capacity of the EEG to identify properties unique to the epileptic condition. Consequently, correlative electrophysiological measurements are likely to continue to be important for this purpose, despite the increasing improvement in methods for imaging a variety of aspects of cerebral function.

Acknowledgments

Supported by Department of Energy contract DE-AM03-76-SF00012 and by USPH grants 7R01-GM-24839, 1P01-NS-15654 and 2P50-NS-02808.

We thank P H Crandall MD, E J Hoffman PhD, S C Huang DSc, N S MacDonald PhD, G D Robinson Jr PhD, J Barrio PhD, J Miller NMRT, F Aguilar NMRT, R Sumida NMRT, E Carr AB, A Ricci AB, M Williams REEGT and D Quinonez REEGT for their assistance.

References

1   Engel J Jr, Crandall PH, Rausch R. In Rosenberg RN, Grossman RG, Schochet S et al, eds. *The Clinical Neurosciences 1982;* In press. New York: Churchill Livingstone
2   Engel J Jr, Rausch R, Lieb JP, Crandall PH. *Ann Neurol 1981; 9:* 215–224
3   Gloor P. *Adv Neurol 1975; 8:* 59–106
4   Hougaard K, Oikawa T, Sveinsdottir E et al. *Arch Neurol 1976; 33:* 527–535
5   Ingvar DH. In Engel A, Larsson T, eds. *Stroke. Thule International Symposia 1966;* 105. Stockholm.
6   Ingvar DH. In Langfitt TW, McHenry LC Jr, Reivich M, Wollon H, eds. *Cerebral Circulation and Metabolism 1975;* 361. New York: Springer-Verlag
7   Lavy S, Melamed E, Portnoy Z, Carmon A. *Neurol 1976; 26:* 418–422
8   Sakai F, Meyer JS, Naritomi H, Hsu M-C. *Arch Neurol 1978; 35:* 648–657
9   Kuhl DE, Edwards RQ, Ricci AR, Reivich M. *J Nucl Med 1973; 14:* 196–200
10   Kuhl DE, Barrio JR, Huang SC et al. *J Nucl Med;* In press
11   Phelps ME. *Semin Nucl Med 1977; 7:* 337–365
12   Phelps ME, Hoffman EJ, Mullani NA, Ter-Pogossian MM. *J Nucl Med 1975; 166:* 210–224
13   Phelps ME, Hoffman EJ, Huang SC, Kuhl DE. *J Nucl Med 1978; 19:* 635–647
14   Phelps ME, Huang SC, Hoffman EJ et al. *Ann Neurol 1979; 6:* 371–388
15   Reivich M, Kuhl DE, Wolf A et al. *Circ Res 1979; 44:* 127–137
16   Huang SC, Phelps ME, Hoffman EJ et al. *Am J Physiol 1980; 238:* E69–82
17   Sokoloff L, Reivich M, Kennedy C et al. *J Neurochem 1977; 28:* 897–916
18   Phelps ME, Hoffman EJ, Raybaud C. *Stroke 1977; 8:* 694–702
19   Phelps ME, Huang SC, Kuhl DE et al. *Stroke 1981; 12:* 607–619
20   Ackerman RH, Correia JH, Alpert MN et al. *Arch Neurol 1981; 38:* 537–543
21   Frackowiak RSJ, Pozzilli C, Legg NJ et al. *Brain 1981; 104:* 753–778

22 Huang SC, Phelps ME, Hoffman EJ, Kuhl DE. *J Cereb Blood Flow Metabol 1981; 1:* 391–402
23 Engel J Jr, Brown WJ, Kuhl DE et al. Pathological findings underlying focal temporal lobe hypometabolism in partial epilepsy. Submitted to Ann Neurol
24 Engel J Jr, Kuhl DE, Phelps ME. In Delgado-Escueta AV, Wasterlain CG, Treiman DM, Porter RJ, eds. *Status Epilepticus: Mechanisms of Brain Damage and Treatment 1982;* In press. New York: Raven Press
25 Engel J Jr, Kuhl DE, Phelps ME. *Neurol 1981; 31:* 130
26 Engel J Jr, Kuhl DE, Phelps ME. *Trans Am Neurol Assoc 1981; 105:* 74–76
27 Engel J Jr, Kuhl DE, Phelps ME, Crandall PH. Localisation of the epileptic focus in partial epilepsy with PCT and EEG. Submitted to Ann Neurol
28 Engel J Jr, Kuhl DE, Phelps ME, Mazziotta JC. Characteristics of interictal local cerebral glucose metabolism in partial epilepsy. Submitted to Ann Neurol
29 Engel J Jr, Kuhl DE, Phelps ME. In Akimoto H, Kazamatsuri H, Seino M, eds. *Advances in Epileptology-1981 1982;* In press. New York: Raven Press
30 Engel J Jr, Kuhl DE, Phelps ME et al. *Metabolic Correlates of 3 per Second Spike and Wave Absences.* Presented at the annual meeting of the American EEG Society, Chicago, June 1981 (abstract)
31 Kuhl DE, Engel J Jr, Phelps ME, Selin C. *Ann Neurol 1980; 8:* 348–360
32 Ido T, Wan CN, Casella V et al. *J Label Compds Radiopharm 1978; 14:* 175–183
33 Barrio JR, MacDonald NS, Robinson GD Jr et al. *J Nucl Med 1981; 22:* 372–375
34 Hoffman EJ, Phelps ME, Huang SC et al. *IEEE Trans Nucl Sci 1981; NS-28:* 99–103
35 Sheibel ME, Crandall PH, Scheibel AB. *Epilepsia 1974; 15:* 55–80
36 Matsumoto H, Ajmone Marsan C. *Exp Neurol 1964; 9:* 286–304
37 Prince DA, Wilder BJ. *Arch Neurol 1967; 16:* 194–202
38 Engel J Jr, Wolfson L, Brown L. *Ann Neurol 1978; 3:* 538–544
39 Collins RC. *Brain Res 1978; 150:* 487–502
40 Collins RC. *Brain Res 1978; 150:* 503–518
41 Collins RC, Caston TV. *Neurol 1979; 29:* 705–716
42 Collins RC, Kennedy C, Sokoloff L, Plum F. *Arch Neurol 1976; 33:* 536–542
43 Caveness WF, Kato M, Malamut BL et al. *Ann Neurol 1980; 7:* 213–221
44 Hosokawa S, Iguchi T, Caveness WF et al. *Ann Neurol 1980; 7:* 222–229
45 Kato M, Malamut BL, Caveness WF et al. *Ann Neurol 1980; 7:* 204–212
46 Watson RE Jr, Siegel A. In Ben-Ari Y, ed. *The Amygdaloid Complex. INSERM Symposium No 20 1981;* 453. Amsterdam: Elsevier/North Holland Biomedical Press
47 Ben-Ari Y, Tremblay E, Riche D et al. *Neurosci 1981; 7:* 1361–1391
48 Brown WJ. In Brazier MAB, ed. *Epilepsy: Its Phenomena in Man 1973;* 341. New York: Academic Press
49 Margerison JH, Corsellis JAN. *Brain 1966; 89:* 499–530
50 Woodbury DM, Kemp JW. In Mrsulja BB, Rakic ZM, Klatzo I et al, eds. *Pathophysiology of Cerebral Energy Metabolism 1977;* 313. New York: Plenum
51 Ackermann RF, Finch DM, Babb TL, Engel J Jr. *Soc Neurosci Abst 1981; 7:* 457
52 Crandall PH, Engel J Jr, Rausch R. Indications for depth electrode recordings in complex partial epilepsy and subsequent surgical results. This volume
53 Walter RD. *Adv Neurol 1975; 8:* 49–58
54 Lombroso CT. *Arch Neurol 1967; 17:* 52–59
55 Hawkes RC, Holland GN, Moore WS, Worthington BS. *J Comput Assist Tomogr 1980; 4:* 577–586
56 Brownell GL, Budinger TF, Lauterbur PC, McGeer PL. *Science 1982; 215:* 619–626
57 Oldendorf WH. *Ann Neurol 1981; 10:* 207–213
58 Phelps ME, Hoffman EJ, Mullani NA, Higgins CS. *IEEE Trans Nucl Sci 1976; NS-23:* 516–522

35

THE PSYCHOLOGICAL MANAGEMENT OF EPILEPSY

T A Betts

Since modern clinical interest in epilepsy developed it has been known that psychological methods of treatment have been of use in stopping some fits in some people with epilepsy. It is also known that psychological events are sometimes responsible for increasing seizure frequency or can even directly precipitate fits. Apart from anecdotal accounts, however, and a few case reports, little scientific study has been made of the best form of psychological management to use in epilepsy. What little is known has been reviewed recently by Fenwick [1], Lubar and Deering [2] and Betts [3].

The reflex epilepsies are probably of the greatest historical interest. In these a specific sensory or psychological stimulus triggers off an epileptic fit in a susceptible individual, and does so consistently at each presentation. The importance of the reflex epilepsies in terms of the psychological management of epilepsy is twofold. Firstly they can often be treated by psychological means rather than using anticonvulsants. Secondly study of them suggests that in many of them it is the emotional response that the individual has to the triggering stimulus that is the most important factor in causing the fit. Thus it is usually the emotional association with the music that seems to be the trigger in musicogenic epilepsy rather than, say, the particular note or pitch of the music.

The reflex epilepsies teach us that emotional factors may be important in the precipitation of fits. Although emotions are probably not often a *direct* cause of fits, it is well established that changes in arousal, either upwards (as in anxiety) or downwards (as in boredom) may markedly increase seizure frequency. The evidence for this is reviewed by Betts [3]. Manipulating arousal levels toward the optimum level of arousal for a particular individual may therefore be beneficial in terms of reducing seizure frequency. It may be, indeed, that whatever they are supposed to do a great many of the current psychological methods of treatment for epilepsy either remove the patient's fear of his attacks or change his arousal levels to a more optimum level.

315

It may also be true that those patients who can control their own seizures by an effort of will do so by increasing or decreasing arousal levels. What proportion of patients can actually do this is unknown. The older literature suggests about five per cent of people with epilepsy can, but there have been recent suggestions [1] that perhaps the proportion is much higher.

It is also true that, just as some people can stop their attacks by an effort of will, so some can induce them at will. This is particularly common in children. Induced seizures are usually brief absences or myoclonic starts brought on by deliberately contrived flickering light: occasionally other mechanisms such as *deliberate* hyperventilation are used. *Unconscious* hyperventilation may be one of the main precipitants of those seizures that occur more frequently during times of heightened arousal.

Again the psychological treatments of epilepsy that I will be describing, whatever they are supposed to do, may be no more than measures to control hyperventilation.

Review of the literature suggests that one of the problems in assessing the impact of psychological treatments on epilepsy is that the majority of patients thus treated are chosen for treatment because they have intractable or atypical forms of epilepsy, or may be simulating their attacks. So far as I know no attempt has ever been made to assess the effect of psychological treatments on fresh untreated cases of epilepsy. Most of the literature consists of single case studies: there have been few properly controlled trials. When such trials have been conducted (it is possible to do this even in a single case study) the effect of such treatment has been markedly less than in uncontrolled studies, suggesting a placebo element in psychological treatments. The placebo effect, of course, is also a psychological effect and it is pertinent to enquire what it was the placebo actually did to the patient's brain to stop his fits.

One other factor that tends to confound the assessment of results in this area is the rivalry that exists between the medical profession (who look with distaste and distrust on psychological manipulation) and behavioural practitioners (mostly psychologists) who tend to see their every success in modifying or controlling epilepsy by psychological means as driving another nail in the medical coffin. The management of epilepsy is a partnership, not a battleground, and anyone who knows epilepsy well should be aware of how physical factors in epilepsy affect emotional ones and vice versa. Several methods have been described and employed for the psychological control of fits.

Willpower

Some people with epilepsy by an effort of will or concentration, by repeating a particular phrase to themselves again and again ("No, no, no!", "Stop it!") or by forcing their mind to go blank or by rapidly shifting their attention onto something else, or by rapidly inducing a feeling of calm or well-being, seem able to

316

abort their attacks. They usually discover their particular technique by accident and are not invariably successful. Sometimes the technique is used to delay an attack to a more convenient time rather than to stop it. Some people, if they do not eventually allow the attack to occur, will feel uncomfortable.

Most patients are loath to tell their doctor that they can control attacks because to reveal such control might imply the faking of attacks. "Can you do anything to stop the attacks?" should be a standard question all patients should be asked as, particularly in intractable epilepsy, developing such control or delaying skills may be important. We should study more carefully what it is such patients do to abort their attacks (it is likely that more than one mechanism is involved) as this information might be valuable to all patients.

Willpower, then, although effective for some, remains an individual and idiosyncratic method which has not been put to formal test. Fenwick [1] describes the reverse of these methods in those patients that with an effort of will can actually induce seizures. Such invoked seizures he calls 'true psychogenic seizures' although the term has been more loosely applied to people who imitate seizures rather than having genuine ones.

Various behavioural methods of treatment have been used to control individual seizures. The field was exhaustively reviewed by Mostofsky and Balaschak [4] and updated by Fenwick [1], Lubar and Deering [2] and Betts [3]. Behaviour therapy uses various techniques to directly change a person's observable behaviour and is thus different from psychotherapy which is directed toward enlightening the patient as to why he is feeling or behaving in a certain way. Behavioural methods have a slight aura of unpopularity because they are mistakenly associated in the lay mind with experiments on animals such as rats in cages receiving electric shocks. There is no doubt, however, that they are successful and appropriate methods of treatment for many conditions in psychiatry, particularly neurotic conditions.

Several workers have applied behavioural methods of treatment to the extinction of epilepsy, although there are many confounding variables in assessing results. Almost all reports of the use of behavioural methods in treating epilepsy are based on individual case studies. There is little doubt that behavioural methods do work in individual patients and, in those case reports which have used a long base line period before treatment and which have employed placebo periods in the treatment design, there is evidence of therapeutic effect (providing they are carefully controlled in this way, single case studies can be valuable).

Although various behavioural methods of treatment look promising, they have not been tested in defined groups of patients with defined types of epilepsy in the same way that clinical trials of new anticonvulsant drugs are carried out. They have not been used in fresh cases of epilepsy previously untreated, as is required in a drug trial, but are largely reserved for intractable epilepsies, or are used in subnormal children who also have behavioural disturbances, or are employed in patients who are particularly anxious or are frightened of their epilepsy.

My own observations over the years [3] would support those of Mostofsky

317

and Balaschak [4] who advise applying caution to the analysis of results of behavioural treatment of epilepsy. One has to be certain that it really was epilepsy that the experimenters were treating. Pseudoseizures (simulated seizures) are common, particularly in patients with supposedly intractable epilepsy. Pseudo-seizures are easily extinguished by behavioural methods (which is the treatment of choice for them). One would also have to be certain that it was not just the general ambiance of the behavioural programme (particularly one using relaxation or one in which a great deal of attention was paid to the patient) which was the effective therapeutic agent. There is evidence that even in biofeedback programmes, which will be described later, such placebo factors are important. A placebo response in a behavioural method of treating epilepsy does not imply that psychological mechanisms are not operating to control the patient's attacks — indeed it implies exactly the reverse — but that the particular behavioural method itself is not important in the control of the attacks.

Extinction and habituation techniques

Habituation and extinction techniques (which are rather 'old hat' as far as psychologists are concerned) have been applied to epilepsy particularly sensorily precipitated epilepsy. Forster [5] is the principle exponent of this method, which consists of continually exposing the patient to the precipitating stimulus until the epileptic response habituates (i.e. disappears). There is no doubt that in some patients repeated exposure (after initially leading to an increase in seizure frequency or of a convulsive EEG response) eventually leads to extinction of the response and, providing the patient practises with the precipitating stimulus a sufficient number of times in the future, the habituation remains so that the patient loses his attacks. The analogy with the massed practice techniques of dealing with tics and habit spasms is a fairly close one and the method, although tedious to use, is applicable to such medical rarities as musicogenic epilepsy or voice induced epilepsy.

Another method of behavioural control in evoked epilepsy is to apply a distracting stimulus when the evoking stimulus is applied which 'turns off' the response. Efron [6] first described such a method in a patient who had learnt that she could abort her partial seizures, in which an olfactory aura occurred, by inhaling smelling salts at the right moment. After a time she learnt to use not the salts themselves but the image of them to suppress her attacks. In the same way distracting stimuli applied at the right time may prevent an evoked response as has been described with reading epilepsy [5]. I am treating a boy with reading epilepsy at the moment, using a distracting method and it is interesting that in this patient learning a controlling technique (merely automatically tapping his knee whenever he sees a particular common word in whatever he is reading) not only works at a physiological level but has also given him a strong psychological boost as he now feels that he has control over his own condition. This illustrates what Mostofsky and Balaschak [4] point out "it is extremely difficult, if not impossible, to examine any one procedure independently from influences of other current conditions".

Classical conditioning procedures then have been very valuable in the treatment of certain kinds of epilepsy and should always be thought of in patients with reflex epilepsy. Fenwick [1] gives cogent reasons why this term, although still in common use, should be abandoned for the expression 'evoked seizures' as first coined by Symonds [7]. Distracting techniques might be applied to other forms of epilepsy than evoked seizures.

Operant conditioning

Operant conditioning implies either consistent reward ('positive reinforcement') of a piece of behaviour or consistent punishment of it ('negative reinforcement') until it is either enhanced and becomes permanent, or it disappears. Most psychologists nowadays feel that reward is more effective than punishment. In treating epilepsy reward is applied to seizure free periods in the hope that they will become longer and eventually continue as permanent. Punishment is applied to actual seizures. Various methods have been used particularly in children or in the subnormal (reviewed by Fenwick [1] and Mostofsky and Balaschak [4]). Reward may be the earning of tokens which can be later exchanged for sweets, toys, etc., or it may be the giving of affection or the giving of praise, while punishment is usually not giving a reward or not giving praise, although a few workers have occasionally used a mild electric shock as a punishment or have even shouted at or shaken the child when it appeared to be about to have a seizure (although this may of course be a distraction technique).

Review of various case reports suggests the most effective method may be that of positive reinforcement of seizure free behaviour if, without making judgements, parents (or nurses) give a child praise the longer he goes without a seizure: seizures are studiously ignored if they occur (so that they are not inadvertently rewarded). This is good parental or nursing practice, anyway. We all know that, if we are not careful, exactly the reverse of this can happen so that a child who has a seizure (in class for instance) gains a great deal of attention and seizure frequency may increase. Unfortunately for evaluating the results of operant conditioning methods in treating seizures this method works particularly well in pseudoseizures. It is not often clear from the literature whether patients treated with such methods were actually suffering from pseudoseizures rather than from the real thing. Any prospective trial of such methods (which might be particularly suitable in children) would have to be very carefully controlled to make sure that it really was epilepsy that was being treated. Operant conditioning — rewarding seizure free behaviour and ignoring 'attacks' — is the method of choice for treating pseudoseizures.

Desensitisation

As has been mentioned above there is no doubt that many people with epilepsy become anxious about their attacks and, as Mostofsky and Balaschak [4] have pointed out and, as I have learnt from my own experience [3], general methods of anxiety reduction — particularly those employing relaxation — can be effective in reducing seizure frequency because high levels of anxiety in many patients lead to an increased number of seizures. Although a small number of patients with epilepsy find relaxation techniques somewhat threatening (and this may even increase seizure frequency) the majority of patients find this helpful and all my in-patients with epilepsy are taught a specific relaxation technique. It should be emphasised, for those unfamiliar with psychological techniques, that relaxation is very much more than just sitting down in a chair and letting the cares of the world drop away from one. Relaxation is an *active* technique which involves the patient's whole concentration and it has to be learnt and practised until the patient is proficient at it. Various methods are employed, but variants of methods using progressive muscular tension and relaxation are most usually taught. We help our patients by using a videotape to teach them the skills required [17] and a nurse or medical student then supervises the patient's training in the method.

Relaxation is an integral part of a more elaborate technique of behavioural management known as *desensitisation* in which, having taught the patient a good relaxation technique so that he can quickly turn on calmness and relaxation, the therapist introduces him to easy stages to the feared stimulus. In this way, the patient gradually adapts to the feared stimulus until he can face it without fear. This procedure is much used for treating phobic anxiety and similar conditions and is very successful.

It has been applied to epilepsy for patients who particularly fear their fits (i.e. the housewife with epilepsy who is afraid of making a spectacle of herself in the local supermarket). Used for the individual patient who particularly fears epilepsy, the technique is successful and leads not only to a reduction in the patient's anxiety but also, as has been described by one or two therapists [3, 8], to a reduction in the patient's attacks as well. It is easy to see why a reduction in anxiety, with concurrent reduction of hyperventilation — an almost invariable component of anxiety — can reduce seizures. What is not known is whether a similar technique to that employed by Standage [8] would work if the patient was not particularly anxious about his seizures. Would getting a patient, in a state of relaxation, to imagine himself having a fit — the basis of desensitisation method of treating seizure anxiety — work in any patient? This has not been put to formal test; I think it should as I have a sneaking suspicion it might help some patients, and is a quite easy technique to learn.

It is possible to help someone overcome his anxiety in a particular feared situation not by gradually desensitising him, but by exposing him to it and holding him in it until the anxiety response extinguishes. Although apparently a cruel method, 'flooding' or 'implosion' as it is called, does work in some anxiety conditions extremely well. It paradoxically increases the patient's morale as he realises that anxiety does not last and can be overcome. Such techniques would seem difficult to apply to epilepsy, although they have been applied to the anxiety surrounding epilepsy [9].

However, an interesting study in the United States [10] points to a possible way that flooding could be used. They showed a group of patients their own seizures on videotape, the hypothesis being that if, on seeing the videotape, the patients could recall the thoughts in their mind immediately before the seizure, they might then be able to talk about those thoughts and their feelings about them and which might lose their emotional importance so as not to trigger off further seizures. Feldman and Paul therefore took a somewhat psychotherapeutic view of their procedure (as is in Trimble's chapter). After being shown their seizures the patients underwent a significant reduction in seizure frequency: my view is that this was a form of behavioural treatment analogous to flooding. It may be that showing a patient his own seizure repeatedly on videotape when relaxed may be an acceptable behavioural method of treating seizures in many patients.

In my experience it is difficult to record an individual patient's seizures on videotape. (The TV studio seems to be one of the most effective anticonvulsants I know.) In my department we have been experimenting with showing the patient not his own seizure, but a similar one to his on videotape.

It must be a common experience for many of us to find that, if one of our patients accidentally sees someone else having a similar seizure to himself, he is often vastly relieved, saying such things as "Is that all I do?"; my guess is that many more patients than actually declare it are anxious and concerned about their seizures and fearfully fantasise about what they do during their period of unconsciousness. Certainly in my own department we have found that a videotape film made for the instruction of medical students and nurses about what epilepsy actually looks like [11] has been very successfully shown to patients and their relatives and seems to have a desensitising function and is a method which needs exploring further.

What has not been shown yet is whether general methods of anxiety reduction like relaxation training (which are easy to learn) would be enough in both patients with ictal anxiety and patients without it, or whether more specific desensitisation is necessary, and whether such time consuming treatment would have specific or general application.

Biofeedback

Biofeedback is a form of operant conditions in which a physiological variable (such as heart rate, muscle tension or EEG rhythm), which is not normally identifiable to the individual who possesses it, is converted into an electronic signal which can be recognised by the individual and can then be altered and controlled by him. An electromyograph (EMG), for instance, can be converted into a sound signal which rises and falls in pitch according to the degree of intensity of the original signal: this can be consciously altered by the subject. Biofeedback is clinically useful, the two most useful methods are probably EMG biofeedback (which is much used in treating muscular tension) and hand temperature biofeedback which is used in treating migraine. Attempts have been made to feedback such variables as heart rate, blood pressure, etc., although this is much more difficult to achieve and indirect methods such as EMG biofeedback can be just as successful in reducing blood pressure as direct feedback itself.

The electroencephalograph (EEG) is a biological signal which is convertible to biofeedback and as such has been used and experimented with extensively, particularly in the United States. Alpha rhythm and theta rhythm feedback trainers are available. Alpha feedback unfortunately obtained an unwarranted quasi-religious reputation and theta feedback, although useful for some patients with tension problems, is more difficult to achieve than the easier EMG method. It was fairly obvious that some attempt would be made to try to use biofeedback principles in the inhibition of seizures and, indeed, there is now a vast literature on this subject. Recent reviews of this literature are Fenwick [1] and Lubar and Deering [2].

Sterman and MacDonald [12] were the first to report the development of biofeedback methods for treating epilepsy. With operant conditions they increase the amount of 14-16 Hertz activity over the sensorimotor cortex in both animals and man. They claim to be able to inhibit seizure activity and have had some clinical success with this method, and suggest that they have merely invoked a normal inhibiting mechanism in the brain. The problem with this method of feedback is that the training is long and arduous for the patient and therefore it has only been used in those patients with intractable seizures: even after training in the laboratory some kind of practice and homework is necessary if improvement is to be maintained. Other workers have not had the success with this method that Sterman and MacDonald claim. By and large British experience [13] suggests that placebo factors may be very important in this particular method. Other methods of biofeedback apart from enhancing sensorimotor rhythm have been employed, including alpha feedback, and feedback of other rhythms such as fast low voltage activity and beta rhythm and some success has been reported.

The problem of evaluating the results of biofeedback is that in many of the studies there has been not enough baseline information and, whilst training has been going on, other changes have been taking place in the patient's life or in his medication. Placebo periods (using false feedback) have usually not been employed and allowance has not been made for the very strong placebo effect that paying frequent attention to a patient has. If a patient is seen frequently and has great interest taken in him and becomes part of an enthusiastic research team then it is not just the team that has an emotional involvement in getting good results. It would be true to say that enthusiasm for biofeedback as a means of treating epilepsy is much stronger in America than it is in this country where reports of its efficiency are far less convincing. Many methods of biofeedback probably reduce anxiety levels and this may be an important factor when it is successful.

However, although some doubt can legitimately be cast on the early enthusiastic reports of its efficiency in treating epilepsy, I feel that research should continue into ways of learning how to control and enhance the inhibiting rhythms in the brain which we know exist. Whether this is done by biofeedback or by other methods (even such techniques as meditation) is unimportant, providing people with epilepsy benefit from such experiments and providing the experimenters tease out from the tangle of factors which are involved in any improvement those factors which really are important. Those experimenters who dismiss any therapeutic effects as merely placebo effect, should be asking themselves what is it that the placebo is actually doing.

Counselling

I have not mentioned in this review anything about psychotherapy which is a specific psychological technique. As with the other therapies in this chapter, psychotherapy is, apart from anecdotal descriptions, of unproven scientific value. Non-specific factors such as interest, attention paying, etc., are probably important in any therapeutic success which is claimed for psychotherapy (as for biofeedback).

Counselling for patients with epilepsy [3] so that they are given full information about their condition and are allowed to work through feelings of denial, grief and anger which appear when they first learn their diagnosis (plus necessary similar counselling work with their families) is regarded as an important part of the management of people with epilepsy, but has never been properly evaluated. Undoubtedly many patients fully and properly counselled (with their family) lose their fear of epilepsy and attack frequency may diminish. But which particular element in the counselling is important and how much should be done and by whom is unknown.

To allow a patient to ask questions, to answer them, to allow him to express his feelings and to give him information is a part of psychotherapy and a part of many of the behavioural methods outlined above (even in biofeedback). It is possible that all psychological methods work merely because they involve good counselling of the individual patient. We should be looking to discover the best way of counselling patients with epilepsy and try to tease out the more important elements in the counselling process. The more I see people with epilepsy and their families, the more I realise how often factors of overprotection, of unresolved anger and unresolved grief are important, not only in indirectly increasing seizure frequency, but also in altering the entire life style of the patient unnecessarily; proper management is not just attempting to control seizures but also helping the person to live a full life even if his seizures continue. In my department we have been trying to automate as much as possible the necessary counselling techniques using videotape [11, 14—16]. We have some evidence that such efforts are successful, both in improving lifestyle and also in reducing seizure frequency.

It is interesting that since Mostofsky and Balaschak's immense review paper in 1977 [4], although other reviews exist, little has been added to the literature of direct relevance, except in the field of biofeedback, and such reports that have been published since remain mainly at an anecdotal level. There is little doubt that in the individual patient, particularly perhaps if he is anxious about his seizures, behavioural methods have a part to play in the management of epilepsy.

Whether behavioural methods applied to the great mass of people with epilepsy would be of use remains an open question. Some of the more complex behavioural techniques require the skills of a clinical psychologist or a fully equipped neurophysiology laboratory and therefore probably will always remain only a minor method of treatment necessary for a few individual patients. Some of the more easy to learn methods, however, such as simple operant conditioning in children (which can be carried out by parents) or relaxation methods or counselling techniques might have perhaps a far wider application and it is in this area that some kind of formal clinical trial could take place. With modern methods of communication like videotape the use of such methods could be taught early and widely and I think might be a benefit. It is time we stopped reviewing each other's anecdotes and got down to serious scientific study.

References

1   Fenwick P. In Reynolds EH, Trimble MR, eds. *Epilepsy and Psychiatry 1981.* Edinburgh: Churchill Livingstone
2   Lubar JF, Deering WM. *Behavioural Approaches to Neurology 1981.* New York: Academic Press
3   Betts TA. In Laidlow J, Richens A, eds. *A Textbook of Epilepsy 2nd edition 1982.* Edinburgh: Churchill Livingstone
4   Mostofsky DI, Balaschak BA. *Psychol Bull 1977; 84, No. 4:* 723—759
5   Forster FM. *Int J Neurol 1972; 9:* 73—86
6   Efron R. *Brain 1956; 79:* 267—281
7   Symonds CP. *Brain 1959; 82(2):* 133—146
8   Standage KF. *Guys Hospital Reports 1972; 121:* 217—219
9   Pinto R. *Br J Psychiat 1972; 121:* 257—258
10   Feldman RG, Paul NL. *J Nerv Ment Dis 1976; 162:* 345—353
11   Betts TA, Birtle J. *Epilepsy — What exactly is it? Videotape Number 0654, 1981.* Birmingham, England: University of Birmingham Television and Film Service
12   Sterman MB, MacDonald LR. *Electroenceph Clin Neurophysiol 1974; 37:* 418—423
13   Guy RJ, Hutt SJ, Forrest S. *Biol Psychol 1979; 9:* 129—149
14   Betts TA, Raffle AE. *It's Only a Fit — Nothing to Worry About: a film about becoming a person with epilepsy. Videotape Number 0637, 1980.* Birmingham, England: University of Birmingham Television and Film Service
15   Betts TA, Birtle J. *A Compendium of Fits. Videotape Number P0001, 1981.* Birmingham, England: Psychiatry Television, Department of Psychiatry, University of Birmingham

16   Betts TA. *Three People with Epilepsy. Videotape Number 0643, 1980.* Birmingham, England: University of Birmingham Television and Film Service

17   Betts TA, Pidd SA, Harvey PG. *Relaxation and Biofeedback. Videotape Number 0463, 1976.* Birmingham, England: University of Birmingham Television and Film Unit

36

KETOGENIC DIETS IN THE MANAGEMENT OF CHILDHOOD EPILEPSY

Ruby H Schwartz, Jane Eaton, A Aynsley-Green, B D Bower

Since Wilder [1] first suggested in his very brief report that a high fat diet might be helpful in the treatment of childhood epilepsy, ketogenic diets have been used in the management of children with intractable epilepsy. Although when initially introduced they were frequently used, with the advent of the modern anticonvulsant drugs they became a specialised treatment restricted to a few centres. When compared with the ease of taking of drugs they form an expensive, strict and some claim unpalatable, treatment. However, interest has again been focused on the diets as it is now recognised that a large number of children are not controlled even with high doses of one or more anticonvulsant drugs and there has been concern about the long term effects of these drugs.

The exact mode of action of diets, if indeed it is a single action, still remains to be elucidated. In an effort to establish the way in which they work and also to assess the clinical efficacy of this form of treatment, an extensive study of the clinical, metabolic, EEG, social and dietary aspects has been undertaken at the John Radcliffe Hospital in Oxford over the last three years. During this period we have gained considerable experience in the use of these diets and this chapter presents the clinical results obtained from 63 studies carried out on 57 patients with intractable epilepsy; in addition, the details of the diets used and the problems encountered are discussed.

In all ketogenic diets the ratio of fat to carbohydrate and protein is raised. This fat is metabolised in the liver to produce ketone bodies, which have been shown to act as brain fuels during starvation in adults. These are subsequently excreted in the urine where they can easily be detected with the use of ketostix, a useful monitoring technique which can be carried out daily by patient or parents. In children the diets produce metabolic changes which are not dissimilar to those seen in adults who are starved as part of the treatment for obesity, only these patients are using up their endogenous fat supply whereas these children metabolise an exogenous fat.

Two diets were initially used in our study, the classical 4:1 diet and the medium chain triglyceride (MCT) ketogenic diet. We have subsequently introduced a third diet and the details of all these are as follows:

The classical diet used in Oxford is worked out on the same principle as that recommended by Livingston [2] in Baltimore and is based on an estimated daily requirement of 75 cals/kg body weight. Eighty per cent of these calories are given as fat and the remaining 20 per cent are provided by protein and carbohydrate. Adequate protein is given each day to prevent catabolism. Thus there is a ratio of four parts fat to one part protein and carbohydrate, and each of the three meals given daily conforms to this ratio. On this diet the fats are mainly long chain saturated and unsaturated fats, eg butter and cream, incorporated during cooking or added directly to the food.

The MCT diet followed is identical to that used at the Royal Manchester Children's Hospital [3]. On this diet the total daily calories are based on the recommended daily intake for the child's age, which is obtained from the dietetic tables and are distributed between fat, protein and carbohydrate (ie 60 per cent calories MCT oil, 10 per cent calories protein, 10 per cent calories carbohydrate, 11 per cent calories saturated fat). The number of calories obtained from the three different food types differs from the classical diet but attempts to make the two identical would have either resulted in the loss of the ratio or would have made the MCT diet totally unpalatable. On this diet the major fat source is medium triglyceride oil which is fractionated coconut oil containing predominantly C_8 and C_{10} saturated fatty acids. It is incorporated into the diet as an emulsion in skimmed milk and also as an oil used for cooking. There is also a small proportion of saturated fats which occur naturally in protein and carbohydrate foods. The diet is worked out on two exchange systems, one for fat and protein and one for carbohydrate and fat. Food is not restricted to three meals a day as on the classical diet but is distributed throughout the day making the diet less rigid.

Despite attempts to devise individual and palatable diets for all children established on the original two ketogenic diets, problems have been encountered as the number of children on each diet has increased and the age range changed. Originally we restricted our studies to children under the age of seven, but now we have extended the work to see the effect of the diet in older children with intractable epilepsy. The rigidity and the somewhat more limited amounts of protein and carbohydrate foods permitted have proved a problem with the classical diet, while many of the children on the MCT diet have found the MCT emulsion unpalatable after a few days. Alternatively they have been unable to tolerate the full amounts through nausea, vomiting and upper abdominal pain. Reduction in the daily dose of MCT oil in some of these children has resulted in increased well-being but loss of ketosis.

However the greatest problem has been an economic one. Although MCT oil is available on prescription, cream and butter are not recognised medicines and their cost in the shops has increased very rapidly over recent years, so that whereas

327

initially we were able to report that the 4:1 diet was only slightly more expensive than a normal diet we are no longer able to do so.

This has led us to devise a modified diet which we have called the John Radcliffe II or J.R.II diet. It works on the same principles as the MCT diet, ie it is based on the child's recommended daily intake, is worked out on two exchange systems and the food can be distributed throughout the day, but the fats come from a combination of the two fats used in the other diets. There are smaller volumes of MCT oil than on the pure MCT diet and we have also incorporated some long-chain saturated fats like cream and butter, which most of the children in the Oxford area enjoy. Initially 30 per cent of the calories come from MCT oil and 30 per cent from long-chain fats though these percentages can be varied in each child according to tolerance. In addition, we have been able to incorporate into our new diet several foods which appear essential to British children such as baked beans, fish fingers, beef burgers and ice cream and, by doing this, have provided a palatable and acceptable diet for the children. At the same time we have attempted to help the parents with the cost by reducing the daily amount of cream and butter. The flexibility of the diet enables other ethnic specialities to be incorporated making it possible to treat children throughout the world.

Is it worth the effort of establishing children on ketogenic diets and maintaining them, sometimes for several years, on these diets? In order to answer the question we present the results obtained from the intensive study of 57 patients who have all been established on one of the diets for more than four months. This group consists of 54 children, age range 6/12 to 15 years at the time of starting the diet, 12 of whom were more than 10 years old. In addition the diet has been tried on three adults attending the adult neurology clinic. There were 27 males and 30 females and all had been suffering from intractable epilepsy for six or more months which had failed to respond to conventional treatment with one or more anticonvulsant drugs used either singly or in combination. Most were having multiple seizures each day.

The major type of seizure experiences is summarised in Table I though many

TABLE I. Type of epilepsy

Children	Drop attacks	25
	Partial seizures	9
	Infantile spasms	7
	Absences	8
	Tonic-clonic seizures	5
Adults	Tonic-clonic	2
	Complex partial	1

suffered from more than one type. Two of the three adults had tonic-clonic seizures. In 46 cases the aetiology was unknown but identifiable conditions were present in the remainder of the cases and these included microcephaly, congenital CMV, a chromosome disorder, Alper's disease, tuberose sclerosis, encephalitis, cerebrovascular accidents and trauma in the case of one of the adults.

In all but one of the children ketosis was established within three weeks of starting the diet and in this case the diet was probably not adhered to at home. Establishment of ketosis was more difficult in the adults and older patients and only one of the three adults obtained significant levels. The mean level of ketosis, ie β-hydroxybutyrate and acetoacetate at different times during the day is shown on the normal, JRII, MCT and classical diets (Figure 1). All the diets induce a significant degree of ketosis but the levels are higher on the classical than on the MCT and JRII diets. This difference is in part due to the fact that more older patients were established on these diets. From our studies we have shown that, using the same principles and same percentages of fat, lower levels of ketosis are induced in older patients. The highest degree of ketosis was seen in the late afternoon and on the classical 4:1 diet, the levels being similar to those seen in diabetic precoma.

In the majority of patients, attempts to correlate the degree of ketosis with the clinical response have been unsuccessful, but the level does appear to be critical in some children. In these the fits recur if the urinary ketone levels fall and they are only maintained in a seizure-free state when the urine contains two or more pulses of ketones.

Overall 41 per cent of our patients have shown a greater than 90 per cent reduction in their seizure frequency within 1 month of starting the diet. All medication was left unaltered over this period but subsequently anticonvulsant dosages have been reduced and in some cases discontinued completely without loss of seizure control. In 81 per cent of the cases a greater than 50 per cent reduction in seizure frequency occurred and only 19 per cent of the patients failed to show any significant change. This group included the only child studied who had tuberose sclerosis and also two of the three adults. Although the remaining adult appeared to improve initially with a reduction in seizure frequency, improvement of mood and more alertness, this effect was not sustained.

In addition to better seizure control many of the children have become more alert and responsive and, in several, school performance has improved.

The diets appeared to be of greatest benefit to children suffering from partial seizures where all those studied had a >50 per cent reduction in seizure frequency and 75 per cent showed a >90 per cent reduction. Eighty-five per cent of the 25 children with drop attacks had a >50 per cent reduction in seizure frequency but this degree of improvement was only seen in 60 per cent of the children with infantile spasms. Only 20 per cent of these had a >90 per cent reduction in seizures.

The relative benefits of each diet are shown in Table II. The results of 63

329

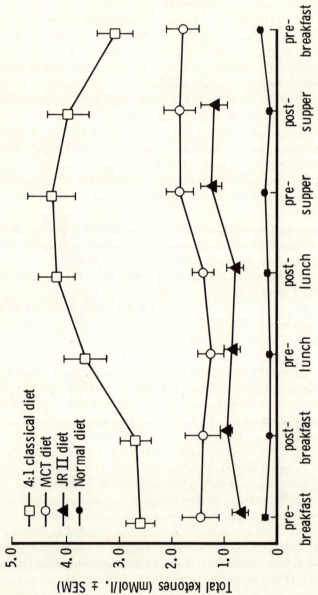

Figure 1

330

TABLE II. Results – three diets

Number of studies	MCT 27	4:1 24	JRII 12
Seizure reduction			
> 90%	10	11	5
50–90%	11	11	3
< 50%	6	2	4

studies are shown as some of the children were established on more than one diet. As can be seen, each diet has had its successes and failures. If one considers a worthwhile result as reducing seizure frequency by more than 50 per cent, the best results have been obtained using the classical diet (92% cases) and the modified diet appears so far to be less effective (67%), though it has been tried in fewer patients. These results do not reach statistical significance. More recent work assessing the clinical, but not biochemical, data suggests that it is equally as effective as the other diets. Review of the clinical response in 31 children now established on the modified diet shows that 77 per cent show a >50 per cent reduction in seizure frequency and this is now our diet of first choice.

Apart from the dietary problems already mentioned, several other problems have been encountered. These include:

1 Nausea and vomiting which is particularly noticeable on the MCT-based diets and can be overcome by reducing the amount of oil and then increasing it again slowly. Also it is less of a problem if the patient sips the oil slowly and takes small amounts through a meal instead of gulping it down in one swallow.

2 Diarrhoea occurs in some children and it is related to the MCT content of the diet, but interestingly does not occur in children suffering from pre-existing constipation. In these children the constipation appears to worsen on the diet.

3 Steatorrhoea occurs when the fat content of the 4:1 diet is not tolerated.

4 Drowsiness has been seen in about half of the patients studied, is usually apparent in the first few weeks after starting the diet and improves spontaneously. This does not appear to be related to the total blood drug levels but may be related to the altered drug binding.

5 Fluctuations in daily ketone levels may occur and this is particularly important in children who are dependent on the level of ketones as fits tend to persist in the early hours of the morning when levels are lowest. Excessive fluid intake may also reduce ketone levels. Many children also show a drop in ketone levels prior to the onset of an intercurrent illness.

6 Some children appear to respond to the diets initially but control is then lost,

but this does not appear to be related to ketone levels or drug manipulation.

Disorders of growth have been reported in other series but have not been apparent in our children. In addition we find that it is easier to manage these children in a home setting than in an institutional environment where it is more difficult to give the personal attention and strict supervision necessary if the diet is to be followed exactly.

We therefore conclude that ketogenic diets do have a place in the management of intractable epilepsy of childhood but we have been unable to show a similar improvement in the limited number of adults studied. The classical 4:1 ketogenic diet appears to be most successful in our children but has both practical and financial limitations. The diets are of particular benefit in children with partial seizures and drop attacks but may help children with other types of epilepsy and may also enable drug dosages to be reduced and drug regimes to be simplified. With careful dietetic advice and regular help and reassurance, parents are able to master the management of the diet but parental motivation is essential before this type of treatment is considered.

References

1   Wilder RM. *Mayo Clin Bull 1921; 2:* 307
2   Livingston S. In *Comprehensive Management of Epilepsy in Infancy, Childhood and Adolescence;* 378–405. Springfield Ill: Charles C Thomas
3   Gordon NS. *Develop Med Child Neurol 1977; 19:* 535–544

37

MECHANISMS OF ACTION OF ANTICONVULSANT DRUGS

B S Meldrum

Introduction

More than 20 drugs are in clinical use as anticonvulsants i.e. they are administered chronically to patients with epilepsy with the intention of reducing the incidence of seizures. On the basis of their molecular structure they can be classified into eight groups (Figure 1). Some of these drugs are also used as 'antiepileptics' in other ways. They are administered acutely to patients in *status epilepticus* in order to terminate seizure activity. They are also administered to patients during and after neurosurgical procedures, or after cerebral insults (trauma, ischaemia/hypoxia), with the intention of preventing early seizures and diminishing the probability of the development of later epilepsy. This chapter is concerned with the cellular and molecular mechanisms by which anticonvulsant drugs diminish the incidence of seizures in patients with epilepsy. Similar mechanisms may operate when the drugs are used in other circumstances.

In considering the eight groups of compounds, emphasis may be placed on effects common to all or most groups, or alternatively on effects unique to one group. Pharmaceutical chemists have repeatedly commented upon the similarities in molecular structure among anticonvulsant drugs [1]. Emphasis has been placed on analogies in the heterocyclic rings (5, 6 or 7 membered) of barbiturates, benzodiazepines, hydantoins, dibenzazepines, oxazolidinediones and succinimides (Figure 1).

In terms of selectivity of clinical action, anticonvulsant drugs fall into at least three categories:

1. Drugs selective for primary generalised seizures of the absence type, e.g. succinimide and trimethadione;

2. Drugs selectively active against partial seizures, either simple or complex, e.g. hydantoins and carbamazepine; and

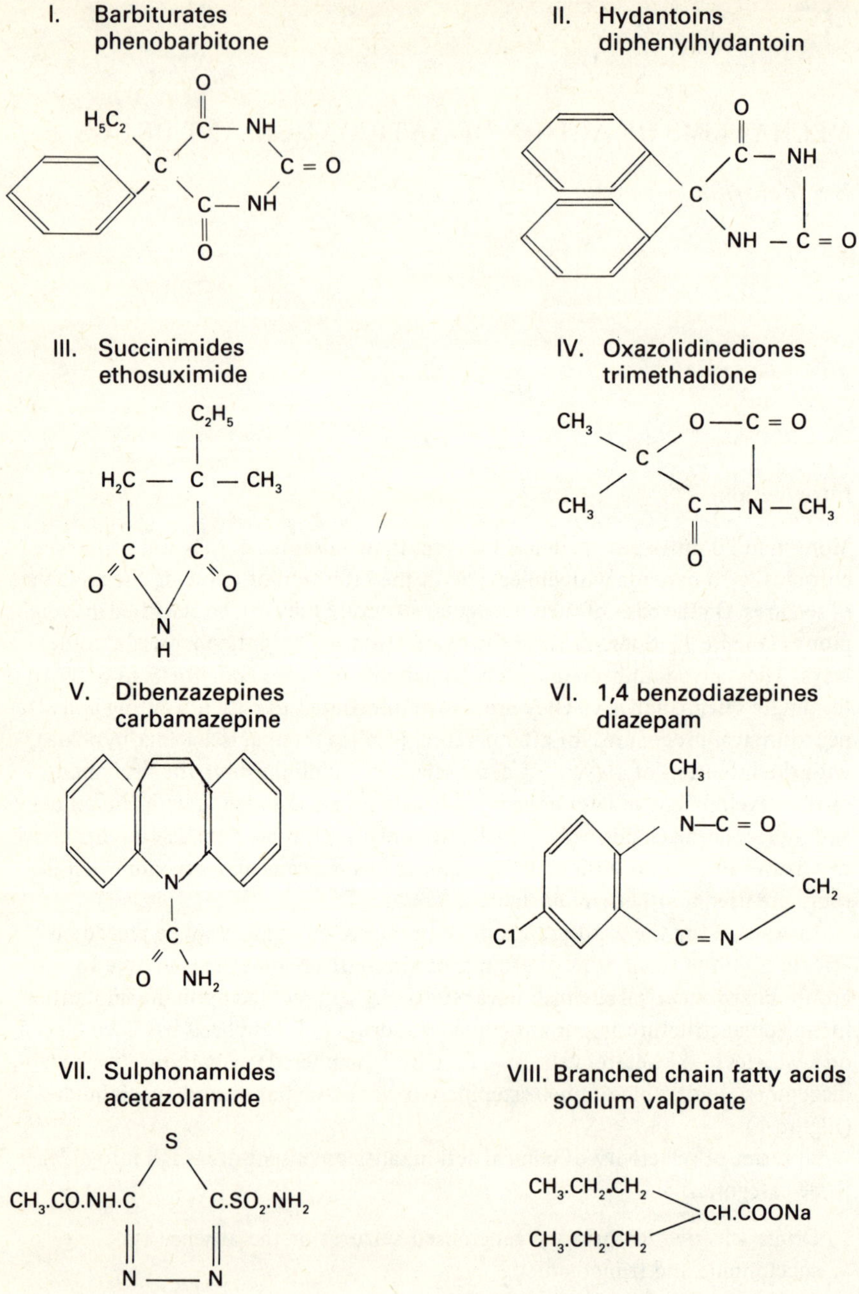

Figure 1. Classification of anticonvulsant drugs on the basis of molecular structure

3. Drugs with limited selectivity, acting against primary generalised seizures of absence and tonic clonic types and against partial seizures (e.g. benzodiazepines and branched chain fatty acids).

These data provide an argument for either three mechanisms of action or for two mechanisms possessed in common by anticonvulsants in variable proportion.

Compounds within any one of the eight chemical categories of anticonvulsant can have many different actions. Among the barbiturates, some have predominantly sedative and anaesthetic actions, some are potent anticonvulsants with only weak anaesthetic actions, and some have central excitant or convulsant actions. Very many different biochemical and neurophysiological actions of barbiturates have been described [2]. A guide to the probable contribution to anticonvulsant action of these different effects is provided by comparison of relative potency of different barbiturates: 1) against specific animal models of epilepsy (where accurate assays are possible), and 2) in biochemical or neurophysiological test systems.

The use of animal models of epilepsy for the quantitative assay of anticonvulsant potency yields rank orders that differ according to the model used. The marked differences in relative potency found utilising maximal electroshock (abolition of tonic-extension) and threshold pentylenetetrazol seizures in rodents [3] provide strong evidence for two different and largely independent mechanisms of action (Table I). Hydantoin and carbamazepine are the prime exemplars of the

TABLE I. Comparative potency of anticonvulsant drugs in acute animal models

	Maximal ECS (mice)	Pentylenetetrazol (mice)	Photic epilepsy (Papio papio)
Clonazepam	27.4	0.003	0.04
Diazepam	6.7	0.06	0.35
Phenobarbital	8.6	5.2	6.5
Primidone	5.2	4.2	45
Carbamazepine	3.7	not active	(17)
Diphenylhydantoin	3.5	not active	(18)
Valproate	162.4	88.9	138
Trimethadione	438	24	
Ethosuximide	not active	0.9	70

Figures indicate intraperitoneal ED_{50} (mice) or minimal intravenous dose abolishing myoclonic responses (baboons) in 10^{-5} moles/kg (data from [3–7]). Table reproduced from Meldrum [46] with permission

anticonvulsant mechanism demonstrated in the maximal electroshock test, and benzodiazepines are the corresponding exemplars for the mechanism responsible for giving protection against threshold pentylenetetrazol seizures. However, some benzodiazepines manifest the 'hydantoin maximal electroshock' mechanism, as well as the pentylenetetrazol mechanism — falling into a rank order in the ECS test (with diazepam more potent than clonazepam) that is different from that in the pentylenetetrazol test (with clonazepam more potent than diazepam). This provides a method for linking molecular actions with specific anticonvulsant effects.

Tests with animal models have provided a further key piece of evidence in the evaluation of mechanisms of anticonvulsant drug action. It has frequently been hypothesised that secondary effects of anticonvulsant drugs (e.g. on metabolism, on the endocrine system or slowly altered ionic distributions) contribute to altered seizure thresholds. However studies in a primate model of epilepsy, photosensitive myoclonus in the baboon, *Papio papio* [4,5] show that acutely administered anticonvulsant drugs are effective when plasma levels are closely similar to levels that are effective during chronic administration in man. This is true for the majority of antiepileptic drugs indicating that a direct pharmacological action on a receptor or on membranes is more likely to be involved than an indirect effect. It is not true for compounds where an active metabolite plays a crucial role (as in the case of clobazam) [6]. It is also not true for sodium valproate for which acute anticonvulsant effects in animals require a higher plasma concentration than is obtained in man [7]. Also anticonvulsant effects with chronic, interrupted administration of valproate are still detectable in animals and man when the plasma concentration has fallen to very low levels [8].

Other central actions of anticonvulsant drugs may provide clues to common or divergent mechanisms of action. Thus the anxiolytic action of benzodiazepines is at least partially shared by valproate and barbiturates. The most striking common feature of anticonvulsant drugs however is their acute cerebellar toxicity, manifest clinically as nystagmus, dysarthria and ataxia. This syndrome is also seen acutely in animals (ataxia in rodents, nystagmus in baboons). Drugs most potent in this respect are hydantoins, carbamazepine and barbiturates.

The most attractive hypotheses about the cellular mechanism of action of anticonvulsant drugs concern three possibilities: 1) enhancement of inhibitory transmission, 2) impairment of excitatory transmission or 3) neuronal membrane 'stabilisation' which acts presynaptically to reduce neurotransmitter release, or post-synaptically to diminish the abnormal excitatory potentials ('paroxysmal depolarising shifts') that are the characteristic substrate of epileptic neuronal discharges. Evidence relating to these three possible mechanisms is summarised below.

Enhanced inhibitory transmission

The highly important role of inhibition mediated by GABA in epileptic phenomena has been emphasised in previous reviews [9,10].

Anticonvulsant effects can be produced in animal models of epilepsy by the use of pharmacological tools that act specifically on GABAergic systems [10,11]. In particular, compounds that prolong the post-synaptic inhibitory action of

336

GABA, by impairing its reuptake into neurones and glia, have significant anticonvulsant actions [12].

Neurophysiological evidence that certain anticonvulsants can enhance GABA-ergic inhibitory transmission is of two kinds:

1. In vitro, principally intracellular (and extracellular) records from spinal neurones in tissue culture with the anticonvulsant applied in the bathing solution, and

2. In vivo, principally extracellular records of single unit firing with the anticonvulsant given intravenously (or focally). Reports of studies of these types are summarised in Table II.

TABLE II. Neurophysiological evidence for enhanced GABAergic inhibition

---

1 In vitro test system

a) Cultured mammalian spinal neurones

BARBITURATES   - increased lifetime of Cl^- channels opened by GABA
- direct increase in Cl^- conductance

BENZODIAZEPINES   - increased frequency of Cl^- channel opening by GABA

VALPROATE   - enhanced conductance increase due to GABA

b) Invertebrate preparations – (Crayfish stretch receptor)

HYDANTOIN   - prolongs IPSP, delays Cl^- channel closing

c) Hemisected frog spinal cord

BENZODIAZEPINES   - (low doses) – enhance primary afferent depolarisation
- enhance GABA-induced hyperpolarisation

d) Hippocampal slices

BENZODIAZEPINES

2 In vivo test systems (Post-synaptic inhibition)

	Iontophoresis of GABA	Stimulation of GABA-ergic pathways
HIPPOCAMPUS	BENZODIAZEPINES	BENZODIAZEPINES BARBITURATES
NEOCORTEX	BENZODIAZEPINES VALPROATE	BENZODIAZEPINES
BRAIN STEM	BENZODIAZEPINES VALPROATE	
CEREBELLUM		BENZODIAZEPINES
CUNEATE NUCLEUS		BENZODIAZEPINES BARBITURATES

In vitro benzodiazepines, at clinically relevant concentrations, enhance the inhibitory (hyperpolarising) effect of GABA applied iontophoretically to mouse

337

spinal neurones. This enhancement is due to an increase in the frequency of Cl^- channel activation by GABA [13]. Barbiturates at concentrations at or above those found clinically have two inhibitory effects, one is a direct effect of Cl^- ionophores increasing conductance (stabilising or enhancing the resting membrane potential), the other is an increase in the lifetime of Cl^- channels opened by GABA [13–15]. The former effect may be responsible for anaesthetic actions of barbiturates. The effect of GABA induced Cl^- conductance changes is produced by phenobarbitone but requires concentrations higher than are normally found clinically. Valproate applied iontophoretically enhances the inhibitory effect of GABA in spinal neurones [16] but this effect is not seen with valproate in the bathing solution at a concentration exceeding that found in clinical use (1mM) (Barker 1982, personal communication).

In vivo studies of single cell firing rates (in various brain regions) (Table II) have established that benzodiazepines (given intravenously at anticonvulsant doses) enhance GABA-mediated inhibition. This enhancement is seen when exogenous GABA is applied iontophoretically or when endogenous GABA is applied by electrical stimulation of a known GABAergic pathway (Table II). There is less detailed evidence relating to the enhancement of physiological GABAergic inhibition (in the hippocampus and cuneate) following barbiturates, and for iontophoretic application of GABA in neocortex and brain stem following valproate.

These physiological studies indicating an enhancement of GABA-mediated inhibition produced by benzodiazepines and barbiturates (and possibly also by sodium valproate) are supported by studies of the binding of radioactive ligands to brain membrane preparations [17].

In particular, diazepam and other benzodiazepines enhance the binding of GABA to fresh synaptosomal brain membrane preparations [18,19], the main effect being an enhancement of the low-affinity sodium-independent GABA binding site. Such an effect is consistent with the increase in the frequency of Cl^- channel openings due to GABA in the presence of benzodiazepines. Further evidence for interaction between membrane sites reacting with GABA and those reacting with benzodiazepines is provided by the observation of enhanced high-affinity benzodiazepine binding to washed membrane preparations in the presence of GABA or GABA agonists [20].

The biochemical effects of sodium valproate are reviewed by Chapman (see this volume). The significance for anticonvulsant activity of the possible inhibition of the three enzymes concerned with the further metabolism of GABA (GABA-transaminase, succinic semi-aldehyde dehydrogenase and aldehyde reductase) remains to be established. Inhibition of the NADPH linked aldehyde reductase, interconverting succinic semialdehyde and 4-hydroxybutyrate, is shown in vitro by a wide range of anticonvulsants including hydantoin, barbiturates, benzodiazepines and valproate [21,22].

The other effect on cerebral amino acid metabolism that is shown by a wide range of anticonvulsant drugs is a reduction in the rate of synthesis, or turnover, of GABA (see Chapman, this volume). This could be a causal link in anticonvulsant action, or it could be a secondary consequence of some other functional effect, either a post-synaptic action enhancing GABAergic inhibition (decreasing activity in GABAergic neurones by negative feedback) or an action decreasing excitatory inputs to GABAergic neurones (such as blockade of aspartergic transmission).

Impaired excitatory transmission

Excitation due to the dicarboxylic amino acids, aspartate and glutamate, probably plays an important role in the spread of seizure activity. Studies using various analogues with agonist and antagonist properties indicate that there are three or four excitatory amino acid receptors, with kainic acid, quisqualic acid, N-methyl-D-aspartic acid and glutamic acid as the preferential agonists [23,24] (Figure 2). The focal injection of excitatory amino acids acting on any of the receptors can induce local seizure activity.

In a recent study utilising a number of selective antagonists of excitatory amino acids we have shown that compounds that block excitation due to N-methyl-D-aspartate protect mice against sound-induced seizures [25]. The most potent such substance, 2-amino-7-phosphonoheptanoic acid, also protects mice against a variety of chemically induced seizures (Czuczwar and Meldrum, unpublished). This evidence that blockade of one type of excitatory transmission, possibly that due to aspartate, has a potent anticonvulsant effect gives a new significance to the observations to be outlined below concerning the actions of known anticonvulsant drugs on excitatory amino acid transmission.

Evidence that barbiturates impair excitatory transmission has been obtained in a wide variety of mammalian and other preparations [2]. Iontophoretic studies in which glutamate is applied to spinal neurones, either in vitro or in vivo, [26–28] have shown a marked depression of excitatory responses in the presence of barbiturates. This effect was originally described with pentobarbitone and was thought to correlate more with anaesthetic than with anticonvulsant action. However it is seen with 'anticonvulsant' concentrations of phenobarbitone and appears to be relevant to reduction of paroxysmal activity produced by barbiturates [29]. This post-synaptic antagonism of excitatory amino acids is not a general property of anticonvulsant drugs.

Although flurazepam antagonises glutamate induced depolarisation in the frog spinal cord [30], and excitation produced by glutamate or aspartate in the cat cerebral cortex [31], benzodiazepines in general do not block excitation induced by amino acids. Thus diazepam or chlordiazepoxide do not block glutamate-induced excitation in cultured mouse spinal cord neurones [32].

However there are effects on the release and on the metabolism of excitatory amino acids that are common to several groups of anticonvulsant. These may be

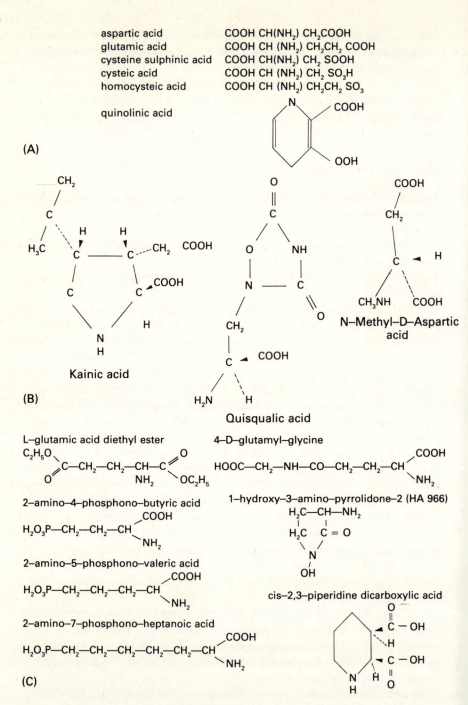

aspartic acid COOH CH(NH₂) CH₂COOH
glutamic acid COOH CH (NH₂) CH₂CH₂ COOH
cysteine sulphinic acid COOH CH(NH₂) CH₂ SOOH
cysteic acid COOH CH (NH₂) CH₂ SO₃H
homocysteic acid COOH CH (NH₂) CH₂CH₂ SO₃

quinolinic acid

(A)

Kainic acid

Quisqualic acid

N–Methyl–D–Aspartic acid

(B)

L–glutamic acid diethyl ester

4–D–glutamyl–glycine

HOOC—CH₂—NH—CO—CH₂—CH₂—CH（COOH）（NH₂）

2–amino–4–phosphono–butyric acid

H₂O₃P—CH₂—CH₂—CH（COOH）（NH₂）

2–amino–5–phosphono–valeric acid

H₂O₃P—CH₂—CH₂—CH₂—CH（COOH）（NH₂）

2–amino–7–phosphono–heptanoic acid

H₂O₃P—CH₂—CH₂—CH₂—CH₂—CH₂—CH（COOH）（NH₂）

1–hydroxy–3–amino–pyrrolidone–2 (HA 966)

cis–2,3–piperidine dicarboxylic acid

(C)

Figure 2. Molecular structures of (A) endogenous excitant amino acids; (B) non-endogenous excitants which act selectively on different classes of receptors; and (C) antagonists of excitation due to dicarboxylic amino acids or their analogues

a consequence of general effects on membranes (as discussed in section below *'Neuronal membrane effects'*) but they may also be more specific consequences of actions at presynaptic receptors or on specific ionic channels in nerve terminals.

Specific selective effects on excitatory amino acid release have been described for barbiturates and for benzodiazepines. Thus in rat cerebral cortex slices pentobarbitone inhibits potassium-evoked release of exogenous D-aspartate [33]. Using electrical stimulation of the lateral olfactory tract, in rat olfactory cortex slices, a decrease in stimulus evoked endogenous aspartate release is seen in the presence of chlordiazepoxide [34]. In vivo, both phenobarbitone and diazepam increase cortical aspartic acid concentration and decrease cortical glutamic acid concentration [35,36]. These changes may be indicative of primary actions on excitatory amino acid transmission, but they may also be secondary to actions on other aspects of cerebral function.

The changes in cerebral dicarboxylic amino acid concentrations after sodium valproate are in the opposite direction to those after barbiturates and benzodiazepines, thus glutamic acid content is increased and aspartate markedly decreased [37, and Chapman, this volume]. These changes may arise from a primary action on metabolism. Nevertheless a secondary reduction in the quantity of aspartate available for synaptic release could influence the spread of seizure activity. In our recent studies with specific antagonists of excitation due to N-methyl-D-aspartate, or aspartic acid [25], we have observed that the most potent and specific such agent (2-amino-7-phosphono-heptanoic acid) has toxic side effects in rodents very similar to those associated with GABA agonists or GABA-mimetics [10]. The excitatory input to cerebellar cyclic GMP concentration in cerebellar slices induced by aspartate is potently blocked by 2-amino-7-phosphonoheptanoic acid [39]. Thus it appears that signs of cerebellar toxicity (ataxia, etc) can be equally well produced by drugs that enhance the inhibitory effect of the GABAergic input to Purkinje cells, and by drugs that diminish the excitatory input to the same cells. Thus the fact that various anticonvulsant drugs share identical toxic side effects cannot be used as an argument in favour of a common mechanism of action.

Neuronal membrane effects

A very wide range of effects of anticonvulsant drugs on neuronal membranes have been described, especially for phenytoin [40,41]. Some of the effects of phenytoin on neuronal physiology have been linked to sodium and potassium movements. Two mechanisms contribute to the elevation of resting membrane potential and of threshold for impulse generation, and to the decreases in repetitive firing and in post-tetanic potentiation after hydantoin. One is activation of membrane Na/K ATPase activity increasing outward sodium transport. The other is a reduced sodium influx due to blockade of Na^+ channels [42]. The inward movement of Ca^{++} associated with neuronal activity is also reduced by phenytoin and this may be important in membrane stabilisation and in reducing the quantity of neurotransmitter released from synaptic endings [40].

In brain membrane or synaptosomal preparations, a Ca^{++} calmodulin activated phosphokinase phosphorylates certain proteins. Phosphorylation of three of these proteins is depressed in the presence of anticonvulsant concentrations of diphenylhydantoin, carbamazepine, or benzodiazepines [43,44]. This phenomenon correlates with anticonvulsant action evaluated with maximal electroshock seizures (abolition of tonic-extensor phase), both in terms of type of anticonvulsant drug, and relative potency in a series of benzodiazepines [44].

This phenomenon also appears to correlate with an in vitro reduction of neurotransmitter release, that shows no selectivity between excitatory and inhibitory amino acids (de Belleroche, this volume). However Skerritt and Johnston [33,45] have described selective effects of barbiturates and trimethadione, which depress aspartate release preferentially to GABA release. This effect on neurotransmitter release is not shown by carbamazepine, and does not correlate with potency for inhibition of Ca^{++} calmodulin activated protein kinases.

Conclusions

Most major classes of anticonvulsant drug have at least two mechanisms of action.

The best established mechanism of anticonvulsant action is enhancement of the post-synaptic inhibitory effect of GABA by benzodiazepines. This involves a site related to the GABA-receptor, and leads to an increased frequency of opening of Cl^- channels by GABA. It correlates with anticonvulsant activity evaluated in the threshold pentylenetetrazol test. Benzodiazepines also manifest a different anticonvulsant mechanism, in common with hydantoin and barbiturates.

Barbiturates enhance inhibitory mechanisms (i) by prolonging the opening time of Cl^- channels opened by GABA, and (ii) by a direct action opening Cl^- channels. They also decrease excitatory transmission, both by a pre-synaptic action and a post-synaptic action.

The precise role of the many actions of hydantoin on ionic movements across the neuronal membrane is uncertain, but impaired neurotransmitter release probably contributes to the anticonvulsant action.

Sodium valproate has actions on the cerebral metabolism of GABA and of aspartate, but the precise molecular mechanisms remain to be established.

Some potential new anticonvulsant drugs currently under investigation have more specific actions on inhibitory or excitatory neurotransmission than existing drugs. They may therefore contribute to understanding of anticonvulsant drug mechanisms as well as to therapeutic success in epilepsy.

Understanding the different actions of anticonvulsant drugs may provide a basis for the rational use of polypharmacy.

References

1   Vida JA, Gerry EH. In Vida JA, ed. *Anticonvulsants 1977.* 151–291. New York: Academic Press
2   Prichard JW. In Glaser GH, Penry JK, Woodbury DM, eds. *Antiepileptic Drugs. Mechanisms of Action 1980;* 553–562. New York: Raven Press
3   Krall RL, Penry JK, White BG et al. *Epilepsia 1978; 19:* 409–428
4   Meldrum BS, Horton RW, Toseland PA. *Arch Neurol 1975; 32:* 289–294
5   Meldrum BS, Anlezark G, Balzano E et al. In Meldrum BS, Marsden CD, eds. *Advances in Neurology 1975; 10:* 119–128. New York: Raven Press
6   Meldrum BS, Croucher MJ. *Drug Dev Res 1982; Suppl 2:* 33–38
7   Meldrum BS, Anlezark GM, Ashton GG et al. In Majkowski J, ed. *Post-traumatic Epilepsy and Pharmacological Prophylaxis 1977;* 138–153. Warsaw: Polish Chapter of the International League Against Epilepsy
8   Lockard JS, Levy RH. *Epilepsia 1976; 17:* 477–479
9   Meldrum BS. *Internat Rev Neurobiol 1975; 17:* 1–36
10   Meldrum B. In Sandler M, ed. *Psychopharmacology of Anticonvulsant Drugs 1982;* 62–78. London: Oxford University Press
11   Meldrum B. In Frey HH, Janz D, eds. *Antiepileptic Drugs, Handbook of Experimental Pharmacology 1982.* Berlin: Springer-Verlag
12   Meldrum BS, Croucher MJ, Krogsgaard-Larsen P. In Okada Y, Roberts E, eds. *Problems in GABA Research 1982;* 182–191. Amsterdam: Excerpta Medica
13   Study RE, Barker JL. *Proc Nat Acad Sci 1981; 78:* 7180–7184
14   Barker JL, Ransom BR. *J Physiol 1978; 280:* 355–372
15   MacDonald RL. *Brain Res 1979; 167:* 323–336
16   MacDonald RL, Bergey GK. *Brain Res 1979; 170:* 558–562
17   Olsen RW. *J Neurochem 1981; 37:* 1–17
18   Guidotti A, Toffano G, Grandison L, Costa E. In Fonnum F, ed. *Amino Acids as Chemical Transmitters 1978;* 517–530. New York: Plenum Press
19   Skerritt JH, Johnston GAR. *Clin Exp Pharmacol Physiol.* In press
20   Karobath M, Placheta P, Lippitsch M, Krogsgaard-Larsen P. *Nature 1979; 278:* 748–749
21   Erwin VG, Deitrich RA. *Biochem Pharmacol 1973; 22:* 2615–2624
22   Javors M, Erwin VG. *Biochem Pharmacol 1980; 29:* 1703–1708
23   Watkins JC, Evans RH. *Ann Rev Pharmacol Toxicol 1981; 21:* 165–204
24   Teichberg VI, Goldberg O, Luini A. *Mol Cell Biochem 1981; 39:* 281–295
25   Croucher MJ, Collins JF, Meldrum BS. *Science 1982; 216:* 899–902
26   Barker JL, Gainer H. *Science 1973; 182:* 720–722
27   Barker JL, Ransom BR. *J Physiol 1978; 280:* 355–372
28   Lambert JDC, Flatmman JA. *Neuropharmacol 1981; 20:* 227–240
29   MacDonald RL, McLean MJ. *Neurology 1982;* In press
30   Nistri A, Constanti A. *Neuropharmacology 1978; 17:* 127–135
31   Nestoros JN, Nistri A. *Can J Physiol Pharmacol 1979; 57:* 1324–1329
32   MacDonald RL, Barker JL. *Nature 1978; 271:* 563–564
33   Bornstein JC, Willow M, Johnston GAR. *Neurosci Lett 1980; 18:* 185–190
34   Collins GGS. *Brain Res 1981; 224:* 389–404
35   Chapman AG, Nordström CH, Siesjö BK. *Anesthesiology 1978; 48:* 175–182
36   Carlsson C, Chapman AG. *Anesthesiology 1981; 54:* 488–495
37   Chapman AG, Riley K, Evans MC, Meldrum BS. *Neurochemical Res 1982; 7:* 1089–1105
38   Wiklund T, Toggenbuurger G, Cuenod M. *Science 1982; 216:* 78–80
39   Roberts PJ, Foster GA, Sharif NA, Collins JF. *Brain Res 1982; 238:* 475–479
40   Delgado-Escueta AV, Horan MP. In Glaser GH, Penry JK, Woodbury DM, eds. *Antiepileptic Drugs. Mechanisms of Action 1980;* 377–398. New York: Raven Press
41   Woodbury DM. In Glaser GH, Penry JK, Woodbury DM, eds. *Antiepileptic Drugs. Mechanisms of Action 1980;* 447–471. New York: Raven Press
42   De Weer P. In Glaser GH, Penry JK, Woodbury DM, eds. *Antiepileptic Drugs. Mechanisms of Action 1980;* 353–361. New York: Raven Press
43   De Lorenzo RJ. In Glaser GH, Penry JK, Woodbury DM, eds. *Antiepileptic Drugs. Mechanisms of Action 1980;* 399–414. New York: Raven Press
44   De Lorenzo RJ, Burdette S, Holderness J. *Science 1981; 213:* 546–549
45   Johnston GAR, Skerritt JH. *Proc Int Congr Biochem West Austr 1982;* In press

38

MOLECULAR INTERACTIONS BETWEEN ANTICONVULSANT DRUGS AND SPECIFIC NEUROTRANSMITTER RECEPTOR SYSTEMS

R H Lowe, P T Lascelles

Anticonvulsant-neurotransmitter system interactions

Despite the wide range of clinically useful anticonvulsant drugs, the mechanisms underlying their pharmacological activities remain, for the large part, obscure. It is likely, however, that studies of their effects upon specific neurotransmitter systems will lead to an understanding of their modes of action at a molecular level. In particular, interactions of anticonvulsant drugs within the GABA-ergic system assume a special relevance in view of:

(i)   the role of GABA as a major inhibitory neurotransmitter in mammalian CNS [1];

(ii) the involvement of GABA-ergic processes in the maintenance of seizure threshold [1]; and

(iii) the numerous reported effects of anticonvulsant drugs on GABA-ergic pharmacology [2–8].

As the synaptic effects of GABA are determined both by the concentration of the transmitter at its receptor recognition sites and by the magnitude of the responses mediated by the receptor in response to a given transmitter concentration, it is possible to identify several potential loci of anticonvulsant interaction at the synaptic level (Figure 1). Thus, we may distinguish between anticonvulsant drug interactions occurring with respect to:

(a)   the processes of GABA synthesis, uptake, release and degradation which influence GABA turnover and metabolism; and

(b)   those occurring at the GABA receptor.

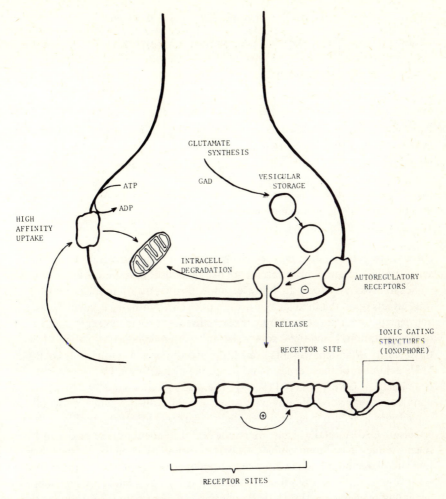

Figure 1. Potential loci of anticonvulsant action at the synaptic level

(a) Effect of anticonvulsants on GABA turnover and metabolism

A number of recent studies have reported the effect of a range of anticonvulsants on the total tissue content of GABA and other selected transmitters on a regional basis in brain [9–12]. Data from a representative study, in rat brain [13], are given in Table I. It is clear from these data that the anticonvulsants phenytoin, phenobarbitone, ethosuximide and sodium valproate have marked effects upon the total tissue levels of both GABA and glutamate, but this type of data is subject to interpretational ambiguities. In particular, the effects of transmitter compartmentation are difficult to assess, as it has been demonstrated that the

345

TABLE I. Effect of anticonvulsants on brain neurotransmitter content

| Drugs | NEUROTRANSMITTERS | | | |
| | Glutamate | | GABA | |
	Cerebral cortex	Cerebellum	Cerebral cortex	Cerebellum
Control	7.78 ± 0.87	7.64 ± 0.76	2.90 ± 0.47	3.32 ± 0.53
Phenytoin	9.32 ± 1.49	7.41 ± 0.47	2.37 ± 0.26	2.26 ± 0.69
Phenobarbitone	7.67 ± 0.87	7.93 ± 0.31	7.88 ± 0.97	4.48 ± 0.23
Ethosuximide	6.23 ± 0.17	6.17 ± 0.35	2.50 ± 0.79	2.82 ± 0.33
Sodium valproate	11.32 ± 1.95	8.75 ± 1.86	7.12 ± 0.90	4.80 ± 0.68

Data from five experimental animals (nmoles/mg wet wt) [13]

correlations between drug induced changes in total tissue GABA levels and its synaptically relevant concentrations are markedly drug specific [14].

Separate assay systems do, however, allow the investigation of anticonvulsant drug effects upon the individual processes of GABA synthesis, uptake, release and degradation. Data derived from these studies are also less subject to ambiguities of interpretation. Using these approaches it has been demonstrated that, whilst the majority of anticonvulsants exert little effect upon the synthesis of GABA [15], a number of these drugs do influence the high-affinity, Na^+-dependent component of GABA uptake [15, 16]. These effects are markedly dependent upon both the region of brain investigated, and the tissue preparation used. Prior convulsions have also been demonstrated to markedly affect the profile of drug effects on GABA uptake. Thus, whilst the Na^+-dependent uptake of GABA into synaptosomes from hippocampal cortex is *decreased* by phenobarbitone, phenytoin and diazepam, the same drugs have been observed to *increase* uptake into synaptosomes derived from the cerebral cortex, with post-ictal tissue demonstrating opposing characteristics [17]. By contrast, an *increase* in GABA uptake has been observed into crude synaptic fractions from whole rat brain in response to phenytoin and phenobarbitone [16], whilst GABA uptake into rat brain slices has been reported to be *unaffected* by phenytoin, diazepam and a variety of other anticonvulsants too, including ethosuximide, methosuximide, phensuximide and trimethadione [18]. Even allowing that the glial and neuronal uptake mechanisms for GABA [19] may exhibit differential drug selectivity and that regional and morphological factors may play a role in explaining the diversity of these effects, it is nonetheless difficult to reconcile these results and their drug specificity with either a similar or consistent mechanism of anticonvulsant drug action. Similar conclusions are also reached in reviewing the effects of the anticonvulsants on the processes of GABA release and degradation. Thus, whilst a number of anticonvulsants have been demonstrated to exert effects upon the release of GABA

346

[15, 20, 21], these effects are similarly drug specific [15].

Few anticonvulsant drugs have been demonstrated to affect the degradation of GABA with the notable exception of valproic acid, which has been shown to inhibit the degradatory enzymes GABA transaminase EC 2.6.19 and succinic semi-aldehyde dehydrogenase EC 1.2.1.16 with Ki values of 42mM and 0.5—1.5mM respectively [22, 23]. The total therapeutic plasma concentrations of valproate are, however, nominally in the range 0.2—0.6mM [24] with up to 95 per cent of the drug bound to plasma protein [25] suggesting that extensive inhibition of GABA degradation in vivo would be unlikely.

Thus, the observed increase in total GABA content induced by valproate [10, 12, 13] is not directly explicable on this basis.

These various reported data have, therefore, clearly demonstrated that whilst some anticonvulsant drugs do indeed exert effects upon GABA turnover and metabolism, such properties are markedly drug-specific. In addition, many of the reported effects require higher than therapeutic concentrations of drug for their demonstration. Whilst these properties undoubtedly contribute to the overall pharmacological profile of the individual compounds, the diversity of effects is in striking contrast to the observation of similar chemical structures amongst the majority of these drugs [26—29] with the exception of valproate. This in turn strongly suggests that a major component of the anticonvulsant effect of these compounds is specifically mediated at structurally sensitive sites other than those affecting the metabolism or turnover of GABA. The GABA receptor complex provides such a locus of drug action and we shall, therefore, now examine the evidence supporting the GABA receptor as a target for anticonvulsant drug action.

Evidence for anticonvulsant drug interaction at the GABA receptor complex

Following its synaptic release and subsequent recognition at its receptor sites, GABA is known to exert its effects by selectively increasing the membrane permeability of the target neurone to chloride ions [30]. The competitive antagonist bicuculline and the non-competitive antagonist picrotoxinin are in turn both capable of inhibiting these responses [31] and this provides the basis for their convulsant properties in vivo. Many categories of anticonvulsant drug including the barbiturates, hydantoins, the benzodiazepines and valproate also have the ability to either indirectly induce increases in membrane chloride ion permeability, or to potentiate the chloride ion mediated hyperpolarisations induced by GABA in a variety of tissues [2—8]. Significantly, these properties are demonstrated under conditions whereby the effects of these anticonvulsants on GABA metabolism or turnover are either unable or unlikely to account for the observed responses. These drug induced increases in chloride ion permeability have also been demonstrated to be inhibited by both bicuculline and picrotoxinin [32, 33]. In addition, a number of anticonvulsant barbiturates including phenobarbitone are also capable of reversing the antagonism induced by either bicuculline or picrotoxinin to the effects of GABA, both in superior cervical ganglion and in intact neurones [34]. Similarly, phenytoin has been reported to be capable of reversing the GABA antagonism induced by picrotoxin in the crayfish stretch receptor [35].

Much experimental data, therefore, suggests a site of anticonvulsant interaction at the GABA receptor. Further evidence for the involvement of a specific recognition process in the mechanism of action of these drugs is also provided by the observation that minor modifications of structure, within all of the major chemical categories of anticonvulsant drugs, results in the appearance of marked *convulsant* rather than anticonvulsant properties [27]. This structurally dependent reversal of pharmacological profile is also mirrored by a parallel reversal of the GABA-potentiating or mimetic properties of the parent anticonvulsant [36]. These opposing properties have also been noted between the enantiomers of the same chemical compound, e.g. the barbiturate 1,3 dimethyl-butyl barbiturate, (+)DMBB, which possesses potent picrotoxinin-like convulsant properties whilst the corresponding (–)enantiomer, (–)DMBB has anticonvulsant properties [37].

This behaviour serves to emphasise the extreme sensitivity of the putative receptor interaction to the absolute stereochemistry of the anticonvulsant drug and is also suggestive of an agonist/antagonist type of dichotomy.

Overall, therefore, the experimental evidence clearly warrants further investigation into the nature of the interaction of anticonvulsant drugs with the GABA receptor complex, particularly with respect to the mechanisms and sites of interaction with picrotoxinin and similar convulsants.

(b) Potential sites of anticonvulsant drug interaction within the GABA receptor complex

A number of functionally distinct sites at which anticonvulsant drug interactions may occur within the receptor complex can be distinguished:

(i) *Primary recognition sites* which are associated with the GABA receptor macromolecule and provide the required molecular selectivity to allow both the recognition of, and subsequent interaction between, molecules of GABA vicinal to the receptor.

(ii) *The effector sites* which serve to mediate the selective increases in neuronal permeability to chloride ions following the successful interaction of transmitter molecules at the primary recognition sites.

(iii) *Receptor-effector coupling mechanisms.*

(iv) *Regulatory sites* which, by analogy with the mechanisms of enzyme regulation sites, are capable of modulating the affinity or the efficacy of the primary transmitter recognition. It may be postulated that regulatory sites may also be associated with effector or ionophore structures.

(i) The direct investigation of anticonvulsant drug interactions with at least some components of the receptor complex have been made possible by the application of suitable radioligand binding techniques [38, 39]. Thus, a number of competitive receptor assays using ^{3}H GABA as ligand have failed to provide any evidence for a direct interaction between anticonvulsant drugs and the GABA recognition sites [40,41], which have been demonstrated to exist as a heterogeneous population differing in terms of their stoichiometry and affinity dependent upon the tissue preparation used [38, 39, 52, 55]. Picrotoxinin and other non-competitive GABA antagonists are also without direct effects upon these sites [40, 41]. It is unlikely therefore that direct interactions of anticonvulsant drugs occur at the primary recognition site for GABA, at least in the tissue preparations investigated.

(ii) and (iii) In view of the GABA potentiating and mimetic properties of the anticonvulsants, and of the demonstrated inactivity of these drugs at the GABA recognition site, it is likely that these drugs exert effects upon either the receptor ionophore coupling or on the ionophore itself. Similarly, the lack of effect of the non-competitive antagonist picrotoxinin on GABA recognition sites also suggests that this compound may mediate its effects at the same sites as the anticonvulsants, especially as it is also capable of inhibiting the chloride ion mediated responses induced by these drugs [32, 33]. This assertion has recently been open to direct experimental investigation following the synthesis of 8,9 ^{3}H dihydro-picrotoxinin, a radioactive picrotoxinin analogue which has subsequently allowed the demonstration of a saturable population of binding sites in mammalian brain [42, 43]. Whilst these sites have been demonstrated to be insensitive to GABA and its analogues [42, 43], a range of convulsant non-competitive GABA antagonists has been demonstrated to inhibit this binding. Further, it has been noted that the displacing potencies of the latter group correlate well with pharmacological potencies as convulsants. This activity is also associated with a distinct structure activity relationship [44]. A number of anticonvulsant drugs, including phenytoin, phenobarbitone, primidone and the benzodiazepines are also capable of displacing dihydropicrotoxinin from its recognition sites [45]. This, in turn, is consistent with the previously noted ability of these anticonvulsants to reverse the GABA antagonism induced by picrotoxinin [34].

Overall, these results strongly imply that specific recognition sites for a number of anticonvulsant and convulsant drugs exist within the GABA receptor complex and that these recognition sites are functionally associated with the mechanisms of receptor-effector coupling.

(iv) The mechanism by which benzodiazepines exert their pharmacological effect has recently been demonstrated to involve a specific population of recognition sites within the CNS. The observed affinity of a series of benzodiazepines for this site has also been shown to be highly correlated with anticonvulsant potency [46, 47]. Prior to the demonstration of such recognition sites, the effects of these drugs had been widely suggested to involve GABA-ergic mechanisms [48]. This appeared consistent with their bicuculline and picrotoxinin sensitive GABA potentiating properties [8] although it had been demonstrated that these drugs were incapable of inhibiting specific GABA binding [38, 40]. Subsequently, neither bicuculline or picrotoxinin have been demonstrated to have significant direct inhibitory effects upon benzodiazepine binding [46], although GABA has recently been demonstrated to enhance benzodiazepine binding by increasing the affinity of its recognition sites [49, 50], an effect possibly mediated by a novel GABA recognition site [51] but one nonetheless capable of inhibition by bicuculline.

A close functional link between the recognition sites for GABA and the benzodiazepines is also suggested on the basis of much other experimental data, including the observation that the benzodiazepines are capable of modifying the apparent affinity and heterogeneity of GABA binding to its recognition sites in synaptic membrane preparations [52, 53] and that the benzodiazepines enhance the extent of GABA binding [54]. It has been suggested that these effects occur as a result of interactions between the benzodiazepines and an endogenous peptide at closely adjacent recognition sites [52, 55]. This peptide (GABA modulin) has in turn been mooted to serve a role in the regulation of GABA receptor function by modulating the affinity for GABA at its primary recognition sites [52, 55]. Further evidence for a benzodiazepine involvement within the GABA-ergic system is provided by the observation that the benzodiazepine recognition sites are closely associated with chloride ion channels [56]. The benzodiazepines also appear to interact with picrotoxinin sensitive sites as evidenced by their ability to inhibit dihydropicrotoxinin binding [45], whilst picrotoxinin itself has little effect on benzodiazepine binding [46,47]. This strongly suggests that the benzodiazepine recognition sites are heterogeneous, with the majority of benzodiazepine effects mediated at the picrotoxinin insensitive recognition sites. A close similarity of recognition requirements between these sites is, however, suggested on the basis of the observation that RO 5-3663, a convulsant benzodiazepine which, whilst only weakly inhibiting flunitrazepam binding, potently inhibits dihydropicrotoxinin binding [45]. This is a directly opposing profile of activity from that demonstrated by the anticonvulsant benzodiazepines. Consistent with these proposals is that few other non-benzodiazepine anticonvulsant drugs interact directly with the benzodiazepine recognition site as revealed by their inability to inhibit benzodiazepine binding except at high concentration [57]. A number of convulsant compounds with little effect on ^{3}H dihydropicrotoxinin binding have also been observed to be capable of inhibiting benzodiazepine binding [57], suggesting that these sites may also act as loci for the expression of both anticonvulsant and convulsant activity. Indirect anticonvulsant drug interactions with the benzodiazepine recognition sites are supported by several lines of experimental evidence. Thus, the barbiturates are capable of stimulating both benzodiazepine [58] and GABA binding [59], these effects being strongly chloride ion dependent and also picrotoxinin sensitive. It has also been demonstrated that phenytoin treatment in rats results in an increase in the apparent number of benzodiazepine receptors [60]. Moreover a specific involvement of these recognition sites in seizure mechanisms has recently been suggested following the separate reports of anomalous benzodiazepine binding characteristics in epileptic brain [61] and the demonstration that increases in benzodiazepine binding, specifically localised in dentate granule cells, occur following kindling [62].

On the basis of these data it is possible that the benzodiazepine anticonvulsants exert their effects by interacting with a discrete population of recognition sites associated within the GABA receptor complex apparently functionally coupled with, but largely distinct from, the picrotoxinin sensitive recognition sites for the non-benzodiazepine anticonvulsants.

The overall nature of the functional interactions occurring between these various recognition sites (i) – (iv) discussed above still, however, remain unclear and warrant further investigation.

Pharmacophores within the GABA receptor complex

Regardless of the specific site of drug interaction within this receptor complex, the observation of molecular specificity in ligand recognition implies that certain criteria require to be satisfied before successful interaction can occur. These criteria effectively represent the ability of the drug to 'fit' a specific recognition site within the complex and hence relate to the degree of molecular complementarity between the drug and its recognition site. Thus, for a series of drugs sharing the same sites of recognition, isosterisms of structure must, by definition, exist. This in turn provides the rationale for studies of structure-activity-relationships. These molecular isosterisms relate both to:

(i)   the spatial characteristics of the ligand, and hence its overall structure and conformation as considered in simple structure-activity-relationship (SAR) studies and

(ii)   the electronic characteristics which determine the specific distribution of charge in the vicinity of the molecule.

It is, therefore, possible by reviewing the overall electronic and spatial properties of a series of drugs which express activity at the same molecular site to define a recognition *pharmacophore* or a specific pattern of charge distribution having the ability to satisfy the recognition criteria at this defined site. Conversely, by demonstrating similarities in the overall spatial and electronic properties of compounds suspected of having a common recognition site, evidence supportive, or otherwise, of this proposal may be gained.

These investigations are made possible by the application of theoretical quantum chemical techniques and specifically by the use of molecular orbital calculations

351

[63] which allow investigation into both the overall conformational and the electronic properties of the molecules studied.

Using these approaches to study a selection of GABA analogues it has, for example, been reported that the GABA agonist pharmacophore is defined by two highly charged regions (-0.6e and +0.6e) separated by approximately 5Å [64]. Thus, the GABA analogues in Figure 2 are, despite differences in functional groupings, all capable of presenting this pharmacophore. Molecular orbital calculations

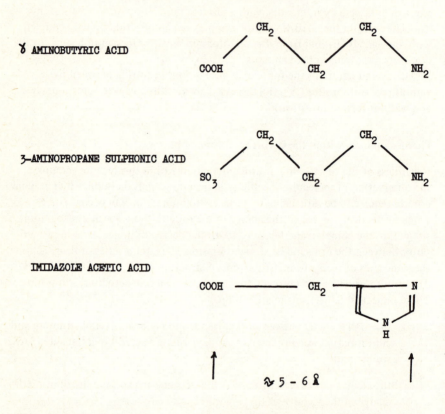

Figure 2. A selection of GABA analogues with electronically isofunctional terminal groups

of some benzodiazepines have also allowed the observation with the directional electronic charge associated with p_y orbital of the aromatic carbon adjacent to the amide nitrogen is highly correlated with anticonvulsant activity [65]. This therefore suggests that the specific charge distribution surrounding this molecular feature comprises part of the recognition pharmacophore required for mediation of the anticonvulsant properties of the benzodiazepines.

Molecular orbital calculations on non-benzodiazepine anticonvulsants

As previously discussed, the possibility exists based on:

(i) the closely similar molecular structures of the majority of non-benzodiazepine anticonvulsants [27] (Figure 3) differing mainly in terms of substituents (Figure 4), and

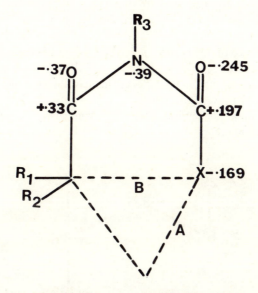

Figure 3. The common structural features associated with the majority of anticonvulsant drugs depicted with CNDO/2 derived charges (fractional e values) which represent an anticonvulsant pharmacophore

DRUG NAME	R_1	R_2	A	B	X	R_3
Phenobarbitone	C_2H_6	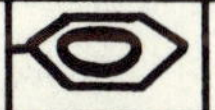 ⬡	✓	—	N	H
Diphenylhydantoin	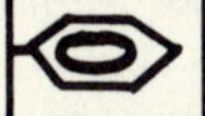 ⬡	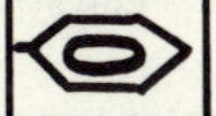 ⬡	—	✓	N	H
Trimethadione	CH_3	CH_3	—	✓	O	CH_3
Ethosuximide	C_2H_5	CH_3	—	✓	CH_2	H
Pheneturide	C_6H_5	C_2H_5, H	—	✓	NH_2	H

Figure 4. Drug specific features associated with the common structural moiety of Figure 3 for a representative selection of anticonvulsant drugs

353

(ii) the observed inhibition of ^{3}H dihydropicrotoxinin binding by a variety of anticonvulsants [45] including phenobarbitone and phenytoin

that picrotoxinin and these drugs may share the same molecular locus of recognition [66].

It was, therefore, decided to conduct theoretical molecular orbital calculations using the CNDO/2 methods [67] to compare the recognition features, and hence the effective pharmacophores, of picrotoxinin (the active component of picrotoxin) and the anticonvulsants phenobarbitone and phenytoin. The use of molecular orbital calculations is particularly relevant to this study in view of the possibility that the compounds may present similarities of charge distribution whilst nonetheless having markedly dissimilar overall chemical structures, a situation in which conventional SAR studies are inapplicable, but which applies to the compounds under investigation.

The results of these calculations, depicted as summarised descriptions of their charge distribution are represented in Figure 3 and Figure 5. The absolute values

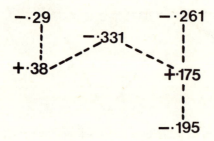

Figure 5. The putative picrotoxinin recognition pharmacophore (charges quoted in fractional e values)

of charge at specific points are quoted in fractional electronic charges (e). From these results it is observed that electronic isosterisms exist between the proposed picrotoxinin pharmacophore (Figure 5) and those for phenobarbitone and phenytoin (summarised as Figure 3).

Further, as the relevant electronic charges are associated with structural features common to the majority of non-benzodiazepine anticonvulsants (Figure 3), these results in turn suggest that both phenobarbitone and phenytoin, and indeed the majority of other non-benzodiazepine anticonvulsant drugs (with the exception of valproate), will display a similar overall pharmacophore and hence share the same recognition site. Thus the recognition site associated with the anticonvulsant pharmacophore is also potentially capable of recognising and mediating the convulsant properties of picrotoxinin and other pharmacologically similar convulsants. It is likely, therefore, that these pharmacophores described for picrotoxinin and both phenobarbitone and phenytoin directly determine only the primary recognition phase of interaction, whilst the overall steric properties of each drug ultimately determine whether anticonvulsant or convulsant properties are expressed [68].

It is now possible to summarise the proposed molecular sites of anticonvulsant interaction within the GABA receptor complex:

(i)   The non-benzodiazepine anticonvulsants, having the structural isosterisms depicted in Figure 3, are likely to interact with specific recognition sites functionally associated with the GABA receptor capable of modulating coupling to the associated chloride ionophore. This site also appears capable of recognising picrotoxinin and a variety of other similar convulsants.

(ii) The benzodiazepine anticonvulsants are likely to exert the majority of their anticonvulsant properties by interacting at a recognition site distinct in its pharmacophore requirements but nonetheless coupled to that proposed in (i), functionally linked to the chloride ion channel and capable of modifying the kinetics of GABA interaction, possibly by displacement of, or competition with, endogenous regulators of synaptic function. Experimental data supports a functional interaction between (i) and (ii) [60] and also supports an association of both sites with the chloride ionophore [69].

Receptor model

In order to attempt to reconcile the apparent diversity of recognition sites within the GABA receptor complex and their interactions, a receptor model is proposed [70] which is of utility in describing both the proposed sites of anticonvulsant drug recognition and in indicating some possible mechanisms of receptor regulation.

The GABA receptor is envisaged as capable of existing in a discrete number of stable, or metastable, conformational states (Figure 6). Interaction of GABA with these receptor conformers may, therefore, occur with differing affinities or slightly modified agonist pharmacophores. Such interactions are in turn likely to induce conformational changes in the receptor macromolecule which are postulated to result in the exposure of additional GABA recognition sites. Following the recognition of a specific number of GABA molecules, which for ease of illustration has been depicted as 4 in Figure 6, it is proposed that the resulting structure initiates an increase in membrane conductance to chloride ions by specifically interacting with the membrane associated ionophore.

It is also proposed that a number of additional sites with distinct pharmacophore requirements are associated with each conformational state of the receptor, each of which is capable of allowing the recognition of a variety of secondary

355

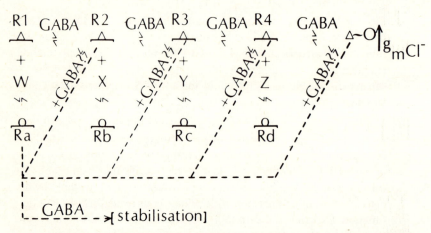

Figure 6. The proposed receptor model. R1, R2, R3 and R4 represent receptor conformations adopted following the serial recognition of the primary ligand (GABA). T represents the antagonist preferring state. W, X, Y and Z refer to secondary binding sites interacting respectfully to yield new conformations, Ra, Rb, Rc and Rd. gmCl⁻ refers to the chloride ionophore

ligands (W–Z, Figure 6) which may either be of endogenous or exogenous origin.

Following recognition, the resultant conformational change of the receptor macromolecule may result in:

(a) the gating of the chloride ionophore, and hence membrane hyperpolarisation associated with a reduced requirement for GABA, leading to a decrease in the apparent co-operativity of the GABA-receptor interaction. This would result in potentiation of GABA-ergic responses.

(b) ligand induced conformational changes which stabilise the receptor, causing the macromolecule to adopt an energetically favourable conformation. This behaviour would in turn prevent the exposure of additional recognition sites for GABA and prevent gating of the ionophore resulting in functional, but non-competitive, GABA antagonism.

It is suggested that the benzodiazepine and non-benzodiazepine anticonvulsant drugs exert activity of type (a) by interacting with distinct accessory recognition sites associated with separate conformational states of the GABA receptor. Similarly, it is proposed that the convulsant compounds capable of separately inhibiting the binding of either the benzodiazepines or dihydropicrotoxinin exert effects of type (b) at the appropriate accessory recognition site.

This model would imply that endogenous ligands of the accessory recognition sites serve a receptor regulatory function. It is significant in this context that a wide variety of endogenous ligands for the benzodiazepine recognition site have been proposed [52, 55, 71−74], possessing either anticonvulsant [74] or convulsant [75] properties, whilst GABA modulin, also proposed as an endogenous ligand of this site, has additionally been demonstrated to modify the kinetics of GABA recognition [52, 55]. Similarly, evidence for existence of an endogenous ligand for the picrotoxinin sensitive site in rat brain has been reported [76].

The conformational properties of membrane molecules are strictly dependent upon the dielectric properties of their environment and are affected by the charge distribution pattern of vicinal structures. In neuronal membranes these properties are, therefore, likely to be largely determined by the stacking patterns of membrane phospholipids. Thus, the absolute conformational properties of the receptor protein, particularly the total number of stable conformations capable of presenting recognition sites and hence the overall co-operativity of the GABA-receptor interactions, may be critically dependent upon the membrane environment.

This is consistent with the observation that phospholipids have pronounced effects upon GABA-ergic receptor function [77] and that altered phospholipid metabolism in certain disease states may alter GABA receptor characteristics [78]. It follows that CNS regional differences of membrane environment may affect both the co-operativity of the GABA-receptor interaction and the absolute stoichiometry of the various recognition sites discussed. Thus, the anticonvulsants may be capable of exerting regionally specific effects in the CNS as a result of regional changes in the stoichiometry, and hence the apparent concentration of their recognition sites.

These drugs would also be expected to demonstrate markedly different pharmacological properties from those induced by classical GABA agonists, and this is observed [79]. Valproic acid is of special relevance in this context as a result of its lipophilic nature and the fact that it does not present the characteristic anticonvulsant pharmacophore but has nevertheless been reported to potentiate responses to GABA in preparations in which the inhibition of GABA metabolism was unlikely to account for the observed activity [7]. It is proposed, therefore, that valproate exerts these properties, and hence a component of its anticonvulsant activity, by affecting the local environment of the GABA receptor reducing the co-operativity of the GABA-receptor interaction leading to potentiation of responses to GABA.

In conclusion, it is proposed that the GABA-ergic system is likely to provide a large number of molecular substrates capable of mediating anticonvulsant activity and that drug interactions at the GABA-receptor complex are associated with specific pharmacophores. Further investigation of these pharmacophores and of the steric properties of the anticonvulsants should provide a deeper insight into the precise molecular mechanism underlying anticonvulsant drug activity at the GABA receptor.

Acknowledgments

We would like to acknowledge the generous financial support provided both by the Boots Co Ltd and the Brain Research Trust.

We would also like to thank Kami Amin for her skilled preparation of the manuscript.

References

1   Roberts E, Chase TN, Tower DB. *GABA in Nervous System Function 1976*. New York: Raven Press
2   Ayala G, Jonston FD, Lin S, Dichter H. *Brain Res 1977; 121:* 259–270
3   Deisz RA, Lux HD. *Neurosci Lett 1977; 5:* 199–203
4   Macdonald RL, Barker JL. *Brain Res 1979; 167:* 323–326
5   Haefely W, Polc P, Schaffner R, et al. In Krogsgaard–Larsen P, Scheel-Kruger J, Kofod H, eds. *GABA Neurotransmitters 1979;* 357. Copenhagen: Munksgaard
6   Nicoll RA, Eccles JC, Oshima TC, Rubia F. *Nature 1975; 258:* 625–627
7   Gent JP, Phillips NI. *Brain Res 1980; 197:* 275–278
8   Macdonald RL, Barker JL. *Nature 1978; 271:* 563–564
9   Vernaetakis A, Woodbury DM. In Roberts E, ed. *Inhibition in the Nervous System and Gamma-aminobutyric Acid 1960;* 242. New York: Macmillan
10   Simler SC, Gensburger L, Ciesielski L, Mandel P. *Commun Psychopharmacol 1978; 2:* 123–130
11   Saad SF. *J Pharm Pharmacol 1972; 24:* 839–840
12   Iadarola MJ, Raines A, Gale K. *J Neurochem 1979; 27:* 1119–1123
13   Patsalos PN, Lascelles PT. *J Neurochem 1981; 36:* 688–695
14   Wood JD, Russell MP, Kurylo E, Newstead JD. *J Neurochem 1979; 33:* 61–68
15   Olsen RW, Ticku MK, van Ness PC, Greenlee D. *Brain Res 1978; 139;* 277–294
16   Weinberger J, Nicklas WJ, Berl S. *Neurology 1976; 26:* 162–166
17   Essman WB, Essman EJ. *Brain Res Bull 1980; 5: Suppl 2:* 821–824
18   Iversen LL, Johnston GAR. *J Neurochem 1971; 18:* 1939–1950
19   Sellström A, Hamberger A. *J Neurochem 1975; 24:* 847–852
20   Julien RM, Halpern LM. *Epilepsia 1972; 13:* 387–400
21   Coleman-Riese D, Cutter RWP. *Neurochem Res 1978; 3:* 423–429
22   Fowler LJ, Beckford J, John RA. *Biochem Pharmacol 1975; 24:* 1267–1270
23   van der Laan JW, de Boer TH, Bruinvels J. *J Neurochem 1979; 32:* 1769–1780
24   Meldrum B. *Brain Res Bull 1980; 5 (Suppl 2):* 579–584
25   Loschler W. *J Pharmacol Exp Therap 1978; 204:* 255–261
26   Close WJ, Spielman MA. In Hartung WH, ed. *Medicinal Chemistry 1961*. New York: John Wiley and Sons Inc
27   Mercier J. In Radouco-Thomas C, ed. *International Encyclopedia of Pharmacology and Therapeutics 1973;* 203. Oxford: Pergamon Press
28   Jones PG, Kennard O. *J Pharm Pharmacol 1978; 30:* 815–817
29   Camerman A, Camerman N. In Bergman E, Pullman B, eds. *Molecular and Quantitative Pharmacology 1974;* 213. Holland: D Reidel
30   McBunney RN, Barker JL. *Nature 1978; 274:* 596–597
31   Krnjević K. *Physiol Rev 1974; 54:* 418–540
32   Nicoll RA. *Proc Nat Acad Sci USA 1975; 72:* 1460–1463

33   Choi DW, Farb DH, Fischbach GD. *Nature 1977; 269:* 342—344
34   Bowery NG, Dray A. *Nature 1976; 266:* 276—278
35   Deisz RA, Lux HD. *Neurosci Lett 1977; 5:* 199—203
36   Schlosser W, Franco S. *J Pharm Exp Therap 1979; 211:* 290—295
37   Downes H, Perry RS, Ostlund RE, Karler R. *J Pharmacol Exp Therap 1970; 175:* 692—699
38   Zukin SR, Young AB, Snyder SH. *Proc Nat Acad Sci USA 1974; 71:* 4802—4807
39   Enna SJ, Snyder SH. *Brain Res 1975; 100:* 81—97
40   Olsen RW, Ticku MK, van Ness PC, Greenlee D. *Brain Res 1978; 139:* 277—294
41   Olsen RW, Greenlee D, van Ness PC, Ticku MK. In Krogsgaard-Larsen P, Scheel-Kruger J, Kofod U, eds. *GABA-Neurotransmitters 1979;* 165—178. Copenhagen: Munksgaard
42   Ticku MK, Ban M, Olsen RW. *Mol Pharmacol 1978; 14:* 391—402
43   Ticku MK, van Ness PC, Haycock JW, et al. *Brain Res 1978; 150:* 642—647
44   Ticku MK, Olsen RW. *Neuropharmacology 1979; 18:* 315—318
45   Olsen RW, Leeb-Lundberg F, Napias C. *Brain Res Bull 1980; 5 (Suppl 2):* 217—221
46   Squires RF, Braestrup C. *Nature 1977; 266:* 732—734
47   Möhler H, Okada T. *Science 1977; 198;* 849—851
48   Costa E, Guidotti A, Mao CC. In Roberts E, Chase TN, Tower DB, eds. *GABA in Nervous System Function 1976;* 413. New York: Raven Press
49   Tallman JF, Thomas JW, Gallager DW. *Nature 1978; 274;* 383—385
50   Karobath M, Sperk G. *Proc Nat Acad Sci USA 1979; 76:* 1004—1006
51   Karobath M, Placheta P, Lippitsch M, Krogsgaard-Larsen P. *Nature 1979; 278:* 748—749
52   Guidotti A, Toffano G, Costa E. *Nature 1978; 275:* 553—555
53   Meiners BA, Salama AI. *Soc Neurosci Abstr 1980; 6:* 189
54   Johnston GAR, Willow M. In Costa E, di Chiara G, Gessa GL, eds. *Advances in Biochemical Psychopharmacology; GABA and Benzodiazepine Receptors 1981; Volume 16:* 191—198. New York: Raven Press
55   Guidotti A, Massotti M, Costa E. In Yamamura HI, Olsen RW, Usdin E, eds. *Psychopharmacology and Biochemistry of Neurotransmitter Receptors 1980;* 665. New York: Elsevier
56   Costa T, Rodbard D, Pert CB. *Nature 1979; 277:* 315—317
57   Antoniadis A, Muller WE, Wollert V. *Neuropharmacology 1980; 19:* 121—124
58   Leeb-Lundberg F, Snowman A, Olsen RW. *Proc Nat Acad Sci USA 1980; 77 (No. 12):* 7468—7472
59   Asano T, Ogasawara N. *Eur J Pharmacol 1982; 77:* 355—357
60   Gallager DW, Mallorga P, Tallman JF. *Brain Res 1980; 189:* 209—220
61   Squires R, Naquet R, Riche D, Braestrup C. *Epilepsia 1979; 20:* 215—221
62   Valdes F, Dsheiff RM, Birmingham F, et al. *Proc Nat Acad Sci USA 1982; 79 (1):* 193—197
63   Kier LB, ed. *Molecular Orbital Theory in Drug Research 1971.* New York: Academic Press
64   Warner D. *PhD Thesis 1975.* London: The City University
65   Lucek RW, Garland WA, Dairman W. *Fed Proc 1979; 39(2):* 541
66   Steward EG, Lowe RH. In Ryall *Iontophoresis and Transmitter Mechanisms in the Mammalian Central Nervous System 1978;* 394. Amsterdam: Elsevier/North Holland Biomedical Press
67   Pople JA, Segal GA. *J Chem Phys 1965; 43:* 5136
68   Andrews PR, Jones GP, Lodge D. *Eur J Pharmacol 1979; 55:* 115—120
69   Olsen RW. *J Neurochem 1981; 37 (1):* 1—13
70   Lowe RH, Lascelles PT. *J Theor Biol.* In press
71   Marangos PJ, Paul SM, Goodwin FK, Skolnick P. *Life Sci 1979; 25(13):* 1093—1102
72   Braestrup C, Nielsen M, Olsen CE. *Proc Nat Acad Sci USA 1980; 77(4):* 2288—2292
73   Davis LG, Cohen RK. *Biochem Biophys Comm 1980; 92:* 141—148
74   Möhler H, Polc P, Cumin R, et al. *Nature 1979; 278:* 563—565
75   Cowen PJ, Green AR, Nutt DJ. *Nature 1981; 290:* 54—55

76   Olsen RW, Leeb-Lundberg F. *Eur J Pharmacol 1980; 65:* 101–104
77   Lloyd KG, Beaumont K. *Brain Res Bull 1980; 5 (Suppl 2):* 285–290
78   Lloyd KG, Davidson L. *Science 1979; 205:* 1147–1149
79   Pedley TA, Horton RW, Meldrum BS. *Epilepsia 1979; 20:* 409–416

39

MECHANISM OF ACTION OF ANTICONVULSANT DRUGS WITH SPECIAL REFERENCE TO THEIR ACTIONS ON AMINO ACID RELEASE

J de Belleroche

Introduction

Anticonvulsant drugs are a heterogeneous group which act in a variety of ways to prolong or facilitate the action of the inhibitory neurotransmitter, gamma-amino-butyric acid (GABA). GABA-mediated inhibition is brought about by an increase in chloride permeability, the chloride channel being operated by the GABA recep-tor. Prolongation of GABA action may occur, for example by sodium valproate, by inhibiting the enzyme GABA-transaminase by which GABA is catabolised. Alternatively, agents such as benzodiazepines and barbiturates, which bind to two distinctive receptor sites associated with the GABA receptor and linked chloride channel [1,2] and enhance the action of GABA [3], may be effective through this action at the GABA receptor complex. This emphasis on stimulating GABA activity in drug treatment of seizures is also supported by a number of clinical and pharmacological observations where impaired GABA production or action, or conversely, where excess release of the excitatory neurotransmitter, gluta-mate, are associated with seizure activity. Thus, GABA antagonists such as picrotoxin are convulsants and, in animal models, epileptic discharges are ac-companied by a large rise in the release of glutamate from cerebral cortex [4]. Furthermore, it has also been reported that GABA levels are low in the cerebro-spinal fluid (CSF) of patients with intractable epilepsy [5].

There is also a good correlation in dogs between CSF GABA levels and clonic seizure threshold values in response to pentylenetetrazol, low GABA levels corresponding to a lower threshold of excitability [6].

Although substantial evidence is accumulating that anticonvulsants such as barbiturates and benzodiazepines have a defined action at the GABA receptor complex, it is of importance to determine whether this interaction is responsible for their anticonvulsant action in man. Benzodiazepines have a range of actions, being anxiolytic, muscle relaxant and sedative as well as

361

anticonvulsant and these may not necessarily be ascribed to the same mechanism. A good starting point for an assessment of this kind is to compare the relative potencies of anticonvulsant drugs in reducing seizure activity and their action at GABA receptors. Two useful animal models of seizure activity for testing anticonvulsant action are maximal electroshock seizure and pentylenetetrazol seizure threshold. Anticonvulsant drugs in general terms can be divided into two groups according to the test against which they are most effective [7]. Drugs that are used clinically against absence seizures such as ethosuximide, clonazepam and valproate are most active or only active (eg ethosuximide) against pentylenetetrazol seizures whereas drugs such as carbamazepine and phenytoin used in grand mal and focal epilepsy are only active against maximal electroshock seizures. An interesting anomaly arises with the benzodiazepines for, although clonazepam is an order of magnitude more potent against pentylenetetrazol seizures than diazepam, diazepam is four times more potent against maximal electroshock seizures. The relative potency of these two agents against pentylenetetrazol seizures is in keeping with the affinity of these agents for the benzodiazepine receptor, the Ki (inhibition of specific binding of (^3H)-diazepam) for clonazepam and diazepam being 1.5nM and 6.3nM respectively [8]. A correlation between the Ki values (similarly determined as above) of 32 benzodiazepines has been shown with both inhibition of pentylenetetrazol convulsions in rat and cat muscle relaxant effects [9], an action that may operate through the benzodiazepine receptor. Other behavioural actions of benzodiazepines, such as antianxiety in man and attenuation of experimentally induced anxiety (conflict) in animals, corresponds well with the relative affinity of the drug for this receptor. A comprehensive correlation incorporating 15 benzodiazepines was shown between rat anticonflict potency and Ki values for inhibition of specific (^3H)-diazepam binding [10]. Despite these clear correlations between binding to benzodiazepine receptors and protection against pentylenetetrazol induced seizures and hence, treatment of absence seizures, the action of anticonvulsants such as phenytoin, carbamazepine, phenobarbitone and diazepam against grand mal, focal epilepsy and status epilepticus requires further explanation. These four anticonvulsants require high plasma concentrations (10^{-5} to 10^{-4}M) for therapeutic efficacy [11–13] reaching levels of 4×10^{-5}, 5×10^{-5} and 1.8×10^{-4}M for carbamazepine, diazepam, phenytoin and phenobarbitone respectively. These concentrations are well above the nanamolar concentrations of diazepam, for example, needed to saturate benzodiazepine receptors and further support the need to find an alternative mechanism of action. This prompted us to look at the actions of these drugs on glutamate and GABA release in cerebral cortex to investigate other aspects of neurotransmission than the GABA receptor chloride channel complex. Further, we concentrated on extracellular concentrations of drugs close to their therapeutically efficacious levels.

362

The effect of anticonvulsants on the release of glutamate and GABA

The release of transmitters of the cerebral cortex such as glutamate, GABA and acetylcholine has been successfully studied in in-vitro preparations such as tissue slices and synaptosomes for a number of years. Depolarisation-induced release may be elicited by square wave electrical pulses, depolarising concentrations of K^+ and by depolarising alkaloids such as veratridine, and has the characteristics seen in more intact preparations of being calcium dependent and associated with a stimulation of transmitter synthesis [14,15]. In-vitro preparations such as these have been shown to actively oxidise substrates such as glucose for the synthesis of ATP and phosphocreatine necessary to maintain membrane potentials, and to respond to depolarising stimuli [16].

The experimental design was as follows: top slices of rat cerebral cortex (0.3mm thick) were taken and incubated in an oxygenated physiological saline, Krebs-bicarbonate medium containing 10mM glucose, at 37°C. Tissue slices were preloaded with low concentrations of radioactively labelled transmitters

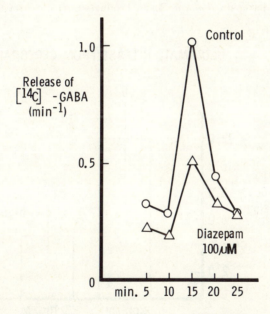

Figure 1. Effect of diazepam (100μM) on the release of (^{14}C)-GABA from tissue slices of rat cerebral cortex. Tissue slices were preincubated for 10 minutes in the presence 0.4μM (^{14}C)-GABA and 100μM amino-oxyacetic acid, transferred through four consecutive washes of incubation medium for one, five, five and five minutes respectively and then incubated for five minute periods, from which samples were taken. Diazepam was present in the first three samples (lower trace only). Elevated medium K^+ (33nM) was present in sample three. Release of (^{14}C)-GABA is expressed as the fractional release coefficient, min^{-1}, which is the release as a percentage of the average tissue stores during the period of release. Further details in reference [25]

363

eg (^{14}C)-glutamate and (^{14}C)-GABA. When using (^{14}C)-GABA, the inhibitor of GABA-transaminase, amino-oxyacetic acid (10^{-4}M), was included to prevent metabolism of GABA. We and other authors have previously shown that the labelle material released by depolarisation from tissue slices labelled in this way is principally GABA and that the conditions are suitable for monitoring transmitter release [17]. After a period of washing with incubation medium, tissue slices were incubated in serial samples of incubation medium for five minutes. The cortical slice from one hemisphere seved as the control for the other hemisphere, to which drugs were applied. The release of GABA was stimulated three to four fold by 33nM K$^+$ (Figure 1) and this evoked release was significantly depressed by the presence of a number of anticonvulsants shown here for diazepam. The resting release of (^{14}C)-GABA was not significantly affected by the range of anticonvulsants examined in this study. Experiments carried out with (^{14}C)-glutamate, showed that a similar depression of the K$^+$-evoked release was also produced in the presence of both phenytoin and diazepam (Figure 2).

A detailed examination of the inhibitory effect of phenytoin (*Epanutin*, Parke-Davis and Co), diazepam (*Valium*, Roche Products Ltd), clonazepam (*Rivotril*,

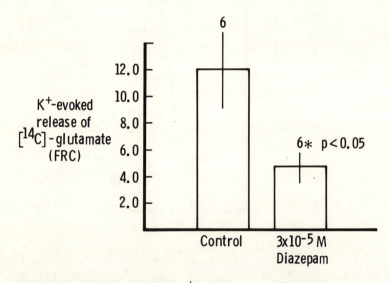

Figure 2. Effect of diazepam on 33nM K$^+$-evoked release of (^{14}C)-glutamate from rat cerebral cortex. Tissue slices were incubated as described for Figure 1 and in the text. The K$^+$-evoked release only is shown for control and diazepam (30μM) conditions. Values of fractional release/five minute period are means ± SEMs for six experiments. * Indicates that diazepam caused a significant inhibition of release p < 0.05. Data are taken from reference [25]

Roche Products Ltd), and phenobarbitone (Macarthys Ltd) on the K^+-evoked release of (^{14}C)-GABA was carried out. Significant inhibition of transmitter release was seen at concentrations of those drugs that are found to be therapeutically effective in man. The inhibitory action of diazepam on GABA release seen in this study confirms previous reports using similar methodology [18,19]. The drug concentrations at which the evoked release of (^{14}C)-GABA is reduced by 50 per cent, IC_{50} values, are given in Table I. The order of potency of anticonvulsants was found to be diazepam>clonazepam>phenytoin>phenobarbitone, which is in keeping with the potency of these drugs in antagonising maximal electroshock induced seizures (see below).

TABLE I. Inhibition of K^+-evoked GABA release from rat cerebral cortex

	IC_{50} values	
Trifluoperazine	1	$\times 10^{-5}$ M
Diazepam	4.7	$\times 10^{-5}$ M
Clonazepam	7	$\times 10^{-5}$ M
Phenytoin	2.8	$\times 10^{-4}$ M
Phenobarbitone	7.9	$\times 10^{-4}$ M

Data from (de Belleroche, Wyrley-Birch and Dick [25])

If drugs such as diazepam were having their effect by facilitating GABAergic transmission at the GABAreceptor linked to a chloride channel, then GABA mimetics would be expected to have a similar action, but the potent GABA agonist, muscimol, was found to be devoid of an inhibitory action of transmitter up to a concentration of 3μM. Since K^+ is known to have a direct depolarising action on nerve terminals, it is therefore likely that nerve terminals are not responsive to muscimol and that a classical GABA receptor is not present on the nerve terminals contained in the cortical slice.

In agreement with these results, picrotoxin was without effect on the inhibitory action of the anticonvulsants tested. In connection with these results, it is also interesting that GABA mimetics have not been shown to be beneficial in reducing seizure activity. For example, intracisternally applied muscimol and GABA (1mg) do not antagonise clonic convulsions induced by pentylenetetrazol whereas diazepam and flurazepam are effective [10]. Similarly, induced myoclonic epilepsy in baboons are not prevented by muscimol, although benzodiazepines are effective [10]. The possibility cannot be precluded, however, that the ineffectiveness of muscimol was due to the lack of a specific effect at a critical population of synapses capable of controlling seizure activity.

A number of studies have provided evidence that anticonvulsants such as phenytoin may produce their effects by altering Ca^{2+} or K^+ conductance (see for example Chapter 10 by Lux and Heinemann in this volume). We investigated whether the effects on transmitter release were the result of drug action on calcium transport within the neurone. This was carried out in two ways, firstly, by studying the effect of drugs on the action of the calcium binding protein, calmodulin, and secondly by looking at the calcium dependence of drug action.

Calmodulin is a major intracellular calcium binding protein, widespread in occurrence, and particularly abundant in the brain, making up 0.6 to 1.0 per cent of the total brain protein [21]. This protein, bound to Ca^{2+}, has been implicated as an activator involved in a number of enzyme systems such as adenyl-cyclase, phosphodiesterase, Ca^{2+}dependent ATPase, Ca^{2+} dependent protein kinase, phospholipase A2 and also in transmitter release. Calmodulin is specifi-

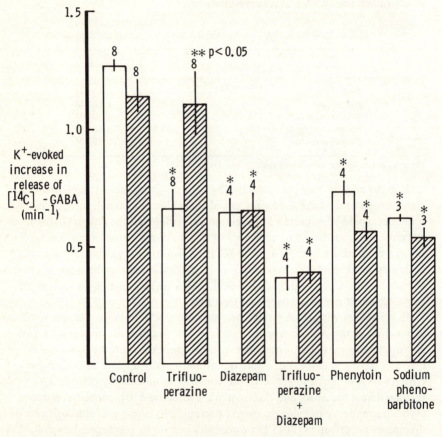

Figure 3. Effect of calmodulin on the inhibition of K^+-evoked release of (^{14}C)-GABA by trifluoperazine, diazepam, phenytoin and sodium phenobarbitone. Tissue slices were incubated as described in the legend to Figure 1. Drugs were present as indicated at the following concentrations, trifluoperazine (10μM), diazepam (100μM), phenytoin (300μM) and sodium phenobarbitone (1mM), and all caused a significant depression of the K^+-evoked release of (^{14}C)-GABA, $p<0.01$, Students t-test. Incubations carried out in the presence of calmodulin significantly increased $p<0.05$ the release of (^{14}C)-GABA in the presence of 10μM trifluoperazine. Values are means ±SEMs for the number of experiments indicated. Data B taken from reference [25]

366

cally complexed by trifluoperazine and the effect of this agent was therefore examined in our test system. (^{14}C)-GABA release was found to be markedly reduced by the presence of trifluoperazine (*Stelazine*, Smith, Kline and French Laboratories Ltd), K$^+$-evoked release being reduced by 50 per cent at 10^{-5}M trifluoperazine (Figure 3). This inhibition could be overcome by adding extracellular calmodulin (0.6μg calmodulin per 15mg tissue slice of cerebral cortex). Hence calmodulin was capable of restoring release, which is likely to have occurred following entry to the neurone and coupling with internal Ca^{2+}. Previous studies have shown that a range of extracellular markers with large molecular weight, such as horseradish peroxidase and dextran, have been shown to be internalised within the neurone following depolarising stimuli, probably occurring by an *endocytotic* process [22].

The present results provide support for the idea that the calcium dependent, K$^+$-evoked release of GABA utilises calmodulin in the process. The inhibition of GABA release by diazepam or by the combination of both diazepam and trifluoperazine or by either phenytoin or phenobarbitone was however *not* countered by adding back calmodulin. These results, together with the observation that the

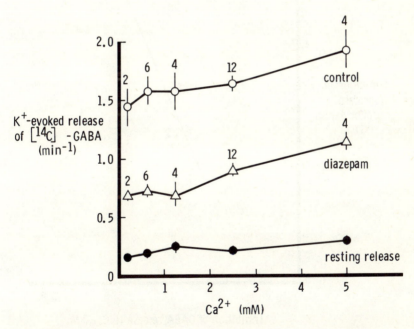

Figure 4. Effect at varying calcium concentrations on the inhibitory effect of diazepam on the K$^+$-evoked release of (^{14}C)-GABA. Tissue slices were incubated as described in the legend to Figure 1 in the presence of varying concentrations of Ca^{++} (0.2 to 5mM). Data are taken from reference [25]. Values (FRC min^{-1}) are means, ± SEMs with the number of experiments indicated above

inhibition by diazepam and trifluoperazine were approximately additive, support the conclusion that the two agents were acting at two separate sites and that the inhibition by diazepam was later in the sequence of events leading up to transmitter release.

One mechanism by which drugs such as anticonvulsants might reduce the calcium dependent release of transmitter is by limiting the calcium influx. To explore this possibility, the effect of varying the external calcium concentration was tested on the degree of inhibition caused by diazepam. However, the effect of diazepam did not vary with calcium concentration (0.2 to 5mM) (Figure 4) although, if diazepam directly affected calcium transport a greater inhibition would be expected at submaximal calcium concentrations.

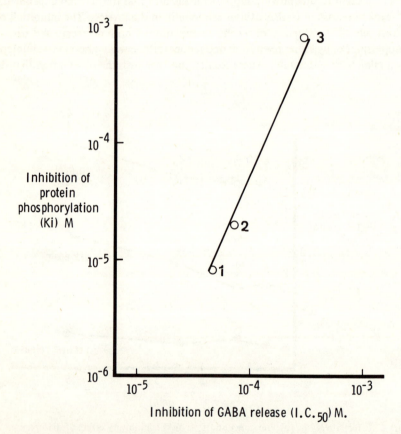

Figure 5. Correlation between inhibition of protein phosphorylation (Ki) and inhibition of K$^+$-evoked release of (^{14}C)-GABA (IC$_{50}$). Data for Ki values are taken from references [23 and 24] and for IC$_{50}$ values from reference [25]. Points 1, 2 and 3 correspond to diazepam, clonazepam and phenytoin respectively

Taking these results together, it appears that inhibition of transmitter release, for example by diazepam, is not brought about by direct interaction with calcium flux or with calmodulin but is more likely to be at a later stage in which the calcium-activated calmodulin molecule is involved, for example an enzyme for which this serves as a prosthetic group. An indirect effect of the drug on calcium flux may however subsequently occur. One particularly relevant contender for this function is a protein kinase studied by De Lorenzo et al [23] that phosphorylates a number of proteins present in synaptic membranes by a calcium activated calmodulin dependent reaction. Furthermore the activity of this enzyme has been shown to be inhibited by a range of benzodiazepines as well as phenytoin [24] and the rank order of potency of inhibition of phosphorylation by drugs is the same as that found in the present study for inhibition of the K^+-evoked release of (^{14}C)-GABA. The close correlation between these actions is shown graphically in Figure 5. A number of other properties are common to both systems, for example trifluoperazine inhibits both transmitter release and phosphorylation and while the trifluoperazine inhibition can be overcome by adding back exogenous calmodulin, the inhibition by the anticonvulsants tested cannot be overcome by calmodulin in either system.

Summary

In conclusion, the results from these experiments indicate that the anticonvulsant agents tested, namely phenytoin, diazepam, clonazepam and phenobarbitone can have a very marked inhibitory action on the depolarisation induced release of neurotransmitters at therapeutically effective drug concentration. Both the excitatory transmitter, glutamate and the inhibitory transmitter, GABA were found to be affected. This mechanism of action could be responsible for the reduction in spread of epileptic discharge seen with drug treatment.

Drug-induced inhibition appears to act as a calcium activated reaction. The rank order of potency of inhibition of transmitter release correlates well with both the therapeutic efficacy of anticonvulsants in grand mal and focal epilepsy, maximal electroshock seizure activity in animals and their inhibition of calmodulin activated phosphorylation of synaptic membranes shown by De Lorenzo et al [23].

Acknowledgments

I am grateful to Mr A Dick and Miss Wyrley-Birch who took part in this project, when in receipt of intercalated BSc awards from the Medical Research Council, whom we thank. I am also grateful to the Mental Health Foundation for financial support.

References

1 Braestrup C, Nielsen M. *Drug Res 1980; 30:* 852–857
2 Olsen RW. *J Neurochem 1981; 37:* 1–13
3 MacDonald R, Barker JL. *Nature 1978; 271:* 563–564
4 Koyama I. *Canad J Physiol Pharmacol 1972; 50:* 740–752
5 Wood JH, Hare TA, Glaeser BS et al. *Neurology 1979; 29:* 1203–1208
6 Loscher W. *J Neurochem 1982; 38:* 293–295
7 Krall RL, Penry JK, White BG et al. *Epilepsia 1978; 19:* 409–428
8 Mohler H, Okada T. *Science 1977; 198:* 849–851
9 Braestrup C, Squires RF. *Europ J Pharmacol 1978; 48:* 263–270
10 Sepinwall J, Cook L. *Federation Proc 1980; 39:* 3024–3031
11 Fowler TJ. In *Epilepsy 1980;* 25. London: Update Books Ltd
12 Glaser GH, Perry JK, Woodbury DM. In *Antiepileptic Drugs: Mechanisms of Action 1980.* New York: Raven Press
13 Bond AJ, Hailey DM, Lader MH. *Br J Clin Pharmacol 1977; 4:* 51–56
14 de Belleroche J, Bradford HF. *J Neurochem 1972; 19:* 585–602
15 de Belleroche J, Bradford HF. *J Neurochem 1972; 19:* 1817–1819
16 de Belleroche J, Bradford HF. *Progress in Neurobiology 1973; 1:* 275–298
17 Nadler JV, White WF, Vaca KW et al. *J Neurochem 1977; 29:* 279–290
18 Olsen RW, Lamar EE, Bayless JD. *J Neurochem 1977; 28:* 299–305
19 Mitchell PR, Martin IL. *Neuropharmacology 1978; 17:* 317–320
20 Pedley TA, Horton RW, Meldrum BS. *Epilepsia 1979; 20:* 409–416
21 Cheung WY. *Science 1980; 207:* 19–27
22 Fried RC, Blaustein MP. *Nature 1976; 261:* 255–256
23 De Lorenzo RJ, Burdette S, Holerness J. *Science 1981; 213:* 546–549
24 De Lorenzo RJ, Emple G, Glaser GH. *J Neurochem 1977; 28:* 21–30
25 de Belleroche J, Dick A, Wyrley-Birch A. Anticonvulsants and Trifluoperazine Inhibit the Evoked Release of GABA from Cerebral Cortex of Rat at Different Sites. Submitted 1982

40

THE EFFECT OF VALPROATE ON CEREBRAL AMINO ACID METABOLISM AND ITS RELATIONSHIP TO ANTICONVULSANT EFFECT

Astrid G Chapman

Sodium valproate, or di-n-propyl acetate, is a short branched-chain fatty acid with a broad-spectrum anticonvulsant action against both clinical seizures and experimental animal seizures [1–3]. The uptake distribution and pharmacokinetics of valproate, the time course of its anticonvulsant effect and the anticonvulsant potency of the valproate metabolites have previously been reviewed [2–7]. Following the administration of a single dose of valproate (200–600mg/kg) in rodents, the protection against different types of seizure models normally lasts for 1–3 hours. Maximum protection against electroshock-induced convulsions in rats is apparent within two min of the i.p. injection of 400mg/kg valproate [8], while the same acute dose of valproate affords two hours of protection against audiogenic seizures in mice [9]. The plasma level of valproate attained following the administration of a single anticonvulsant dose of valproate in mice is around 150–400µg/ml, while the corresponding brain valproate level is 30–120µg/g, or approximately 0.2–0.8mM [10].

GABAergic mechanism of anticonvulsant action

There is a large body of evidence implicating the GABA-mediated inhibitory system in the mechanism of action of both convulsant and anticonvulsant compounds [11–14]. Thus, inhibitors of the GABA metabolising enzyme, GABA transaminase, such as γ-vinyl-GABA, γ-acetylenic GABA, gabaculine, aminooxyacetic acid and ethanolamine-o-sulfate, produce large increases in the cerebral GABA levels and have potent anticonvulsant action in a number of animal models [14]. Benzodiazepines and barbiturates are believed to exert their anticonvulsant action through an interaction at separate sites, with a postsynaptic GABA-receptor-complex, thereby enhancing the inhibitory action of GABA [12,13]. The GABAergic mechanism of these compounds, however, is not revealed in an increased brain GABA concentration as shown in Table I. There

TABLE I. Effect of some anticonvulsants on cortical neurotransmitter amino acid concentrations

		GABA	ASP	GLUT	Reference
Diazepam	(1–2mg/kg)	→	↑ 20%	↓ 6%	15
Flurazepam	(10mg/kg)	→	↑ 30%	→	*
Phenobarb	(150mg/kg)	→, ↓ 15%	↑ 35%	↑ 7%	16
Valproate	(400mg/kg)	↑ 32%	↓ 22%	↑ 14%	17
γ-vinyl-GABA	(1g/kg)	↑ 200%	→	→	17

*   Riley, Chapman and Meldrum, unpublished observations

are no changes in the cortical GABA concentration following the administration of anticonvulsant doses of diazepam or flurazepam [15], while high doses of phenobarbital have no initial effect on the cortical GABA level and only produce a slight fall in the level three hours after the barbiturate administration [16]. The group of anticonvulsants listed in Table I have no single, consistent effect on the cortical levels of the excitatory transmitters, aspartate and glutamate.

Valproate and the GABA system

GABA levels

It was early established that valproate administration lead to an elevation of cerebral GABA levels in rodents [18], and that the period of GABA elevation following acute valproate administration coincides with the period of protection against audiogenic seizures [9,19]. Subsequent studies have shown that valproate exhibits anticonvulsant action against audiogenic seizures at doses insufficient to raise brain GABA levels [20], and that the protection by valproate against electroshock-induced convulsions is established before (at 2 min) brain GABA levels have increased [6,8]. Nevertheless, in light of the GABAergic features shared by most anticonvulsant compounds, it is not surprising that the major research emphasis in elucidating the mechanism of action of valproate has focused on the GABAergic system. There has been a large number of studies that have included measurements of cortical or whole brain GABA levels during the first hour following acute valproate administration (200–600mg/kg in rodents) (Table II). These studies all support the early observation by Mandel's group [18] in showing a 17–60 per cent valproate-induced rise in GABA concentration [9,17,20–23]. Following daily (5–14 days) valproate administration the GABA rise following the final injection appears larger than that observed following acute valproate administration [25,34–37], but the subsequent return of GABA to control levels following valproate administration appears to be similar for chronic and acute treatment [37]. Valproate administered orally to rats for seven days causes no increase in the brain GABA level [26].

372

TABLE II. Effect of valproate on cortical or whole brain acid levels in rodents

	Acute	Reference	Chronic	Reference
GABA	17– 60% ↑	9,17–33	33–225% ↑	25,34–37
Aspartate	11– 48% ↓	5,9,17,18,25,26	51% ↑	36
Glutamate	→, 14% ↑	17,18,25,28	13– 46% ↑	35,36
Glutamine	→	17,18,25	18% ↑	35
Glycine	→	17,18,25	→	*
Taurine	→	17	22– 80% ↑	35,36
Tryptophar	33–150% ↑	25,38,39	→, 32% ↑	38

Amino acid levels were determined 15–60 min after acute administration of valproate
(200–600mg/kg), or 3–120 min after the last injection of chronically administered
valproate (5–21 days; 300–400mg/kg daily).
* Karobath M, unpublished results

Attempts have been made to identify valproate-induced effects on the functional 'transmitter-pool' of GABA by isolating synaptosomes from rats treated
with valproate or valproate metabolites [31,32,40,41]. In some studies [32,41]
there appears to be a correlation between anticonvulsant activity and elevation
of synaptosomal GABA levels; in others not [31]. Another attempt at selectively
studying 'transmitter-pool' GABA involves lesioning the GABA projection to the
substantia nigra with a subsequent disappearance of 'neurotransmitter GABA'
in the lesioned nigra [30]. Nerve terminal GABA is then calculated as the difference in concentration between the intact and lesioned hemispheres. The calculated elevation in nerve terminal GABA (39%) following valproate administration
(300mg/kg, 30 min) is very similar to the elevation observed in total intact
nigra GABA (36%), providing little evidence for a selective sensitivity of transmitter GABA levels to valproate treatment.

GABA-related enzymes

The synthesis and metabolism of GABA via the GABA-shunt are shown in Figure 1.
GABA is synthesised by the GAD-catalysed decarboxylation of glutamate, and
subsequently metabolised to succinic semialdehyde in the reversible, GABA-T
catalysed reaction. Succinic semialdehyde (SSADH) can be further metabolised
either by SSADH-catalysed oxidation to succinate, or by aldehyde reductase-
catalysed reduction to γ-hydroxybutyrate (Table III). Although the activity of
total aldehyde reductases is comparable to the SSADH activity in ox brain homogenates [45], the major route of succinate semialdehyde metabolism is undoubtedly that of oxidation to succinate. The conversion of GABA to γ-hydroxybutyrate
via the aldehyde reductase reaction has recently been shown to occur in rat brain
homogenates [50], but only at a rate of approximately 1nmole/min/g brain

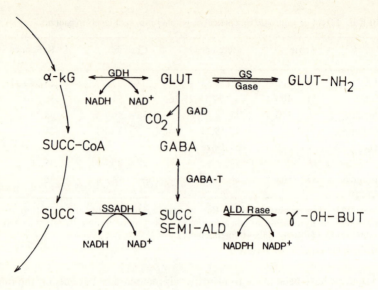

Figure 1. The 'GABA-shunt' and associated reactions

GDH	=	glutamate dehydrogenase (EC 1.4.1.2)
GS	=	glutamine synthase (EC 6.3.1.2)
Gase	=	glutaminase (EC 3.5.1.2)
GAD	=	glutamate decarboxylase (EC 4.1.1.15)
GABA-T	=	GABA transaminase (EC 2.6.1.19)
SSADH	=	succinic semialdehyde dehydrogenase (EC 1.2.1.16)
ALD. Rase	=	NADPH-linked aldehyde reductase (EC 1.1.1.2)

TABLE III. Enzyme inhibition by valproate

Enzyme	K_i in-vitro	Reference	In-vivo effect, rodents	Reference
GAD	81mM	42	↑ 20−30% synaptosomal GAD	31,41
			↓ 20%, chronic valproate	34
GABA-T	10−100mM	42−46	↓ 0−30%	20,24,31, 32,34
SSADH	0.5−4.8mM	20,44−47	−	
Ald. reductase	0.07−0.08mM	45,48	−	
(liver) Glycine cleavage	~ 3mM	49	↓ 50%, chronic valproate	49

(37°) which is about 0.1−0.3 per cent of the rate reported for the SSADH reaction in brain homogenates [20,45]. The effect of valproate on the activities of GABA-related enzymes is shown in Table III.

In-vitro inhibition of GAD activity in mouse brain homogenates is only observed in the presence of extremely high valproate concentrations (K_i = 81mM) [42]. The in-vivo effect of valproate on GABA synthesis needs to be clarified. In brain homogenates and synaptosomes prepared from mice given an acute valproate injection (125–290mg/kg, i.p.) 30 min previously, there are 20–25 per cent increases (statistically significant) in the synaptosomal GAD activity in all doses of valproate tested [31,41], which lead Löscher to propose that the valproate-induced rise in brain GABA level is partially due to an enhanced rate of GABA synthesis. The GAD activity in the whole brain homogenate is only significantly (25–35%) elevated following the administration of 170–200mg/kg, i.p. valproate [31,41]. A lower (125mg/kg) valproate dose causes no rise in whole brain GAD activity, while a higher dose (290mg/kg) causes an apparent (non-significant) 10 per cent rise in whole brain GAD activity [31]. Following chronic administration of valproate (21 days; 200mg/kg, i.p. daily or seven days; 400mg/kg, i.p. daily) to rats, there is an apparent 20 per cent decrease (non-significant) in the GAD activity of the cortical homogenate [34].

There is better agreement about the ability of valproate to inhibit the further metabolism of GABA. Although unphysiologically high valproate levels are required to obtain significant inhibition of GABA-T activity in vitro (K_i values of 10–100mM reported) [42–46] or in vivo (0–15 per cent inhibition of GABA-T activity observed after administration of 125–400mg/kg valproate [20,24,31, 32,34], 30 per cent inhibition observed after 600mg/kg valproate [20]) the subsequent enzyme in the GABA metabolising pathway, SSADH, is much more sensitive to valproate inhibition (K_i values of 0.5–4.8mM) [20,44–47] leading to a cumulative inhibition of GABA oxidation by valproate which might account for the increased brain GABA level observed following valproate administration.

Thus the results from the in-vitro and in-vivo studies on GABA-related enzymes point to a reduction in the rate of GABA metabolism in the presence of valproate, but do not give any conclusive answer about the effect of valproate on the rate of GABA formation. Alternative approaches have therefore been devised to establish the effect of valproate on the rate of GABA turnover in brain.

Rate of GABA turnover

There are two main methods for estimating in-vivo GABA turnover rates (Table IV). Each method gives internally consistent results, but there is an unexplained, approximate 10-fold difference in GABA turnover rates estimated by these two methods. One of the methods depends on determining the rate of accumulation of GABA following a supposed complete and irreversible inhibition of GABA-T by potent GABA-T inhibitors. This method assumes an undiminished rate of GABA formation in the presence of a complete blockage of its subsequent metabolism. An approximately linear rate of GABA accumulation observed at least for a certain time period following the administration of the GABA-T

TABLE IV. Effect of acute valproate administration on GABA turnover in rodent brain

| | Cortical GABA turnover (μmoles/min/g brain) | | | |
	GABA-T inhibition method	Reference	Rate of ^{14}C-labelling method	Reference
Control	0.03–0.1	33,51–53	0.6–0.9	28,51,54
Valproate (200mg/kg)	0.02	33	–	
Valproate (350mg/kg)	–		0.56	28
% of control	25%		74%	

inhibitors γ-vinyl-GABA [52], AOAA or gabaculine [53] seems to support this assumption. We have also recently shown [17] that the rate of GABA formation (^{14}C-labelling of GABA) is not affected by the prior administration of a dose of γ-vinyl-GABA (1g/kg) sufficient to cause an 80 per cent inhibition of GABA-T [52] and three-fold increase in cortical GABA level, again strengthening the above assumption. Fonnum [51] has compiled some of the values for cerebral GABA turnover rates estimated by this method (and these are included in Table IV). Similar GABA turnover values are obtained in the presence of a number of different GABA-T inhibitors. This rate of GABA turnover is estimated to be 0.03–0.1 μmole/min/g brain [33,51–53], which corresponds to only 2–6 per cent of the total glucose utilised by rat brain (CMR_{gl} = 0.8μmoles/min/g [17]) being oxidised through the GABA shunt. A similar rate of GABA turnover (0.11μmoles/min/g) is obtained by estimating the initial rate of *post-mortem* GABA accumulation (due to inhibition of the SSADH reaction by NAD^+ depletion) [55].

However, when GABA turnover is estimated from the rate of ^{14}C incorporation into glutamate and GABA from labelled precursors (usually ^{14}C-glucose), much higher estimates for GABA turnover are obtained. This method leads to GABA turnover rates of 0.6–0.9μmoles/min/g [28,51,54], which represents 35–55 per cent of the total glucose utilised being oxidised via the GABA shunt. These calculations are hampered by a lack of knowledge of the size of the amino acid pools actually being labelled. The experimentally determined total cortical amino acid concentrations are necessarily used for the calculations although it is known that glutamate, glutamine and GABA exist in at least two kinetically distinct compartments in the brain [28,51,54,55].

Despite the large discrepancy in GABA turnover rates obtained with these two methods, it is interesting to note that valproate appears to inhibit the GABA turnover estimated by either method. Using the GABA-T inhibition method (gabaculine), a 60–80 per cent inhibition of GABA turnover is reported in animals given 60–600mg/kg valproate [33]. However, it needs to be established that valproate does not partially reverse the gabaculine inhibition of GABA-T under the conditions used since the method requires a complete blockade of further

GABA metabolism. Wood and co-workers have shown that valproate (400mg/kg) injected simultaneously with AOAA (6.6mg/kg) into mice reduces the AOAA-induced inhibition of GABA-T activity in the brain homogenate by about one-half [32], whereas the gabaculine-induced inhibition of GABA-T was much less affected by valproate administration.

Using an acute, anticonvulsant dose of valproate (350mg/kg) that has little or no effect on the overall rate of cerebral glucose utilisation [17,28], Cremer and co-workers [28] studied the rate of labelling of glutamate and GABA 2–20 min following the i.v. injection of 2-^{14}C-glucose, and found that valproate reduced the estimated rates of GABA formation from 0.76 to 0.56μmoles/min/g. A similar experiment, shown in Figure 2, shows that valproate (400mg/kg) has no effect on the rate of labelling of cortical glutamate following an i.v. injection of 2-^{14}C-glucose, whereas valproate significantly depresses the initial rate of cortical GABA labelling, supporting a reduced rate of GABA formation in the presence of valproate [17].

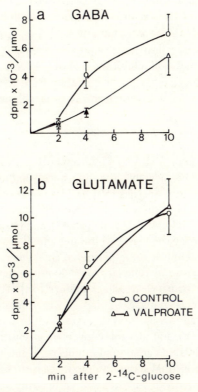

Figure 2. Rate of labelling of cortical GABA (2a) and glutamate (2b) from a 2-^{14}C-glucose (80μCi/kg) precursor injected i.v. in control rats and rats given valproate (400mg/kg i.p.; 30 min) [17]

377

There have been two other studies examining the effect of valproate on the ^{14}C-labelling of brain amino acids. In one early study [18] only one late time point (30 min) was used, and there was no difference between the experimental and the control groups under these steady state conditions. The other study [56] compared ^{14}C incorporation into cortical amino acids five min after U-^{14}C-glucose was injected directly into the 3rd ventricle. In rats treated with 100mg/kg valproate there was a 90 per cent increase in the amount of ^{14}C incorporated into GABA. This increase was less apparent (a 35% non-significant increase) when a higher dose (200mg/kg) of valproate was used. One possible explanation for the difference in results could be that higher doses of valproate (350–400mg/kg) are required for the inhibition of GABA formation, and that the apparent activation of GABA labelling observed at a low valproate dose (100mg/kg) might be related to the previously discussed activation of GAD activity by valproate. However, the enhancement of synaptosomal GAD activity was similar (20–25%) throughout the range of valproate doses used (125–290mg/kg) [31,41], whereas there was no activation of whole brain GAD activity following the administration of a dose of valproate (125mg/kg) [31] comparable to that dose (100mg/kg) causing the increased ^{14}C-incorporation into GABA reported above.

Thus it seems quite conclusive that valproate, when administered acutely in high anticonvulsant doses, will inhibit the rate of GABA formation. The effect of lower doses of valproate and any possible relation to the reported valproate-induced activation of GAD-activity remains to be established.

The aldehyde reduction reaction

The possible conversion of GABA to γ-hydroxybutyrate via succinic semialdehyde (Figure 1) has received considerable attention since γ-hydroxybutyrate has been shown to have convulsant properties [57] and also since one of the aldehyde reductase isozymes has been shown to be extremely sensitive to inhibition by valproate (K_i = 0.07–0.08mM; Table III) [45,48] and most other anticonvulsant drugs such as benzodiazepines, barbiturates and hydantoins [48,58,59]. However, the most potent class of inhibitors of aldehyde reductase, the flavonoids (K_i values in the low micromolar range) do not possess any anticonvulsant activity against maximal electroshock in mice [58]. The physiological function of aldehyde reductase is unclear. It has, however, recently been shown that GABA can be converted to γ-hydroxybutyrate in rat brain homogenates albeit at a slow rate (see above), and that this conversion is sensitive to inhibition by the same anticonvulsants that are potent inhibitors of aldehyde reductase in vitro [50]. For instance, 1mM sodium valproate causes a 67 per cent inhibition of the conversion of GABA to γ-hydroxybutyrate in the homogenate preparation. Despite the very potent inhibitory effects of valproate and other anticonvulsants on aldehyde reductase, it is not known how this relates to the anticonvulsant action of valproate.

378

Functional effects of valproate on GABAergic transmission

Valproate enhances the inhibitory action of GABA when the latter is applied iontophoretically to neurons in tissue culture [60]. Similar effects of valproate have been described in cerebral cortex and brain stem of the rat [8,61,62]. These effects have a very short latency (< 2 min) and indicate an action on the post-synaptic membrane, presumably at a site within or intimately related to the GABA receptor/chloride ionophore/benzodiazepine complex. Attempts to establish a molecular basis for a functional interaction of valproate with GABAergic synapses have so far mostly been negative. There is no evidence for an interaction of valproate with the GABA recognition site or the benzodiazepine site [42,64]. However, high levels of valproate have been shown to inhibit the binding of ^{3}H-dihydropicrotoxinin ($IC_{50} = 0.5$mM) to its receptor [65]. It has therefore been suggested that valproate might enhance GABAergic inhibitory transmission by acting at the picrotoxinin site and prolonging the open phase of the chloride channels.

Valproate and other cerebral amino acids

Aspartate

The administration of acute doses of valproate (200—400mg/kg, i.p.) leads to significant reductions in cerebral aspartate levels in rats and mice (Table II) [5,9,17,18,25,26]. It has been shown that the time course for the decrease in aspartate concentration correlates with the period of valproate-induced protection against audiogenic seizures in DBA/2 mice [9]. The aspartate decrease also coincides with the increase in brain GABA levels [9]. We have recently shown (Table V) that the decreases observed in aspartate concentrations following valproate administration (400mg/kg i.p., 30 min) are general to all regions studied (cortex, striatum, hippocampus, cerebellum) in contrast to the valproate-induced rise in the GABA level which we only observe in the cortex [17] (Table V).

This consistent decrease in the level of an excitatory amino acid during anticonvulsant treatment with valproate has received relatively little attention. Recently, a new class of excitatory amino acid antagonists (blocking excitation due to aspartate or to N-methyl-D-aspartate) has been shown to have potent anticonvulsant properties [66] but, at present, there is no evidence for an interaction between valproate and an aspartergic transmitter system. The metabolic mechanism for the decrease in aspartate level is also unknown; the possibilities include a direct effect of valproate on enzymes involved in aspartate synthesis (e.g. aspartate transaminase or pyruvate carboxylase), or it could be a consequence of a possible diminished synaptic release of aspartate in the presence of valproate.

Glutamate, glutamine, taurine

The concentrations of the putative neurotransmitters, glutamate, glutamine and taurine, are all increased in most brain regions examined following the chronic

379

TABLE V. Regional amino acid concentrations in control rat brains and following valproate (400mg/kg i.p., 30 min) administration. Data from Chapman et al [17]

	Cortex	Striatum	Hippocampus	Cerebellum
Glutamate				
control	11.37 ± 0.35	10.42 ± 0.30	11.42 ± 0.53	7.86 ± 0.38
valproate	13.01 ± 0.37**	9.37 ± 0.34*	9.63 ± 0.37*	9.17 ± 0.40*
% control	114%	90%	84%	117%
Glutamine				
control	5.94 ± 0.27	6.37 ± 0.29	5.70 ± 0.27	4.49 ± 0.46
valproate	6.79 ± 0.34	6.57 ± 0.36	6.13 ± 0.40	5.39 ± 0.39
% control	114%	103%	108%	120%
Taurine				
control	4.41 ± 0.34	3.33 ± 0.43	4.37 ± 0.48	3.63 ± 0.29
valproate	4.17 ± 0.48	2.81 ± 0.32	4.36 ± 0.44	3.40 ± 0.20
% control	95%	84%	100%	94%
Aspartate				
control	3.42 ± 0.16	2.69 ± 0.22	3.04 ± 0.26	2.26 ± 0.24
valproate	2.69 ± 0.15**	2.34 ± 0.29	2.13 ± 0.13**	1.77 ± 0.16
% control	79%	87%	70%	78%
GABA				
control	1.89 ± 0.10	2.61 ± 0.23	2.30 ± 0.15	1.96 ± 0.19
valproate	2.50 ± 0.15**	2.64 ± 0.16	2.18 ± 0.13	1.78 ± 0.14
% control	132%	101%	95%	91%
Glycine				
control	1.74 ± 0.20	–	–	–
valproate	1.81 ± 0.17	–	–	–
% control	104%	–	–	–
Serine				
control	1.13 ± 0.13	–	–	–
valproate	1.02 ± 0.16	–	–	–
% control	90%	–	–	–

Values are expressed as mean ± SEM, μmoles/g wet wt
Statistically significant differences as evaluated by the Student's t-test are denoted as
*p < 0.05; **p < 0.01

administration of valproate (300mg/kg/day for five or 10 days) [35,36], but no changes are observed in regional taurine or glutamine levels following acute administration of valproate (Table V and Table II).

Whole brain glutamate levels have been reported to be unaffected (2–8% non-significant increases in levels) by acute valproate administration (350–400mg/kg) [18,25,28], which is in general agreement with the mean of our regional glutamate determination (Table V), where cortical and cerebellar glutamate levels are increased 14 per cent and 17 per cent respectively by valproate, and striatal and hippocampal glutamate levels are decreased 10 per cent and 16 per cent. The reason for this regional variation in response to valproate treatment is unclear.

Glycine

Elevated levels of the putative inhibitory transmitter glycine have been demonstrated in serum and urine of rats receiving chronic valproate (rats : 500mg/kg/day for 20 days [49]. Valproate has been shown to inhibit the glycine cleavage system in rat liver both in in-vitro and in-vivo experiments (Table III). The resulting rise in serum glycine is not associated with an increase in glycine levels in rat brain either following acute valproate administration [17,18,25] or after chronic valproate treatment (M Karobath, unpublished results) (Table II).

There have been suggestions that the valproate-induced hyperglycinaemia is linked with impairment of fatty acid oxidation. These arguments have been reviewed recently by Hammond and co-workers [3] and they may be relevant to the cases of liver failure reported during valproate treatment.

Tryptophan

There are large increases in the brain concentrations of tryptophan and of the acidic monoamine metabolite 5-hydroxyindoleacetic acid (5-HIAA) following acute [24,25,38,39] or chronic [38] valproate administration. Valproate displaces tryptophan from serum proteins. This results in an increased serum concentration of free tryptophan and hence an increased cerebral tryptophan uptake with a resulting decrease in total serum tryptophan [25,38].

Horton and co-workers [24] have shown that the anticonvulsant action of valproate is not correlated with monoamine concentrations. They could block the increase in 5-HIAA by use of inhibitors of monoamine synthesis without affecting the protective action of valproate against audiogenic seizures in mice.

Summary

Valproate, when administered acutely in doses (200–400mg/kg i.p.) offering significant protection against most experimentally induced seizures, has a number of effects on cerebral amino acid metabolism.

Valproate enhances cerebral uptake of tryptophan, increasing brain tryptophan concentration and thereby affecting the monoamine metabolism in the brain, but blocking this change does not affect the anticonvulsant action of valproate.

Glycine metabolism is inhibited systemically in the presence of valproate (partially due to the inhibition by valproate of the hepatic glycine cleavage system) leading to increased serum and urine levels of glycine, but apparently without affecting the brain glycine levels.

Brain aspartate concentrations are substantially reduced in several regions following valproate administration, and the change in aspartate level coincides with the protective action of valproate against seizures. The mechanism responsible for these decreases is not known.

Regional brain glutamate concentrations are also somewhat affected by valproate administration, with small increases observed in cortical and cerebellar glutamate levels and small decreases in hippocampal and striatal levels. Again,

381

the mechanism for these changes and for the heterogeneity of regional response remains unclear.

The effect of valproate on the GABA system is well documented. Valproate administration leads to increased GABA levels, at least in the cortex. The time-course for the concentration change correlates generally with the protective action of valproate against seizures, although anticonvulsant effect of valproate has been observed in the absence of an increased brain GABA level. The increased GABA concentration is probably a consequence of a cumulative inhibitory effect by valproate on the two enzymes, GABA-T and SSADH, involved in the oxida-tive metabolism of GABA. In addition, the rate of GABA turnover is reduced in the presence of valproate, as indicated by a reduced rate of ^{14}C-labelling of GABA from glutamate in valproate-treated rats. The reductive conversion of GABA to γ-hydroxybutyrate is also inhibited by valproate, probably through the inhibi-tion of aldehyde reductase by valproate.

Biochemical data alone do not necessarily favour a GABAergic mechanism of action of valproate over one involving for instance aspartate. The commonly accepted working-hypothesis of a GABAergic mechanism of action of valproate is partly reinforced by analogy with the mechanism of action of other anticon-vulsant compounds, and partly by electrophysiological data, since it has been shown that valproate, at least in high concentrations, directly augments the inhibitory activity of GABA.

References

1   Simon D, Penry JK. *Epilepsia 1975; 16:* 549–573
2   Bruni J, Wilder BJ. *Arch Neurol 1979; 36:* 393–398
3   Hammond EJ, Wilder BJ, Bruni J. *Life Sci 1981; 29:* 2561–2579
4   Schobben AFAM. *Stichting Studentenpers Nijmegen 1979*
5   Meldrum B. *Brain Res Bull 1980; 5 Suppl 2:* 579–584
6   Kerwin RW, Taberner PV. *Gen Pharmac 1981; 12:* 71–75
7   Löscher W. *Arch Int Pharmacodyn 1981; 249:* 158–163
8   Kerwin RW, Olpe HR, Schmutz M. *Br J Pharmac 1980; 71:* 545–551
9   Schecter PJ, Tranier Y, Grove J. *J Neurochem 1978; 31:* 1325–1327
10   Lacolle JY, Ferrandes B, Eymard P. In Meinardi H, Rowan AJ, eds. *Advances in Epileptology 1977;* 162–167. Amsterdam: Swets and Zeitlinger
11   Meldrum BS. *Int Rev Neurobiol 1975; 17:* 1–36
12   Haefely W, Polc P, Schaffner R, et al. In Kroggsgaard-Larsen P, Scheel-Krüger J, Kofod H, eds. *GABA-Neurotransmitters 1979;* 357–375. Copenhagen: Munksgaard
13   Olsen RW. *J Neurochem 1981; 37:* 1–13
14   Meldrum BS. In Sandler M, ed. *Psychopharmacology of Anticonvulsants 1982.* Oxford: Oxford University Press
15   Carlsson C, Chapman AG. *Anesthesiology 1981; 54:* 488–495
16   Chapman AG, Nordström C-H, Siesjö BK. *Anesthesiology 1978; 48:* 175–182
17   Chapman AG, Riley K, Evans MC, Meldrum BS. *Neurochem Res 1982;* In press
18   Godin Y, Heiner L, Mark J, Mandel P. *J Neurochem 1969; 16:* 869–873
19   Simler S, Ciesielski L, Maitra M et al. *Biochem Pharmac 1973; 22:* 1701–1708
20   Anlezark G, Horton RW, Meldrum BS, Sawaya MCB. *Biochem Pharmac 1976; 25:* 413–417
21   Ciesielski L, Maitre M, Cash C, Mandel P. *Biochem Pharmacol 1975; 24:* 1055–1058

22   Simler S, Gensburger C, Ciesielski L, Mandel P. *Comp Rend Soc Biol 1976; 170:* 1285–1288

23   Lust WD, Kupferberg HJ, Passonneau JV, Penry JK. In Legg NJ, ed. *Clinical and Pharmacological Aspects of Sodium Valproate (EPILIM) in the Treatment of Epilepsy 1976:* 123–129. Tunbridge Wells: MCS Consultants

24   Horton RW, Anlezark GM, Sawaya MCB, Meldrum BS. *Europ J Pharmacol 1977; 41:* 387–397

25   Kukino K, Deguchi T. *Chem Pharm Bull 1977; 25:* 2257–2262

26   Perry TL, Hansen S. *J Neurochem 1978; 30:* 679–684

27   Simler S, Gensburger C, Ciesielski L, Mandel P. *Commun in Psychopharmacol 1978; 2:* 123–130

28   Cremer JE, Sarna GS, Teal HM, Cunningham VJ. In Fonnum F, ed. *Amino Acids as Transmitters 1978;* 669–689. New York and London: Plenum Press

29   Iadarola MJ, Raines A, Gale K. *J Neurochem 1979; 33:* 1119–1123

30   Gale K, Iadarola MJ. *Science 1980; 208:* 288–291

31   Löscher W. *Biochem Pharmacol 1981; 30:* 1364–1366

32   Wood JD, Kurylo E, Tsui S-K. *J Neurochem 1981; 37:* 1440–1447

33   Bernasconi R, Maitre L, Martin P, Schmutz M. *Abstracts, International Society of Neurochemistry, Eighth Meeting, Nottingham 1981;* 175

34   Emson PC. *J Neurochem 1976; 27:* 1489–1494

35   Williams RJH, Patsalos PN, Lowe R, Lascelles PT. In Royal Society of Medicine International Congress and Symposium No. 30. *The Place of Sodium Valproate in the Treatment of Epilepsy 1980:* 95–101. London: Academic Press and Royal Society of Medicine

36   Patsalos PN, Lascelles PT. *J Neurochem 1981; 36:* 688–695

37   Simler S, Ciesielski L, Klein M, Mandel P. *Neuropharmac 1982; 21:* 133–140

38   Hwang EC, Van Woert MH. *Neuropharmacol 1979; 18:* 391–397

39   MacMillan V. *Can J Physiol Pharmacol 1979; 57:* 843–847

40   Seiler N, Sarhan S. *Prog Clin Biol Res 1980; 39:* 425–439

41   Löscher W, Böhme G, Schäfer H, Kochen W. *Neuropharmac 1981; 20:* 1187–1192

42   Löscher W. *J Neurochem 1980; 34:* 1603–1608

43   Fowler LJ, Beckford J, John RR. *Biochem Pharmacol 1975; 24:* 1267–1270

44   Maitre M, Ossola L, Mandel P. *FEBS Lett 1976; 72:* 53–57

45   Whittle SR, Turner AJ. *J Neurochem 1978; 31:* 1453–1459

46   Van Der Laan JW, De Boer TH, Bruivels J. *J Neurochem 1979; 32:* 1769–1780

47   Harvey PKP, Bradford HF, Davison AN. *FEBS Lett 1975; 52:* 251–254

48   Javors M, Erwin VG. *Biochem Pharmacol 1980; 29:* 1703–1708

49   Mortensen PB, Kølvraa S, Christensen E. *Epilepsia 1980; 21:* 563–569

50   Whittle SR, Turner AJ. *J Neurochem 1982; 38:* 848–851

51   Fonnum F. In Pycock CJ, Taberner PV, eds. *Central Neurotransmitter Turnover 1981;* 105–124. London: Croom Helm, Baltimore: University Park Press

52   Schechter PJ, Tranier Y, Jung MJ, Böhlen P. *Europ J Pharmacol 1977; 45:* 319–328

53   Bernasconi R, Maitre L, Martin P, Raschdorf F. *J Neurochem 1982; 38:* 57–66

54   Bertilsson L, Mao CC, Costa E. *J Pharmacol Exp Ther 1977; 200:* 277–284

55   Patel AJ, Johnson AL, Balázs R. *J Neurochem 1974; 23:* 1271–1279

56   Taberner PV, Charington CB, Unwin JW. *Brain Res Bull 1980; 5: Suppl 2:* 621–625

57   Marcus RJ, Winters WD, Mori K, Spooner CE. *Int J Neuropharmacol 1967; 6:* 175–185

58   Whittle SR, Turner AJ. *Biochem Pharmacol 1981; 30:* 1191–1196

59   Erwin VG, Deitrich RA. *Biochem Pharmacol 1973; 22:* 2615–2624

60   MacDonald RL, Bergey GK. *Brain Res 1979; 170:* 558–562

61   Gent JP, Phillips NI. *Brain Res 1980; 197:* 275–278

62   Baldino F, Geller HM. *J Pharm Exp Ther 1981; 217:* 445–450

63   Olsen RW, Ticku MK, Greenlee P, Ven Ness P. In Krogsgaard-Larsen P, Scheel-Krüger P, Kofod H, eds. *GABA – Neurotransmitters 1979;* 165–178

64   Ross SM, Craig CR. *J Neurochem 1981; 36:* 1006–1011

65   Ticku MK, Davis WC. *Brain Res 1981; 223:* 218–222

66   Croucher MJ, Collins JF, Meldrum BS. *Science 1982;* In press

41

ASPECTS OF THE METHODOLOGY OF CLINICAL ANTICONVULSANT TRIAL DESIGN AND A BIBLIOGRAPHY OF PHENYTOIN AND CARBAMAZEPINE STUDIES

S D Shorvon

Introduction

The poor quality of previous clinical studies of anticonvulsant efficacy was first emphasised by Coatsworth in his NINDS monograph of 1971 [1] in which were demonstrated a variety of omissions in design, execution and reporting. Following this review there have been a few publications concerned with anticonvulsant trial design [2–6], but each has touched only briefly, if at all, on certain important and difficult practical aspects of the problem. The ILAE commission on anti-epileptic drugs [5] laid out general principles for clinical anticonvulsant drug testing in which the division of anticonvulsant trials into three phases was proposed. Phase I comprises clinical studies in 'normal' volunteers. Phase II preliminary clinical studies in patients with epilepsy, and Phase III the definitive clinical studies in populations of patients with epilepsy ('long-term studies of efficacy and safety').

This chapter will deal exclusively with certain specific methodological problems encountered in the design and analysis of Phase III studies. Neither the results of these investigations nor other aspects such as toxicity will be considered and I will concentrate on selected problems, particularly applicable to the study of epilepsy, and not the more general problems of any clinical trial in any area of medicine (eg methods of selection, randomisation, data collection, etc) as these have been well reviewed elsewhere [7,8]. The problems to be considered are:

Numerical and statistical problems:
  Sample size
  Duration of follow-up
  Seizure frequency
  Statistical evaluation
Documentation of prognostic factors

384

The handling of Adjunctive Anticonvulsant Medication:
  Withdrawal
  Addition

Anticonvulsant serum level estimations

Studies of newly diagnosed patients

Compliance with medication.

A survey of the published reports of treatment with phenytoin and carbamazepine

To illustrate this discussion, I have attempted to survey the whole of the English language literature and the most important foreign papers (until January 1980) on the efficacy of phenytoin and carbamazepine, I have included in this review any article in which is given original clinical data showing the results of seizure control of treatment with either drug (Table I). These papers are listed in Appendix I.

One hundred and seventy-one reports were identified, presenting the results of treatment with phenytoin in 67, carbamazepine in 94 and with both drugs in 10. The results of 11 of these studies were presented in more than one report (in one case in four publications) and the analysis that follows is therefore of 155 studies, 65 of phenytoin, 85 of carbamazepine and 5 of both drugs.

TABLE I. Survey of published reports of treatment with phenytoin and carbamazepine

		Phenytoin	Carbamazepine
Number of Studies		77	104
Published:	1938–1949	47	-
	1950–1959	7	-
	1960–1969	6	41
	1970–1979	17	63

(Included all reports in which original clinical data regarding the efficacy of phenytoin and/ or carbamazepine are given)

Numerical and statistical problems

In any comparative anticonvulsant trial, numerical considerations relating to the population size, the duration of follow-up and the measurements of seizure frequency are of crucial importance. These stem from two basic problems. First, that the anticonvulsant drugs are of generally similar efficacy and that any differences noted are likely to be slight. Thus, in the statistically adequate studies

in which phenytoin has been compared with carbamazepine [9—18], with phenobarbitone [9—13, 19—28], with primidone [20,28] and valproate [29], no one
drug was shown to be significantly more efficacious than any other drug. As will
become clear, there are serious methodological problems in these studies which
may well have obscured real difference. Nevertheless, on present evidence at least,
it seems that difference in efficacy may be small. The second problem derives
from the inherent inter- and intra-individual variability of seizure frequency.
Examples of intra-individual variation are given by Turner [30] who showed
that amongst 1000 severe institutionalised cases 5 per cent had remissions of
2 years or more, Annergers et al [31] who found 50 per cent of patients followed
for 20 years since diagnosis to be in terminal remission of at least 5 years and
Rodin [32] who evaluated 71 patients on two occasions and found seizure frequency distributions of less than one attack per year and more than one attack
a week in 10 per cent and 27 per cent respectively on the first evaluation and
42 per cent and 4 per cent on the second. Similarly a marked inter-individual
variation is shown in all population surveys, for instance, Gowers [33] in 1222
cases found 36 per cent of patients suffering from more than one attack a week
and 22 per cent less than one a month, Turner [30] in 316 outpatients, 43 per
cent more than one attack per week and 26 per cent less than one attack a
quarter and Lowry [34] a range of seizures amongst children of 3—36,000 per
year.

Sample size The narrow differences in efficacy of anticonvulsant drugs have
important implications for sample size. In any comparative study, it is possible
to calculate the numbers of patients required to demonstrate a particular difference at any given significant level (p = 0.05 for instance) and at any given probability (power). This is best illustrated by numerical example:
    Let us suppose that we wish to compare the efficacy of new treatment A with
established treatment B in a population of patients on a between patient basis,
and treatment A reduces seizure frequency by 20 per cent more than treatment
B. (This is the order of magnitude of effect claimed in many comparative studies).
i)   If seizure frequencies are normally distributed: If on treatment B the mean
seizure frequency is one attack a month and the seizure frequencies are normally
distributed with a standard deviation of 0.4 attacks a month (i.e. 68 per cent of
the patients will have a seizure frequency between 0.6 and 1.4 a month and 95
per cent between 0.2 and 1.8 a month), to have an 80 per cent chance of observing a difference between the two treatments at a level of significance of 5 per
cent using a t-test, one would need to include 128 patients.
ii)   If the distribution of seizure frequencies is positively skewed: The assumption that seizure frequencies are normally distributed is unlikely to be valid except
in selected groups. If, as is more likely, we assume that the variance is proportional
to the mean and that as an approximation the variance is twice the mean (this

fits best to data personally collected), in the population with a mean seizure frequency of one attack a month on treatment A and 0.8 attacks a month on treatment B, to have an 80 per cent chance of observing a difference at a significance level of 5 per cent one would need to include a total of 158 patients.

iii)   Non-parametric test: To avoid any assumption at all about the distribution of seizure frequencies in the population one could observe changes in the proportion of patients with a seizure frequency above a certain figure on the two treatments. In our 'typical' population therefore we could see 50 per cent of the patients on treatment B and 30 per cent of the patients on treatment A with a seizure frequency above one a month. Using the binomial test it is estimated that to have an 80 per cent chance of observing a difference at a significance level of 5 per cent one would need to include a total of 186 patients.

Duration of follow-up and seizure frequency It was assumed that the units of measurement of drug efficacy are easily formulated. This is, unfortunately, not the case, and there are methodological difficulties which stem from the inherent variability in the occurrence of seizures. Efficacy can be assessed using a continuous variable such as seizure frequency or non-continuous variables such as the number of patients rendered seizure free, the number with a 50 per cent reduction in attacks and so on but, whichever is used, the duration of follow-up is of crucial importance.

Let us consider the measurement of seizure frequency: If seizures occurred absolutely regularly, then seizure frequency could be calculated after only two attacks, but of course this is rarely the case. One is therefore faced with the problem of trying to decide after how many attacks can a fair estimate of seizure frequency be made. Clearly the longer the period and the more frequent the attacks the more accurate the assessment becomes, but what can be taken as an acceptable minimum? As there are no published data quantifying 'natural' variations in the occurrence of seizures any attempt at mathematical analysis is necessarily arbitrary.

To illustrate this take the following examples: In a study set up to estimate seizure frequency, it was decided that five attacks per patient should be observed . In the population described above (example ii) in which the mean seizure frequency is one attack a month and the seizure frequencies distribution is positively skewed to observe five attacks in 75 per cent of the patients the group would have to be followed for 8 months. If the mean seizure frequency is one attack every three months, with the same distribution, the length of follow-up is prolonged to 25 months. It might be concluded therefore that the more frequent the seizures the more suitable the patients, but, as is common clinical experience, patients with very frequent seizures are often intractable to any treatment (almost by definition), and this group will therefore be unsuitable for many types of study. A compromise must be made but, in the absence of clear guidance from the literature, this must be decided on empirical grounds. Similar problems arise using measures other than seizure frequency (number of patients seizure free, number of patients with a 50 per cent reduction in attacks and so on), and the essential point to make is that in the design of all anticonvulsant studies, the duration of follow-up and the severity of the epilepsy are interrelated factors which require the most careful consideration, and upon which the validity and the success of the investigation will often heavily depend.

One hundred and fifty-five studies of phenytoin and carbamazepine treatment:

On reviewing the 155 reports it becomes immediately apparent that these numerical difficulties have often been overlooked. Sample size is shown in Table II. As can be seen approximately one-third of the studies were of 30 patients or less and only 15 per cent were of more than 100 patients. The duration of follow-up was often inadequate as shown in Table III. It was not mentioned at all in 28 per cent of the studies (21% of the phenytoin and 31% of the carbamazepine reports), and in those studies in which this information was available it took various forms. The documentation of seizure frequency is shown in Table IV. In 56 per cent of the 155 studies no seizure frequencies or numbers were reported, (and when given were often incomplete). Moreover, in within patient studies in which the treatment phase was compared with some previous period (81 reports) the seizure frequency or number of this earlier phase was given in only 46 per cent.

TABLE II. 155 studies: sample size

No of Patients	Phenytoin (n=70)		Carbamazepine (n=90)		Total (n-155)	
	n	%	n	%	n	%
Less than 30	24	34	29	32	49	32
30–59	22	31	35	39	56	36
60–99	12	17	14	16	26	17
100 or more	12	17	12	13	24	15

Statistical evaluation As the documentation of much of the essential numerical data has been so poor it is not surprising to find that few of the 155 reports received adequate statistical evaluation. In only 16 (10%) of the patients (10% of both the phenytoin and carbamazepine reports) were statistical methods, other than the simple calculation of percentage change (or its equivalent), employed. These consisted of:

i)   Non parametric tests (Fisher's exact probability, Wilcoxon, Spearman Rank Correlation) in 7 cases, and in general, these were correctly applied and carried out (although the null hypothesis was seldom specified).

ii)   Student t-test was used in 3 studies and in each case its use was of doubtful

TABLE III. 155 studies: the duration of follow-up on phenytoin or carbamazepine

Duration of follow-up	Phenytoin (n=70)	Carbamazepine (n=90)		Total (n=155)
Not specified	15 (21%)	28	(31%)	43 (28%)
Fixed period[1]	10 (14%)	14	(16%)	21 (14%)
Mean + Range[2]	9 (13%)	10	(11%)	17 (11%)
Range only	27 (39%)	20	(22%)	47 (30%)
Mean only	4 (6%)	7	(8%)	11 (7%)
Other[3]	5 (7%)	11	(12%)	16 (11%)

1 Fixed period: Same for each subject
2 Mean + Range: Included here are reports in which the duration of follow-up for each individual subject is specified
3 For example group frequency distribution

TABLE IV. 155 studies: seizure number, frequency and duration

Documentation/ Details given of*	Phenytoin	Carbamazepine	Total
1 Test treatment phase- Seizure frequency/	(n=70)	(n=90)	(n=155)
Number	46%	40%	44%
2 Pre-treatment phase** Seizure frequency/	(n=41)	(n=46)	(n=81)
Number	56%	41%	46%
Duration	41%	33%	33%

*Any information, however sketchy or incomplete, is included
** Pre-treatment phase: In within patient and cross over studies, the period with which the test treatment is compared

value as the data (seizure frequency and number measured) were not shown to be normal and the variance in each treatment group to be similar.
iii)   Other methods of the analysis of variance (latin square designs etc) were used in 6 studies and again their application was often misconceived.

Finally, there was no indication that the 'power' of the statistical analysis (which depends on sample size, duration of follow-up and seizure frequency) was considered in more than a handful of these studies.

389

Anticonvulsant drug action is not equal in all types of epilepsy or in every patient population. There are a number of factors of known or imputed influence on response to treatment. I say imputed influence for there is considerable disagreement about the importance of many of these which makes both the construction and analysis of controlled studies difficult. Again there has been little attention paid to this in previously published reports. In Tables V and VI are shown 9 such factors and the proportion of studies in which these were documented or correlated with the results of treatment.

The problem is further compounded by the fact that documentation may itself be difficult because of problems of definition and measurement.

TABLE V. 155 studies: the proportion in which there was a failure to document or specify prognostic factors

Factors	Phenytoin Studies (n=70)		Carbamazepine Studies (n=90)		Total (n=155)	
	n	%	n	%	n	%
Aetiology of epilepsy	57	81%	71	79%	123	79%
Seizure type	31	44%	8	9%	36	23%
Seizure frequency	44	63%	60	67%	102	66%
Age of onset	67	96%	84	93%	146	94%
Duration of seizures	43	61%	60	67%	100	65%
Age of the patient	35	50%	24	26%	55	35%
Sex of the patient	51	73%	37	41%	85	55%
Additional handicaps	47	67%	66	73%	110	71%
Setting	23	33%	48	53%	68	44%

The influence of aetiology on the responses to treatment can be taken as an example. The literature is almost equally divided between those authors who find idiopathic epilepsy to have a better prognosis than symptomatic epilepsy [33, 35—43] and those who find the prognosis to be similar [30, 31, 44—49]. Such divergence of opinion arises partly from the fact that the designation of 'aetiology' depends on various factors which are often not explicitly stated. The extent of investigation is obviously important here since, the more refined or extensive the investigation, the higher is the yield of aetiological factors. Angeleri et al [50], for instance, found a structural lesion in 72% of cases of partial epilepsy investigated by CT scanning and this included many cases previously diagnosed as 'idiopathic', and similar findings were noted by others [51—54]. The incorporation of EEG data into diagnostic categories, as recommended by the

TABLE VI. 155 studies: the proportion in which attempts were made to correlate prognostic factors with the results of treatment

Factor	Phenytoin Studies (n=70)		Carbamazepine Studies (n=90)		Total (n=155)	
	n	%	n	%	n	%
Aetiology of epilepsy	0	0%	1	1%	1	1%
Seizure type*	29	41%	66	73%	92	59%
Seizure frequency	2	3%	3	2%	3	2%
Age of onset	0	0%	2	2%	2	1%
Duration of seizures	0	0%	1	1%	1	1%
Age of the patient	0	0%	3	3%	3	2%
Sex of the patient	1	1%	1	1%	2	1%
Additional handicaps	0	0%	1	1%	1	1%

*Less than 10% specified according to the International Classification (Gastaut, 1969). The problem of poor definition of seizure type is dealt with in the text

(Setting is not considered as in no trial were patients in two settings directly compared)

Committee of the International League against Epilepsy [55] in their deliberations concerning classification, similarly alters the aetiological perspective. A further complication is that the production of epilepsy depends on an interplay of environmental and constitutional factors. It is well recognised, for instance, that patients with a family history of epilepsy are more likely to develop seizures after head injury than those with no such predisposition [56]. In view of this, when can we accept a factor as 'causative'? When, for instance, does a history of birth asphyxia or of minor head injury become significant or when is it to be ignored? If different studies use different criteria then different conclusions may well be reached.

Similar difficulties are experienced in the documentation, definition and measurement of other prognostic factors and, as shown in Table V, these have been largely overlooked in previous reports. The problem is further complicated by the interrelation of factors (eg age and duration of epilepsy) and by the varying importance of individual factors in different circumstances.

The handling of adjunctive anticonvulsant medication

In most reports of anticonvulsant efficacy the test drug has been added to previously established anticonvulsant medication, and this may itself produce serious methodological complications. Having introduced the test drug, the previous regime can be either withdrawn or maintained at a fixed or variable dose and each of these alternatives is attended by specific problems (Table VII).

391

TABLE VII. 155 reports: design problems

	Phenytoin (n = 70)		Carbamazepine (n = 90)		Total (n = 155)	
	n	%	n	%	n	%
Adjunctive Medication:						
Withdrawn[1]	25	36%	13	14%	33	21%
Maintained[2]	34	49%	62	69%	95	61%
Test drug monotherapy	19	27%	11	12%	26	27%
Serum levels specified	16	23%	19	21%	30	19%
Previously untreated patients[3]	1	1%	0	0%	1	1%

1 Withdrawal of some or all of adjunctive medication. In other reports withdrawal may have occurred but this was not specified
2 Maintenance of adjunctive medication at a dosage which was either variable or not stated
3 Studies wholly of newly diagnosed and previously untreated patients

Additional medication withdrawn Withdrawal of medication can affect seizure frequency in several ways. First, there is a risk of precipitating 'withdrawal seizures' (in spite of the fact that in the absence of any features differentiating withdrawal seizures from 'ordinary' attacks it is difficult accurately to assess this risk) but, in view of this, most authors advise a gradual withdrawal, although the time recommended is very variable [43, 46, 57—59]. Second, it appears that, in some patients, multiple drug therapy may actually perpetuate seizures and that the reduction of therapy may for this reason alone reduce the seizure frequency. In a study of 40 patients, followed for two years, in whom reduction of therapy from two or three drugs to single drug treatment was achieved, 55 per cent experienced a decrease in seizure frequency on single drug therapy [60]. Similar results were found in the studies of the Milano Collaborative Group [61] who reduced the drug intake of institutionalised patients from 2.5 to 2 drugs and observed a 50 per cent reduction in seizure frequency. Thirty-three (21%) of the 155 reports reviewed included patients whose previous medication was definitely withdrawn, but in none of these reports were those problems considered. (It is, moreover, probable that in a number of other studies anticonvulsant withdrawal occurred but the documentation is too brief to be certain).

Additional medication maintained at a fixed dose In studies in which the established medication is continued, the assumption is made that the addition of the drug can confer additional anticonvulsant action. Surprisingly, there is little evidence to support this and indeed it seems more likely that in the majority of cases a single drug used optimally is just as effective (or ineffective) as a combination of drugs, and this is particularly so since the advent of serum level monitoring which has allowed the individual drugs to be used in a more rational fashion [62]. There have, in fact, been only a small number of studies which have been specifically designed to compare single drug with combination therapy. It is widely held, for instance, that there is a synergism between the actions of phenytoin and phenobarbitone but, in spite of this, there appear to be only four studies [63–66] in which this proposition has been specifically tested, and in only one of these was combination therapy clearly superior. There is a single experimental study in which phenytoin was administered to animals already on effective doses of tridione, phenobarbitone or mesantoin and tested against metrazol-induced seizures; the combination therapy provided no extra protection against these seizures than was afforded by the single drug [67]. A final point to make is that even if the previous medication is continued at an unchanged dosage, the introduction of a new anticonvulsant may well alter the serum levels and this effect is unpredictable [68, 69]. If the test drug is to be accurately assessed in this situation, therefore, the serum level of the other anticonvulsants should be monitored and the dose manipulated to provide steady levels. This is, in practice, extremely difficult and it is not surprising that it was stated to have been achieved in only one of the 155 reports.

Additional medication maintained at a varying dose If the dose (or serum level) of the concomitant medication is not carefully stabilised then controlled assessment of the test drug is impossible. It is surprising to note that in 95 (61%) of the 155 studies the handling of the adjunctive medication was either variable (and depending, for instance, on response to treatment) or simply not documented.

Monotherapy As I hope will have become by now clear, it is highly desirable in most situations to assess the efficacy of a test drug with that drug used alone. It is indeed remarkable to see how often a test drug is added to a previous regime, often of several drugs and often varying from patient to patient, and it is doubtful whether an accurate assessment of anticonvulsant efficacy or a comparison between drugs can be made in this situation.

In only 26 (17%) of the studies reviewed were all the patients taking the test drug alone (27% of the phenytoin and 13% of the carbamazepine studies), and they were usually of small numbers of patients followed for short periods of time (Table VIII). In a further 40 (26%) studies there were some patients on monotherapy although this proportion was usually small and in only a few cases were the results analysed separately for this group.

Anticonvulsant serum level estimations

The ability to measure the concentration of anticonvulsant drugs in plasma has been of major importance to the more rational and efficient prescribing of these

393

TABLE VIII. 155 studies: reports of patients on monotherapy

Number of Patients			Duration of follow up (Months)		
	n	%		n	%
1–29	14	54	Not stated	4	15
30–59	10	38	1–6	11	42
60–99	2	8	7–12	6	23
Over 100	0	0	Over 12	2	8
			Variable	3	12

drugs [68–70]. With this increasing pharmacokinetic understanding, there has developed the view that there is an 'optimum range' of anticonvulsant serum levels, at which the anticonvulsant actions of the various drugs are at their maximum. Although there are important qualifications to the acceptance of this view [69, 71], there is general agreement that the response to treatment is related, even if loosely, to serum levels for most anticonvulsant drugs in most patients. In all comparative clinical trials, therefore, serum anticonvulsant measurements should be utilised for several reasons. First, it is important to ensure that the drugs are being compared and tested on 'equal terms'. Second, at least in some patients, a higher serum level of a drug will succeed in controlling attacks where a lower level has failed and the measurement of the seizure frequency therefore should always be qualified by a serum level. Third, the measurement of serum levels is the most effective way of checking on (and improving!) compliance and avoiding toxicity. Finally, as pointed out by Richens [6], in any research study, the correlation between serum level and effect (therapeutic or toxic) of any drug is 'sound evidence that the effect is really due to the drug'. The analysis of the results of clinical trials utilising serum level estimations is of course more complicated than of those with no such measurements. The same problems of control, selection, comparison of varying durations of follow up and so on which are so difficult to deal with in the comparison of different drugs apply just as tightly to the use of the same drug at different serum levels, and it is striking to find how few statistically satisfactory within or between patient analyses have been made utilising serum level measurements.

Of the 155 reports, serum levels were measured in only 19 per cent and in only 2 of these was the protocol for adjusting dose according to levels given. The serum levels were related to the results of treatment in 10 per cent of the reports, but in almost none of these reports were the serum levels manipulated in a controlled or independent fashion, and their statistical validity is doubtful.

Studies of newly diagnosed and previously untreated patients

As will have become clear from much of the above, the great majority of anticonvulsant trials have taken place amongst chronic (often intractable!) epileptics, who have almost invariably received other anticonvulsant drugs. An alternative, which has received surprisingly little attention, is to study newly diagnosed and previously untreated patients. There are obvious and attractive advantages to this: there are no pharmacological complications (withdrawal, addition, carry over effects or drug interaction for instance); the patients can receive sophisticated pre-treatment assessment and documentation; the clinical, electrophysiological and biochemical data can be prospectively monitored before and during treatment; patient compliance is probably better. It should be recognised however that the response to treatment in this group may not be applicable to other categories of patients (this is true for any selected population) and, indeed, it has been claimed the prognosis for seizure control is better amongst new than more chronic cases [30, 32, 33, 35, 48, 49, 58].

Twenty-one (14%) of the 155 trials (10% of the phenytoin and 16% of the carbamazepine studies) included some data on previously untreated patients, although only a single (and eccentric) study was exclusively of such patients.

Compliance with medication

One of the results of the introduction of serum anticonvulsant level measurements has been the realisation that a significant proportion of patients on chronic anticonvulsant medication are failing to take these drugs regularly. This was first pointed out by Buchthal et al [72], who estimated that 50 per cent of ambulant patients complied poorly, and first systematically investigated by Lund et al [73] who found a poor compliance rate of 66 per cent in ambulatory patients and Kutt et al [74] who similarly found a poor compliance rate of 75 per cent in a group of 'refractory' patients. More recently, Sherwin et al [75] found a non-compliance rate of about 38 per cent in 70 young patients with absence seizures, Wannamaker et al [76] a rate of 37 per cent in 30 regular outpatients in South Carolina and Gibberd et al [77] a rate of 42 per cent in a prospective outpatient study in London, and similar findings have been found by others [78–81]. When compliance was improved there was an improvement in seizure control in every study in which this was measured. It seems probable that irregular tablet taking is a leading cause of poor seizure control at least in the outpatient clinics and this is clearly important in the analysis of longitudinal anticonvulsant trials.

Patient compliance can probably be improved in a number of ways. The introduction of serum level monitoring itself is probably important in this respect [75, 80, 82, 83]. Increasing the frequency of clinic visits has also been shown to improve compliance [76, 77, 84] and other methods include the simplification of the medication regime and repeated education and explanation [73, 85]. Of the 155 reports of phenytoin and carbamazepine treatment the problems of compliance were directly discussed in only two studies, serum levels were measured in only 22 per cent of the studies, and the frequency of clinic visits was reported in only 9 per cent of the reports.

Acknowledgments

I would like to thank Dr EH Reynolds for his helpful advice and Dr AJ Johnson for statistical assistance in the preparation of this chapter.

References

1   Coatsworth J. *NINDS monograph No 12*. Washington DC: US Government Printing Office
2   Cereghino J, Penry J. In Woodbury D, Penry, J, Schmidt R, eds. *Anti-epileptic Drugs 1972;* 63–73. New York: Raven Press
3   Coatsworth J, Penry J. In Woodbury D, Penry J, Schmidt R, eds. *Antiepileptic Drugs 1972;* 87–95. New York: Raven Press
4   Millichap J. In Woodbury D, Penry J, Schmidt R, eds. *Antiepileptic Drugs 1972;* 75–80. New York: Raven Press
5   International League Against Epilepsy: Commission on Antiepileptic Drugs. *Epilepsia 1973; 14:* 451–458
6   Richens A. In Laidlaw J, Richens A, eds. *Textbook of Epilepsy 1976;* 185–247. Edinburgh, London and New York: Churchill Livingstone
7   Hill A. *Controlled Clinical Trials 1960*. Oxford: Blackwell
8   Hill A. *Principles of Medical Statistics 1966*. London: Lancet
9   Benassi E, Loeb C, Besio G, Tanganelli P. In Johannessen S, Morselli P, Pippenger C et al, eds. *Anti-epileptic Therapy: Advances on Drug Monitoring 1980;* 195–200. New York: Raven Press
10   Cereghino J, Brock J, Van Meter J et al. *Neurology 1974; 24:* 401–410
11   Cereghino J, Brock J, Van Meter J et al. *Clin Pharmac Ther 1975; 18:* 733–741
12   Cereghino J, Van Meter J, Brock J. *Neurology 1972; 22:* 409
13   Cereghino J, Van Meter J, Brock J et al. *Neurology 1973; 23:* 357–366
14   Simonsen N, Olsen P, Kuhl V et al. *Acta Neurol Scand 1975; Suppl 60:* 39–42
15   Simonsen N, Olsen P, Kuhl V et al. *Epilepsia 1975; 17:* 169–178
16   Troupin A, Green J, Halpern L. *Acta Neurol Scand 1975; Suppl 60:* 13–26
17   Troupin A, Green J, Levy R. *Neurology 1974; 24:* 863–869
18   Troupin A, Ojemann L, Halpern L et al. *Neurology 1977; 27:* 511–519
19   Cohen B, Showstack N, Myerson A. *J Am Med Ass 1940; 114:* 480–484
20   Gruber C, Brock J, Dyken M, Gibson M. *Clin Pharmac Ther 1962; 3:* 23–28
21   Gruber C, Mosier J, Grant P, Glen R. *Neurology 1956; 6:* 640–645
22   McLendon S. *Sth Med J (Nashville) 1943; 36:* 303–306
23   Merritt H, Putnam T. *Am J Psychiat 1940; 96:* 1023–1027
24   Robinson L, Osgood R. *J Am Med Ass 1940; 114:* 1334–1337
25   Ruskin D. *Am J Psychiat 1950; 107:* 415–421
26   Thorne F. *Am J Psychiat 1948; 104:* 570–574
27   Tullidge G, Tylor Fox. *Lancet 1942; ii:* 6–9
28   White P, Plott D, Norton J. *Arch Neurol (Chicago) 1966; 14:* 31–35
29   Shakir R, Johnson R, Lambie D et al. *Epilepsia 1981; 22:* 27–33
30   Turner W. *Epilepsy – A Study of the Idiopathic Disease 1907*. London: Macmillan
31   Annegers J, Hauser W, Elveback L. *Epilepsia 1979; 20:* 729–737

32   Rodin EA. *The Prognosis of Patients with Epilepsy 1968.* Springfield: Charles Thomas
33   Gowers W. *Epilepsy and Other Chronic Convulsive Disease: Their Causes, Symptoms and Treatment 1881.* London: Churchill
34   Lowry E. *Jl Lancet 1941; 61:* 178–180
35   Haabermas S. *Allg ZF Psychiat 1901; 58:* 243–253
36   Alstroem C. *A Study of Epilepsy in its Clinical Social and Genetic Aspects 1950.* Copenhagen: Munksgaard
37   Livingston S. *The Diagnosis and Treatment of Convulsive Disorders in Children 1954.* Springfield: Thomas
38   Strobos R. *Arch Neurol (Chicago) 1959; 1:* 216–221
39   Lennox W. *Epilepsy and Related Disorders 1960.* Boston: Little
40   Fukuyama Y, Arima M, Nagahata M, Okada R. *Epilepsia 1963; 4:* 207–224
41   Juul-Jensen P. *Epilepsy: A Clinical and Social Analysis of 1020 Adult Patients with Epileptic Seizures 1963.* Copenhagen: Munksgaard
42   Gudmundsson G. *Acta Neurol Scand 1964; Suppl 25;* 91–99
43   Oller-Daurella L, Marquez J. *Epilepsia 1972; 13:* 161–170
44   Kirstein L. *Acta Med Scand 1942; 112:* 515–523
45   Arieff A. *Dis Nerv Syst 1951; 12:* 19–22
46   Yahr M, Sciarra D, Carter S, Merritt H. *J Am Med Ass 1952; 150:* 663–667
47   Putnam R, Rothenberg S. *J Am Med Ass 1953; 152:* 1400–1406
48   Kiorboe E. *Acta Psychiat Scand 1961; 36 Suppl 150:* 166–178
49   Trolle E. *Acta Psychiat Scand 1961; 36 Suppl 150:* 187–199
50   Angeleri F, Provinciali L, Salvolini U. In Canger R, Angeleri F, Penry J, eds. *Advances in Epileptology. The XIth Epilepsy International Symposium 1980;* 53–64. New York: Raven Press
51   Gastaut H, Gastaut J-L. In Penry J, ed. *Epilepsy. The VIIIth International Symposium 1977;* 5–15. New York: Raven Press
52   Gawler J, Bull J, Du Boulay G, Marshall J. *Lancet 1974; ii:* 419
53   Cala L, Mastaglia F, Woodings T. *Proc Aust Ass Neurol 1977; 14:* 237–244
54   Yang P, Berger P, Cohen M, Duffner P. *Neurology 1979; 29:* 1084–1088
55   Gastaut H. *Epilepsia 1969; 10 Suppl 2:* 1–28
56   Caveness W. In Vinken P, Bruyn G, eds. *The Epilepsies Vol XV. Handbook of Neurology 1974;* 274–294. Amsterdam: North Holland Publishing Co
57   Juul-Jensen P. *Epilepsia 1964; 5:* 352–363
58   Holowach J, Thurston D, O'Leary J. *N Engl J Med 1972; 286:* 169–174
59   Rodin E, John G. In Wada J, Penry J, eds. *Advances in Epileptology. The Xth Epilepsy International Symposium 1980;* 183–186. New York: Raven Press
60   Shorvon S, Reynolds E. *Br Med J 1979; 2:* 1023–1025
61   Advancini G, Baruzzi A, Bordo B et al. In Gardner-Thorpe C, Janz D, Meinardi H, Pippenger C, eds. *Anti-epileptic Drug Monitoring 1976;* 197–213. Tunbridge Wells: Pitman Medical
62   Reynolds E, Shorvon S. *Epilepsia 1981; 22:* 1–10
63   Pratt C. *J Ment Sci 1939; 85:* 986–998
64   Cohen B, Shoestack N, Myerson A. *J Am Med Ass 1940; 114:* 480–484
65   Merritt H, Brenner C. *J Nerv Ment Dis 1942; 96:* 245–250
66   Blair D. *Br Med J 1942; 2:* 171–174
67   Weaver L, Swinyard C, Goodman L. *J Am Pharm Ass 1958; 47:* 645–648
68   Eadie M, Tyrer J. *Anticonvulsant Therapy 1980 2nd Edn.* Edinburgh, London and New York: Churchill Livingstone
69   Laidlaw J, Richens A. *A Textbook of Epilepsy 1982 2nd Edn.* Edinburgh, London and New York: Churchill Livingstone
70   Woodbury D, Penry J, Schmidt R. *Antiepileptic Drugs 1972.* New York: Raven Press
71   Reynolds E. *Pharmac Ther 1981; 8:* 217–235
72   Buchthal F, Svensmark O, Schiller P. *Arch Neurol (Chicago) 1960; 2:* 624–630
73   Lund M, Jorgensen R, Kuhl V. *Epilepsia 1964; 5:* 51–58
74   Kutt H, Haynes J, McDowell F. *Arch Neurol (Chicago) 1966; 14:* 489–492
75   Sherwin A, Robb J, Lechter M. *Arch Neurol (Chicago) 1973; 28:* 178–181

76   Wannamaker B, Morton W, Gross A, Saunders S. *Epilepsia 1980; 21:* 155–162
77   Gibberd F, Dunne J, Handley A, Hazelman B. *Br Med J 1970; 1:* 147–149
78   Haerer A, Grace J. *Acta Neurol Scand 1969; 45:* 18–31
79   Gardner Thorpe C, Parsonage M, Smethurst P, Toothill C. *Acta Neurol Scand 1972; 48:* 213–221
80   Booker H. In Woodbury D, Penry J, Schmidt R, eds. *Antiepileptic Drugs 1972;* 329–334. New York: Raven Press
81   Blackwell B. *N Engl J Med 1973; 289:* 249–252
82   Dawson K, Jamieson A. *Arch Dis Childh 1971; 46:* 386–388
83   Kutt H, Penry J. *Arch Neurol (Chicago) 1974; 31:* 283–288
84   Lund L. *Arch Neurol 1974; 31:* 289–294
85   Sackett D, Haynes R. *Compliance with Therapeutic Regimes 1976.* Baltimore: Johns Hopkins Press

Appendix 1: Bibliography of Studies of Phenytoin and Carbamazepine Efficacy (to January 1980)

Phenytoin treatment

Black N. *Psychiat Q 1939; 13:* 711–720
Blair D. *J Ment Sci 1940; 86:* 888–927
Blair D. *Br Med J 1942; 2:* 171–174
Blair D, Bailey K, McGregor J. *Lancet 1939; ii:* 363–367
Bonafede V, Nathan R. *Psychiat Q 1940; 14:* 603–611
Borofsky L, Louis S, Kutt H, Roginsky M. *Pediat Pharmac Ther 1972; 81:* 995–1002
Bray P. *Pediatrics 1959; 23:* 151–161
Buchanan R, Allen R. *Neurology 1971; 21:* 866–871
Buchthal F, Svensmark Q, Schiller P. *Arch Neurol Psychiat (Chicago) 1960; 2:* 624–632
Burrows R. *J Ment Sci 1947; 93:* 778–784
Butter A. *J Neurol Neurosurg Psychiat 1945; 8:* 49–51
Cohen B, Showstack N, Myerson A. *J Am Med Ass 1940; 114:* 480–484
Coope R. *Lancet 1939; i:* 180–181
Coope R, Burrows R. *Lancet 1940; i:* 490–492
Davidson D, Berman B. *J Am Med Ass 1956; 160:* 766–769
Davidson S, Sutherland J. *Br Med J 1939; 11:* 720–721
Dawson K, Jamieson A. *Arch Dis Childh 1971; 46:* 386–388
Dickerson W. *Am J Psychiat 1942; 93:* 515–523
Doltolo J, Bennett C. *Psychiat Q 1940; 14:* 595–602
Feely M, Duggan B, O'Callaghan M, Callaghan N. *Ir J Med Sci 1979; 148:* 44–49
Fetterman J. *J Am Med Ass 1940; 114:* 396–400
Fetterman J, Shallenberger W. *Dis Nerv Syst 1941; 2:* 383–389
Foster F. *J Am Med Ass 1951; 145:* 211–215
Frankel S. *J Am Med Ass 1940; 114:* 1320–1321
Frost I. *J Ment Sci 1939; 85:* 976–981
Gardner W. *Med Bull Veterans' Adm 1941; 17:* 372–375
Gruber C, Brock M, Dyken M, Gibson M. *Clin Pharmac Ther 1962; 3:* 23–28
Gruber C, Mosier J, Grant P, Glen R. *Neurology 1956; 6:* 640–645
Hawke W. *Canad Med Ass J 1940; 43:* 157–159
Hawke W. *Canad Med Ass J 1941; 45:* 234–236
Hodgeson E, Reese H. *Wisconsin Med J 1939; 38:* 968–971
Ives E. *J Am Med Ass 1951; 147:* 1332–1335
Johnson H. *Psychiat Q 1940; 14:* 612–618
Keith H. *Jl Lancet 1947; 67:* 449–450
Keith H. *Am J Dis Child 1947; 74:* 140–146
Kimball O. *J Am Med Ass 1939; 112; ii:* 1244–1249

Kimball O, Horan T. *Ann Intern Med 1939; 13:* 787–793
Laws J. *Br Med J 1939; 2:* 725–726
Lowry E. *Jl Lancet 1941; 61:* 178–180
Lund L. *Arch Neurol (Chicago) 1974; 31:* 289–294
McCartan W, Carson J. *J Ment Sci 1939; 85:* 965–970
McLendon S. *Sth Med J (Nashville) 1943; 36:* 303–306
Marburg O, Helford M. *J Nerv Ment Dis 1946; 104:* 465–473
Merritt H, Brenner C. *J Nerv Ment Dis 1942; 96:* 245–250
Merritt H, Putnam T. *J Am Med Ass 1938; 111:* 1068–1073
Merritt H, Putnam T. *Am J Psychiat 1940; 96:* 1023–1027
Millichap J, Ortez W. *Neurology 1967; 17:* 162–165
Petersen J, Keigh H. *Canad Med Ass J 1940; 43:* 248–250
Pratt C. *J Ment Sci 1939; 85:* 986–998
Prudhomme C. *Med Bull Veterans' Adm 1941; 18:* 148–152
Robinson L. *Am J Psychiat 1942; 99:* 231–237
Robinson L, Osgood R. *J Am Med Ass 1940; 114:* 1334–1337
Ross A, Jackson V. *Ann Intern Med 1940; 14:* 770–774
Ruskin D. *Am J Psychiat 1950; 107:* 415–421
Schmidt D. In Johannessen S, Morselli P, Pippenger E et al, eds. *Anti-epileptic Therapy: Advances in drug Monitoring 1980;* 221–228. New York: Raven Press
Schmidt D. *Proceedings of XIth Epilepsy International Symposium 1980.* To be published
Shakir R, Johnson R, Lambie D et al. *Epilepsia 1981; 22:* 27–33
Steel J, Smith E. *Lancet 1939; ii:* 367–369
Thorne F. *Am J Psychiat 1948; 104:* 570–574
Tullidge G, Tylor Fox. *Lancet 1942; ii:* 6–9
Viukari N. *J Ment Defic Res 1969; 13:* 212–218
Weaver O, Harrell D, Arnold G. *Va Med Mon 1939; 66:* 522–527
Weinberg J, Goldstein W. *Am J Psychiat 1940; 96:* 1029–1034
White P, Plott D, Norton J. *Arch Neurol (Chicago) 1966; 14:* 31–35
Williams D. *Lancet 1939; ii:* 678–681
Yahr M, Sciarra D, Carter S, Merritt H. *J Am Med Ass 1952; 150:* 663–667
Ying-K'un F, Ying-Kuei H. *Chin Med J 1941; 59:* 508–525

Both phenytoin and carbamazepine treatment

Benassi E, Loeb C, Besio G, Tanganelli P. In Johannessen S, Morselli P, Pippenger C et al, eds. *Anti-epileptic Therapy: Advances on Drug Monitoring 1980;* 195–200. New York: Raven Press
Cereghino J, Brock J, Van Meter J et al. *Neurology 1974; 24:* 401–410
Cereghino J, Brock J, Van Meter J et al. *Clin Pharmac Ther 1975; 18:* 733–741
Cereghino J, Van Meter J, Brock J, Penry J. *Neurology 1972; 22:* 409
Cereghino J, Van Meter J, Brock J et al. *Neurology 1973; 23:* 357–366
Simonsen N, Olsen P, Kuhl V et al. *Acta Neurol Scand 1975; Suppl 60:* 39–42
Simonsen N, Olsen P, Kuhl V et al. *Epilepsia 1975; 17:* 169–178
Troupin A, Green J, Halpern L. *Acta Neurol Scand 1975; Suppl 60:* 13–26
Troupin A, Green J, Levy R. *Neurology 1974; 24:* 863–869
Troupin A, Ojemann L, Halpern L et al. *Neurology 1977; 27:* 511–519

Carbamazepine treatment

Aquilar-Quiro F. *Tegetol en la Epilepsia Temporal 1967.* Barcelona: Librode Becas Geigy
Arieff A, Mier M. *Neurology 1966; 16:* 107–110
Armbrust-Figueinedo J. *Archos Neuro Psiquiat (S Paulo) 1968; 26:* 223–228
Barot M. In Roberts F, ed. *Tegretol in Epilepsy 1977;* 50–54. Macclesfield: Geigy

399

Bird C, Griffin J, Miklaszewska J, Galbraith A. *Br J Psychiat 1966; 112:* 737–742

Blomberg L, Buren A, Dahlqvist L. *Lakartidningen 1970; 67:* 4305–4311

Bonduelle M. In Wink C, ed. *Tegretol in Epilepsy 1972;* 80–88. Manchester: Nicholls

Bonduelle M, Bourgues P, Sallou C, Chemaly R. In Bradley P, Flugel F, Hoch P, eds. *Proceedings of the IIIrd Meeting of the Collegium Internationale Neuro-Psycho-pharmacologium 1964;* 312–316. Amsterdam: Elsevier

Bonduelle M, Bourgues P, Sallou C, Chemaly R. *Electroenceph Clin Neurophysiol 1964: 17:* 716–723

Boucaud P, La Roche R, Brison J. *Progres Med 1966; 94:* 255–259

Callaghan N, O'Callaghan M, Duggan B, Feely M. *J Neurol Neurosurg Psychiat 1978; 41:* 907–912

Calderon M, Mellan S. *Prensa Med Mex 1971; 36:* 350–353

Dalby M. *Epilepsia 1971; 12:* 325–334

Dalby M. In Wink C, ed. *Tegretol in Epilepsy 1972;* 98–106. Manchester: Nicholls

Dalby M. *Skand Epilep Arsmode 1972; 9:* 22–24

Dallos V, Heathfield K. In Wink C, ed. *Tegretol in Epilepsy 1972;* 89–94. Manchester: Nicholls

Dam M, Christiansen J. In Janz D, ed. *Epileptology 1976.* Stuttgart: Thieme

Dam M, Jensen A, Christiansen J. *Acta Neurol Scand 1975; Suppl 60;* 33–38

Daneel A. *S Afr Med J 1967; 41:* 772–775

Davis E. *Med J Aust 1964; 1:* 150–152

Dreyer R. *Nervenarzt 1965; 10:* 442–445

Eichelbaum M, Bertilsson L, Lund L et al. *Eur J Clin Pharm 1976; 8:* 417–421

Feely M. In Roberts F, ed. *Tegretol in Epilepsy 1977;* 79–89. Macclesfield: Geigy

Ferrar-Vidal L, Subater-Tobella J, Oller-Daurella L. In Birkmayer W, ed. *Pain: An International Symposium 1976;* 165–174. Berne: Huber

Fishsel H, Heyer R. *Dtsch Med Wschr 1970; 95:* 12367–12374

Da Fonseca F. Ribeiro C. Rodrigues C. In *Coloquio Sobre Uso Clinico do Tegretol 1967;* 29–33. Basel: Geigy

Franzen G. *Nord Psykiat T 1976; 30:* 3–13

Fukushina Y, Tarabe F, Nishizaka H. *New Drugs and Clin Eval 1965; 14:* 558–562

Galindo S, Limon G, Gonzalez D. *Prensa Med Mex 1969; 34:* 388–390

Gamstorp I. *Dev Med Child Neurol 1966; 8:* 296–300

Gamstorp I. *Acta Paediat Scand 1970; 206: Suppl 1:* 96–97

Gamstorp I. In Wink C, ed. *Tegretol in Epilepsy 1972;* 6–11. Manchester: Nicholls

Gamstorp I. In Penry J, Daly D, eds. *Advances in Neurology 11 1975.* New York: Raven Press

Gamstorp I. In Roberts F, ed. *Tegretol in Epilepsy 1977;* 1–3. Macclesfield: Geigy

Giroire M. *Ouest-Med 1965; 7:* 414–417

Grant R. In Wink C, ed. *Tegretol in Epilepsy 1972;* 16–24. Manchester:Nicholls

Grant R. In Birkmayer W, ed. *Pain: An International Symposium 1975;* 104–110. Berne: Huber

Gupta R, Jolly S. *Indian Practnr 1972; 25:* 399–404

Hanke N. *Ganeesk Gids 1970; 1:* 329–331

Harper W, Roberts J, McCandless A, Horne J. In Roberts R, ed. *Tegretol in Epilepsy 1977;* 8–10. Macclesfield: Geigy

Hassan M, Parsonage M. In Penry J, ed. *Epilepsy. The VIIIth International Symposium 1977.* 135. New York: Raven Press

Hildebrand H. *Aerztl Praxis 1965; 17:* 2221–2222

Jeavons P. In Roberts R, ed. *Tegretol in Epilepsy 1977;* 45–49. Macclesfield: Geigy

Jongmans J. *Epilepsia 1964; 5:* 74–82

Kanbiah V, Saldina L. *Transactions of the Leningrad Nanch-Issledovat Institute im VM Bechterava 1970; 55:* 243–250

Kanjijal G. In Wink C, ed. *Tegretol in Epilepsy 1972;* 63–68. Manchester: Nicholls

Kanjijal G. In Roberts F, ed. *Tegretol in Epilepsy 1977;* 55–59. Macclesfield: Geigy

Marjerrison G, Jedlicki S, Keogh R et al. *Dis Nerv Syst 1968; 29:* 133–136

Marques-Assis L. In Birkmayer W, ed. *Pain: An International Symposium 1976;* 89–90. Berne: Huber

Mehta P, Parsonage M. In Roberts F, ed. *Tegretol in Epilepsy 1977;* 68–78. Macclesfield: Geigy

Moene Y, Courjon J. *Lyon Med 1969; 14:* 817–825

Monaco F, Riccio A, Benna P et al. *Neurology 1976; 26:* 936–943

O'Donohoe N. In Roberts F, ed. *Tegretol in Epilepsy 1977;* 10–14. Macclesfield: Geigy

Paredes Cencillo C de. *Tegretol Comoantiepileptico y psicotropo. Libro de Becas Curso 1968/1969;* 159–168. Barcelona: Geigy

Parsonage M. In Wink C, ed. *Tegretol in Epilepsy 1972;* 69–79, 135. Manchester: Nicholls

Parsonage M. In Penry J, Daly D, eds. *Complex Partial Seizures and their Treatment 1975.* New York: Raven Press

Poch G. *Prensa Med Argent 1969; 56:* 1263–1266

Pryse-Phillips W, Jeavons P. *Epilepsia 1970; 11:* 263–273

Rajotte P, Jilek W, Jilek L et al. *Medical Canada 1967; 96:* 1200–1206

Rey-Bellet J, Martin F, Tchicaloff M, Beboux J. *Revue Med Suisse Romande 1966; 86:* 439–455

Reyer Armijo E. *Prensa Med Mex 1968; 33:* 136–141

Riccio A, Monaco F. In Birkmayer W, ed. *Pain: An International Symposium 1976;* 111–119. Berne: Huber

Rodin E, Rim C, Kitano H et al. *J Nerv Ment Dis 1976; 163:* 41–46

Rodin E, Rim C, Rennick P. *Epilepsia 1974; 15:* 547–561

Roedenbeck S, Santos J. *Revue Neuro psiquiat 1967; 30:* 290–310

Schain R, Ward J, Guthrie D. *Neurology 1977; 27:* 476–480

Scheffner D, Schiefer I. *Epilepsia 1972; 13:* 819–838

Scheffner D, Schiefer I. *Follow up Studies of Epileptic Children Treated with Carbamazepine. Presented at the Vth European Symposium on Epilepsy, London 1972*

Schneider H. In Penry J, ed. *Epilepsy: The VIIIth International Symposium 1977;* 57–62. New York: Raven Press

Schneider P, Burner M, Pagani J. *Encephale 1965; 54:* 433–439

Simpson G, Kunze E, Watts T. *Proceedings of IVth International Congress of Neuropsychopharmacology 1964;* 442–448. Amsterdam: Elsevier

Singh A, Saxena B, Germain M. In Penry J, ed. *Epilepsy. VIIIth International Symposium 1977;* 47–56. New York: Raven Press

Singhal B, Desai H. *Indian Practnr 1968; 21:* 293–298

Singhal B, Hansotio P, Parekh C, Hawalder P. *Bombay Hospital J 1972; 14:* 41–47

Smyth V. In Wink C, ed. *Tegretol in Epilepsy 1972;* 48–53. Manchester: Nicholls

Stràndjord R, Johannessen S. *Carbamazepine as the only Drug in Patients with Epilepsy. Serum Levels and Clinical Effect 1978. Presented at the Xth Epilepsy International Symposium in Vancouver*

Strandjord R, Johannessen S. In Johannessen S, Morselli P, Pippenger C et al, eds. *Anti-epileptic Therapy: Advances in Drug Monitoring 1980;* 229–236. New York: Raven Press

Tchicaloff M, Pennett F. *Schweiz Med Wschr 1963; 93:* 1664–1666

Van der Drift. *Med T Geneesk 1967; 11:* 483–485

Vasconcelos D. *Nervenarzt 1967; 38:* 506–509

Vasquez C. *Sem Med 1968; 133:* 1599–1595

Vigoroux R. *Lyon Med 1968; 26:* 1–4

Vorchenko A, Morozov A. *Transactions of the Leningrad Nauchn-Issledovat Institute im VM Bechtereva 1970; 55:* 251–257

Wolf P. In Wink C, ed. *Tegretol in Epilepsy 1972;* 95–97. Manchester: Nicholls

Wulfsohn M. *S Afr Med J 1972; 31:* 1091–1092

42

TWO CLOBAZAM STUDIES

A Wilson, A Herxheimer, F Clifford Rose

Introduction

This chapter describes the problems experienced at the Charing Cross Hospital in the design and execution of two studies of clobazam as an antiepileptic drug. Clobazam is a 1,5 benzodiazepine which differs from diazepam only in that it has a nitrogen atom in the 1 and 5 position, and a ketogroup in the 4 position (Figure 1).

Potential as antiepileptic drug

Clobazam is an effective anxiolytic agent, but causes less sedation and muscle relaxation than do the 1,4 benzodiazepines, and less impairment of psychomotor and motor performance [1–3]. In animal studies clobazam shows a clear potential as an antiepileptic drug, raising the threshold of audiogenic seizures in mice,

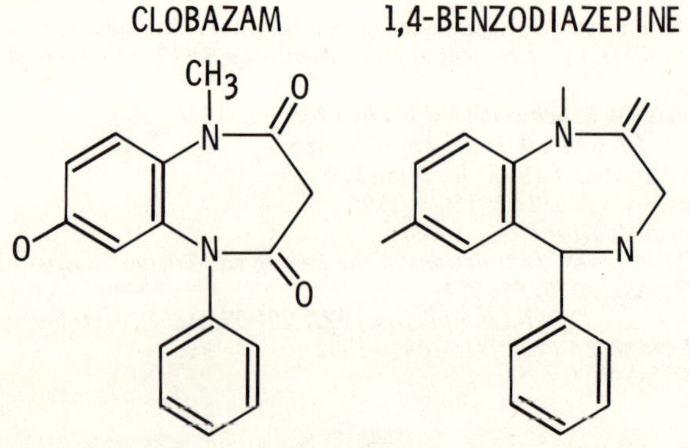

CLOBAZAM   1,4-BENZODIAZEPINE

Figure 1

light-induced seizures in baboons [4], and the threshold of electroshock and chemical seizures in rats and mice [5]. It is thus active in all animal models of epilepsy tested.

In the last three years some twelve clinical studies have been performed on in-patients with epilepsy, four of which have been published [6–9]. These studies suggest that clobazam may protect against seizures, at least for a period, before tolerance develops [6,7]. Eleven of the studies were 'adjunctive', ie clobazam was added to pre-existing medication in an attempt to achieve better control of seizures but only one of these was double blind [9]. The one study in new patients was controlled, but no conclusions were drawn (Del Pesce, unpublished). It is not possible to assess the efficacy of clobazam as an antiepileptic drug from these studies since the methods of assessment were inadequately described, but no serious problems have arisen. The interactions of clobazam with other antiepileptic drugs were described in only three studies, so that further evaluation of clobazam as an antiepileptic drug is therefore required.

Two trials at Charing Cross Hospital

The efficacy of clobazam is being tested on out-patients in two studies, the first being an adjunctive study where clobazam or placebo is added to pre-existing medication; the effects of clobazam on the plasma concentration of other anti-epileptic drugs are recorded. The second study on new patients aims to establish whether clobazam alone has any antiepileptic activity, and compares this with the effect of phenytoin given to provide serum levels within the therapeutic range. In both studies records are kept of side effects and of haematological and biochemical variables. Both studies are double blind, patients being allocated at random to concurrent treatment periods. Fit frequency is recorded as 'fit days'. (Sometimes it is not possible for the patient to remember how many fits have occurred in a particular period. Therefore if any single or multiple event occurs in a twenty-four hour period, this is recorded as 'fit day'). All treatment failures such as drop outs and those suffering intolerable side effects will be included in the final analysis. Compliance is maximised by frequent outpatient visits, tablet counts at each visit and a once daily tablet regime.

Problems

Duration of trial

The factors affecting the duration of a trial are chiefly the rate of referral, the rate of recruitment, and the duration of financial support [10]. The rate at which patients are referred for the trial depends on the notification, and enthusiasm, of general practitioners as well as hospital colleagues. As with other centres, Charing Cross Hospital has lacked reliable data from which to predict recruitment.

Estimates based on size of catchment area indicated that eight patients a month would be referred to the adjunctive study, and four patients a month to the new patient study.

In ten months since inception, 128 referrals have attended the epilepsy clinic. Of these, 28 have met the criteria for inclusion in the studies, twenty-three being recruited to the adjunctive study and five to the new patient study. The shortfall in both studies is large but both trials have proved valuable as pilot, or 'Phase 2', studies as described in the previous chapter. The principal reason for the difference between referral and recruitment is that better control was achieved by simply altering or even simplifying the regime of current medication, a mandatory manoeuvre written into the protocol. Thus greater interest engendered by separating patients into an epilepsy clinic, and by a research project, can itself lead to more effective therapy. Most epileptics of recent onset were excluded from the new patient study because they had been started on medication by their general practitioners prior to their first attendance at the clinic, a mandatory exclusion written into the protocol (In future trials such exclusion should be avoided since there is no ethical objection to changing the medication of patients referred who give their fully informed consent).

The funding of the two Charing Cross studies was based on the assumption that they could be completed in two years, but the current rate of patients entering the trials in the first ten months makes it unlikely that an adequate sample size and duration of follow up could be achieved within this time limit, since no statistically useful conclusions would be possible at the end of the two-year period.

Estimate of seizure frequency

Seizure frequency occurring in the adjunctive study has to be compared with that previously occurring during a defined period. All retrospective studies lack accuracy since documentation of past seizure frequency in hospital notes are not uniform and often inaccurate. Patients cannot be relied on to record their seizures accurately so that general practitioners as well do not have this information. With both retrospective and prospective studies, seizure frequency is recorded with a diary card, filled in by the patient, or the patient's relatives. Since it is not possible to predict seizure frequency in epileptics of recent onset, a six months' duration of treatment in a new patient study is not long enough to show any significant effect.

Deciding between competing projects

Since the resources in investigators, patients and facilities for clinical trials in epilepsy are limited, it is important to use them in the most productive way to find answers to major questions of treatment. The first task is to specify precisely the questions, and then to decide on their relative importance. If this is done then the questions asked by the clinical study of new drugs can be given their proper scientific priority. It is necessary to rank the pressing therapeutic problems that need trials in epilepsy.

Summary

The previous chapter [10] has described the deficiencies of clinical trial methods in previous antiepileptic drug studies. The trials we are attempting at Charing Cross Hospital to assess the potential of clobazam as an antiepileptic drug illustrate the problems described. It is suggested that for useful results to accumulate, new patient studies in epilepsy should be multicentre and that they will need to be of many years duration.

References

1   Bugat R, Fourcade J. *Comparative Effects of Benzodiazepine on Human Behaviour. RSM International Congress Symposium Series 43; 1981:* 41–43
2   The effects of benzodiazepines on psychomotor performance. *J Clin Pharmacol 1967; 7 (Suppl 1):* 61S
3   Psychomotor drug use and driving risk: review and analysis. *J Safety Res 1970; 2:* 73
4   Chapman B, Horton, Meldrum. *Epilepsia 1978; 19:* 293–299
5   Fielding and Hoffman. *Br J Clin Pharmacol 1979; 7 (Suppl 1):* 7S–15S
6   Gastaut H, Low MD. *Epilepsia 1979; 20:* 437–446
7   Gastaut H. *The Effect of Benzodiazepine or Chronic Epilepsy in Man. RSM International Congress Symposium Series 43; 1981:* 141–150
8   Martin P. *The Antiepileptic Effects of Clobazam: a Long Term Study in Resistant Epilepsy. RSM International Congress Symposium Series 43; 1981:* 151–157
9   Critchley E et al. *Double Blind Clinical Trial of Clobazam in Refractory Epilepsy and the Effect of Clobazam on Blood Levels of Phenobarbitone, Phenytoin and Carbamazepine. RSM International Congress Symposium Series 43; 1981:* 159–163
10 See chapter 41

43

MONOTHERAPY WITH SODIUM VALPROATE AND CARBAMAZEPINE

P M Jeavons

Monotherapy is not new but has become increasingly fashionable following the publication of Reynolds et al [1] and the increasing knowledge of the pharmaco-kinetics of antiepileptic drugs, especially in relationship to drug interactions and serum levels. In the past, paediatricians used monotherapy with troxidone or ethosuximide for absences, and phenobarbitone has been used as a single drug by physicians for many years. It is regrettable that there was a tendency for patients to be treated *ab initio* with a combination of phenytoin and phenobarbitone, a combination still used despite the numerous publications on phenytoin mono-therapy. Polytherapy is encouraged by the availability of tablets or capsules in which two antiepileptic drugs are combined. Furthermore, polytherapy is likely to follow the introduction of any new antiepileptic, because such drugs are evaluated initially in patients with long-standing epilepsy whose seizures have not yet been controlled and in whom any new drug will be added to their current medication. If seizures are thereby controlled, the patients and the physician may be unwilling to withdraw the previous medication. However, even the most enthusiastic proponents of monotherapy are beginning to admit that polytherapy may have a place. Monotherapy is most likely to be effective in the primary generalised epilepsies, in newly diagnosed patients with a short history, and in patients without psychiatric or neurological signs or symptoms. Poor results are likely in patients whose seizures are symptomatic of cerebral damage or disease, in complex partial seizures and in myoclonic astatic epilepsy (Lennox syndrome), and in patients with several types of seizure. The advantages and disadvantages of monotherapy and polytherapy have recently been evaluated by Gastaut [2] who rightly points out that both monotherapy and polytherapy have their proper place and should not be regarded as alternatives.

Reports on monotherapy with sodium valproate are rare [3–10] as are those for carbamazepine [11–13].

For many years we have used sodium valproate as the drug of choice, for

406

primary generalised epilepsy and myoclonic astatic epilepsy, and carbamazepine for partial epilepsies. Half the patients seen at the epilepsy clinics have primary generalised epilepsy, 43 per cent have partial epilepsy, and 7 per cent have myoclonic epilepsy. As is to be expected, the patients referred to a special clinic for epilepsy tend to have a long history, and only 27 per cent of those with primary generalised epilepsy had a history of less than two years duration, whilst 45 per cent had had seizures for more than six years. An even longer history was given by those with partial epilepsy, 56 per cent of whom had seizures for more than 10 years. Of the patients with myoclonic astatic epilepsy 39 per cent had a history extending over six years or more. At the time of the original referral to the clinics, seizures occurred daily or several times each week in 52 per cent of those with primary generalised epilepsy, in 59 per cent of those with partial epilepsy and in 95 per cent of those with myoclonic astatic epilepsy. A further indication of the intractable nature of the patients' epilepsy is indicated by the fact that 56 per cent of patients with primary generalised epilepsy and partial epilepsy had been treated previously by other physicians, as had 80 per cent of those with myoclonic astatic epilepsy.

Sodium valproate was given as the initial drug in 100 patients and in 140 patients all previous medication was withdrawn. Ninety-six patients received sodium valproate in combination with other drugs. Only 16 patients were treated *ab initio* with carbamazepine, but previous medicine was withdrawn from 99 patients and 42 remained on co-medication. If a patient did not respond to initial therapy with sodium valproate or carbamazepine, either the patient was given the alternative drug, or the two drugs were combined, this combination being used in 112 patients.

Thus, 357 patients (59 per cent) have been treated with monotherapy using sodium valproate or carbamazepine.

Early experience with sodium valproate [14] indicated that it was effective in the primary generalised epilepsies but less so in partial epilepsies, hence the relatively small number of patients with partial seizures (Table I). The number of

TABLE I

	SODIUM VALPROATE		CARBAMAZEPINE	
	Total cases	Monotherapy: no seizures	Total cases	Monotherapy: no seizures
Absences	70	43 61%		
Myoclonic	62	43 69%		
Photosensitive	61	42 69%		
Primary tonic-clonic	67	49 73%	21	15 71%
Secondary tonic-clonic	18	9 50%	32	18 56%
Simple partial	(9)	(2) (22%)	17	10 59%
Complex partial	(11)	(5) (45%)	85	39 46%
Myoclonic astatic	38	7 18%	(2)	(1)
TOTAL	336	200 59%	157	83 53%

patients with primary tonic-clonic seizures treated with carbamazepine is also small, because sodium valproate was originally preferred, but in recent years an increasing number of such patients have been treated with carbamazepine, and in female patients carbamazepine may be preferred at times because of the greater tendency of sodium valproate to cause an increase in weight in females compared to males [15].

Sodium valproate was originally introduced at a daily dose of 400mg [8, 14], increased to 600mg daily after three days and daily dosage was subsequently increased by 200mg every one or two weeks, administration of the plain tablet being twice daily, at meal times. More recently the 500mg enteric coated tablet has been used, with initial dosage of 500mg daily for a week, followed by 500mg increments each week. Since 1978 enteric coated medication has been administered once daily [4, 16]. Therapy with sodium valproate has been easier since the introduction of the 200mg enteric coated tablet which is easier for young children to swallow and which facilitates dosage adjustment.

Carbamazepine was introduced more slowly than sodium valproate, to avoid transient side effects. The initial daily dose was 100mg for children and 200mg for adults. The daily dose was increased by 100 or 200mg every two weeks, since weekly increases tended to induce side effects. Administration was twice daily, with the largest dose at night. Dosage was increased until seizures ceased, or transient side effects (diplopia or dizziness) occurred about two hours after the morning dose. Experience showed that this was a more reliable indication of maximum tolerable dose than serum levels. If side effects occurred after the morning dose, three divided doses were given, or the total daily dose was reduced by 100 or 200mg. The introduction of the 400mg tablet of carbamazepine has helped those patients who are receiving a high dosage, and who tended to be daunted by having to take six or eight tablets a day.

Compliance improved, particularly in the adolescent, with once daily administration of sodium valproate, and the use of the 500mg tablet of sodium valproate and the 400mg tablet of carbamazepine.

On original referral to the clinics 60 per cent of patients were receiving barbiturates and 50 per cent phenytoin. Once seizures were controlled following the introduction of sodium valproate, other medication was withdrawn one drug at a time, always starting with phenobarbitone. Reduction of barbiturates was in decrements of 15mg of phenobarbitone or 125mg of primidone every two weeks, phenytoin being withdrawn in doses of 25mg every two weeks.

Serum levels were assessed only when the response of the patient to therapy was not that which was to be expected. For example, if control of seizures was not achieved by a daily dose of 30mg/kg or more of sodium valproate, or 20mg/kg of carbamazepine, or if there was evidence of side effects, serum levels were assessed. Once control of all seizures had been achieved by monotherapy with either drug, serum levels were assessed in order to gain some idea of effective levels. Blood sampling was at the time of usual clinic attendance, rather than before the morning dose, since in practice this was more convenient.

The length of follow-up before the final assessment of results of therapy varied according to the type of seizure and the frequency of attacks before the introduction of sodium valproate or carbamazepine, follow-up being longer with the former drug. The follow-up was longer than three years in 78 per cent of patients treated with sodium valproate and in 43 per cent of those receiving carbamazepine. Short periods of follow-up occurred either in patients who failed to show any response after four to six months of therapy, or in a few whose attacks had occurred many times a day but ceased after one or two months therapy. The latter patients might be assessed after one year's therapy. In no patient was the epilepsy regarded as controlled unless the period of freedom from seizures was longer than had occurred before the introduction of the new drug. Patients were classified according to the most common type of seizures which they experienced. Thus patients with frequent complex absences and rare tonic-clonic seizures were classified as complex absence seizures. Those with simple absences only had this one type of seizure. All patients with complex partial or simple partial seizures were grouped together, whether or not they had secondary tonic-clonic seizures. Patients with primary tonic-clonic seizures had no other type of seizure. Those classified as secondary tonic-clonic seizures had partial seizures with secondary generalisation as evidenced by an aura or focal onset, or clear EEG evidence of a focus.

Patients with photosensitive epilepsy included those whose fits were induced by TV or flickering sunlight, and also patients with eyelid myoclonia [17].

Results (Table I)

Of 240 patients who received sodium valproate alone, 71 per cent became free from all seizures, the response being equally good in the 140 from whom other drugs had been withdrawn as in the 100 who received sodium valproate as initial therapy. The response to monotherapy with carbamazepine was essentially similar, 73 per cent becoming free from fits, whether other drugs were withdrawn or carbamazepine had been given alone from the start.

Simple absences responded well to monotherapy with sodium valproate, all attacks ceasing in 11 of 12 patients. With complex absences co-medication was needed more often and only 36 of 52 patients received sodium valproate alone, 32 becoming free from all seizures. No patients with myoclonic absences responded to monotherapy. Of the 70 patients with simple, complex or myoclonic absences, 61 per cent became free from seizures with sodium valproate as sole antiepileptic drug.

Fifty of 62 patients with myoclonic epilepsy of childhood or myoclonic epilepsy of adolescence, with or without photosensitivity, received sodium valproate alone and 43 ceased to have any seizures.

Forty-two patients whose seizures occurred only when watching television, or in the presence of flickering sunlight were all treated with sodium valproate as sole antiepileptic drug. The results of therapy were assessed on the responses to intermittent photic stimulation (IPS) since seizures are very rare in these patients; in all patients IPS evoked abnormal discharges, commonly spike-wave, prior to therapy. In 76 per cent all EEG abnormality disappeared.

Patients with eyelid myoclonia and absences [17] are difficult to treat. The absences and rare tonic-clonic seizures often respond rapidly to therapy with sodium valproate, but the jerking of the eyelids and the photosensitivity may not respond to monotherapy. Of 19 patients, five needed a combination of sodium valproate and ethosuximide and of the 14 on monotherapy with sodium valproate only 10 (53 per cent) became free from seizures and had a normal EEG.

Of 88 patients with primary generalised tonic-clonic seizures, 82 per cent received monotherapy with sodium valproate or carbamazepine and responded equally well to either drug, complete control of fits occurring in 73 per cent of those receiving sodium valproate and in 71 per cent of those treated with carbamazepine. Twenty-two of the patients with primary tonic-clonic seizures showed abnormality in the EEG provoked by IPS, but responded equally well as those without photosensitivity.

Partial epilepsy responded less well to monotherapy than primary generalised epilepsy. Of 50 patients with secondary tonic-clonic seizures (partial seizures with secondary generalisation), 14 had received sodium valproate alone, and 26 received carbamazepine alone. Complete control of seizures was achieved in 50 per cent of those on monotherapy with the former drug, and in 56 per cent of those on the latter.

Only three patients with simple partial seizures were treated with sodium valproate alone, and in two all fits ceased. Monotherapy with carbamazepine was used in 13 of 17 patients with simple partial seizures, 10 of whom ceased to have seizures.

Sodium valproate was rarely used for treating complex partial seizures, because of initial experience [14], but it was given to patients who developed severe side effects when first treated with carbamazepine. Only five patients received initial monotherapy with sodium valproate, but in all five complete control was achieved. Monotherapy with carbamazepine was used in 55 of 85 patients with complex partial seizures and in 39 seizures ceased. Complex partial seizures proved to be the most difficult type of seizure to treat with a single drug (apart from myoclonic absences) and only 46 per cent were completely controlled by monotherapy, an additional 10 per cent being controlled by a combination of carbamazepine and other drugs, usually phenytoin.

Myoclonic astatic epilepsy was treated mainly with sodium valproate in combination with other drugs. Monotherapy was used in 13 of the 40 patients and was successful in 8 (20 per cent), 7 of whom received sodium valproate. Four of the latter had a history of epilepsy of less than two years.

Effective dosage

The establishment of effective daily dosage, frequency of administration, effective serum levels, and toxic levels can only be assessed with any reliability in patients whose seizures are completely controlled by monotherapy. Experience with sodium valproate resulted in administration of sodium valproate twice daily, and then once daily [4, 16]. Comparison of twice daily administration with once daily showed that the latter resulted in improvement without increase in daily dose [4]. It has been shown that higher dosage is needed to achieve an adequate serum level of sodium valproate when other antiepileptic drugs are combined [5], mainly because of induction of liver enzymes. In our patients receiving monotherapy with sodium valproate the mean daily dose of those aged 11 years or more was 23 ± 5mg/kg, serum levels being 89 ± 22mg/L. Children aged less than 11 years received higher daily dosage, usually between 15 and 50mg/kg. In most patients treated successfully with sodium valproate monotherapy the range of serum levels was 60–120mg/L.

With carbamazepine the effective mean daily dose in monotherapy was 15mg/kg, the range being 4–24mg/kg, indicating considerable individual variation. There was also considerable fluctuation and variation in serum levels, the mean being 11mg/L regardless of time of sampling, the range being 4–17mg/L.

Side effects with monotherapy

Side effects with monotherapy with sodium valproate have already been reported [15]. In two-thirds of the 240 patients there were no unwanted effects. Temporary loss or thinning of hair or changes from straight to wavy hair occurred in 11 per cent. Sedation was uncommon (2 per cent). The most frequent side effect was increase in weight (18 per cent), not always associated with increase in appetite. Other reports confirm the frequency of this side effect [18, 19].

Although there is evidence that sodium valproate reduced the platelet count and thrombocytopenia was found in 6 per cent [15] no patient showed significant clinical signs. An abnormal SGOT result was found in 3 per cent of 109 patients on sodium valproate alone, but none showed any clinical evidence of hepatic disorder. From the literature it seems probable that side effects are more likely if the daily dose of sodium valproate exceeds 50mg/kg or the serum level exceeds 120mg/L [20].

Side effects in patients receiving monotherapy with carbamazepine have also been rare, the most common being transient diplopia (14 per cent) or dizziness (6 per cent), as a result of the method of therapy. The most serious side effect of carbamazepine is a skin rash, which occurred in 3 per cent, and resulted in withdrawal of the drug. In 71 per cent there were no unwanted effects. Sedation (2 per cent) was as rare as with sodium valproate. Low osmolality occurred in eight patients, only six of whom showed clinical symptoms, five responding to reduction in daily dose of carbamazepine.

Because of the lack of serious side effects sodium valproate and carbamazepine have been the drugs of choice for the therapy of all forms of epilepsy, and monotherapy has been effective in many cases.

Acknowledgment

I am grateful to my colleagues Dr J E Clark, A Convanis and A K Gupta for their collaboration over many years in the epilepsy clinics.

References

1   Reynolds EH, Chadwick D. Galbraith AW. *Lancet 1976; i:* 923–926
2   Gastaut H. *Le Concours Medical 1981; 103:* 36, 5618–5633
3   Briant RH, Foote SE, Wallis WE. *NZ Med J 1978; 88:* 479–482
4   Covanis A, Jeavons PM, Gupta AK. In Dam M, Gram L, Penry JK, eds. *Advances in Epileptology: XIIth Epilepsy International Symposium 1981;* 527–532. New York: Raven Press
5   Henriksen O, Johannessen SI. In Johannessen SI, Morselli PL, Pippenger CE, Richens A, Schmidt D, Meinardi H, eds. *Anti Epileptic Therapy: Advances in Drug Monitoring 1980;* 253. New York: Raven Press
6   Jeavons PM, Covanis A, Gupta AK. In Canger R, Angeleri F, Penry JK. eds. *Advances in Epileptology: XIth Epilepsy International Symposium 1980;* 415–418
7   Jeavons PM, Covanis A, Gupta AK, Clark JE. In Parsonage MJ, Caldwell ADS, eds. *The Place of Sodium Valproate in the Treatment of Epilepsy 1980;* 53. London Royal Society of Medicine
8   Jeavons PM, Clark JE, Maheshwari MC. *Dev Med Child Neurol 1977; 19:* 9–25
9   Lagenstein I, Stenowsky HJ, Blaschke E, et al. *Arch Psychiat Nervenkr 1978; 226:* 43–55
10   Suzuki M, Maruyama H, Ishibashi Y, et al. *Med Prog 1972; 82:* 470–488
11   Callaghan N, O'Callaghan M, Duggan B, Feely M. *J Neurol Neurosurg Psychiatry 1978; 41:* 907–912
12   Shorvon SD, Galbraith AW, Laundy M, et al. In Johannessen SI, Morselli PL, Pippenger CE, Richena A, Schmidt D, Meinardi H, eds. *Anti Epileptic Therapy: Advances in Drug Monitoring 1980;* 253. New York: Raven Press
13   Strandjord RE, Johannessen SI. *Epilepsia 1980; 21:* 655–662
14   Jeavons PM, Clark JE. *Br Med J 1974; ii:* 584–586
15   Clarke JE, Covanis A, Gupta AK, Jeavons PM. In Parsonage MJ, Caldwell ADS, eds. *The Place of Sodium Valproate in the Treatment of Epilepsy 1980;* 133. London Royal Society of Medicine
16   Covanis A, Jeavons PM. *Dev Med Child Neurol 1980; 22:* 202–204
17   Jeavons PM. *Dev Med Child Neurol 1977; 19:* 3–8
18   Dam M, Gram L. In Dam M, Gram L, Pedersen B, Ørum H, eds. *Valproate in the Treatment of Seizures 1981;* 83. Hvidore, Danish Epilepsy Society
19   Egger J, Brett EM. *Br Med J 1981; 283:* 577–581
20   Jeavons PM. In Woodbury DM, Penry JK, Pippenger CE, eds. *Antiepileptic Drugs 1982;* In press. New York: Raven Press

44

A COMPARISON BETWEEN SODIUM VALPROATE AND PHENYTOIN IN THE TREATMENT OF ADULT ONSET EPILEPSY

D M Turnbull, M D Rawlins, D Weightman, D W Chadwick

Introduction

The role of sodium valproate (sodium di-n-propylacetate) in the treatment of adult onset epilepsy is uncertain. There have been few studies reporting the use of valproate alone [1,2], or comparing it with more conventional anticonvulsants as single drug therapy in adults.

We recently reported the results of a comparative study of the first year's treatment with valproate or phenytoin in adult epileptic patients [3]. In this chapter, we report the results of a two year follow-up of a group of 83 patients.

Methods

The patients included in this study were over the age of 16 years, with a history of two or more epileptic seizures in the previous three years. After stratification for age, sex and type of seizure, they were randomised to therapy with either sodium valproate or phenytoin. Three age groupings were used ie 16–25, 26–65, 66 or older. Patients were allotted to the tonic-clonic seizure group if there was no positive *clinical* evidence of a focal onset or aftermath to the seizure. Other groups consisted of simple partial seizures with or without generalisation. Inclusion in the first group does not indicate that all patients had 'primary generalised epilepsy' and, indeed, some of these patients had focal EEG abnormalities.

All patients were routinely investigated with skull X-ray and electroencephalogram (EEG). Further neurological investigation was undertaken as clinically indicated. Prior to therapy, estimations of haemoglobin, white cell count, platelet count, MCV, serum B_{12} and folate, and red cell folate were carried out. Plasma urea, creatinine, serum calcium and alkaline phosphatase, bilirubin, aspartate transaminase and serum albumin and globulin concentrations were also measured. Patients were commenced on therapy with either sodium valproate (600mg

413

per day, in three divided doses) or phenytoin (300mg per day, in three divided doses). Follow-up was at one month after initiation of therapy, then at three-month intervals if seizure free. At each visit the occurrence of seizures or side-effects was documented and plasma anticonvulsant levels estimated. Compliance was estimated by counts of tablets returned to pharmacy. At six-month intervals following the commencement of therapy haematological and biochemical screening were repeated.

If further seizures occurred during the follow-up period the dose of anticonvulsant was increased. Patients who had further seizures whilst taking valproate received sequential increments to 1.2g/day, 2.1g/day and 3g/day (in three divided doses) until there were no seizures or until unacceptable adverse effects occurred. No reference was made to the plasma anticonvulsant level when the medication was increased. For patients receiving phenytoin, the daily dose was increased by 50mg if the previous plasma level was below $10\mu g/ml$ (40mmol/L) and by 25mg if the level was $10\mu g/ml$ (40mmol/L) or greater. Increments were administered until seizures were controlled or clinical signs of intoxication occurred irrespective of the plasma level.

An individual drug was only regarded to have 'failed' if the patient suffered unacceptable adverse effects, or if seizures continued at doses up to those which caused dose-related toxicity.

Results

Ninety-seven patients were entered into the study 24 months or more before the date of analysis. Forty-eight of these were allocated to therapy with valproate and 49 to therapy with phenytoin. Ten patients were lost to follow-up, 6 from the valproate group and 4 from the phenytoin group. These patients had all been seizure free when lost to follow-up. Four patients died within the follow-up period, 2 from intracranial tumours diagnosed after randomisation, one from stroke and one from myocardial infarction. Of these 4 patients two had been allocated to therapy with valproate and 2 to phenytoin. Of the remaining 83, 49 had a history of tonic-clonic seizures without focal features (23 were treated with valproate and 26 with phenytoin) and 28 patients had complex partial seizures with or without secondary generalisation (13 received therapy with valproate and 15 with phenytoin). Six patients had symptoms of simple partial seizures with or without secondary generalisation (4 received valproate and 2 phenytoin). For the present analysis these have been included with the complex partial group.

Tonic-clonic seizures without focal features

Table I illustrates that there is no difference in the sex, age and EEG abnormalities of patients in the two therapeutic groups. There were no significant differences between valproate and phenytoin groups for the length of history of epilepsy,

414

TABLE I. Patients with tonic-clonic seizures (without focal features)

	Sex		Age (± SD)	EEG		
	M	F		N	G	F
Valproate	11	12	32 (± 17)	17	3	3
Phenytoin	14	12	34 (± 16)	18	4	4

N = normal or non-specific abnormality

G = generalised paroxysmal abnormality

F = focal paroxysmal abnormality

the frequency of seizures, and the number of seizures prior to therapy (Mann-Whitney U Test).

Table II illustrates the outcome of drug therapy in this group of patients. Sixteen (69%) of patients receiving valproate remained seizure-free during the first two years of therapy. Seven (31 per cent) had further seizures at 3–12 (mean 9) months after the initiation of therapy and required an increase in dosage; 4 patients were controlled on the first dosage increment of valproate (1.2g/day) for periods of between 15 and 18 (mean 16.5) months. One patient

TABLE II. Outcome of therapy — patients with tonic-clonic seizures

	Fit-free	Further fits	Failed	Early withdrawal	Total
Valproate	16 (69%)	6 (26%)	1 (5%)	0	23
Phenytoin	17 (65%)	5 (19%)	2 (8%)	2 (8%)	26

Fit-free v Further fits p > 0.2 not sig.
Fit-free v Further fits + failed p > 0.2 not sig.

Further fits	- seizures occurring after the commencement of therapy but subsequently controlled on an increased dose
Failed	- continued seizures in spite of increases in dosage sufficient to cause toxicity
Early withdrawal	- drug induced side-effects

had a further seizure 3 months after the first dosage increment of valproate and a further seizure 12 months after treatment at a dose of 2.1g/day; this patient has been seizure free for 9 months on the final dose increment 3g/day. One patient had a further seizure 3 months after first dosage increase but has been seizure-free on 2.1g/day for 9 months. One patient developed tremor and irritability on valproate 1.2g/day, although remaining seizure free on this dose. In this group, 11 seizures occurred in the 24 months of therapy compared with approximately 73

415

in the 12 months prior to treatment.

Seventeen (65 per cent) phenytoin-treated patients remained seizure-free. Seven (27 per cent) required an increase in phenytoin dosage because of further seizures occurring 1 to 18 (mean 8.3) months after the start of therapy. Three patients remained seizure free on the first dosage increment for 9–21 (mean 15) months. Two patients have subsequently been followed up for 6 and 21 months on a dosage of 400mg/day, with no recurrence of seizures. Two patients continued to have seizures despite doses sufficient to cause acute phenytoin toxicity (ataxia, dysarthria and nystagmus). Two patients were withdrawn from therapy shortly after commencement, in one case because of maculo-papular rash, and in the other because of acute erythroderma, associated with jaundice and disturbed liver function tests.

In this group there were 30 seizures in 24 months (15 in one patient) compared with approximately 73 in the 12 months prior to therapy.

Partial seizures (with or without secondary generalisation)

Table III illustrates that there is no difference in sex, age and the EEG findings in the patients in the two treatment groups. The groups do not differ significantly for the number of seizures, the length of history and the frequency of seizures in the 12 months prior to treatment (Mann-Whitney U Test).

TABLE III. Patients with partial seizures

	Sex		Age (± SD)	EEG		
	M	F		N	G	F
Valproate	8	9	38 (± 16)	8	-	9
Phenytoin	10	7	37 (± 15)	10	-	7

N = normal, or non-specific abnormality
G = generalised paroxysmal abnormality
F = focal paroxysmal abnormality

Table IV documents the response to therapy with valproate and phenytoin in patients with partial seizures. Of 17 patients treated with valproate 4 (24%) remained seizure-free on the initial dose of valproate and 13 (76%) experienced further seizures. These occurred at 1 to 18 months after the initiation of therapy (mean 5.5 months). Five of these patients have subsequently been controlled on an increased dose of 1.2g/day of valproate for between 7 and 30 months (mean 18.2). One of these patients, however, developed hair loss and was withdrawn from valproate in spite of good seizure control. Eight patients continued to have seizures despite receiving valproate 1.2g/day. These seizures occurred at 1 to 6

TABLE IV. Outcome of therapy – patients with partial seizures

	Fit-free	Further fits	Failed	Early Withdrawal	Total
Valproate	4 (24%)	7 (41%)	6 (35%)	0	17
Phenytoin	5 (29%)	9 (53%)	3 (18%)	0	17

Fit-free v further fits + failed p > 0.2 not significant
Fit-free + further fits v failed p > 0.2 not significant
Fit-free v further fits   p > 0.2 not significant

Further fits - seizures occurring after the commencement of therapy but subsequently controlled on an increased dose

Failed   - continued seizures in spite of increases in dosage sufficient to cause toxicity

(mean 2.6) months following the dosage increment to 1.2g/day. One patient remained seizure-free for 6 months following a second dosage increment but developed hair-loss necessitating valproate withdrawal. Two patients have been controlled on valproate 3g/day for 6 and 12 months respectively and 1 patient controlled on 2.1g/day for 6 months. Four patients (24% of whole group) have continued to have seizures in spite of doses of valproate of 2.1g/day in 2 patients and 3g/day in 2 patients which caused the development of a characteristic syndrome of intoxication.This consisted of a fine postural tremor, motor restlessness and irritability, and in 3 female patients, excessive weight gain. Thus, some 6 (35%) patients with partial seizures treated with valproate have been withdrawn from the drug during the first twelve months of treatment because of either failure of seizure control or the development of untoward side-effects at doses necessary to achieve seizure control.

In the 24 months after commencement with valproate there were 80 partial seizures compared with approximately 293 in the 12 months prior to treatment. Of the 13 patients experiencing further seizures on valproate, only 6 had a total of 9 secondary generalised seizures during the 24 months of treatment. This compares with 31 such seizures in the 12 months prior to treatment for the whole group. Eight patients who had tonic-clonic seizures prior to treatment had no such attacks whilst taking valproate.

Of the 17 patients with partial seizures treated with phenytoin, 5 (29%) have remained seizure-free during the 24 months of follow-up. Twelve (71%) had further seizures at between 1 and 18 (mean 5.2) months after the initiation of therapy. An initial dose increase of phenytoin to 350mg daily resulted in control in 3 more patients for periods of 15 and 24 (mean 19) months. Nine patients experienced further seizures between 1 and 12 (mean 5.2) months after the dose increase to 350mg daily. Of these 9 patients further increase in dosage up to 375 or 400mg of phenytoin daily, resulted in control in 4 patients for periods of between 6 and 27 months. Two patients are being followed-up taking doses of greater than 400mg daily. Three patients (18% of the whole group —phenytoin-treated group) have continued to have seizures up to doses of 375, 400 and 475mg daily, which caused symptoms and signs of phenytoin intoxication.

In this group of patients there were 75 partial seizures in the 24 months after commencement of phenytoin compared with approximately 134 in the 12 months prior to treatment. Of the 12 patients with further seizures only 2 patients had a total of 5 generalised seizures. Twelve patients who had tonic-clonic seizures prior to therapy had no such attacks on treatment.

Haematological and biochemical parameters

Changes in haematological and biochemical parameters were examined by comparison of pre-treatment values with values obtained after one year on treatment using Student's paired 't' test. Statistically significant changes were seen in the case of phenytoin where there was increase of mean cell volume ($p > 0.01$), alkaline phosphatase ($p > 0.005$) and aspartate transaminase ($p > 0.005$); and reductions in red cell folate ($p > 0.001$), serum folate ($p > 0.005$) and calcium ($p > 0.001$). For valproate there was statistically significant reduction in red cell folate ($p > 0.001$), in serum alkaline phosphatase ($p > 0.001$) and calcium ($p > 0.005$). The only patient with markedly abnormal biochemical parameters was the single patient with phenytoin induced hepatotoxicity.

Discussion

The quality of studies reporting the efficacy of anticonvulsant therapy in epileptic patients is historically poor. Most studies have been poorly controlled and have been undertaken in patients with severe, drug resistant epilepsy [4]. All too often these studies have been of short duration and interpretation has been complicated by patients receiving multiple drug therapy. More recently, the long-term efficacy of anticonvulsants used as monotherapy has been documented in patients with less severe, adult-onset epilepsy [5].

We still possess very little information on the comparative efficacy of single anticonvulsants in man. This requires long-term studies following randomisation to individual drugs, ideally in patients who have not received previous anticonvulsant therapy. The present study was designed to enable the comparison of sodium valproate with phenytoin, a well established anticonvulsant agent.

The groups of patients randomised to valproate and phenytoin are comparable in all major respects, ie for age, sex, proportion of patients with EEG abnormalities, length of history and the severity of epilepsy prior to treatment. Also, the follow-up periods which have been compared were identical enabling statistical analysis of our data.

The results at two years are strikingly similar to those obtained following one year's therapy [3]. Very few patients who were controlled at one year relapse at a later date. This finding is in keeping with that reported by Shorvon and Reynolds [6], in a similar group of patients treated with either phenytoin or carbamazepine.

This study shows valproate to be an effective anticonvulsant in adult-onset epilepsy. Its spectrum of action appears to be similar to phenytoin in that both are highly effective in the control of seizures in patients who have only tonic-clonic attacks without a significant aura. Both are less effective in controlling partial seizures. Twice as many patients taking valproate experienced continued seizures at doses up to those causing adverse reactions, as did patients taking phenytoin. There were fewer secondary generalised seizures in fewer patients in the phenytoin treated group. Whilst these differences are not statistically significant, further study may yet reveal that phenytoin is more effective in this group of patients.

Valproate, in doses ranging from 1.2–3g/day, caused a number of adverse reactions, including alopecia, weight gain, tremor and irritability. Such symptoms were seen in patients with plasma valproate levels greater than 90μg/ml (630 mmol/L) [7]. We have not seen evident hepato-toxicity in any patients receiving valproate, but such a reaction did occur in one patient receiving phenytoin.

Thus, after two years' follow-up there seem few differences in the efficacy of valproate and phenytoin in previously untreated adult epileptic patients. Similar long term comparisons of individual anticonvulsant drugs are necessary to allow more rational use of both old and new anticonvulsant drugs.

Acknowledgments

We are grateful to all those physicians who kindly referred patients for inclusion in the study and to Labaz for financial support. Also we thank Professor D A Shaw and Dr E H Reynolds for their helpful criticism and advice.

D M T is in receipt of an MRC Training Fellowship.

References

1 Pinder RM, Brogden RN, Speight TM, Avery GS. *Drugs 1977; 13:* 81–123
2 Shakir RA, Johnson RH, Lambie DG et al. *Epilepsia 1981; 22:* 27–33
3 Turnbull DM, Rawlins MD, Weightman D, Chadwick DW. *J Neurol Neurosurg Psychiat;* In press
4 Coatsworth JJ. *NINDS Monograph No 12 1971*
5 Reynolds EH, Shorvon SD. *Epilepsia 1981; 22:* 1–10
6 Reynolds EH, Shorvon SD. *Personal communication 1982*
7 Turnbull DM, Rawlins MD, Weightman D, Chadwick DW. *Plasma Valproate Concentrations: Correlation with Seizure Control and Toxicity.* In preparation

419

45

CHRONIC TOXICITY ON SINGLE DRUG TREATMENT

C I Dellaportas, S D Shorvon, E H Reynolds

Epilepsy is commonly a disorder of early life or adolescence, but at any age of onset requires long-term drug treatment. An increasing number of chronic toxic effects of anticonvulsant therapy have been recognised in the last 15 years [1,2]. Almost every system can be affected including subtle effects on mental and peripheral nerve function. Metabolic disturbances which have been widely recognised include: a fall in serum and red blood cell folate, occasionally leading to megaloblastic anaemia; a fall in calcium and phosphate levels, and a rise in alkaline phosphatase, sometimes associated with metabolic bone disease and evidence of altered vitamin D metabolism; a fall in serum bilirubin levels due to increased bilirubin conjugation in the liver; subtle effects on protein, lipid and endocrine metabolism. The drugs most commonly incriminated have included barbiturates such as phenobarbitone and primidone, and hydantoins such as phenytoin. However, the relative importance of the different drugs in producing these effects has been difficult to assess because all previous studies of chronic toxicity have been undertaken in groups of chronic patients of whom most, if not all, have been on polytherapy.

We have recently been examining the potential for single drug therapy in epilepsy by prospective studies, assisted by drug level monitoring, in previously untreated referrals to a neurological department [3—5]. This has given us the opportunity to investigate prospectively the evolution of chronic toxic effects in patients treated with different individual drugs. We here report and compare the effects of phenytoin and carbamazepine monotherapy on metabolic indices of chronic toxicity and on peripheral nerve function.

Patients and methods

These are reported in detail elsewhere [6,7]. All were participating in the studies of single drug therapy in new referrals with epilepsy reported by Shorvon et al

420

[3,4] who describe the design of the studies, details of drug administration and blood level monitoring, and outcome for seizure control. All the patients were followed prospectively with regular monitoring of drug levels. No other drugs were administered during the study.

For the metabolic studies 30 patients (median age 26, range 13–62) on phenytoin alone were compared with 33 patients (median age 28, range 8–68) on carbamazepine. Each drug had been administered prospectively for 2 years.

For the peripheral nerve studies, 32 patients (median age 25, range 15–68) on phenytoin were compared with 19 patients (median age 27, range 10–59) on carbamazepine. Each drug had been administered prospectively for 1–5 years.

Haemoglobin (Hb) and Mean Cell Volume (MCV) were measured with the Coulter S Counter; serum and red blood cell (RBC) folate by the standard *Lactobacillus casei* microbiological assay; calcium, phosphate, alkaline phosphatase, protein, albumen and total bilirubin on a Technicon SMAC Analyser. Sensory action potentials and conduction velocities of the median and sural nerves were measured according to the method of Burke et al [8]. Serum phenytoin and carbamazepine were measured by the gas chromatographic techniques of Kupferberg [9] and Toseland et al [10] respectively. No patient was intoxicated or had a serum phenytoin level greater than $30\mu g/ml$ at the time of testing.

Results

Metabolic

Table I summarises the means and standard errors for all the variables before and after 2 years of treatment with either phenytoin or carbamazepine. For both groups there was a significant rise in MCV on treatment, although in no patient did this exceed $96cu^3$. In the phenytoin group both serum and RBC folate fell significantly but although a similar trend was seen for carbamazepine this was not significant. In only 4 patients on phenytoin and one on carbamazepine did the serum folate fall below 2.5ng/ml. For both drugs we observed a significant fall in serum calcium and phosphate and elevation of alkaline phosphatase. In 5 patients on phenytoin and 3 on carbamazepine the latter rose above 90IU/L. In both groups total bilirubin fell, significantly with carbamazepine, but just short of significance for phenytoin. There were no changes in haemoglobin or albumen levels but a significant fall in total protein on carbamazepine. There were no significant differences between the effects of the two drugs on any of the variables.

Table II summarises the percentage of patients in whom the mean drug level during the course of follow-up over 2 years was in the optimum range. Approximately twice as many patients on carbamazepine compared to phenytoin were in the optimum range.

TABLE I. Indices of chronic toxicity before and after two years on treatment

	PHENYTOIN				CARBAMAZEPINE			
	Number of patients	Before treatment	After 2 years on treatment	p	Number of patients	Before treatment	After 2 years on treatment	p
Haemoglobin (g/100ml)	22	14.2 ± 0.3	14.4 ± 0.3	NS	22	14 ± 0.3	13.9 ± 0.3	<0.05
Mean cell volume (fl)	20	86 ± 1	89 ± 1	<0.001	20	85 ± 1	88 ± 1	<0.005
Serum folate (ng/ml)	18	4.6 ± 0.3	3.2 ± 0.3	<0.005	23	6.7 ± 0.8	5.4 ± 0.7	NS
Red cell folate (ng/ml)	15	443 ± 47	318 ± 32	<0.05	19	396 ± 44	338 ± 31	NS
Total protein (g/L)	19	73 ± 1	72 ± 1	NS	18	75 ± 1	72 ± 1	<0.05
Albumin (g/L)	19	41 ± 1	44 ± 1	NS	19	44 ± 1	45 ± 1	NS
Total bilirubin (µmol/L)	17	8 ± 1	6 ± 1	NS	19	9 ± 1	5 ± 1	<0.005
Calcium (µmol/L)	17	2.47 ± 0.02	2.42 ± 0.02	<0.05	20	2.54 ± 0.02	2.42 ± 0.05	<0.05
Phosphate (µmol/L)	16	1.08 ± 0.06	0.95 ± 0.05	<0.01	18	1.12 ± 0.04	1.00 ± 0.04	<0.01
Alkaline phosphatase* (IU/L)	13	61 ± 4	78 ± 5	<0.005	13	68 ± 8	82 ± 17	<0.0005

* Patients below 18 years old were excluded

TABLE II. Mean drug levels — over 2 years

	Number	Mean ± SE (μg/ml)	Range	% of patients in optimum range*
Phenytoin	30	9.2 ± 0.7	5.2–16.5	37%
Carbamazepine	33	5.8 ± 0.4	2.5– 8.1	75%

* Optimum range for phenytoin 10–20μg/ml; for carbamazepine 4–8μg/ml

Peripheral nerve

There was no clinical evidence of neuropathy in any of the patients on phenytoin or carbamazepine. There were no electrophysiological abnormalities associated with carbamazepine but 6 out of the 32 patients on phenytoin showed slight electrophysiological changes (Table III). The sural sensory action potential was

TABLE III. Electrophysiological findings in normal controls and patients on carbamazepine or phenytoin

	Number	Age	Sural nerve		Median nerve	
			CV (m/sec)	SAP (μV)	CV (m/sec)	SAP (μV)
Control	20	36 (21–65)	48 ± 4.1	15.3 ± 3.8	56 ± 5.2	18 ± 6.4
Carbamazepine	19	30 (10–59)	49 ± 3.6	18 ± 5.5	53 ± 4.5	18 ± 5.1
Phenytoin						
a) Electrophysiologically normal	26	30 (10–67)	48 ± 6.6	16 ± 4.5	58 ± 5.5	21 ± 5.6
b) Electrophysiologically abnormal	6	35	–	Absent	57	36
		17	42	8	55	22
		21	50	8	50	18
		33	42	8	55	22
		60	38	5	39	10
		24	48	5	54	14

Data is presented as mean ± SD, except for individual data of the 6 abnormal patients on phenytoin

CV = conduction velocity
SAP = sensory action potential

abnormal in six cases, with abnormal sural conduction velocity in one, and reduced median nerve conduction in one.

In Table IV, the 26 patients on phenytoin with normal and the six with abnormal electrophysiological findings are compared. At the time of testing no significant differences were found in the serum phenytoin, serum or red cell folate levels although there were trends towards higher phenytoin and lower folate levels in the electrophysiologically abnormal group. However, the number of patients in the two subgroups with *previous* exposure to high phenytoin levels, or to low folate levels, were significantly different. Sixty-seven per cent of those with abnormal, and 14 per cent of those with normal, electrophysiological findings had been previously exposed to high serum phenytoin levels ($p = 0.01$ x^2 Yates correction); 83 per cent of those with abnormal and 17 per cent of those with normal electrophysiological findings had been exposed to subnormal folate levels ($p = 0.001$ x^2 Yates correction). There was no significant relationship of age, sex or duration of treatment to the electrophysiological findings.

TABLE IV. A comparison of patients on phenytoin with normal and abnormal electrophysiological findings

	At time of electrophysiological examination			Prior to electrophysiological examination	
	Serum phenytoin Mean (range) μg/ml	Serum folate Mean (range) ng/ml	Red blood cell folate Mean (range) ng/ml	Serum phenytoin %	Subnormal folate* %
Normal (n = 26)	9.6 (3.1–26.2)	4.1 (1.4–9.9)	346 (185–683)	14%	17%*
Abnormal (n = 6)	12.5 (3.5–26.7)	3.2 (1.9–7.3)	270 (130–396)	67%	83%
Significance	ns	ns	ns	p = 0.01	p = 0.001

* Subnormal folate: serum folate below 2.0ng/ml and/or red blood cell folate below 160ng/ml

* n = 23

Discussion

After 2 years of single drug therapy in previously untreated epileptic patients the direction of change in the haematological and metabolic indices of chronic toxicity conforms to previous studies in chronic patients on polytherapy [1,2].

These include a rise in MCV and alkaline phosphatase; and a fall in serum and red cell folate, calcium, phosphate and bilirubin. However, in this population the degree of change so far is slight as evidenced by the fact that with the exception of alkaline phosphatase in 8 patients (5 on phenytoin, 3 on carbamazepine) and serum folate in 5 patients (4 on phenytoin, 1 on carbamazepine) none of the variables has deviated from the normal range for our laboratory. Furthermore, we are unaware of any clinical effects of these changes.

Although phenytoin and carbamazepine are structurally very different anti-convulsants it is interesting that so far we have found no significant differences between their effects on any of the metabolic variables examined. This may per-haps be in keeping with the postulated liver enzyme inducing mechanisms for both drugs on bilirubin, vitamin D and folate metabolism [11]. However, it should be noted that the effect of carbamazepine on folate metabolism appears to be less marked than that of phenytoin, especially bearing in mind that twice as many patients on the former drug than the latter were in the optimum range. Other mechanisms, including gut or hormonal effects, have been proposed to account for the influence of anticonvulsants on folate [1,12] and on calcium and vitamin D [1,13] metabolism.

Previous reports of anticonvulsant neuropathy have suggested that the incidence of clinical neuropathy varies between 0–33 per cent and of electrophysiological neuropathy between 0–89 per cent [7]. The possible reasons for these discordant conclusions include: 1) the failure to recognise the reversible slowing of conduction associated with toxic phenytoin levels [7,14]; 2) the study of selected groups of chronic patients on polytherapy without allowing for the possible contribution of other drugs, e.g. barbiturates [7]; and 3) failure to study other factors associated with prolonged therapy, e.g. folate deficiency [15]. In this study we found no clinical evidence of neuropathy in our patients on monotherapy with phenytoin or carbamazepine. However, although there were no electrical changes in patients on carbamazepine, 18 per cent of those on phenytoin had slight electrophysiological abnormalities.

In the patients on phenytoin monotherapy some interesting differences emerged when the six patients with electrophysiological abnormalities were compared with the remaining 26 without such changes (Table IV). The abnormal subgroup had significantly more past evidence of exposure to toxic levels of the drug and to low folate levels. This suggests the possibility that permanent neuropathy due to this drug (and perhaps barbiturates) may result from pro-longed or repeated episodes of intoxication or folate deficiency. This would be consistent with the studies reporting a high incidence of clinical neuropathy in chronic epileptic patients who had a frequent history of past toxicity or high drug levels at the time of testing [7]. There is evidence that severe folate deficiency in non-epileptic subjects may lead to peripheral neuropathy, amongst other neuropsychiatric complications [16,17], and the relationship of the gener-ally milder prolonged anticonvulsant induced folate deficiency to neuropathy

425

in epileptic patients is discussed elsewhere [15].

The relatively trivial and clinically insignificant metabolic and peripheral nerve changes noted so far in these studies contrast with the more widespread and florid abnormalities reported in chronic patients [1,2]. We have argued elsewhere on the basis of our clinical studies in both new referrals and chronic patients that there is much undesirable and unnecessary polytherapy in the treatment of epilepsy [5,18,19]. Although further prolonged follow-up will be of interest the present findings are in keeping with our view that it is possible to greatly reduce the incidence of chronic toxicity by careful monitoring of single drug treatment.

Summary

Metabolic indices of chronic anticonvulsant toxicity (MCV, serum and RBC folate; calcium, phosphate and alkaline phosphatase; bilirubin, protein and albumin) have been measured before and after 2 years of prospectively monitored single drug treatment with phenytoin or carbamazepine. Peripheral nerve function was investigated after 1–5 years treatment with the same individual drugs.

The direction of change of the metabolic indices was in agreement with previous reports of chronic patients on polytherapy but the degree of change was slight and clinically insignificant. There were no significant differences between the metabolic effects of the two drugs. Peripheral nerve function was normal in patients on carbamazepine but 18 per cent of patients on phenytoin had slight electrophysiological abnormalities. The occurrence of the electrophysiological abnormalities was possibly related to previous exposure to high phenytoin and/or low folate levels. Chronic anticonvulsant toxicity can be greatly reduced by careful monitoring of single drug treatment.

Acknowledgments

We are grateful to Drs I Chanarin, A Galbraith, W Marshall and J Payan for help and advice; to Mr M Laundy and Mr L Vydelingum for technical assistance and Dr AL Johnson for statistical advice.

References

1   Reynolds EH. *Epilepsia 1975; 16:* 319–352
2   Reynolds EH. *Irish Med J 1980 (Suppl); 73:* 45–51
3   Shorvon SD, Chadwick D, Galbraith AW, Reynolds EH. *Br med J 1978; 1:* 474–476
4   Shorvon SD, Galbraith AW, Laundy M et al. In Johannessen SI, Morselli PL, Pippenger CE et al, eds. *Antiepileptic Therapy: Advances in Drug Monitoring 1979;* 213–219. New York: Raven Press
5   Reynolds EH, Shorvon SD. *Epilepsia 1981; 22:* 1–10
6   Dellaportas CI, Shorvon SD, Galbraith AW et al. *J Neurol Neurosurg Psychiat 1982.* In press
7   Shorvon SD, Reynolds EH. *Br med J 1982.* In press

8   Burke D, Skuse N, Lethlean A. *J Neurol Neurosurg Psychiat 1974; 37:* 647−652
9   Kupferberg HJ. *Clin Chimi Acta 1970; 29:* 283−288
10   Toseland PA, Grove J, Berry DJ. *Clin Chim Acta 1972; 38:* 321−328
11   Perucca E. In Laidlaw J, Richens A, eds. *A Textbook of Epilepsy 1982.* Edinburgh: Churchill Livingstone
12   Chanarin I. *The Megaloblastic anaemias 1980.* Oxford: Blackwell
13   Stamp TCB. In Preger L, ed. *Induced Disease, Drug Medication and Occupation 1980.* New York: Grune and Stratton
14   Birket-Smith E, Krogh E. *Acta Neurol Scand 1971; 47:* 265−271
15   Shorvon SD. In Botez MI, Reynolds EH, eds. *Folic Acid in Neurology, Psychiatry and Internal Medicine 1979;* 335−346. New York: Raven Press
16   Shorvon SD, Reynolds EH. In Botez MI, Reynolds EH, eds. *Folic Acid in Neurology, Psychiatry and Internal Medicine 1979;* 413−421. New York: Raven Press
17   Shorvon SD, Carney MWP, Chanarin I, Reynolds EH. *Br med J 1980; 281:* 1036−1038
18   Shorvon SD, Reynolds EH. *Br med J 1977; 1:* 1635−1637
19   Shorvon SD, Reynolds EH. *Br med J 1979; 2:* 1023−1025

46

THE INFLUENCE OF ANTICONVULSANT DRUGS ON COGNITIVE FUNCTION AND BEHAVIOUR

M R Trimble, P J Thompson

Cognitive function

The relative part that anticonvulsants play in the production of cognitive disabilities and mental deterioration in epileptic patients has not been much explored. Lennox [1] suggested that such drugs were responsible for intellectual deterioration in 15 per cent of his patients, although later he reduced this to 5 per cent [2]. A recent review of the subject has emphasised not only that few of the drugs used in treatment have been evaluated, but also that most of the studies were carried out prior to the availability of serum anticonvulsant estimations [3]. In order to explore further the interrelationships of anticonvulsant blood levels to cognitive function a series of studies has been carried out on patients with epilepsy, and volunteers.

STUDY 1

Methods

Three hundred and twelve of 314 epileptic children resident at a hospital school received a neuropsychiatric examination. Information on their cognitive abilities was provided by the school psychologist. A number of children (207) had been assessed on more than one occasion while at the school, and it was possible to detect from these a group of children whose IQ (WISC or equivalent) had fallen. The criteria taken for intellectual deterioration were a sustained fall in IQ of more than 10 points occurring in two tests over one year apart. Blood was taken from the children for assessment of blood levels of phenytoin, primidone, phenobarbitone and carbamazepine. Information about a variety of other parameters such as seizure type, frequency, drugs administered, etc., were obtained from the children's case notes.

428

In order to assess drug effects, the data were analysed in three ways. First, serum levels of children with a fall in IQ were compared with the rest of the children. Secondly, the incidence of deterioration in children with high serum levels (arbitrarily taken as above 60μmol/L for phenytoin, above 80μmol/L for phenobarbitone, above 20μmol/L for primidone and above 24μmol/L for carbamazepine) was compared to the children with below such values. Finally, Pearson correlation coefficients between individual IQ scores and the serum levels of the drugs were calculated on children with an IQ > 70.

Results

Of the 312 children studied 219 were males. Of 204 children who had two or more measurements of IQ, 31 (= 15.2 per cent) had a fall in IQ. In the majority of these the fall was more than 15 points, and in some considerable (range 10 to 48 points).

TABLE I. Mean serum levels ± standard deviations (number in brackets)

	Phenytoin μmol/L	Primidone μmol/L	Phenobarbitone μmol/L	Carbamazepine μmol/L
Fall in IQ:				
Present	39.2 ± 28.5* (19)	23.4 ± 3.8** (10)	80.5 ± 40.9 (13)	15.5 ± 2.6 ((3)
Absent	28.4 ± 22.2* (166)	19.5 ± 13.8* (63)	68.8 ± 38.3 (97)	16.7 ± 7.6 (48)

't' test present v absent: * $p < 0.05$; ** $p < 0.01$

TABLE II. Fall in IQ in patients with high serum levels of anticonvulsants (μmol/L)

	Phenytoin < 60	Phenytoin > 60	Primidone < 20	Primidone > 20	Phenobarbitone < 80	Phenobarbitone > 80	Carbamazepine < 24	Carbamazepine > 24
Fall in IQ:								
Present	26	5	21	10	24	7	0	2
Absent	229	11	199	41	203	37	8	42
x^2	5.58*		4.15*		0.4		0.4	

* x^2 result $p < 0.05$

Table I shows the mean serum levels of anticonvulsant drugs in those children with a fall in IQ, compared with the rest of the children. Table II shows the numbers of children with such a fall having high serum anticonvulsant levels compared to those with lower levels.

429

These results indicate that children with a fall in their IQ have significantly higher levels of serum phenytoin and primidone than the other children in the study. The mean level for phenytoin is within the accepted tolerance limits for the drug. Similarly, children with higher levels of phenytoin and primidone have a higher incidence of deterioration than children with lower levels. Table III shows the Pearson correlation coefficients between IQ estimates and serum levels in children with an IQ > 70. It indicates negative correlations between all full-scale estimates and performance scale estimates of IQ and the serum levels of the drugs under study. Significant negative correlations are noted between phenytoin and the full-scale IQ, and phenytoin and phenobarbitone and the performance scale IQ. A trend towards significance is noted with primidone and the performance IQ.

TABLE III. Correlation coefficients between IQ estimates and serum anticonvulsant levels (IQ > 70 only) (number in brackets)

	Phenytoin	Phenobarbitone	Primidone	Carbamazepine
IQ Full-scale	−0.20 (86)	−0.20 (46)	−0.22 (35)	−0.22 (18)
p	<0.06	NS	NS	NS
IQ Verbal scale	−0.17 (84)	+0.12 (43)	+0.08 (33)	−0.25 (18)
p	NS	NS	NS	NS
IQ Performance scale	−0.22 (84)	−0.36 (43)	−0.30 (33)	−0.13 (18)
p	<0.04	<0.02	<0.10	NS

No relationship was found between seizure frequency and fall in IQ. There was no age or sex difference between the children on the drugs under study. Neither was there any difference between the numbers of children on the drugs under study that had gross brain damage, frequent seizures, or any particular type of epileptic discharge as recorded on the electroencephalogram.

TABLE IV. Mean serum levels (μmol/L) of anticonvulsants ± standard deviations and fall in IQ (number in brackets)

	PHENYTOIN Present	Absent	PRIMIDONE Present	Absent
< 10 seizures per month	41.8 ± 26.0 (13)*	28.6 ± 23.0 (114)*	22.6 ± 3.9 (5)	20.5 ± 13.7 (40)
IQ > 70	46.4 ± 31.2 (7)**	26.5 ± 20.9 (75)**	21.0 ± 2.0 (4)	21.5 ± 15.2 (29)
	PHENOBARBITONE Present	Absent	CARBAMAZEPINE Present	Absent
< 10 seizures per month	82.6 ± 43.8 (7)	66.5 ± 35.6 (60)	15.5 ± 2.6 (3)	17.1 ± 5.5 (27)
IQ > 70	69.6 ± 35.7 ((5)	70.4 ± 38.5 (38)	†	†

't' test present vs absent: *p<0.05; **p<0.01
† Numbers too small to analyse

430

In order to rule out some other factors that may be influencing IQ, the mean serum levels were re-examined in populations of children with low seizure frequency (< 10 per month), and in children with higher IQs (> 70) – (Table IV).

Table IV shows that even when these selected populations were examined, the phenytoin levels were still significantly elevated in the children with deterioration of intellectual abilities.

STUDY 2

Interpretation of the above study was difficult since many children were on polypharmacy, seizure frequency was difficult to quantify, and measurement of cognitive function was undertaken using psychological tests standardised for the assessment of intelligence, not for the detection of drug effects. To explore further the relationship between anticonvulsants and cognitive function, preliminary studies were undertaken in non-epileptic volunteers who were prescribed one drug for two weeks. These studies had the advantage of allowing for a carefully controlled and balanced design, including comparison with placebo, which is often not possible in patients with epilepsy for ethical and treatment reasons. For the assessment of cognitive functions a series of tests was designed specifically to monitor drug effects. The psychological measures covered various aspects of cognition in which patients with epilepsy often show difficulty, especially memory which will be discussed here.

In three consecutive trials different groups of subjects were prescribed phenytoin, carbamazepine and sodium valproate respectively. The general design will be described for the phenytoin trial, details of the other two trials being mentioned where they differ from this.

Method

Phenytoin

Subjects Eight non-epileptic male volunteers with a mean age of 23 (range 18 to 32) took part in the study.

Design Subjects were prescribed phenytoin 100mg capsules three times a day for two weeks in a double blind cross-over design with identical placebo capsules. Four subjects received phenytoin in the first treatment period and four in the second treatment period. Psychological testing took place on three occasions: (a) a baseline measure immediately prior to treatment; (b) at the end of the first treatment; and (c) at the end of the second treatment. On completion of the second and third sessions, a blood sample was taken for the measurement of anticonvulsant serum levels and to check compliance.

431

Carbamazepine

Subjects Eight male subjects with a mean age of 23 (range 19 to 28) participated in the study.

Design Subjects were prescribed carbamazepine 200mg tablets three times a day and identical placebo tablets each for a period of two weeks.

Sodium valproate

Subjects Ten male subjects with a mean age of 26 (range 19 to 33) participated in the study.

Design Subjects were prescribed sodium valproate tablets and identical placebo tablets each for a period of two weeks. Dosage of sodium valproate was increased from one tablet a day (200mg) to four tablets a day (800mg) in the first three days of treatment and by an additional tablet to five tablets (1,000mg) in the second week. A one-week 'wash-out' period, during which neither active drug or placebo was taken, was included because of reports of carry-over effects of this drug [4].

Psychological measures

At the beginning of each session, 20 slides of coloured magazine pictures were presented. Individual pictures were exposed for 1.5 seconds with an inter-slide interval of 1.5 seconds. Subjects were told to try and remember the pictures. Following a one-minute retention interval, filled with conversation, immediate recall for the pictures was tested by asking the subjects to describe as many of the pictures as they could. A similar procedure was repeated but with 20 slides of single common words. Delayed recall for both pictures and words was tested an hour later after the administration of other psychological tests. On completion of each recall test a 'Yes'/'No' recognition test took place. For each type of material the original 20 stimulus items were presented again, randomly interspersed with 20 new slides. The subjects were requested to say whether or not they had seen the slides at the beginning of the session. If the subject was in any doubt a guess was encouraged.

A different set of stimulus items and distractors were used on the three sessions. These had been shown to be matched for difficulty.

Analysis of data

To reduce the influence of initial variance in level of performance between subjects, analysis of the results was based on the difference score between the pre-treatment baseline and the drug and the placebo sessions. Three-way analysis of variance was computed on these scores in which treatment effects, session effects and individual differences were the factors.

TABLE V. Means on the memory tests in the three drug trials

	TRIAL 1: Phenytoin N = 8		TRIAL 2: Carbamazepine N = 8		TRIAL 3: Sodium valproate N = 10	
	Phenytoin ($\bar{X}$ 39.4μmol/L)	Placebo	Carbamazepine ($\bar{X}$ 30.4μmol/L)	Placebo	Sodium valproate ($\bar{X}$ = 452.3μmol/L)	Placebo
PICTURES						
Immediate recall (max = 20)	10.9	12.3	12.1	12.9	12.0	12.0
Delayed recall (max = 20)	10.1	12.3*	11.1	12.3	10.7	11.9
Recognition (max = 40)	39.4	39.8	38.6	39.8	39.7	39.7
WORDS						
Immediate recall (max = 20)	6.6	8.8*	7.4	8.8	7.4	8.1
Delayed recall (max = 20)	3.4	6.0	5.3	6.3	6.4	6.3
Recognition (max = 40)	30.6	32.4	31.5	31.6	30.6	31.0

* $p < 0.05$

433

Results

Mean scores on the memory tests in the drug and placebo conditions of the three trials are presented in Table V.

Phenytoin

Fewer pictures were recalled in the phenytoin condition, a significant effect being observed on the test of delayed recall ($F = 7.8$; $p < 0.05$). Scores on the recognition test were not analysed statistically because of the occurrence of a ceiling effect.

Recall of words was also impaired on phenytoin in comparison with placebo and statistical differences were found on the immediate recall test ($F = 6.6$; $p < 0.05$). Performance on the recognition test (total number of correct responses) revealed no significant drug effect.

Serum levels The mean phenytoin serum level of the eight subjects was 39.4μmol/L with a range of 16 to 78μmol/L. The mean value falls just below the commonly quoted therapeutic range, 40 to 80μmol/L [5].

Carbamazepine

There was a consistent trend toward impaired performance on the drug in comparison with placebo, but no significant differences between treatments were observed.

Serum levels The mean serum level of the eight subjects was 30.4μmol/L with a range of 25 to 50μmol/L, a mean figure within the therapeutic range [6].

Sodium Valproate

No statistically significant differences between drug and placebo sessions were observed for sodium valproate, neither was there any tendency of impaired performance on the drug.

Serum levels The mean serum level of the ten subjects was 452.3μmol/L with a range of 265 to 805μmol/L, a mean figure within the therapeutic range of 300 to 600μmol/L [6].

Discussion

The results of the first study suggest that epileptic children with a fall in IQ have significantly higher levels of serum phenytoin than children without such a fall. In addition negative correlations occur between measures of performance IQ and

434

serum levels of all three drugs under study — significant for phenytoin and phenobarbitone. The results for phenytoin lend support for observations of others that a chronic deterioration of intellectual function can occur with this drug [7], and that such an effect may occur at serum levels considered to be within the therapeutic range [8]. This effect is unlikely to be due to seizure frequency, since the results are similar where children having a large number of seizures are omitted from the analysis. We attempted to avoid the problems of measuring IQ at lower levels by examining a population of children with an IQ of more than 70; but the mean levels of phenytoin are still elevated in the population with intellectual deterioration.

In addition these data show negative correlations between serum anticonvulsant levels and actual IQ scores. A review of literature [9] indicates that such effects have been reported by others, although which drugs are most likely to produce this effect has not been adequately explored. The correlations here are stronger for phenytoin and phenobarbitone. A problem of interpretation of this study was that all the children were receiving polytherapy, and interactional effects were impossible to rule out. For this reason the second study was initiated in which volunteers, thus free from factors such as seizures which may interfere with cognitive ability, were used, and drugs were given in a controlled double-blind fashion compared to placebo. This also demonstrated differences between anticonvulsant drugs. Phenytoin interfered with immediate and delayed recall of words and pictures, significantly so in some measures. In comparison carbamazepine resulted in less impairment of performance on these measures, no significant differences being recorded.

These results in volunteers are in keeping with the results of Study 1 with regard to the deleterious effect of phenytoin on cognitive function and the differences between this drug and carbamazepine. It also supports many reports in the literature which suggest that changing patients from phenytoin to carbamazepine is accompanied by beneficial effects on cognition [10]. The results with sodium valproate are also of interest. Although it has been claimed that this drug has psychotropic effects [11], very few studies of its relationship to cognitive function have been undertaken. In this study it is clearly different from phenytoin, producing no deficits in immediate or delayed recall, being similar, therefore, to carbamazepine.

For ethical reasons, the volunteer study was carried out on adults, and similar trials in children are not likely to be undertaken. However, when acknowledging that deleterious effects of such drugs on cognitive function as important in adults, we believe that recognition of such problems in children is of utmost importance, and clearly further studies in such patients are necessary.

Behaviour

There are many studies which anecdotally suggest anticonvulsant drugs adversely influence behaviour, although few have been carried out using appropriate designs with measurement of behavioural change [3]. Results are here presented from our studies with epileptic patients and volunteers.

STUDY 3

Methods

The population was the same as for Study 1. The teachers and the house parents at the school were asked to complete standardised behaviour rating scales on the children [12], and, in those rated as 'deviant', individual items of the questionnaire were extracted to provide scores for either 'neurotic' or 'conduct' deviance. Depending on the resulting category, children were diagnosed as having either 'neurotic' or 'conduct' disorder.

In addition, as part of a more general neuropsychiatric examination, irritability and depression were assessed. The criteria for these were scored on a 0–3 scale. In the final analysis a score of 0 or 1 was taken to indicate the disorder was absent, and a score of 2 or 3 that the disorder was present. In a brief pilot study the inter-observer consistency of these measures was found to be 97.4 per cent and 87.2 per cent respectively. The validity and reliability of the behaviour rating scales have been assessed and found satisfactory [12].

Blood was taken for serum anticonvulsant level monitoring as near as possible to the behaviour rating.

Results

The frequency of the behaviour disorders is given in Table VI which the house-parents' scale is referred to as the 'A' scale and the teachers' scale as the 'B' scale. This indicates that conduct disorder is the commonest category of abnormal behaviour in this population. Depression was recorded in 5.1 per cent of the total sample. No drug appeared to be significantly associated with conduct disorder, but the highest incidence of this pattern of behaviour was recorded with phenobarbitone, 50 per cent of the children on this drug having conduct disorder. It was least associated with carbamazepine and sulthiame.

TABLE VI. Percentage frequency of behaviour disorders

	A scale only	B scale only	Both A & B	Total
Neurotic disorder	13.8	8.7	3.8	26.3
Conduct disorder	17.3	11.9	13.1	42.3
Irritability	2.9			
Depression	5.1			

TABLE VII. Mean serum levels (μmol/L) ± standard deviations for children with and without behavioural side effects (number in brackets)

| | NEUROTIC DISORDER | | CONDUCT DISORDER | |
	Present	Absent	Present	Absent
Phenobarbitone	72.5 ± 40.2 (12)	69.1 ± 38.0 (101)	71.8 ± 34.1 (20)	68.5 ± 38.3 (67)
Phenytoin	35.2 ± 23.5 (28)	30.9 ± 26.0 (157)	34.3 ± 26.8 (37)	29.9 ± 22.0 (122)
Primidone	22.8 ± 17.4 (6)	21.7 ± 13.0 (66)	16.1 ± 13.7 (16)	21.2 ± 14.0 (41)
Carbamazepine	16.0 ± 11.2 (6)	16.1 ± 6.8 (37)	11.5 ± 7.6 (5)	15.8 ± 6.8 (30)

| | IRRITABILITY | | DEPRESSION | |
	Present	Absent	Present	Absent
Phenobarbitone	79.5 ± 37.0 (6)	69.3 ± 39.3 (117)	74.7 ± 20.1 (4)	69.7 ± 39.4 (119)
Phenytoin	22.8 ± 14.6 (6)	31.3 ± 25.5 (206)	29.3 ± 13.2 (13)	31.0 ± 25.5 (199)
Primidone	22.0 ± 3.4 (3)	21.1 ± 13.9 (76)	Insufficient numbers	
Carbamazepine	Insufficient numbers		15.8 ± 10.4 (5)	16.4 ± 7.2 (48)

Table VII shows the mean serum values of the anticonvulsants for the populations of children with and without behaviour abnormalities. This table indicates only non-significant trends towards high serum levels of phenobarbitone in children with irritability and depression, and lower levels of primidone and carbamazepine in patients with conduct disorder.

In an attempt to minimise the effects of brain damage and low IQ on behaviour, the results were re-examined on a population of children who had an IQ greater than 70 points. Table VIII gives the mean serum level results for this population

TABLE VIII. Mean serum levels of drugs (μmol/L) ± standard deviations in children with IQ > 70 and behaviour abnormalities (number in brackets)

| | NEUROTIC DISORDER | | CONDUCT DISORDER | |
	Present	Absent	Present	Absent
Phenobarbitone	44.2 ± 28.5 (4)	74.8 ± 37.5 (45)*	62.8 ± 29.0 (9)	66.0 ± 32.4 (32)
Phenytoin	33.1 ± 27.7 (12)	27.8 ± 21.7 (73)	33.3 ± 20.4 (10)	27.7 ± 21.5 (62)
Primidone	14.3 ± 12.5 (3)	23.3 ± 15.1 (33)	17.5 ± 16.2 (8)	23.5 ± 16.0 (22)
Carbamazepine	Insufficient for analysis		Insufficient for analysis	

* 't' test p < 0.05

for conduct disorder and neurotic disorder (there were insufficient numbers of children with irritability and depression for a meaningful analysis), and Table IX

437

TABLE IX. Spearman correlation coefficients between serum anticonvulsant levels and abnormal behaviour scores (IQ > 70 points)

	Neurotic disorder	Conduct disorder
Phenobarbitone	+0.01 (50)	+0.19 (24)*
Phenytoin	0.00 (20)	+0.04 (50)
Primidone	−0.19 (24)	+0.09 (20)
Carbamazepine	−0.24 (10)	−0.48 (10)*

* Carbamazepine vs phenobarbitone p < 0.05

the correlation coefficients between the serum levels and the actual deviant behaviour score taken from the rating scales in those children who were rated as having abnormal behaviour. These tables indicate lower mean levels of phenobarbitone and primidone (significant at the < 0.05 level for the former) in children with neurotic behaviour disturbances. The direction of the correlation between conduct disorder and serum levels of all drugs except carbamazepine was positive. For the latter the higher the serum level the less the deviance score. The difference between the correlations for conduct disorder and phenobarbitone, and that for carbamazepine is significant (p < 0.05).

In order to rule out other factors, such as seizure frequency, that may influence the behaviour of children, the results were examined in a population of children having infrequent seizures (less than 10 per month), and the results were similar to Table IV, indicating no significant differences between the groups for mean serum level estimations. No significant relationships were detected between seizure frequency and either neurotic or conduct disorder, although children with frequent seizures had a higher incidence of irritability and depression. The distribution of the children with regard to seizure frequency and seizure type, especially with reference to focal epilepsy on the different drugs, revealed no differences except for a tendency for children on sodium valproate to have a higher seizure frequency [13]. Age, sex, or length of time that the children had seizures were similar for all the different drug groups.

STUDY 4

In the three drug trials outlined in Study 2, a Mood Adjective Check List (MACL) adapted from McNair and Lorr [14], was used to measure the affective state of the subject. The MACL consisted of 24 adjectives, descriptive of various mood states, each to be rated on a 4-point intensity scale. At the beginning of each testing session, subjects completed the MACL indicating how they felt at that moment in time.

Results were analysed non-parametrically using Wilcoxon t tests [15].

Phenytoin

On phenytoin, subjects rated themselves as feeling more anxious, less active, more tired, more aggressive and more depressed in comparison with placebo. Differences in ratings were significant only for ratings of tiredness ($p < 0.01$).

Carbamazepine

Differences in mood ratings between carbamazepine and placebo conditions were small and non-significant. All changes in mood observed, however, suggested improvement on carbamazepine.

Sodium valproate

There were no significant differences in ratings between the sodium valproate and placebo conditions. Neither was there any consistent trend in that subjects rated themselves more tired, less active but less aggressive on valproate in comparison with placebo.

Discussion

The children from Study 1 had a variety of types of epilepsy, and were usually on more than one drug. However, they provided a suitable sample for study, in that accurate and careful records of their seizure frequency and drug administration were kept, and behaviour was evaluated using standardised rating scales. The dichotomy between neurotic and conduct disorder used has been evaluated previously, and the scales assessed for both reliability and validity [12]. Although the classification is entirely phenomenological, the scales distinguish adequately between children attending child guidance clinics and the general population, and the individual items used to make up neurotic and conduct disorder categories can be identified clinically [12].

The results suggest that phenobarbitone has different effects on conduct and neurotic disorder, such that this drug may exacerbate the former, but alleviate the latter. This is in keeping with anecdotal reports that phenobarbitone makes impulsive and aggressive behaviour in children worse, although this fact has never before been systematically studied [3], and with the known anxiolytic effect of the barbiturates. Similarly the low incidence of neurotic disorder associated with primidone reflects anecdotal reports. Whether this is due to the phenobarbitone which results from primidone metabolism, or is an independent effect of the primidone is uncertain. The finding that sulthiame is least associated with conduct disorder is in keeping with reports that this drug has been used in the management of behaviour disorders in children [16].

The serum level results on the total sample of patients did not give further help in assessing the behavioural effects of the drugs. The lower mean levels noted of carbamazepine and primidone in children with conduct disorders and higher levels of phenobarbitone in children with irritability and depression support the suggestions made above. Behaviour is influenced by a number of other factors, some of which are probably more liable to produce disturbances than the drug effects, and thus analysis of the total sample may not be expected to detect significant relationships. Neither seizure frequency nor site of focal discharge on the EEG was significantly related to neurotic or conduct disturbances, and re-analysis of the results on the population of children with infrequent seizures produced the same result pattern. By examining only the population of children with an IQ of more than 70 it was possible to minimise the effects of low IQ and gross brain damage on the results. With such an analysis a clearer pattern of drug effects related to mean serum levels emerged. The negative relationship between phenobarbitone and primidone and neurotic disorder suggested from the whole sample analysis was still found, although the correlation coefficients do not suggest this was a dose-related effect. The association between phenobarbitone and conduct disorder was less clear, suggesting that children with higher IQs may be less prone to develop such abnormalities than others. Correlation coefficients support a dose-dependent effect for carbamazepine. Thus a negative correlation coefficient between conduct disorder and the serum carbamazepine level was found, significantly different from the phenobarbitone correlation coefficient, highlighting the differential effects of these two drugs on conduct disorder. This is in keeping with the idea that carbamazepine is psychotropic, an effect often observed clinically but poorly investigated [17]. The fact that this relationship was detected in the brighter children only is important, since some studies that have failed to detect psychotropic properties with this compound have been carried out on subnormal patients in an institutionalised setting (for references see [10]). The volunteer study with adults indicated some possible positive effects on mood for carbamazepine, although these were non-significant. This is not surprising since the subjects were non-depressed. The results are in keeping however with a recent study [18] in which carbamazepine was given in a double-blind trial to 10 manic-depressive patients and found to be superior than placebo in controlling abnormal mood states.

Our studies are an attempt to assess the relative influence of anticonvulsant drugs on both cognitive function and behaviour. Further studies are in progress,

TABLE X. Effects of anticonvulsant drugs on cognition and behaviour

	Negative	Positive
Cognition	Phenytoin ? Phenobarbitone	? Carbamazepine
Behaviour	Phenobarbitone (Conduct, irritability, etc.)	Phenobarbitone (anxiolytic in children) Sulthiame Carbamazepine

not only on volunteers, but also on patients, both adult and children. A tentative summary of the data so far may be given as in Table X but, as our methods of investigation improve, and as newer and hopefully safer anticonvulsant drugs become available, such conclusions must still be regarded as tentative.

Acknowledgments

The authors wish to acknowledge Dr T C Nicol and Dr P Dupré of Lingfield Hospital School for their help; and Miss E A Paul for her guidance with statistics.

The study has been supported by the Shorvon Fund, the Brain Research Trust, and the Thorn Epilepsy Research Fund.

References

1 Lennox WG. *Am J Psychiat 1942; 99:* 174—180
2 Lennox WG, Lennox MA. *Epilepsy and Related Disorders 1960.* Boston: Little Brown
3 Trimble MR, Reynolds EH. *Psychol Med 1976; 6:* 169—178
4 Rowan AJ, Binnie CD, Warfield CA, et al. *Epilepsia 1979; 20:* 61—68
5 Richens A. *Drug Treatment of Epilepsy 1976.* London: Henry Kimpton
6 Eadie MJ, Tyrer JH. *Anticonvulsant Therapy. Pharmacological Basis and Practice 1980.* London: Churchill Livingstone
7 Vallarta JM, Bell DB, Reichert A. *Am J Dis Childh 1974; 128:* 27—34
8 Reynolds EH, Travers R. *Br J Psychiat 1974; 124:* 440—445
9 Trimble MR. In Essman W, Valzelli L, eds. *Current Developments in Psychopharmacology 6, 1981.* New York: Spectrum Publications Inc
10 Trimble MR, Richens A. *Advanc Hum Psychopharmacol 1981; 2:* 183—202
11 Jeavons PM, Clark JE. *Br Med J 1974; 2:* 584—586
12 Rutter M, Graham P, Yule W. *A Neuropsychiatric Study in Childhood 1970.* Philadelphia: Spastics International Medical Publications
13 Trimble MR, Corbett JA. *Irish Med J 1980; Suppl 73:* 21—28
14 McNair DM, Lorr M. *J Abnorm Soc Psychol 1964; 69:* 620—627
15 Siegal S. *Non-parametric Statistics for the Behavioural Sciences 1955.* London: McGraw Hill
16 Moffatt WR, Siddiqui AR, Mackay DN. *Br J Psychiat 1970; 117:* 673—678
17 Trimble MR. *Epilepsia 1978; 19:* 241—250
18 Ballenger JC, Post RM. *Commun Psychopharmacol 1978; 2:* 159—175

47

AUTOMATED PSYCHOLOGICAL TESTING IN THE CONTROL OF ANTICONVULSANT MEDICATION

A Elithorn, A Stavrou, J Powell

Introduction

In clinical work psychological testing is almost invariably undertaken on an individual basis. It is hence time consuming and labour intensive. Psychologists are expensive professional people and the automation of many psychological tests with inexpensive microprocessors can easily be made cost effective. This unfortunately may tend to obscure and delay the development of some of the important improvements which computer techniques can bring to psychological testing.

In this chapter, we argue not just that computer automation will make the clinical psychologist's life much easier but also that computer technology can increase the power and sensitivity of tests in ways which open up a range of novel, important and cost effective applications.

A microprocessor test system to be effective need only be powerful enough to administer a single test or questionnaire on a 'stand alone basis'. The data obtained can then either be transferred to a data bank at a large central computing facility or stored locally on 'floppy discs' or on a larger disc storage unit shared by several test terminals. In a similar way, a library of test programs can be stored either locally or centrally and down-loaded as needed into the test terminal [1]. The system described in this chapter, which is based on this intelligent terminal concept, was first implemented on a PDP8 with the addition of a special interface and keyboard. It is now available on the British made RML 380Z systems and can be adapted to other Z80 based systems such as the North Star Horizon which use the S100 Bus. It will shortly be available on the Apple, using an additional Z-80 card.

The system provides a moderately complex graphic display and the duration of each stimulus and the timing of each inter-stimulus interval is accurately controlled. The subject's responses are timed accurately, to the nearest millisecond. Its operation does not require expert knowledge and it can be operated by nursing staff, receptionists, or by the patient himself.

Epilepsy affects mental functions in two distinct ways. In general, a reduction in fit frequency is followed by an increase in mental efficiency and social competence. Occasionally fit suppression may lead to an increase in inter-ictal abnormal electrical activity and hence to the impairment of the patient's intellectual functions and also his emotional control. However, some anticonvulsants produce fit control by reducing abnormal electrical activity overall while others act primarily by reducing the frequency with which focal discharges erupt in a generalised storm.

The second way in which anticonvulsants affect mental functions is through their side effects. With one or two exceptions anticonvulsants are depressant and in most subjects impair both intellectual and psychomotor performance. However, amphetamine which has an anticonvulsant effect, is a stimulant and stimulant effects have also been recorded with phenytoin and ethosuximide.

Many anticonvulsants produce other unwanted and sometimes dangerous side effects and the use of any particular drug can only be justified if the degree of overall improvement brought about justifies the risks and side effects involved. No physician would dream of treating hypertension without measuring the effect of the treatment on the patient's blood pressure. In treating neurological disorders it is equally desirable to measure and record the effect that treatment has on the patient's mental competence. Attempts to achieve this with conventional psychological tests, even in research trials has been demonstrably unsatisfactory. Thus a review of a number of psychological studies on the effects of Levo-dopa on the mental status of patients suffering from Parkinsonism showed that results from different studies were contradictory [2]. Some workers found that Levo-dopa produced no effect on mental functions, others reported an improvement, whilst a third group claimed that Levo-dopa produced intellectual deterioration. While existing psychological tests may be effective in assessing gross differences between individuals and the relatively large intra-individual changes which accompany maturation and education, they are insensitive to small changes in individual competence and unsuited to the repeated testing of the same individual. This however need not be the case with computer based criterion referenced tests. Computer techniques can also bring to the clinic techniques which previously were only available in psychological laboratories. Thus in a pilot study, John Weinmann and the senior author (AE), using a small battery of automated tests based on a PDP8 system, were able to show that the main changes in intellectual functions produced by Levo-dopa could be related to its arousal or alerting effect and its stimulating action on mood [2].

Tailored testing — the application of process control methodology to psychological test procedures — is one very important development that computer techniques make possible. In tailored testing the subject's performance is continuously assessed and the test items presented are selected according to the pattern of the subject's performance to date. In tailored aptitude testing as developed in the US, a large number of standardised items must be stored by the computer. With performance criterion referenced tests such as the Perceptual Maze Test or the Digit Span Test the subject's performance can be related to a variable such as the size of the maze item or the length of the string of digits presented and it is possible for the computer to generate items randomly using a specification determined by the subject's performance. For example, with the digit span test, each time the subject recalls a string of digits correctly a longer string is generated; if he fails, a shorter string is generated. Such programmed testing has two advantages. Firstly the testing procedure is concentrated at the level of ability appropriate to the subject. This means that less time is wasted presenting items which are either far too simple for that subject or which are much too difficult. Testing is more efficient. Secondly, items which are too easy tend to bore and irritate the more intelligent subject while continual failure frustrates and depresses most people. Tailored testing is therefore more rewarding in terms of success and failure and hence the subject's motivation is greater and again testing is more efficient.

Behavioural fragmentation

A second advantage of automating psychological tests is that computer presentation makes it much easier to control a subject's performance in detail. Not only can the presentation of items and the subject's overall response be timed accurately but different aspects of the subject's performance can be isolated and timed separately. This means that we can extract information about a subject's psychomotor skills from a test which also samples cognitive skill. This facility to analyse test performance in detail means that the psychologist can analyse the different ways in which different subjects attain the same level of performance − their cognitive style [3].

Many psychological tests lend themselves readily to automation and those we have so far programmed include: Digit Span, a Digit Symbol Coding Test, the PMT, a Tracking Task, Memory Tests for words and nonsense syllables, Self-Recording Analogue Scales, a Tapping Test, Visual and Sound Reaction Time Tests, an Adjective Check List, a Stress Questionnaire, Tests of Reading Speed, a Vigilance Test, and a Three Letter Word Recognition Test which has been shown to correlate well with linguistic skill.

Anticonvulsant medication

In the past, the benefits of fit control have often overshadowed the sedative depressant effect which many anticonvulsants have on a range of mental functions, but many modern anticonvulsants overall are less sedative than their predecessors and clinicians have a wider choice and more difficult decisions. In general, it is best to choose the anticonvulsant which is effective and has the least side effects but the choice of a particular treatment regimen should always depend on the balance of advantages and disadvantages to the patient concerned.

In some cases the certainty of a depressant effect must be balanced against the remote possibility of a fatal blood dyscrasia. At a simpler level, it was shown in one study that 12 per cent of all women and in another that 27 per cent of middle-aged women were regular and recent users of tranquillisers [4]. Patients with epilepsy are more likely than control subjects to exhibit anxiety symptoms, though these may be overshadowed by their convulsions. The effects of the sedative depressant action of an anticonvulsant regimen may therefore in some patients be beneficial. In one study of the effects of sedative drugs on car driving, it was shown that, compared with the placebo, clobazam improved the scores of 12 neurotic patients in four out of five of the measures of car driving [5].

Microprocessor-based psychological testing combined with some recently developed methods of statistical analysis now make it practicable to record and analyse day-to-day fluctuations in mental competence which in part may reflect minor changes in an anticonvulsant treatment regime. The value of intervention studies using these techniques for monitoring the use of psychotropic drugs in neurotic and psychotic patients has been reported elsewhere [6] and a validation study of the value of monitoring the sedative and depressant effects of anticonvulsant drugs is currently taking place at the Chalfont Epileptic Centre.

Apart from the depressant — or stimulant — side effects, anticonvulsants affect mental processes in a variety of ways. Fit suppression in general has a psychologically beneficial effect — essentially a psychotherapeutic one. The reduction of abnormal electrical activity, which is usually associated with the therapeutic control of fits, is also often accompanied by an improvement in many mental functions and the effect is sometimes dramatic, but anticonvulsants act in more than one way and occasionally a reduction in fit frequency may be accompanied by an increase in interictal electrical activity. Geier [7] has argued plausibly that "the clinical manifestations of epilepsy are generally briefer than the accompanying EEG paroxysms" but his argument that "all electroclinical correlations are valid only statistically and never on an individual basis. . ." is less cogent. In this chapter we argue, on the basis of studies with two psychiatric patients with focal EEG abnormalities, that drug-induced but minor fluctuations in abnormal electrical activity may at times be accompanied by changes in mental functions which are subclinical merely because our existing techniques for assessing a patient's mental state are too insensitive.

Single subject intervention studies

Two inpatients were tested daily at the same time of day, with a small battery of automated psychological tests. Treatment changes were determined solely by clinical need and were blind to the test system. The results reported here are those obtained with the automated version of the Perceptual Maze Test (PMT). The PMT presents subjects with a complex cognitive and perceptual task which has proved particularly suitable for automation and computer analysis. It is a criterion referenced performance test which has been identified by Butcher [8] as a test which bridges the gap between psychometric endeavour and experimental psychology. It is a relatively pure measure of perceptual speed [9] which is particularly sensitive to both biochemical and physical impairment of right hemisphere functions [10,11]. A sample item from the neuropsychiatric version of the PMT test is presented in Figure 1.

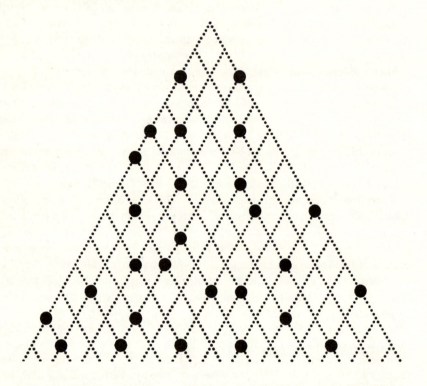

Figure 1. In this test the subject's task is to find a pathway along the background lattice which passes through the greatest number of target dots. At each intersection the path must continue forward, i.e. the subject may fork right or left but must not double back. In general, there is more than one solution. A subject is either told the maximum score he can obtain, or this information is withheld. Conventionally, these two methods of presentation are called the 'with information condition' and the 'without information condition'

In the computer version of the test, the subject using left and right response keys fills in a pathway on a CCTV video display. Additional keys allow the subject to make corrections and indicate when he is ready for the next item. Each key response is timed individually. The analysis of the subject's performance provides a number of indices which reflect different aspects of his performance. Those used in the present study are:

446

1. Search time:	The time from stimulus onset until the first motor response
2. Track time:	The time from the first motor response until the completion of the task
3. Check time:	The time between a subject completing his tracking and his signifying that he is satisifed with his solution
4. Non fatal errors:	Number of corrections per item
5. Fatal errors:	Number of items incorrect
6. Motor index:	Average of fastest 10 per cent of key response
7. Refresh index:	Number of pauses >1 sec during the tracking phase
8. Laterality index:	Percentage of right preferences

The first subject reported is a patient suffering from a severe schizo-affective illness. While on treatment with chlorpromazine, he was found unconscious in the lavatory. Subsequently on five occasions his EEG showed fluctuating activity generally predominantly on the left but on one occasion maximally on the right. His medication was changed to haloperidol. He found this depressing and threatened to discontinue medication, but agreed to the systematic withdrawal of his medication while undergoing daily automated testing. Following the withdrawal of his medication he became progressively more over-active and excitable. With the demonstration that his performance on the tests was deteriorating he agreed however to restart haloperidol at a lower dosage which in the event proved quite adequate. When his psychiatric condition stabilised he agreed on the basis of his nocturnal collapse and the EEG findings to a trial of phenytoin.

The second subject was a 19 year old male with a history of 'minimal brain damage' as a child and a putative diagnosis of schizophrenia, but the final diagnosis remains in doubt. He does not show any schizophrenic process symptoms and the preferred formulation is a severe obsessional neurosis complicated by and perhaps partly determined by brain damage. There is no history of epilepsy but in his EEG recordings there is a persisting but fluctuating preponderance of posterior rhythmic theta activity at 4 c/sec, more obvious and of greater amplitude over the right rather than the left hemisphere.

Statistical methods

A key problem deterring psychologists from developing the methodology of single-person studies, is the difficulty of specifying the degree of confidence to ascribe to intervention effects in such studies, where the data is time-dependent and generally contains auto-regressive components.

In analysing the solution times, search times and motor indices for the first subject we have used a Bayesian Analysis developed by Professor Adrian Smith

[12] which makes it possible to analyse intervention effects in time-series data even though these may contain auto-regressive and learning components. The technique first fits a mathematical model to the series and then sets up the hypothesis that there is a discontinuity in the data and that this would be better represented by two models. A likelihood analysis then calculates for each point the probability that the discontinuity occurs at that point. If there is little likelihood that there is a discontinuity then these probabilities — totalling one — are distributed evenly between the observations. If there is a relatively high probability of a discontinuity at one point, the data are then split at this point and the analysis repeated on each section.

For the analysis of the laterality indices we have used Olmstead's technique, as described on pages 194—195 in the 7th Edition of Documenta Geigy Scientific Tables [13]. For testing the significance of differences between sets of observations we have used standard randomisation tests.

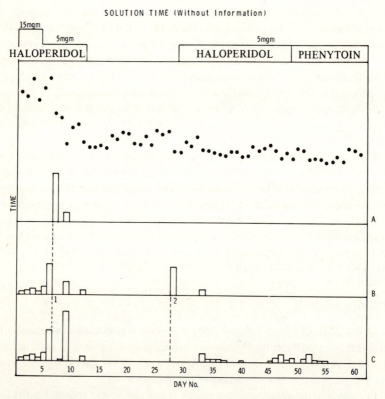

Figure 2.1. Overall performance of subject 1 on the Perceptual Maze Test. Mean time per item (see text)

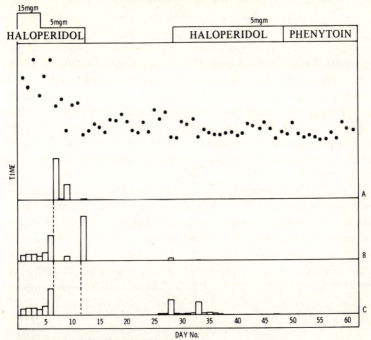

Figure 2.2. Perceptual Indices (search time) for subject 1 derived from the data on 2.1 (see text)

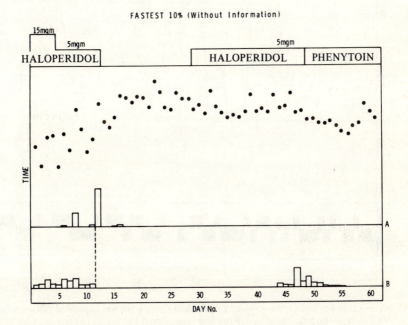

Figure 2.3. Motor Indices for subject 1 derived from data in Figure 2.1 (see text)

449

Results

Some results of the intervention study undertaken with the first subject are presented in Figure 2. In Figure 2.1 the median solution times on the PMT plotted and below this the result of three runs of Professor Smith's program. In run 1 there is evidence for a discontinuity in the period during which his haloperidol was being withdrawn. In run 2 an additional discontinuity occurs at the point where treatment with haloperidol was reintroduced. In run 3 there is some further evidence for the disruption in the performance caused by the withdrawal of the haloperidol.

In Figure 2.2 the data analysed are the search index described for the same test. There is again evidence in all the runs of a disruption of performance during the period of withdrawal and in runs 2 and 3 evidence that this perceptual component of his performance was also affected by the reinstatement of haloperidol.

In Figure 2.3 the motor component of the subject's performance is analysed. This time the initial disruption is more clearly related to the final withdrawal of haloperidol. There is no detectable effect when haloperidol is reintroduced but

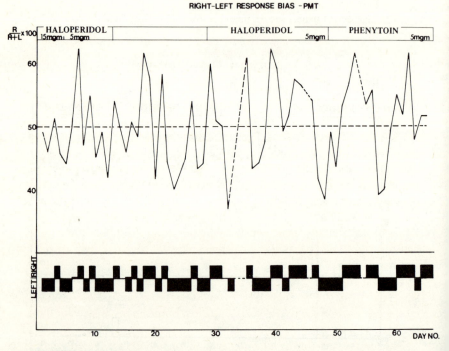

Figure 3. Laterality Indices for subject 1. The blocks below the line represent runs in what the bias is to the left. Those above the line runs is what the bias is to the right (see text)

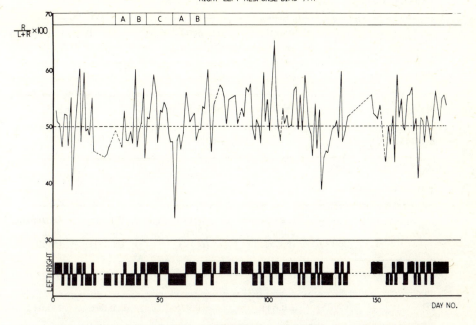

Figure 4. Laterality Indices for subject 2. Conventions as for Figure 3 (see also text). Drug code: A = Placebo; B = Chlorpromazine (50mg); C = Amitriptyline (50mg)

there is unexpected evidence for a speeding of the motor component at the time that treatment with phenytoin is introduced.

Another measure that can be extracted from the PMT is a laterality index. The data for this index for the patient are plotted in Figure 3 together with a block diagram which plots the 'runs' in which sequential recordings showed the same laterality bias. Inspection of the data suggests that there is initially a fluctuating left bias and that following the addition of phenytoin the subject's bias becomes on average right-sided and fluctuates less randomly. The laterality index for the second patient is plotted in Figure 4. There appears to be evidence both for non random fluctuations in laterality preference and changes in the mean values of the laterality index which can be related to the different treatment regimes. Unlike performance scores some indices of cognitive style are relatively immune to practice effects. With the Perceptual Maze Test the subject is unaware of any laterality bias in his performance and there is no a priori reason why this should change as his performance improves. That this is so is borne out by the mean values recorded in the sequential observations made with these patients.

The mean values for the laterality indices for subjects are therefore presented in Tables I and II.

451

TABLE I (see text)

	No drugs (N 16)	Haloperidol (5mg) (N25)	Phenytoin (50mg) (N 15)
$\bar{x}$	0.489	0.503	0.507
SD	± 0.066	± 0.075	± 0.061
P drug v no drugs		P<0.05	P<0.05

TABLE II (see text)

	Placebo (N 14)	Chlorpromazine 50mg (N 15)	Amitriptyline 50mg (N 12)	Diazepam 9mg (N 23)	Diazepam 9mg (N 39)
$\bar{x}$	0.483	0.507	0.524	0.532	0.525
SD	± 0.051	± 0.041	± 0.035	± 0.041	± 0.042
P drug v placebo		P<0.2	P<0.05	P<0.01	P<0.01

For the first subject the drug effects for each drug do not reach a statistically significant level but the changes are in the same direction for both drugs and also in the same direction as the drug effects in the second subject. The effect therefore is probably real. In the second subject the results with diazepam and amitriptyline are highly significant and the effect with chlorpromazine is clearly a real one. That these effects are not due to practice is borne out firstly by the observation that the effect became less marked when the dosage of diazepam was reduced. Furthermore, between the end of treatment with amitriptyline and the beginning of treatment with diazepam there was a period during which the patient was receiving neither drugs nor placebo. For this period the mean value of the laterality index was 49.75 ± 4.49 lower than that recorded in either the preceding or the following drug periods and not significantly different from the placebo values.

In Figures 3 and 4 and from the variances recorded in the tables it is clear that the laterality index fluctuates considerably from day to day and within each drug period. Some of the fluctuation is due to the version of the test used in that the items presented were generated randomly and not 'balanced'. Fluctuations due to the test material would therefore be random and it is appropriate to test the randomness of the runs observed with a test which is independent of the average bias (Documenta Geigy, 7th Edition, page 194). With this test the probability that the runs are random is less than 0.29 for the first subject and less than 0.02 for the second subject.

Conclusion

In this chapter we have presented some results from the proving studies we are undertaking during the development of an automated psychological test system. This system is now sufficiently sensitive and reliable for us to be able to record and analyse daily fluctuations in different aspects of a patient's performance on simple and complex cognitive tasks and to relate those fluctuations to changes in the patient's treatment regime.

Neither of the two patients reported here suffered from epilepsy but both have fluctuations and focal changes in their EEG. In one these were clearly epileptic and the patient was presumed to have had a convulsion precipitated by chlorpromazine. In both cases the changes seen in performance are associated with medication. In the first subject it is reasonable to attribute some of the changes in laterality preference and to fluctuations in the level of focal abnormal electrical activity. It seems likely that these fluctuations were determined both by the changes in medication and by other more random physiological factors. Unfortunately we were not able to record the EEG while our subjects were undertaking their psychological tests and this interpretation is therefore speculative. We hope that it will be possible to undertake such studies and to show convincingly that such subclinical fluctuations in the interictal EEG may affect both the level and pattern of conscious activity. In many patients such minor diminution of the level of conscious skill may be of little or no social significance. In some they may be of considerable importance. Certainly as clinicians we would welcome more accurate methods with which to assess and quantify, not only the depressant action of anticonvulsant drugs, but also the effect that their anticonvulsant action has on cerebration.

Acknowledgments

It is a pleasure to acknowledge the support and encouragement of our colleagues at the Royal Free Hospital and the National Hospital for Nervous Diseases. To Professor Adrian Smith, Dr CD Litton and Dr JA Heady, we are particularly grateful for statistical advice and assistance with the analyses.

References

1   Elithorn A, Powell J, Telford A, Cooper R. In Grimsdale RL, Hankins HCA, eds. *Human Factors and Interactive Displays 1980.* Buckingham: Network
2   Elithorn A, Lunzer M, Weinman JJ. *Neurol Neurosurg, Psychiat 1975; 38 No 8:* 794–798

3   Weinman J, Elithorn A, Farag S. In Friedman M, O'Connor N, Das JP, eds. *Intelligence and Learning 1981.* New York: Plenum Press

4   Edwards FC. In Murray et al, eds. *The Misuse of Psychotropic Drugs 1981.* Gaskell

5   Hindmarch I. In Murray et al, eds. *The Misuse of Psychotropic Drugs 1981.* Gaskell

6   Elithorn A, Cooper R, Lennox R. In Crooks J, Stevenson IH, eds. *Drugs and the Elderly 1979.* London: Macmillan

7   Geier S. *Clin Neurophysiol 1971; 31:* 499–507

8   Butcher HG. *Human Intelligence: its Nature and Assessment 1968.* London: Methuen

9   Beard R. *Br J Educ Physiol 1965; 35:* 2, 210–222

10   Archibald YM. *Cortex 1978; 14:* 1,22–31

11   Carter-Saltzman L. In Wittig NA, Petersen AC, eds. *Sex-related Differences in Cognitive Functioning 1979.* London: Academic Press

12   Smith AFM. In Barra JR et al, eds. *Recent Developments in Statistics 1977.* Amsterdam: North-Holland Publishing Co

13   In Diem K, Lentner G. *Documenta Geigy Scientific Tables, 7th Edition 1970.* Basle: Geigy SA

48

BIOCHEMICAL PHARMACOLOGY OF ANTICONVULSANT DRUG INTERACTIONS

P N Patsalos, P T Lascelles

The administration of more than one anticonvulsant drug to patients with epilepsy as an aid to the management of their fits is common clinical practice. A recent survey by Guelen et al [1] of 11,700 patients showed that each patient was receiving a mean of 3.2 drugs of which 84.3 per cent were anticonvulsants. Due to the chronic long-term nature of epilepsy and consequently its treatment, the possibility of anticonvulsant drug interactions is high. Commonly, most drug interactions have been discovered as a result of unexpected changes in clinical status of patients upon addition to, or withdrawal from, existing medication of a drug. Some interactions depress the blood level of an anticonvulsant and exacerbate seizures while others raise blood levels and precipitate toxicity, while yet other interactions raise levels and increase therapeutic response. The most commonly used anticonvulsant drugs are shown in Table I.

Biochemical basis of interactions

Pharmacokinetic: (a) drug absorption
                         (b) plasma (serum) protein binding
                         (c) liver metabolism (induction and inhibition)
                         (d) elimination or excretion

Pharmacodynamic: The most commonly observed clinically significant interactions can be attributed to interactions at the level of plasma protein binding and liver metabolism.

Numerous pharmacodynamic interactions have been reported but since the possibility of pharmacokinetic type interactions were not fully excluded their significance cannot be interpreted at present.

455

TABLE I. Commonly used anticonvulsant drugs

Group	Drugs
Hydantoins	Phenytoin, albutoin, ethotoin, methoin
Barbiturates	Phenobarbital, primidone, methylpheno-barbital, phenylmethylbarbituric acid
Benzodiazepines	Diazepam, clonazepam, nitrazepam, oxazepam
Iminostilbenes	Carbamazepine
Succinimides	Ethosuximide, methosuximide, phenosuximide
Valproates	Sodium valproate, valproic acid
Acetylureas	Pheneturide, phenocemide
Oxazolidines	Troxidone, paramethadione, aloxidone
Sulphonamide derivates	Sulthiame, acetazolamide

Frequency of interactions

The most frequently observed anticonvulsant drug interactions involve phenytoin. The reasons for this are:

a) It is the most commonly prescribed anticonvulsant.

b) Phenytoin has a narrow plasma therapeutic range and the upper limit of the therapeutic range is very close to the level at which neurological manifestations of phenytoin intoxication are observed.

c) Phenytoin exhibits saturation kinetics within the therapeutic range, i.e. as the blood level of phenytoin is increased the enzyme responsible for its metabolism becomes saturable resulting in a steep dose/blood level relationship.

d) Since phenytoin is highly bound to plasma proteins and has a low apparent volume of distribution, its displacement from plasma protein binding sites can result in highly significant increases in the pharmacologically active free fraction.

Specific interactions

Phenytoin/sodium valproate

Plasma protein binding: Phenytoin and sodium valproate are highly bound (approximately 90%) to plasma proteins and have a low apparent volume of distribution. Displacement of either drug from binding sites can, therefore, result in significantly higher levels of pharmacologically active unbound drug. Sodium valproate, a relatively new anticonvulsant drug, is a short chain branched

456

fatty acid and, like other fatty acids, it can displace phenytoin from its plasma protein binding sites. This interaction is now well documented [2–10] and results in an immediate but transient reduction in total plasma levels and increased excretion of the principal phenytoin metabolite, 5-(p-hydroxyphenyl)-5-phenylhydantoin [6,11–14].

The clinical implication of this interaction is that neurological features of phenytoin intoxication could be precipitated by sodium valproate co-administration which would not be predicted from an estimation of the routine total plasma phenytoin concentration. Presumably neurological intoxication would be precipitated as a result of more unbound phenytoin reaching the brain [2].

Inhibition of liver metabolism: Evidence is accumulating to suggest that in addition to its plasma protein binding interaction with phenytoin, sodium valproate has a separate and opposing effect on phenytoin disposition, namely, inhibition of its metabolism [8,15–17]. This may explain some of the earlier reports in which sodium valproate administration was observed to elevate plasma phenytoin levels [18,20]. Using rat liver microsomal preparations in vitro, sodium valproate has been observed to be an uncompetitive inhibitor (Ki, 1.8×10^{-2} M) of phenytoin metabolism (hydroxylation) [15].

Phenytoin/phenobarbital

Phenobarbital is known to be a strong inducer of liver microsomal enzymes [21]. It would be expected, therefore, that plasma phenytoin levels of patients on chronic treatment with phenytoin would be lowered by the addition of phenobarbital to their regime on a long-term basis. However, occasional instances have been reported [22–25] in which phenytoin levels have either not changed or have been raised by the addition of phenobarbital. The observation that phenobarbital is a strong competitive inhibitor of phenytoin hydroxylation [15,26] (Ki, 9×10^{-4} M) may explain these observations if in the chronic situation the inhibition effect prevails over induction.

The mechanism which determines whether induction or inhibition will prevail is not known but it has been pointed out that induction prevails when the starting phenytoin dose is relatively high [27] and an inhibition when the phenobarbital dose is high [28]. Thus, if a patient is highly induced by administration of either a low concentration of phenobarbital on a long-term basis or a high concentration on a short-term basis, and is also given phenytoin in addition, any augmentation of the phenobarbital dosage might provoke an inhibition of phenytoin hydroxylation and an elevation of phenytoin plasma levels since maximal induction by phenobarbital already exists.

457

Phenytoin/sulthiame

Hansen et al [29] and Houghton and Richens [30] showed that the administration of sulthiame to patients already taking phenytoin produced an elevation of serum phenytoin concentration and an increased half life. These changes were not immediate but occurred over a period of 8–20 days after sulthiame administration probably reflecting the time required for sulthiame to accumulate.

Using 9,000 rat liver microsomal preparations, Patsalos and Lascelles [15] have shown that sulthiame is a potent competitive inhibitor of phenytoin hydroxylation (Ki, 8.8×10^{-4} M), the mechanism being a direct competition between the two drugs for binding to the cytochrome P450 receptor [31]. Whether the metabolites of sulthiame produce any additional inhibition has not been determined but, if they do, it is unlikely to be important since inhibition by sulthiame itself is so profound.

Phenytoin/ethosuximide

Frantzen et al [32], Dawson et al [33] and Lander et al [34] have observed an elevation of phenytoin plasma levels upon the addition of ethosuximide to the regime of epileptic patients. It is not possible from these reports to determine the mechanism of this interaction, but Patsalos and Lascelles [15] have observed in vitro that ethosuximide is a competitive inhibitor (Ki, 1.1×10^{-2} M) of phenytoin hepatic microsomal hydroxylation.

Phenytoin/methosuximide

Rembeck [35] in a study of 94 hospitalised epileptic patients observed that the co-administration of methosuximide and phenytoin resulted in a significant elevation of phenytoin blood levels. It is suggested [35] that the interaction is due to competition by the two drugs for a common hydroxylating enzyme system. In the same study Rembeck [35] also observed that methosuximide raised phenobarbital levels but not to the same degree as that observed with phenytoin, a metabolic interaction again being indicated [35].

Carbamazepine/phenytoin

During chronic administration, carbamazepine is observed to induce its own metabolism resulting in a decrease in half life and a gradual fall in its steady state serum level [36,37]. Carbamazepine has also been reported to induce the metabolism of phenytoin, sodium valproate, clonazepam and ethosuximide [20, 38–40].

Phenytoin, also a strong inducer of hepatic microsomal enzymes, has been consistently reported to lower carbamazepine steady state serum level and to shorten half life when administered in combination [40–42]. Westenberg et al [43] observed that carbamazepine epoxide/carbamazepine ratio was significantly increased in such patients. Since the epoxide of carbamazepine is pharmacologically active it is not possible to assess the significance of their interaction.

This interaction with carbamazepine can be expected when administered in combination with other enzyme inducing anticonvulsants (phenobarbital, primidone, pheneturide) [40,41,44,45].

Phenobarbital/sodium valproate

The addition of sodium valproate to a regime of phenobarbital results in a significant increase in phenobarbital blood levels parallelled by an increase in phenobarbital half life, phenobarbital levels having been reported to be increased by 27–100 per cent [5,11,12,46–49]. This interaction has recently been extensively studied in epileptic patients [44] and in normal subjects [50], and these strongly indicate that the mechanism of sodium valproate induced elevation of plasma phenobarbital levels is inhibition of phenobarbital metabolism. Furthermore, Kapetonovic and Kupferberg [51] have shown, using rat liver microsomal preparations in vitro, that sodium valproate competitively inhibits (Ki, 1.2 x 10^{-3} M) phenobarbital metabolism.

The clinical significance of this interaction is that sedation or even coma may ensue, necessitating a reduction in phenobarbital dosage.

Diazepam/sodium valproate

Dhillon and Richens [52], using human serum albumin in vitro, have observed that over the therapeutic range of sodium valproate (350–700μmol/L) the binding of diazepam was competitively inhibited so that the unbound fraction was increased two fold. Since the free fraction is small (2%) this interaction may cause a significant alteration in diazepam disposition.

Ethosuximide/sodium valproate

Mattson and Cramer [53] in a series of 5 patients observed that the addition of sodium valproate to a regime containing ethosuximide resulted in an approximately 60 per cent increase in serum levels. The resulting intoxication was only eliminated by a reduction of ethosuximide dose. Sodium valproate inhibition of ethosuximide metabolites is suggested to be the mechanism of interaction [53].

Multiple drug interactions

Many epileptic patients are administered three different anticonvulsant drugs as an aid to seizure management. In such situations, pharmacokinetic interactions can be expected to be even more frequent and, in addition, previously insignificant interactions may become clinically important.

Using rat liver microsomal preparations, Patsalos and Lascelles [54] studied the effect of various anticonvulsant combinations on phenytoin hydroxylation. Of the various combinations studied, a significant increase in inhibition of phenytoin hydroxylation was only observed with sulthiame/phenobarbital and ethosuximide/sodium valproate combinations. If these interactions also occur in the in vivo situation, then in the case of ethosuximide/sodium valproate, the interaction may be of importance since singly these anticonvulsants are relatively weak inhibitors of phenytoin metabolism [15].

Conclusions

Due to the traditional practice of treating epileptic patients with more than one drug, the possibility of anticonvulsant drug interactions is high. The clinical importance of the interactions described in this chapter is variable since dose requirements and plasma levels required for a therapeutic or toxic response varies from patient to patient. The knowledge of the possibility of such interactions and the frequent monitoring of plasma levels, can result in a more rational therapeutic approach to seizure management.

References

1   Guelen PJM, Van Der Kleijn E, Woudstra V. In Schneider H, Janz D, Gardner-Thorpe C et al, eds. *Clinical Pharmacology of Antiepileptic Drugs 1975;* 2–10. Berlin: Springer-Verlag
2   Patsalos PN, Lascelles PT. *J Neurol Neurosurg Psychiat 1977; 40:* 570–574
3   Patsalos PN, Lascelles PT. *Lancet 1977; 1:* 50–51
4   Monks A, Boobis S, Wadsworth J, Richens A. *Br J Clin Pharmacol 1978; 6:* 487–492
5   Wilder BJ, Willmore LJ, Bruni J, Villareal HJ. *Neurology 1978; 28:* 892–896
6   Bruni J, Wilder BJ, Willmore LJ, Barbour B. *Neurology 1979; 29:* 904–905
7   Friel PN, Leal KW, Wilensky AJ. *Ther Drug Monitor 1979; 1:* 243–248
8   Perucca E, Hebdige S, Frigo GM et al. *Clin Pharmacol Ther 1980; 28:* 779–789
9   Rodin EA, De Sousa G, Haidukewych D et al. *Arch Neurol 1981; 38:* 340–342
10   Pisani FD, Di Perri R. *Neurology 1981; 31:* 467–470
11   Vakil SD, Critchley EMR, Philips JC et al. In Legg NJ, ed. *Clinical and Pharmacological Aspects of Sodium Valproate (Epilim) in the Treatment of Epilepsy 1975;* 75–77. Tunbridge Wells: MRC Consultants
12   Bruni J, Gallo JM, Lee CS et al. *Neurology 1980; 30:* 1233–1236
13   Adams DJ, Luders H, Pippenger C. *Neurology 1978; 28:* 152–157
14   Sackellares JC, Lee SI, Dreiguss FE. *Epilepsia 1979; 20:* 697–703
15   Patsalos PN, Lascelles PT. *Biochem Pharmacol 1977; 26:* 1929–1933
16   Bruni J, Wilder BJ, Perchalski RJ et al. *Neurology 1980; 30:* 94–97
17   Kock KM, Ludwick BT, Levy RH. *Epilepsia 1981; 22:* 19–25
18   Vajda F, Morris P, Drummer O, Blodin P. In Legg NJ, ed. *Clinical and Pharmacological Aspects of Sodium Valproate (Epilim) in the Treatment of Epilepsy 1976;* 92–100. Tunbridge Wells: MRC Consultants

19   Windorfer A, Sauer W, Gaedeke R. *Acta Paediat Scand 1975; 64:* 771–772
20   Windorfer A, Sauer W. *Neuropediatrie 1977; 8:* 29–41
21   Conney AH. *Pharmacol Rev 1967; 19:* 317–366
22   Kutt H, Winters W, Scherman R, McDowell F. *Arch Neurol 1964; 11:* 649–656
23   Buchanan RA, Heffelfinger JC, Weiss CF. *Paediatrics 1969; 43:* 114–116
24   Kutt H, Hayres M, Verebely K, McDowell F. *Neurology 1969; 19:* 611–616
25   Diamond WD, Buchanan RA. *J Clin Pharmacol 1970; 10:* 306–311
26   Kutt H, Verebely K. *Biochem Pharmacol 1970; 19:* 675–686
27   Cucinell SA. In Woodbury DM, Perry JK, Schmidt RP, eds. *Antiepileptic Drugs 1972;* 319–327. New York: Raven Press
28   Garrettson LK, Dayton PG. *Clin Pharmacol Ther 1970; 11:* 674–679
29   Hansen JM, Kristensen M, Skovsted L. *Epilepsia 1968; 9:* 17–22
30   Houghton GW, Richens A. *Br J Clin Pharmacol 1974; 1:* 59–66
31   Patsalos PN, Lascelles PT. *Res Commun Chem Pathol Pharmacol 1980; 27:* 31–43
32   Frantzen E, Hansen JM, Hansen OE, Kristensen M. *Acta Neurol Scand 1967; 43:* 440–446
33   Dawson GW, Brown HW, Clark BG. *Annals Neurol 1978; 4:* 583–584
34   Lander CM, Eadie MJ, Tyrer JH. *Proc Aust Assoc Neurol 1975; 12:* 111–116
35   Rambeck B. *Epilepsia 1979; 20:* 147–156
36   Rawlins MD, Collste P, Bertilsson L, Palmer L. *Eur J Clin Pharmacol 1975; 8:* 91–96
37   Hansen JM, Siersback-Nielsen K, Skousted L. *Clin Pharmacol Ther 1971; 12:* 539–543
38   Bowdle TA, Levy RH, Cutler RE. *Clin Pharmacol Ther 1979; 26:* 629–634
39   Warren JW, Benmaman JB, Wannamaker BB, Levy RH. *Clin Pharmacol Ther 1980; 28:* 646–651
40   Cereghino JJ, Brock JT, Van Meter JC et al. *Clin Pharmacol Ther 1975; 18:* 733–741
41   Christiansen J, Dam M. *Acta Neurol Scand 1973; 49:* 543–546
42   Johannessen SI, Strandjord RE. In Schneider H, Janz D, Gardner-Thorpe C et al, eds. *Clinical Pharmacology of Anti-Epileptic Drugs 1975;* 201–205. Berlin: Springer-Verlag
43   Westenberg HGM, van der Kleijn E, Oei TT, de Zeeuw RA. *Clin Pharmacol Ther 1978; 23:* 320–328
44   Schneider H. In Schneider H, Junz D, Gardner-Thorpe C et al, eds. *Clinical Pharmacology of Anti-Epileptic Drugs 1975;* 184–195. Berlin: Springer-Verlag
45   Eichelbaum M, Bertilsson L, Lund L et al. *Eur J Clin Pharmacol 1976; 9:* 417–422
46   Richens A, Ahmed S. *Br Med J 1975; 4:* 255–256
47   Schobben F, van der Kleijn E, Gabreels FJM. *Eur J Clin Pharmacol 1975; 8:* 97–105
48   Nesdjian E, Mesdjian JL, Bouyard P et al. In Meinardi H, Rowan AJ, eds. *Advances in Epileptology 1978;* 266–268. Amsterdam: Swets and Zeillinger
49   Kapetonovic IM, Kupferberg HJ, Porter RJ et al. *Clin Pharmacol Ther 1981; 29:* 480–486
50   Patel IH, Levy RH, Cutter RE. *Clin Pharmacol Ther 1980; 27:* 515–521
51   Kapetonovic IM, Kupferberg HJ. *Biochem Pharmacol 1981; 30:* 1361–1363
52   Dhillon S, Richens A. *Br J Clin Pharmacol 1981; 12:* 591–592
53   Mattson RH, Cramer JA. *Ann Neurol 1980; 7:* 583–584
54   Patsalos PN, Lascelles PT. *Gen Pharmacol 1981; 12:* 51–55

49

RECENT DEVELOPMENTS IN THERAPEUTIC DRUG MONITORING

V D Goldberg, N Ratnaraj, A Elyas, P T Lascelles

Introduction

Over the last ten years little in the field of clinical chemistry has been more remarkable than the acceptance of the concept of therapeutic drug monitoring (TDM) as a valuable aid in the care and management of patients receiving drug therapy. There are two major situations where the levels of drugs in the body fluids are estimated, namely overdose or poisoning cases and therapeutically for the control of disease; whereas in the late 1950s virtually all determinations of drug levels in the body fluids were confined to the first case, in 1981 the bulk of drug determinations fell under the heading of TDM [1,2]. For example, in August 1972, forty requests for anticonvulsant drug determinations were processed for patients at the National Hospital; by 1979 the number had risen to two hundred a month. From 1972 to 1981 the proportion of requests for anticonvulsant drug determinations rose from less than 1 per cent to 25 per cent of the Chemical Pathology patient workload.

The use of microprocessor control has made possible the concept of small semi-automatic items of equipment such as the Guilford Stasar III (Corning Medical) used in conjunction with a pipettor dilutor and microcomputer in situations outside the clinical laboratory [3–5]. On the other hand, there is also a tendency running parallel with increasing sophistication of methodology to carry out drug estimations in specialist centres, which means a heavy workload for a comparatively small number of laboratories and puts a further premium on the development of automatic methods [6]. The Drug Analysis Unit at the National Hospital is currently processing 125 patient requests a week for anticonvulsant levels from the hospital and its associated units and other hospitals within the North East Thames Region, amounting to a total of 700–750 tests a week. The workload from all sources has increased by a factor of 10 per cent per annum in the last five years [3]. This explosion in numbers has occurred as clinicians have become more and more convinced of the value of TDM in patient care, and has been accompanied by very real advances in technique [3].

A number of reviews on the subject of TDM have been published recently including those edited by Pippenger et al [7] and Wilder and Bruni [8] about anticonvulsant drugs and by Tognoni et al [9], Richens and Marks [10] and Sadée and Beelen [11] on more general aspects of TDM. It has also been found desirable to publish a journal devoted to TDM and related topics alone [12]. Consequently, this chapter will primarily review developments in the field from 1980 onwards.

Indications for therapeutic drug monitoring (TDM) of anticonvulsant drugs

Numerous reviews of this topic have appeared over the years [13—16], emphasis being given recently to patients during adolescence, in the elderly, during pregnancy and intercurrent illnesses. In children too, the tendency is now to monitor therapy more frequently, especially in those patients on sodium valproate and carbamazepine. Observations of our own (in preparation) suggest that high levels of carbamazepine epoxide are present in children more frequently in those on multiple drug therapy, and these observations are in line with the findings of McKauge et al [17].

By contrast, the introduction of monotherapy has tended to simplify drug treatments of selected subjects by eliminating the complication of drug interactions, an important factor leading to unexpected variation in plasma levels in some patients.

The questions of therapeutic ranges of anticonvulsants is a matter in which there is still a surprising lack of precise scientific data and different authorities quote different ranges. Whilst the lower limit is of use namely in relationship to compliance and the upper limit in defining the beginning of the toxic range, no data at all are available concerning whether the therapeutic range of individual drugs should be different when drugs are used in combination.

Technical advances

There has been one striking new addition to the range of techniques available in the field of TDM in the past five years and that is an assay based on the concept of radioreceptor binding [18]. With this one exception, technical advances in TDM over the last five years have comprised not so much development of new techniques as improvements to existing techniques in a continuing process, so that increasing numbers of drugs can be analysed accurately and speedily. The range at which precise measurements can be carried out accurately has been brought down to the low nanogram level so that drugs, such as the benzodiazepines and tricyclic antidepressants, which are present in serum in very low concentrations can be monitored [19—21], while the microprocessor control of instrumentation which is increasing in scope [6] aids precision, as well as speeding up the calculation of results. Several reviews of these topics have been published recently [19—28], and a new journal has been established to cover the sphere of automation in analytical chemistry [29].

The techniques most commonly employed in TDM at present are gas liquid chromatography (GLC), high performance liquid chromatography (HPLC) and various types of immunoassay [30]. Recent developments in these methods and others less frequently used, such as thin layer chromatography (TLC), will be considered separately.

Gas liquid chromatography

The development of the specialised electron capture and nitrogen specific detectors constituted a major advance in GLC, as they allowed analyses to be carried out at high sensitivity after a simple extraction process. Analysis of drugs could often be performed without derivatisation and there was little or no interference from substances normally present in patients' sera. In addition, sample sizes could be reduced to $200\mu l$ or less. The major drawback to these detectors was their instability. The new generation of pulsed ^{63}Ni-electron capture detectors are linear over a wide range and less easily contaminated than earlier ^{3}H-models [19]. They are now in general use, particularly for the analysis of benzodiazepines such as diazepam [31], clobazam [32] and flurazepam [33] without derivatisation, and bromazepam [34], which is best represented chromatographically as its N-methyl derivative, because of strong absorption on the stationary phases of gas chromatographic columns. Benzodiazepines have also been analysed by a capillary column linked to an electron capture detector [35]. A support-coated open tubular column was used in this case, and the support layer consisted of silanised fumed silica coated with the liquid phases 0.5 per cent PPE-21 and 3 per cent OV17 [35]. Similar techniques to these can be employed in the analysis of triazolam [36,37]. These methods have in common great sensitivity with detection limits for benzodiazepines and related compounds ranging from 500 pg ml^{-1} to 50ng ml^{-1} but, while they are not subject to interference from endogenous substances present in serum, interference from co-prescribed drugs has not always been documented [35—37]. With this proviso, however, methods based on the use of electron capture detection have enormous potential for the future in routine TDM for drugs and metabolites present in serum only in extremely low concentrations.

The new nitrogen-specific detectors consist of a rubidium glass bead which can be heated directly, giving them greater stability and sensitivity than the original large crystals [38], and they have proved particularly useful in the field of anticonvulsant drug analysis [39,40]. Haloperidol [41] and tricyclic antidepressant drugs [20,21] are also suitable compounds for assay with this type of detector if quality control of the detector response is maintained carefully [42], and an important application has been the analysis of theophylline, caffeine and phenobarbitone extracted from 30µl blood spot samples on filter paper [43]. This is of particular relevance in the areas of neonatal and perinatal medicine because the samples can be collected by means of a heel or finger prick [43].

A wall-coated open tubular column coated with liquid phase SE30 has been coupled with a nitrogen specific detector for the analysis of diazepam, meprobamate, phenylbutazone and thioridazone in serum [44]. The main advantages of this technique are the efficiency and short elution time of the column added to the specificity and sensitivity of the detector [44]. Barbiturates are also analysed by capillary column gas chromatography [45].

A new type of detector, the element selective electrolyte conductivity detector (HECD, Hall 700A; Tracor Inc), uses the principle of combustion of organic compounds in a furnace under set conditions to produce ammonia, hydrogen chloride, chlorine or sulphur dioxide, mixing these gases with a deionised liquid such as an isopropanol/distilled water solution in a gas liquid contractor, and measuring conductivity with an A.C. bridge circuit and auxillary recorder [46–48]. It obviously has great potential for measuring drug concentrations in all body fluids, but has been used so far mainly to assay drug levels in urine. It can be set in a 'Sulphur Mode' and this gives it a particular advantage in the analysis of sulphur-containing drugs such as thiopentone, which can be detected in urine at the picogram level [47].

An adaptation of the FID detector (FIDOH) [49], which provides a hydrogen-rich atmosphere with concentric jets for oxygen and the other gases, has been developed to overcome problems of increase in noise level when chlorocarbons are analysed. It has so far not been used for drug analysis, but may have wider application in the future [49].

In recent years a series of specialised column packing materials have been developed for TDM, replacing to some extent the liquid phases such as OV17 and SE30 which have a more general use, and are therefore less specific. These include DC-420 silastic gum which has been used for anticonvulsant drug analysis [50], SP 2510-DA for anticonvulsants [38,51] and clobazam [32] and theophylline [52,53] and SP 2250 and Apolar 87 (Kovats 87) for benzodiazepines [19,31,38]. The use of these specially-prepared liquid phases allows the simultaneous determination of anticonvulsant drugs without derivatisation under isothermal conditions [51]. These are important factors in the design of analytical processes suitable for automatic running of samples [40,51], which is particularly important in the rapidly-growing sphere of anticonvulsant TDM [40,51].

Finally, there is an increasing tendency for gas chromatographs to be designed with complete microprocessor control of operating parameters as well as calculation of results, for example, by Analytical Instruments of Cambridge, and also the Perkin-Elmer Sigma 1 and 2 and the Hewlett-Packard 5880 series. This also has great implications for the future in terms of automatic running of samples with minimal supervision by staff, thus enabling an increasing workload to be processed by, what is indeed, a reliable and widely used technique.

High performance liquid chromatography

HPLC offers an attractive alternative procedure to GLC, and is being increasingly used for TDM in three particular circumstances:

1. In cases where an elaborate 'clean-up' procedure may be necessary to remove interfering substances from serum even when a selective detector is used [54].
2. When drugs or metabolites such as sulthiame, carbamazepine, or chlordiazepoxide and their major metabolites are thermally unstable, or can only be chromatographed with difficulty [19,55,56].
3. When decomposition of metabolites such as 7-aminoclonazepam or promethazine-5-sulphoxide make it difficult to resolve them from their parent compounds [57,58].

New HPLC analyses have recently been devised for a number of drugs and their major metabolites with sensitivity in the low nanogram range and sample sizes less than 500μl. Generally, a reverse-phase or reverse-phase ion-pair mode is used with ultraviolet spectrophotometric detectors (UV detectors) because many drugs absorb strongly in the ultraviolet. The drugs analysed include sulthiame [55], carbamazepine and its epoxide metabolite [17,56], tricyclic antidepressants [59], chlordiazepoxide and diazepam and their major metabolites [54,60,61], anticonvulsants [30,62,63] and theophylline [64]. Care, however, must be taken to use appropriate extraction methods for the preparation of samples, for example, in the case of patients with uraemia [65], and to avoid deproteinisation procedures that lead to poor peak shape [66]. It has also been found that some types of ODS (reverse-phase) columns may cause peak distortion in certain assays [66], and care must be taken in the choice of silica or alumina (i.e. straight phase) columns to avoid interference by endogenous substances present in serum [67].

Detection by UV spectrophotometry has a wide applicability, but interference from extraneous substances present in serum may be difficult to detect in any assay when the UV spectra of two compounds are very similar, even using ratios of peak heights obtained at two different wavelengths [68]. For example, in theophylline assays, paraxanthine, a metabolite of caffeine, which is almost invariably present in serum from adults and from the newborn, may chromatograph with theophylline, unless conditions are adjusted carefully, leading to elevated drug values [68,69]. A number of published HPLC procedures provide little or no information about interference from co-prescribed drugs, or else recommend commonly-prescribed drugs as internal standards rather than substances not normally present in patients serum [56,63,70]. These methods are suitable for TDM if no other drug is being taken or for pharmacokinetic studies under controlled conditions. To avoid problems of interference it is anticipated that fluorimetric detection will be used increasingly. Though pre- or post-column derivatis-

466

ation procedures are usually necessary, a general purpose HPLC fluorimetric detector can be adapted for use with non-fluorescing compounds if the mobile phase is spiked with anilene [71].

Electrochemical detectors are of particular importance in the analysis of compounds like adrenaline or M-dopa but an assay has been developed recently for the determination of sulphanilimides in milk with a detection limit of $10ng/ml^{-1}$ [72], a greater sensitivity than has been achieved for sulphanilimide analysis previously [72]. In an important extension to this technique, Suckow and Cooper [73] have described an analytical procedure for the tricyclic drugs imipramine and desipramine and their metabolites, while Murakami et al [74] have used HPLC with electrochemical detection for the analysis of chlorpromazine and levopromazine in plasma and urine. Work is continuing to adapt this methodology for the analysis of additional drugs in body fluids [75–77], and a related technique now under consideration is the linking of an HPLC column to a polarographic detector [76,77,79]. The theoretical basis of this technique, which may be of particular importance in the analysis of benzodiazepine levels in body fluids [77–79], has recently been discussed in detail [80].

One report has been published recently describing the linking of HPLC columns in straight phase or reverse phase mode to a Hall detector [81]. The design of the HECD makes it possible to handle the effluent from an HPLC column with only minor adjustment, and the method would seem to be suitable for TDM of drugs which cannot easily be examined in other ways [81].

A technique analogous to capillary GLC, 'very fast LC', which employs column packings of 3μ particle size instead of the more usual 5 or 10μ, has been used for the simultaneous analysis of four anticonvulsant drugs (phenobarbitone, primidone, phenytoin and carbamazepine) [82]. Each run takes two minutes instead of the more usual 10 minutes and, in order to handle the very fast throughput with a UV detector, the cell is reduced in size from about 2ml to 0.5ml and the detector is microprocessor controlled [82]. A further development is the use of 'on-column detection' where the HPLC column and UV flow cell are both constructed from fused small-bore silica tubing; this gives a 6nl cell. The flow rate is $1.06\mu l/min^{-1}$ for 50:50 methanol water as opposed to the usual $1-2ml/min^{-1}$ with standard columns [83].

New methods have been devised to prepare samples for analysis by HPLC, for example, disposable SEP-PAK cartridges (Waters Ass) which act like miniature columns retaining protein and other extraneous materials in serum, while allowing drugs such as anticonvulsants to pass through to be collected quantitatively and analysed [84,85]. Though no advantages were claimed for this method in the analysis of thiopentone [86], the sample preparation time was reduced from 150 to 40 minutes in the case of antidepressant drug analysis [87] and it would seem to have advantages where the extraction process is particularly tedious [87]. On the other hand, the 'FAST-LC' system from Technicon comprises a completely automatic extraction and injection system, with $200\mu l$ serum samples treated with buffer and extracted with organic solvents, and evaporated to dryness by being carried on a moving wire along a glass module which is kept warm. The sample is redissolved in methanol, collected in a loop and injected onto a reverse phase column. This system has been used with success for the analysis of anticonvulsant drugs and metabolites, and theophylline [88,89]. FAST-LC has a great potential for routine work because it can handle up to 100 samples completely automatically, but should perhaps be considered as a research tool at present.

In the future, HPLC techniques are likely to be used more frequently on account of their inherent ability to handle the analysis of multicomponent samples containing anticonvulsant drugs [30,63]. The ability of HPLC to accommodate automation is also an important factor in this respect [30].

Thin layer chromatography

This technique has the advantage of being relatively cheap to operate but, in the opinion of some, it inevitably requires great skill and experience from staff to achieve results comparable to other methods in quality control schemes [90], and it is gradually being replaced by other methods [30]. The development of automatic applicators by the firms Merck and Camag and the use of microprocessor control have increased expense, but improved the sensitivity and precision of the method [91]. This new technique, high performance thin layer chromatography (HPTLC), enables nanogram amounts of drugs and metabolites to be accurately quantified [91], and the use both of reverse phase plates (RPTLC) and normal phase plates has been reported recently, for example, Gattavecchia and Tonelli have used RPTLC plates coated with RP-18 to assay the drugs metronidazole and misonidazole and their metabolites [92]. On the other hand, Simona and Grandjean have analysed di-isopyramide and its major N-dealkylated metabolite [93] and Rohdewald and Drehsen have analysed a range of analgesics in saliva to high ng level [94] using Merck HPTLC plates coated with silica gel 60. It is anticipated that the use of RPTLC will increase greatly as more becomes known about the theoretical basis of the method [95].

Mass spectrometry

The use of a mass spectrometer as a detector for a gas chromatograph (GC/MS) is now a well established procedure [22,25]. Selective ion monitoring is the GC/MS method most commonly used in the analysis of drug levels in biological fluids [25]. Of its two applications, single ion monitoring is the more sensitive technique allowing low picogram quantities of drugs or metabolites to be measured; often, deuterated analogues of drugs are used as internal standards. Single ion monitoring has the advantage that scans can be made very rapidly over the same ion, while multiple ion monitoring is less sensitive but more specific in that scans are made of several ions, so that there is less possibility of incorrect identification with extraneous materials in serum. Alternatively, multiple ion monitoring allows a number of different compounds to be quantified in a single analytical run without the requirement that they all possess the same ion [22,25,96].

The technique of GC/MS has such sensitivity that it can be used to assay drugs which are present only in very small amounts in serum, such as tricyclic anti-depressants [20,21,70]. It can also be used to analyse anticonvulsants in $40-60\mu l$ quantities of saliva collected on PKU paper [97]. The technique is limited by the fact that some compounds are difficult to chromatograph by GC, as already discussed (see page 466), and that derivatisation is usually necessary. In these cases a sample 'clean-up' followed by direct injection by probe into the mass spectrometer might be increasingly useful, a technique that has already been applied to the simultaneous analysis of six anticonvulsant drugs using multiple ion monitoring [98]. Another way of solving this problem is by the linking of a liquid chromatograph to a mass spectrometer, a technique still very much in the developmental stage though commercial equipment is available, but at the moment its use is limited by the expense of the equipment. The same limitation applies to other adaptations of mass spectrometry such as field description and metastable ion analysis.

Chemical ionisation mass spectrometry is a technique in which a reaction gas, typically methane, interacts with sample molecules at low pressure to generate mostly ions such as $(M + H)^+$ or $(M + CH_4)^+$. Since many of these ions do not fragment further, unlike the situation in electron impact mass spectrometry, they are abundant enough to be scanned effectively; the technique is very sensitive and many applications have been reported [22,25,98]. The use of gas chromatography — negative ion chemical ionisation mass spectrometry, though less frequently used, is of particular relevance in the analysis of benzodiazepines which have a strong electron capture capability [22,99,100].

The development of bench-top quadropole mass spectrometers, which are much cheaper than the earlier magnetic instruments and more stable in operation, is proceeding rapidly [96]. Together with microprocessor control and the development of improved interfaces between gas chromatograph and mass spectrometer, they will tend to bring the technique of GC/MS more into routine use for its advantages of absolute specificity and sensitivity [96]. Its major application in TDM is the identification of unknowns and as a back-up for other procedures when it is suspected that interfering substances may be present [96,101], since a different pattern of metabolism or the presence of an unknown drug may disturb the course of the other methods. Of the methods under review, only mass spectroscopic techniques offer positive identification of drugs to be analysed or of compounds which have been chromatographed.

469

Polarography

Polarography is a technique with advantages of convenience and speed [76], in particular, since most endogenous materials present in body fluids are polarographically inactive the method can be used for the direct determination of drugs in serum or urine.

Since polarographic techniques have relatively poor selectivity, it may be necessary to separate a drug from its major metabolites by chromatographic methods before analysis, and the technique requires comparatively large quantities of serum [76–78]. While these disadvantages have prevented the wider use of polarography in TDM [76–78], a method has recently been described for the analysis of indomecathin concentrations in body fluids [102] and polarographic techniques continue to be used for the assay of benzodiazepines [78,103]. The recent improvements in apparatus design have allowed full polarographic examination of compounds like the benzodiazepine flurazepam [104], and it is expected that these improvements will increase the scope of polarographic applications [76–79,105], in particular in HPLC analysis (see page 466).

Immunoassay and related techniques

The technique of coupling a drug to a protein carrier, raising up an antibody against the antigen thus formed and then using the antibody in a competitive reaction between free drug and a drug-label conjugate, has become increasingly important in TDM over the past five years. Various techniques have been devised using different types of label and conjugate, and these methods have proved to be particularly well adapted for the production of commercial kits and thence for automation. The small size of sample required, usually less than $50\mu l$ of serum or plasma, is a major advantage over other methods.

Radioimmunoassay was the first immunoassay technique to be adapted for TDM [106]. Reliable commercial kits are now available for certain widely used drugs such as digoxin, gentamicin and phenytoin from a number of sources, such as Amersham International and New England Nuclear, and have proved satisfactory in practical use when compared with chromatographic methods [107]. Assay techniques have recently been published for benzodiazepines such as diazepam [108], loretazepam [109] and flunitrazepam [110], and a wise variety of other drugs including tricyclic antidepressants [21,111]. Recently a double radioimmunoassay method has been developed for vitamin B_{12} and folic acid, and this approach will probably be adopted for TDM [112].

Progress has been made in automation of equipment. A semi-automatic system such as the Union Carbide Centria seems the most satisfactory, with the sample-dilution and reagent addition, physical separation of antibody-bound and free ligand, and the reading of the results in a scintillation counter constituting three separate steps. Using the appropriate kits it is possible to analyse a number of drugs including phenytoin. There are technical difficulties in designing a completely automatic system using the continuous flow principle for assays with long incubation times [112] or when binding is less than 50 per cent, but Ismail et al [113] have described a continuous flow apparatus which will measure bound or unbound antibody separately or combined together. The antibody is covalently linked to porous particles of Sepharose 4B, which are directed into a separation block controlled by a system of valves and then pumped out into a scintillation counter; the whole process, which is completely automatic, is microprocessor controlled. In another approach, Cais and Shimoni [114,115] have reported new mixing devices based on the principle of solvent extraction for the separation step, which is always the most error-filled procedure in RIA.

The major advantages of radioimmunoassay are its extreme sensitivity, which means that it is particularly useful for assaying substances present in serum in low concentration, such as drug metabolites, and the fact that non-specific interference produced by biological materials is minimal because of the nature of the radioactive label [112]. A major disadvantage, which radioimmunoassay shares to some extent with other immunoassays, is the difficulty in producing antibodies entirely specific for the antigen; an unusual metabolite may be found to cross-react even after an assay has been in use for a long period [112]. Ethical considerations also tend to limit the scope of the technique [27].

Enzyme immunoassay The technique of enzyme immunoassay has had enormous impact in the field of TDM mainly because of the development of EMIT, a homogeneous assay system using UV to measure the reaction (SYVA Diagnostics UK Ltd). This system is quite sensitive enough for clinical use and has set the standard for speed and reliabllity to which other assays must aspire [107]. At the present time kits have been developed for the assay of 18 drugs in serum, including the most widely used anticonvulsants, and results obtained by EMIT correlate well with those obtained by other analytical procedures such as GLC, HPLC and radioimmunoassay [3,51, 116, 117]. The EMIT assays for some anticonvulsant drugs can be adapted in the laboratory for the analysis of saliva, tears and cerebrospinal fluid as well as serum, and the correlation with GLC is again satisfactory [118, 119], but there are limitations to its use. Apart from the possibility of interference in an assay by co-prescribed drugs, it has recently been reported that EMIT gives higher results for phenytoin than GLC, by a factor of between two and four in the case of patients with uraemia [120,121]. Although this is caused partly by an increase in the serum level of the major metabolite of phenytoin (5-p-hydroxyphenyl-5-phenylhydantoin) bound to glucuronic acid in these patients [122], the amount of cross-reactivity between the metabolite and the EMIT phenytoin reagent kit may not be sufficient on its own to account for the discrepancy, and there is a possibility that other non-specific interferences are involved [57,123]. New style kits have greatly reduced the scale of the problem [122], and the method of collection of the patient's sample may also have a bearing on the accuracy of the procedure, for example, in the valproic acid assay [116].

One of the advantages of the EMIT system is the possibility of completely automatic analysis of samples, using for example the Guilford System 3500 or Abbott Biochromatic Analyser — 100 [3,124], and these systems can analyse 60 samples an hour. Recently it has been found possible to adapt the EMIT kits satisfactorily for use with several centrifugal analysers such as the Centrifichem 500 and Multistat III with great savings in cost as well as in time for long analytical runs [125]. Between 60 and 100 samples can be processed in an hour even though incubation time has to be increased because the kits are diluted. The major disadvantage of this type of operation is that samples cannot be added once a run has started so that emergency samples are comparatively expensive to run [125].

A drug assay kit procedure based on the ELISA system, which is a heterogeneous enzyme immunoassay, is available for digoxin which is the least sensitive of the EMIT assays and requires 30 minutes for incubation as against 45 seconds for anticonvulsant drugs [107]. It seems that the ELISA procedure, though capable of greater sensitivity than EMIT, is more suitable for semi-quantitative work, such as the checking of compliance in dapsone therapy. This method has great cost advantages over EMIT and RIA in terms of equipment costs and running costs and is very simple to operate, so it is particularly useful for spot-testing where few laboratory facilities are available [107].

Fluoroimmunoassay Fluoroimmunoassay (FIA) is a heterogeneous immunoassay technique which differs from radioimmunoassay only in using a fluorescent label instead of a radioactive label. In specificity and wide application, though not yet in sensitivity, it is comparable with radioimmunoassay [26,27], and anomalous results caused by metabolic disorders have so far not been reported (January 1982).

Recently, Landon and co-workers [126,127] have described several assays using magnetic sedimentation of antibody-bound fluorimetric tracer, followed by removal of the supernatant which contains interfering substances. The antibody-bound tracer is then eluted, and since the fluorescence fluorimetry is carried out at visible wavelengths, disposable plastic tubes can be used. This method has been applied for the analysis of propranolol [126] and phenytoin [127], and results have been shown to be comparable with standard methods; and it is anticipated that assay kits produced by Seward Laboratories will become available for the major anticonvulsant drugs in late 1982. Karnes et al [128] on the other hand have developed a fluoroimmunoassay procedure where bound and free labelled antigen are separated by precipitation with a second antibody.

Another type of fluoroimmunoassay, namely polarisation fluoroimmunoassay, has very great potential for the future and, since it requires less than 5μl of serum, can be carried out using heel-prick quantities of blood, which is of crucial importance in perinatal medicine. The assay depends on the irradiation by polarised-light of a freely moving fluorochrome in solution which will then emit polarised light, while the larger molecules formed by binding the fluorochrome to antibody modify this effect. No separation step is therefore necessary, and the effect is measured on a polarisation fluorimeter [129,130]. Non-specific interference by protein binding may be eliminated by proteolytic digestion of the sample [129,130]. Recently, Jolley et al [131] have devised a completely automated system to carry out fluorescence polarisation assays, which has an additional advantage in that calibration curves stored in the instrument are valid for 10 days. Analysis of each sample takes less than 5 minutes and the results obtained correlate well with other methods. A range of drugs including phenobarbitone and phenytoin have been analysed by this method [131].

Adaptations of immunoassay procedures Two types of homogeneous immunoassay which have been developed by the Ames Division of Miles Laboratories Inc are of particular importance in the field of TDM, because they can be adapted to the new technique of dry reagent chemistry. The first is substrate-labelled fluorescent immunoassay (SLFIA), a procedure in which a drug is conjugated with a fluorophore in such a way that it is freely available for hydrolysis by an enzyme when the drug substrate complex is bound to antibody, but unavailable when it is not bound. In the test procedure, there is competitive binding between free drug and drug-fluorophore conjugate for places on the drug antibody which is in short supply. Therefore, the amount of fluorescence developed during the hydrolysis of the conjugate depends directly on the number of free drug molecules present in the sample analysed and can be measured conveniently in a fluoroscope. The method is comparable to EMIT in speed and sensitivity, and correlates well with RIA, EMIT, GLC and HPLC in the analysis of drugs such as phenytoin and theophylline [132,133]. Kits are now available (Ames TDA) for a number of drugs including phenobarbitone and phenytoin.

Morris et al [134] have applied the same principle to another type of homogeneous immunoassay, prosthetic group label homogeneous immunoassay (PGLIA), which has been used for the estimation of theophylline. In this assay flavin adenine dinucleotide (FAD) is substituted for the fluophore, and the drug-FAD conjugate competes with free drug for binding sites on a limited amount of antibody. The unbound drug-FAD conjugate reconstitutes glucose oxidase apo-enzyme to give active enzyme, and the reaction is quantified by measuring the colour developed in the presence of peroxidase and a chromagen.

Dry reagent chemistry Dry reagent chemistry has only been employed for TDM on a very small scale at the time of writing (January 1982) but the technique will obviously have a great impact in the future as the methodology improves and kits become available. Though reflectance photometry is generally used to

473

quantify dry reagent procedures, there have been two different approaches in method development. The first makes use of multilayered films with a similar configuration to photographic film, which has the advantage that the measured response is independent of solvent volume [135]. On the other hand the second method (reagent strip format) uses the dipstick technology, developed originally for urine analysis, where analytical reagents are successively impregnated on to paper fibre [135,136]. This approach has the advantage that the strips are saturated with specimen, so response is virtually independent of viscosity [135,136], which is an important factor in the application of reagent strip chemistry to analysis of drug levels in serum. Recently, the Ames SLFIA procedure has been modified for reagent strip format [137,138]. The reagents are quantitatively applied to paper strips and the addition of sample activates the assay; only one dilution step is necessary and the volume of serum required is very small. Phenytoin and phenobarbitone have been assayed by this technique, and PGLIA has been modified also to carry out the analysis of phenytoin and theophylline by reagent strip [139]. Work is continuing on the development of a simple reflectance photometer, the Seralyzer, to be used with solid phase applications such as glucose and uric acid analysis [136] and this methodology will probably be adapted for TDM in the future. A solid phase radioimmunoassay kit, the digoxin 'RIA Bead', is in the preliminary stages of development [140].

Nephelometry A variation of this technique, which has a long history of studying antigen-antibody reactions, has been applied to the monitoring of phenytoin and phenobarbitone [141]. The method of competitive inhibition used resembles enzyme immunoassay. It depends on the formation of a drug-protein conjugate, the raising of an antibody against this antigen and competition between free drug in serum and drug conjugate for binding sites on the antibody. The free drug inhibits formation of antigen-antibody complex; and the light scattering induced by the antigen-antibody complex is measured in a nephelometer. The method has been found to correlate well with the EMIT phenytoin and phenobarbitone assays. At the time of writing (January 1982) four drugs including phenytoin can be assayed by this method using kits developed for the ICS semi-automatic analyser (Beckman Instruments Ltd) which is computer-calibrated, so that a single point calibration step only is required for each run in the laboratory. The method will be adapted for the fully automatic ICS analyser later in the year and kits for an additional four drugs may also be available.

Receptor binding assays

A truly major advance in the field of TDM is the introduction of receptor binding assay techniques, which have the advantage that they estimate the active metabolites as well as the parent drug [142,143].

Many commonly prescribed drugs such as carbamazepine and procainamide give rise to therapeutically active metabolites which may be present in serum as well as at the site of action of the drug [17,56, 144–146], and the relative pharmacological activity of parent drug and metabolite may be difficult to evaluate [146]. In these cases, a method which can estimate the total concentration of drug and active metabolites is potentially of great value in the field of TDM. This is so because symptoms of toxicity may occur while the serum level of the parent drug remains well below the quoted upper limit of the drug, either because the level of metabolite has an additive effect, as is suspected in the case of carbamazepine [17,56], or because the adverse effects produced by drug and metabolite differ qualitatively [146].

Receptor binding assays were originally derived from the finding that neuroleptic drugs exert anti-schizophrenic therapeutic effects by blocking brain dopamine receptors [147]. Following the development of phenothiazine radioreceptor assays for clinical purposes [18, 148], Squires and Braestrup [149] and Mohler and Okada [150] observed highly specific receptors for benzodiazepines in rat brain. The increasing sophistication of synthetic radiochemical techniques is now allowing the preparation of tritium-labelled compounds of a very high specific activity [151]. An assay for clobazam using ³H-diazepam has been developed [152], and Duka et al [153] have described the use of ³H-flunitrazepam as a ligand, while Innis et al [154] developed a radioreceptor assay for tricyclic drugs, using the fact that these compounds compete effectively for the binding of ³H-quinuclidinyl benzylate to muscarinic cholinergic receptors in brain membranes.

Recently, a group from Burroughs Wellcome Company and the University of Connecticut have developed a kit for the radioreceptor assay of all neuroleptic drugs and their active metabolites [143], using the principle of competition between unlabelled drug and ³H-spiperone for dopamine receptors on stabilised calf caudate membranes. Another recent development of the greatest importance is the production of commercial preparations of rat brain receptors for benzodiazepines [155] which eliminates the need for a lengthy and tedious extraction process whenever this assay is performed, and makes it a practical proposition for routine use in TDM, as suggested by Lowe [151]. It is known that phenobarbitone and phenytoin specifically and competitively inhibit binding of ³H-picrotoxinin to its receptor sites in the brain. While only 10 per cent of this binding is specific, it is hoped that future developments might include the synthesis of ³H-picrotoxinin analogues with higher affinity for the binding site, which might possibly form the basis of a receptor binding assay for anticonvulsants [151].

Forward look

Recent trends in the field of TDM, particularly of anticonvulsant drugs, include the provision of clinic services, the use of monitoring free drug levels in saliva, and a trend towards monotherapy. These advances in the field of TDM have been made possible by the technical advances already described, especially the introduction of the new rapid methods of drug determination and the use of microprocessors which have speeded the process of calculation of results.

Clinic service

The concept of a rapid turn-around of drug estimation requests has become established in recent years [3–5, 156]. Using EMIT, the estimation of serum levels of selected anticonvulsant drugs can be carried out when the patient arrives at the hospital out-patient clinic, and the results given to the doctor during the consultation with the patient. In this way adjustment of drug regimen can be arranged without the necessity of a further appointment, leading to better fit control. This is particularly important in pregnancy when frequent adjustment of anticonvulsant drug dosage may be necessary, particularly in the last trimester, and it is obviously a very great advantage if these alterations can be made immediately.

If a semi-automatic analyser, such as the Stasar III (Corning Medical), is used to carry out the EMIT procedure in conjunction with a microcomputer, the standard curves for the drugs to be analysed can be prepared before the clinic and stored until needed, the actual analysis of each drug sample in duplicate together with a quality control specimen taking between five and six minutes [156]. The Stasar III is compact enough to be placed on a trolley and wheeled to the out-patient clinic, so that the analyses can be carried out in an annexe to the doctor's consulting room [4,5]. Alternatively, the specimens themselves can be transported to the laboratory for analysis and the completed reports returned to the clinician before the consultation with the patient [156]. The time between the taking of a blood sample and the receipt of the completed report giving the result of the analysis can be as short as 15 to 20 minutes [3,5,156].

Marty et al [4] recently carried out a three month evaluation of a rapid assay service for phenytoin and carbamazepine in an out-patient clinic, and concluded that the service was useful for detecting non-compliers, confirming suspected toxicity and aiding decisions in doubtful cases. This report corresponds well with the authors' own experience over a nine month period, when a rapid clinic service was provided for the anticonvulsants phenobarbitone, phenytoin and carbamazepine [156].

Monotherapy

It is a matter of concern that patients with epilepsy are frequently treated with multiple drugs because most patients take medication for many years or even for a lifetime and there is increasing anxiety about the toxic effects of anticonvulsant drugs [157, 158] (and see Chapter 50). It is now possible to establish firm control over serum levels of phenytoin by increasing the dose of the drug very gradually with frequent determination of serum levels, so that the lowest possible dose necessary to control seizures can be found without toxic symptoms developing. Recent work with both carbamazepine and phenytoin has shown that seizure control can be achieved by monotherapy with frequent monitoring of serum drug levels [157–159].

Reynolds et al [158] have recently reported the results of a five year study of phenytoin monotherapy with previously untreated patients with grand mal and/or partial seizures, and have shown that seizures could be controlled in 80 per cent of cases. In some instances control was achieved with sub-optimal serum levels, and the dose of drug rarely had to be raised above 300mg a day. It was considered that TDM not only allowed the dose of phenytoin to be adjusted to the individual patient's needs, but also contributed to the comparative rarity of acute toxic symptoms in the group. It was also estimated that, without TDM, 72 per cent of the patients in the trial might have had to be given an additional anticonvulsant drug, and that the potential for successful monotherapy would be even greater if the problem of non-compliance with anticonvulsant therapy could be overcome [158].

Gannaway and Maurer [159] have reported a successful transfer from multiple drug therapy to monotherapy with phenytoin in a group of 20 patients. Phenytoin levels of $140\mu mol/L^{-1}$ could be achieved without the appearance of toxic symptoms, though an upper limit of $80\mu mol/L^{-1}$ was considered more satisfactory. An increment even as small as 25mg in the daily dose sometimes proved to be too much, for example, an increase from 400mg per day to 425mg per day caused an excessive rise in the steady state serum level from 67 to $152\mu mol/L^{-1}$ in one patient. A reduction to 400mg and 425mg on alternate days was found to be satisfactory, and the serum level was reduced to $112\mu mol/L^{-1}$. These results could not have been achieved without the degree of fine control provided by TDM [159].

Although these reports confirm that monotherapy is a practicable method of treatment for many patients with epilepsy when TDM facilities are available, there may be occasions when fit control can only be achieved by the addition of another anticonvulsant to the regimen. A recent report has indicated that there is a synergistic action between phenytoin and phenobarbitone in mice, which seems to occur within the nervous system itself since it cannot be explained by changes in the amounts of these drugs entering the brain [160]. A potentiation of the action of phenytoin by phenobarbitone would also explain the findings of Kanematsu et al [161] that the mortality among phenobarbitone- and phenytoin-treated mice exposed to electro-shock was nil, while mice treated with phenytoin alone and exposed to electro-shock had a mortality rate of 15 per cent.

Many drugs are bound to plasma protein to a greater or lesser degree; the proportion of bound drug may be as high as 96 per cent of the total plasma concentration in the case of diazepam or 90 per cent in the case of phenytoin. Since it is accepted that the unbound drug alone is available at the site of action of the drug it follows that the changes in the proportion of bound drug, for example, carbamazepine, may produce toxic symptoms even though the total plasma level (which includes both free and bound drug) indicates that the drug is not present in toxic concentrations [17]. As discussed below (see Chapter 50), TDM of free plasma levels of phenytoin is indicated particularly when 'unbinding' is likely to occur, for example, in pregnancy and infancy or when the patient is suffering from uraemia or when other anticonvulsants are co-prescribed [162]. Much work has been carried out on the estimation of free drug levels, especially of phenytoin and carbamazepine. The separation techniques most frequently used for free and bound fractions of drugs namely equilibrium dialysis, ultracentrifugation, and ultrafiltration have been shown to correlate well [163], but recently doubt has been cast on the performance of the Worthington 'ultrafree' filters which have been shown to give unreliable results when serum rather than plasma samples are used, or when the tests are carried out at $37^{\circ}C$ rather than at ambient temperature [164, 165]. A kit for the determination of free phenytoin levels has recently been introduced by SYVA to be used in conjunction with their EMIT assay; it is at present (January 1982) undergoing trials and it is hoped it will prove satisfactory in clinical practice. The analytical procedures used to determine free drug levels after the separation process include GLC with nitrogen detection and HPLC as well as EMIT [17, 162, 166], which have the sensitivity to analyse drugs present in such low concentration $(1-10\mu\text{mol/L}^{-1}$, approximately in the case of phenytoin).

It is accepted that the concentration of certain drugs in saliva corresponds to the free drug level in plasma [97,162,166]. As discussed below (see Chapter 50) a major advantage of the monitoring of saliva drug concentrations is that the technique is non-invasive and so is particularly useful in paediatric practice. A minor disadvantage is that care must be taken to avoid contamination from the drug preparation itself in tablet or capsule form when it is taken orally, which requires special training of personnel who are generally more used to taking blood samples. The low concentration of drugs such as anticonvulsants in saliva adds to the difficulties in measurement, but the same analytical techniques which have been found satisfactory for free drug levels can be adapted for estimation of drugs in saliva [118, 119, 162, 166]. A particular advantage of HPLC in this connection is its ability to analyse the concentration in saliva of the major epoxide metabolite of carbamazepine which may itself have anticonvulsant properties [166].

478

Summary

The picture emerging from these advances points to the increasing use of multi-system analysis against the background of more systematic use of TDM in epilepsy.

Despite the improvements in techniques for TDM described here, no one method has established itself as superior in every respect to the others, and it is doubtful whether any one method will be found to be the best alternative for all drugs under all circumstances. Nevertheless, it can reasonably be predicted that receptor binding techniques, with their capacity to assay active metabolites as well as the parent drug, will become increasingly important and that improvements in technology will enable these assays to be used on a routine basis [151].

It seems likely that additional dry reagent chemistry assays will be developed for TDM. It is possible that reagent strip format kits used in conjunction with a calibration chart will enable tests to be carried out in the general practitioner's surgery or in health clinics, for example to check compliance — a major problem in anticonvulsant therapy. Recently, however, a warning note has been sounded about the use of test procedures outside the laboratory [123,167], and any such development can only be regarded as a 'back-up' for the full laboratory service for TDM [167].

Finally it can be predicted that the use of automatic methods will continue to expand, and produce more accurate results than manual methods [168, 169]. At the same time it is likely that the accuracy and sensitivity of immunoassay methods will be improved, perhaps to the level of estimating trace quantities of drugs [170–172].

Wilder and Bruni have stated that interaction between the laboratory and the patient's physician will generally improve patient care [173], and it is important that this continues at a high level, so that the expertise available for TDM is used to the best advantage in economic terms as well as in the interests of the patient [174,175].

Acknowledgments

The authors wish to acknowledge the great assistance given by Miss Kami Amin in preparing this manuscript.

Addendum

Neukermans et al [176] have recently (January 1982) described a non-radioactive electron-capture detector using a thermionic source of electrons, which has a greatly increased sensitivity over the present generation of electron-capture detectors.

References

1   Richens A, Marks V. In Richens A, Marks V, eds. *Therapeutic Drug Monitoring 1981; V.* London: Churchill Livingstone
2   Pippenger CE. *SYVA Monitor 1981; 10:* 1–2
3   Goldberg V, Ratnaraj N, Elyas A, Lascelles PT. *Anal Proc 1981; 18:* 313–316
4   Marty J, Fullinfaw R, Tuckett R et al. *Ther Drug Mon 1981; 3:* 253–258
5   Stanley PE. In Richens A, Marks V, eds. *Therapeutic Drug Monitoring 1981;* 54–60. London: Churchill Livingstone
6   Craig TM. *J Aut Chem 1981; 3:* 63–65
7   Pippenger CE, Penry JK, Kutt H et al. *Antiepileptic Drugs: Quantitative Analysis and Interpretation 1978.* New York: Raven Press
8   Wilder BJ, Bruni J. *Seizure Disorders: a Pharmacological Approach to Treatment 1981.* New York: Raven Press
9   Tognoni G, Latini R, Jusko WJ. *Frontiers in Therapeutic Drug Monitoring 1980.* New York: Raven Press
10 Richens A, Marks V. *Therapeutic Drug Monitoring 1981.* London: Churchill Livingstone
11 Sadée W, Beelen GCM. *Drug Level Monitoring – Analytical Techniques Metabolism and Pharmacokinetics 1981.* New York: Wiley - Interscience
12 Pippenger CE. *Ther Drug Mon 1979; 1:* 1–2
13 Lascelles PT. In Peters DK, ed. *Advanced Medicine 1976:* 108–117. London: Pitman Medical
14 Koch-Weser J. *Ther Drug Mon 1981; 3:* 3–16
15 Johannessen SI. *Ther Drug Mon 1981; 3:* 17–37
16 Wilder BJ, Bruni J. In Wilder BJ, Bruni J, eds. *Seizure Disorders: A Pharmacological Approach to Treatment 1981;* 23–45. New York: Raven Press
17 MKauge L, Tyrer JH, Eadier J. *Ther Drug Mon 1981; 3:* 63–70
18 Creese I, Snyder SH. *Nature 1977; 270:* 180–182
19 Greenblatt DJ, Shader RI. In Richens A, Marks V, eds. *Therapeutic Drug Monitoring 1981;* 272–280. London: Churchill Livingstone
20 Braithwaite R. In Richens A, Marks V, eds. *Therapeutic Drug Monitoring 1981;* 239–254. London: Churchill Livingstone
21 Scoggins BA, Maguire KP, Norman TR, Burrows GD. *Clin Chem 1980; 26:* 5–17
22 McCamish M. *Eur J Mass Spect 1980; 1:* 7–31
23 Voller A, Bartlett A, Bidwell D. *Immunoassays for the 80s 1981.* Lancaster: MTP Press Ltd
24 Farwell SO, Gage DR, Kagel RA. *J Chrom Sci 1981; 19:* 358–376
25 Garland WA, Powell ML. *J Chrom Sci 1981; 19:* 392–434
26 Smith DS, Ad-Hakiem MHH, Landon J. *Ann Clin Biochem 1981; 18:* 253–274
27 Schall RF Jr, Tenoso HJ. *Clin Chem 1981; 27:* 1157–1163
28 Rambeck B, Riedmann M, Meijer JWA. *Ther Drug Mon 1981; 3:* 377–395
29 Stockwell PB. *J Aut Chem 1982; 4:* 1
30 Riedmann M, Rambeck B, Meijer JWA. *Ther Drug Mon 1981; 3:* 397–413
31 Dhillon S, Richens A. *Br J Clin Pharmacol 1981; 12:* 841–844
32 Riva R, Tedeschi G, Albani F, Baruzzi A. *J Chrom 1981; 225:* 219–224
33 Riva R, de Anna M, Albani F, Baruzzi A. *J Chrom 1981; 222:* 491–495
34 Klotz U. *J Chrom 1981; 222:* 501–506
35 Jochemsen R, Breimer DD. *J Chrom 1982; 227:* 199–206
36 Jochemsen R, Breimer DD. *J Chrom 1981; 223:* 438–444
37 Greenblat DJ, Divoll M, Moschitto LJ, Shader RI. *J Chrom 1981; 225:* 202–207
38 Toseland PA, Wicks JFC. In Richens A, Marks V, eds. *Therapeutic Drug Monitoring 1981;* 85–109. London: Churchill Livingstone
39 Bente HB, In Pippenger CE, Penry JK, Kutt H, eds. *Antiepileptic Drugs: Quantitative Analysis and Interpretation 1978;* 139–145. New York: Raven Press
40 Rambeck B, Meijer JWA. *Ther Drug Mon 1980; 2:* 385–396

41 Bianchetti G. In Richens A, Marks V, eds. *Therapeutic Drug Monitoring 1981;* 307–319. London: Churchill Livingstone

42 Orsulak PJ, Gerson B. *Ther Drug Mon 1980; 2:* 233–242

43 Brazier JL, Delaye D, Desage M, Bannier A. *J Chrom 1981; 224:* 439–448

44 Debruyne D, Moulin MA, Camsonne R, Bigot MC. *J Pharm Sci 1980; 69:* 835–838

45 Kinberger B, Holmen A, Wahrgren P. *J Chrom 1981; 224:* 449–455

46 Cox V. *Tracor Chrom 1979;* Appl 79–20

47 Anderson JA, MacDonald J. *Tracor Chrom 1979;* Appl 79–29

48 Cox V. *Tracor Chrom 1980;* Appl 80–01

49 Simpson CF, Gough TA. *J Chrom Sci 1981; 19:* 275–282

50 Schaal DE, McKinley SL, Chittwood GW. *J Anal Tox 1979; 3:* 96–98

51 Kulpmann WR, Oellerich M. *J Clin Chem Clin Biochem 1981; 19:* 249–258

52 Schwertner HA. *Clin Chem 1979; 25:* 212–214

53 Schier GM, Eng Tho Gan I. *J Chrom 1981; 225:* 208–212

54 Ratnaraj N, Goldberg VD, Elyas A, Lascelles PT. *Analyst 1981; 106:* 1001–1006

55 Berry DJ, Clarke LA, Vallins GE. *J Chrom 1979; 171:* 363–370

56 Elyas AA, Ratnaraj N, Goldberg VD, Lascelles PT. Routine monitoring of carbamaze-pine and carbamazepine-10-11-epoxide in plasma by high performance liquid chromatography using 10-methoxycarbamazepine as internal standard. Submitted for publication 1982

57 Toseland PA. Personal communication to author 1981

58 Patel RB, Welling PG. *Clin Chem 1981; 27:* 1780–1781

59 Wallace JE, Shimek EL Jr, Harris SC. *J Anal Tox 1981; 5:* 20–23

60 Tjaden UR, Meeles MTHA, Thys CP, van der Kaaz M. *J Chrom 1980; 181:* 227–241

61 Vree TB, Baars AM, Heckster YA, van der Kleijn E. *J Chrom 1981; 224:* 519–525

62 Christofides JA, Fry DE. *Clin Chem 1980; 26:* 499–501

63 Szabo GK, Browne TR. *Clin Chem 1982; 28:* 100–104

64 Broussard LA, Stearns FM, Tulley R. *Clin Chem 1981; 27:* 1931–1933

65 Conlan AM, Tabor KJ, Lesko LJ. *Clin Chem 1981; 27:* 513

66 Jowett DA. *Clin Chem 1981; 27:* 1785

67 Skellern GG. *Analyst 1981; 106:* 1071–1075

68 Miksie JR, Hodes B. *J Pharm Sci 1979; 68:* 1200–1202

69 Edholm L-E. *Eur J Resp Dis (suppl 109) 1980; 61:* 45–53

70 Breutzmann DA, Bowers LD. *Clin Chem 1981; 27:* 1907–1911

71 Yu SY, Jurgensen A, Bolton D, Winefordner JD. *Anal Lett 000; 14A:* 1–6

72 Alawi MA, Russel HA. *Z Anal Chem 1981; 307:* 382–384

73 Suckow RF, Cooper TB. *J Pharm Sci 1981; 70:* 257–261

74 Murakami K, Murakami K, Ueno T et al. *J Chrom 1982; 227:* 103–112

75 Burmicz JS. In Smyth WF, ed. *Electroanalysis in Hygiene, Environmental, Clinical and Pharmaceutical Chemistry 1980:* 309–326. Amsterdam: Elsevier Scientific Publishing Co

76 Rooney R. *Lab Equip Dig 1980; 18:* 75–79

77 Smyth WF. *Anal Proc 1982; 19:* 82–86

78 Brooks MA. In Smyth WF, ed. *Electroanalysis in Hygiene, Environmental, Clinical and Pharmaceutical Chemistry 1980:* 287–298. Amsterdam: Elsevier Scientific Publishing Co

79 Harekamp HB, Voogt WH, Frei RW, Bos P. *Anal Chem 1981; 53:* 1362–1365

80 Kutner W, Debrowski J, Kemula W. *J Chrom 1981; 218:* 45–50

81 Lloyd RJ. *J Chrom 1981; 216:* 127–136

82 Vandemark FL. *Perkin Elmer Liquid Chromatographic Application Note 1982:* CL-3

83 Yang FJ. *J High Res Chrom Comm 1981; 4:* 83–85

84 George RC. *Clin Chem 1981; 27:* 198–199

85 Berg MJ, Lanz RK. *Clin Chem 1981; 27:* 1090 (abstract)

86 Salvadori C, Farinotti R, Duvaldestin PH, Dauphin A. *Ther Drug Mon 1981; 3:* 171–176

87 Narasimhachari N. *J Chrom 1981; 225:* 189–195

88 Dolan JW, can der Wal SJ, Bannister SJ, Snyder LR. *Clin Chem 1980; 26:* 871–880

89   van der Wal SJ, Snyder LR. *Clin Chem 1981; 27:* 1233–1240
90   Pippenger CE, Kutt HP, Penry JK, Daly DD. In Pippenger CE, Penry JK, Kutt HP, eds. *Antiepileptic Drugs: Quantitative Analysis and Interpretation 1978:* 187–197. New York: Raven Press
91   Fenimore DL, Davis CM. *Anal Chem 1981; 53:* 252A–266A
92   Gattavecchia E, Tonelli D, Breccia A. *J Chrom 1981; 224:* 465–471
93   Simona MG, Grandjean EM. *J Chrom 1981; 224:* 532–538
94   Rohdewald P, Drehsen G. *J Chrom 1981; 225:* 427–432
95   Sander LC, Sturgeon RL, Field LR. *J Liquid Chrom 1981; 4 (Suppl 1):* 63–97
96   Agurell S, Lindgren J. In Richens A, Marks V, eds. *Therapeutic Drug Monitoring 1981:* 110–130. London: Churchill Livingstone
97   Horning MG. *Clin Chem 1979; 26:* 1052 (abstract)
98   Schier GM, Eng Tho Gan I, Halpern B, Korth J. *Clin Chem 1980; 26:* 147–149
99   Miwa BJ, Garland WA, Blumenthal P. *Anal Chem 1981; 53:* 793–797
100   Garland WA, Min BH. *J Chrom 1979; 172:* 279–286
101   Cailleux A, Turcant A, Premel-Cabic A, Allain P. *J Chrom Sci 1981; 19:* 163–176
102   Alkayer M, Vallon JJ, Pegon Y, Bichon C. *Anal Lett 1981; B14:* 1047–1070
103   Zimak J, Gasparic J, Volke J. *Cesk Farm (Praha) 1980; 29:* 353–362
104   Groves JA, Smyth WF. *Analyst 1981; 106:* 890–897
105   Ivaska A, Smyth WF. In Smyth WF, ed. *Electroanalysis in Hygiene Environmental, Clinical and Pharmaceutical Chemistry 1980:* 337–347. Amsterdam: Elsevier Scientific Publishing Co
106   Yalow RS, Berson SA. *J Clin Invest 1960; 39:* 1157–1175
107   Marks V. In Richens A, Marks V, eds. *Therapeutic Drug Monitoring 1981:* 155–182. London: Churchill
108   Rutterford MG, Smith RN. *J Pharm Pharmacol 1980; 32:* 449–452
109   Hümpel M, Nieuweboer B, Milius W et al. *Clin Pharmacol Ther 1980; 28:* 673–679
110   Dixon R, Glover W, Earley J. *J Pharm Sci 1981; 70:* 230–231
111   Weinryb I, Shroff JR, Olson DR. *Drug Metab Rev 1979; 10:* 271–283
112   Bolton AE. In Voller A, Bartlett A, Bidwell D, eds. *Immunoassays for the 80s 1981:* 69–83. Lancaster: MTP Press Ltd
113   Ismail AAA, West PM, Goldie DJ, Poole AC. *Ann Clin Biochem 1981; 18:* 287–291
114   Cais M, Shimoni M. *Ann Clin Biochem 1981; 18:* 317–323
115   Cais M, Shimoni M. *Ann Clin Biochem 1981; 18:* 324–329
116   Elyas A, Goldberg VD, Ratnaraj N, Lascelles PT. *Ann Clin Biochem 1980; 17:* 307–310
117   Braun SL, Tausch A, Vogt W et al. *Clin Chem 1981; 27:* 169–172
118   Goldsmith RF, Ouvrier RA. *Ther Drug Mon 1981; 3:* 151–157
119   Piredda S, Monaco F. *Ther Drug Mon 1981; 3:* 321–323
120   Flacks H, Rasmussen JM. *Clin Chem 1980; 26:* 361
121   McDonald DM, Kabra PM. *Clin Chem 1980; 26:* 361–362
122   Aldwin L, Kabakoff DS. *Clin Chem 1981; 27:* 770–771
123   Toseland PA. *Anal Proc 1981; 18:* 391–393
124   Dietzler DN, Hoelting CR, Leckie MP et al. *Am J Clin Pathol 1980; 74:* 41–50
125   Shaw W, McHan J. *Ther Drug Mon 1981; 3:* 185–191
126   Al-Hakiem MHH, White GW, Smith DS, Landon J. *Ther Drug Mon 1981; 3:* 159–165
127   Kamel RS, Landon J, Smith DS. *Clin Chem 1980; 26:* 1281–1284
128   Karnes HT, Gudat JG, O'Donnell CM, Winefordner JD. *Clin Chem 1981; 27:* 249–252
129   Watson RAA, Landon J, Shaw EJ, Smith DS. *Clin Chim Acta 1976; 73:* 51–55
130   McGregor AR, Crookall-Greening JO, Landon J, Smith DS. *Clin Chim Acta 1978; 83:* 161–166
131   Jolley ME, Stroupe SD, Schwenzer KS et al. *Clin Chem 1981; 27:* 1575–1579
132   Wong RC, George R, Yeung R, Burd JF. *Clin Chim Acta 1980; 100:* 65–69
133   Li TM, Benovic JL, Buckler RT, Burd JF. *Clin Chem 1981; 27:* 22–26
134   Morris DL, Ellis DB, Hornby WE et al. *Anal Chem 1981; 53:* 658–665
135   Greyson J. *J Aut Chem 1981; 3:* 66–70
136   Zipp A. *J Aut Chem 1981; 3:* 71–75

137 Walter B. *Clin Chem 1981; 27:* 1086 (abstract)
138 Greenquist AC, Walter B, Li TM. *Clin Chem 1981; 27:* 1614–1617
139 Tyhach RJ, Rupchock PA, Pendergrass JH et al. *Clin Chem 1981; 27:* 1499–1504
140 Ho TT. *Clin Chem 1981; 27:* 1088 (abstract)
141 Finley PR, Dye JA, Williams RJ, Lichti DA. *Clin Chem 1981; 27:* 405–409
142 Lascelles PT. *Psychological Med 1981; 11:* 661–667
143 Patzke J, Lai A, Glueck BC et al. *Clin Chem 1980; 26:* 999–1000 (abstract)
144 Drayer DE. *Clin Pharmacokinet 1976; 1:* 426–443
145 Atkinson AJ Jr, Strong JM. *J Pharmacokinet Biopharm 1977; 5:* 95–109
146 Atkinson AJ Jr, Stec GP, Lertora JJL et al. *Ther Drug Mon 1980; 2:* 19–27
147 Creese I, Burt DR, Snyder SH. *Science 1976; 192:* 481–483
148 Tune LE, Creese I, Depaulo PR et al. *Am J Psych 1980; 137:* 187–190
149 Squires RF, Braestrup C. *Nature 1977; 266:* 732–734
150 Möhler H, Okado T. *Science 1977; 198:* 849-851
151 Lowe R. Personal communication to author 1981
152 Hunt P. *Br J Clin Pharmacol 1979; 7 (suppl 1):* 375–405
153 Duka T, Höllt V, Herz A. *Brain Research 1979; 179:* 147–156
154 Innis RB, Tune L, Rock R et al. *Eur J Pharmacol 1979; 58:* 473–477
155 Lund J. *Scand J Clin Lab Invest 1981; 41:* 275–280
156 Ratnaraj N, Elyas A, Goldberg V. *Med Lab Sci 1982; 39:* 97
157 Reynolds EH, Shorvon SD. *Epilepsia 1981; 22:* 1–10
158 Reynolds EH, Shorvon SD, Galbraith AW et al. *Epilepsia 1981; 22:* 475–488
159 Gannaway DT, Mawer GE. *Br J Clin Pharmacol 1981; 12:* 833–839
160 Masuda Y, Utsui Y, Shiraishi Y et al. *J Pharmacol Exp Ther 1981; 217:* 805–811
161 Kanematsu M, Hisayama T, Asai Y et al. *J Pharm Dyn 1981; 4:* 639–642
162 Knott C, Hamshaw-Thomas A, Reynolds F. *Br Med J 1982; 284:* 13–16
163 Garlock CM, Pippenger CE, Desaulniers CW, Sternberg S. *Clin Chem 1979; 25:* 1117
164 Perucca E, Richens A. *Ther Drug Mon 1981; 3:* 310
165 Ruprah M, Perucca E, Richens A. *Br J Clin Pharmacol 1981; 12:* 753–756
166 MacKichan JJ, Duffner PK, Cohen ME. *Br J Clin Pharmacol 1981; 12:* 31–37
167 Leader. Chemical Pathology on the Ward. *Lancet, February 1981:* 487
168 Northam BE. *Ann Clin Biochem 1981; 18:* 189–199
169 Jansen RTP, Pijpers FW, de Valk GAJM. *Ann Clin Biochem 1981; 18:* 218–225
170 O'Sullivan MJ. *Anal Proc 1981; 18:* 104–108
171 Wiseman A. *Anal Proc 1981; 18:* 359–361
172 Turton T. *Lab News 1982; 248:* 14
173 Wilder BJ, Bruni J. In Wilder BJ, Bruni J, eds. *Seizure Disorders: A Pharmacological Approach to Treatment 1981:* 169–183. New York: Raven Press
174 Lundberg GD. *JAMA 1981; 245:* 1762–1763
175 Levin B, Cohen SS, Birmingham PH. *Am J Hosp Pharm 1981; 38:* 845–851
176 Neukermans A, Kruger W, McManigill D. *J Chrom 1982; 235:* 1–20

50

SALIVA MONITORING OF ANTICONVULSANT DRUGS

Christine Knott, Felicity Reynolds

Treatment of convulsive disorders was largely empirical until the 1940s when methods were developed to measure phenytoin and phenobarbitone concentrations. These methods were laborious, time-consuming, and capable only of measuring very high-to-toxic drug concentrations. During the next 10 to 20 years, spectro-photometric [1, 2] and fluorimetric techniques improved sufficiently for plasma levels within the so-called 'therapeutic range' to be detected. Subsequently, many laboratories reported that clinical effect correlated better with concentration than with dose [3–8].

Phenytoin is perhaps the most difficult anticonvulsant to use in practice because Michaelis-Menten-like saturation of hepatic mixed function oxidases occurs within the narrow optimum range [9], resulting in a curvilinear relationship between steady state plasma concentrations and daily dose [10]. Disproportionately high, and highly variable, increases in plasma concentrations are commonly produced by quite modest (for example 50mg) dose increments [11], and the need to monitor phenytoin therapy is well recognised [12–16].

Methods used to determine phenytoin dose requirements frequently use plasma concentrations as an index of free phenytoin concentrations, and their accuracy therefore depends on constant protein binding. When protein binding is disturbed, as it is in hypoalbuminaemia [17–20], renal failure [21–25], hepatitis [26–29], pregnancy [30, 31], infancy [32–34], and polytherapy with other highly bound drugs [35–37], plasma monitoring is invalidated. With the advent of more sensitive techniques in the early 1970s [38–40], many workers sought a medium which would reflect unbound drug concentrations even in the presence of altered protein binding. Saliva seemed a possible answer.

Saliva collection

Saliva is secreted by the three saliva glands: parotid, submaxillary and sublingual, as well as by the buccal, palatal and labial glands [41]. Many authors eagerly devised exotic and imaginative methods of collecting saliva fractions from individual gland types, to compare the nature and composition of their secretions. Such methods included invasion of the mouth with a variety of suction apparatuses and orthodontic cribs and clasps, cannulation of Stensen's ducts, brushing the gingiva [42], and an assortment of techniques for collecting mixed saliva such as chewing paraffin wax [43], parafilm [44–47] or washed rubber bands [48], spraying citric acid on the dorsum of the tongue [49], and even sucking glass marbles [50], or pebbles [51]. Some of these methods are tedious, uncomfortable, or just plain dangerous and, not surprisingly, interest in saliva monitoring waned.

Our method of saliva collection has always been to ask the patient to spit into a pot.

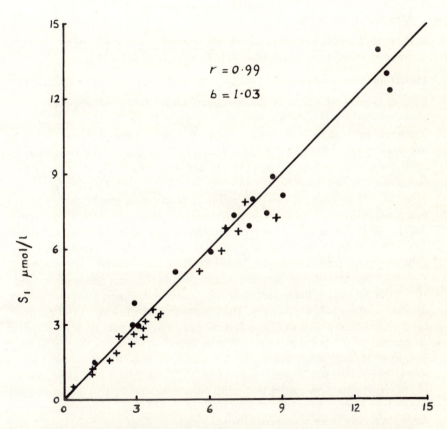

Figure 1. The relationship between paired saliva samples taken 10 minutes apart (●) and between paired stimulated (S_1) and unstimulated (S_2) saliva samples (+) in individual patients

Our initial studies were to compare phenytoin concentrations in whole saliva (which is a mixture of secretions from major and minor glands, and a small amount of gingival fluid) [52], with the less viscous citric acid stimulated mixed saliva [25]. We found that whole saliva concentrations were reproducibly 6 per cent higher than stimulated saliva concentrations, but that paired values correlated highly (r 0.99, Figure 1). Thereafter, we used citric acid stimulated saliva for three main reasons:

1. Large volumes are readily available (without frightening patients away with suction machines, or paraffin flavoured wax);

2. Saliva amylase and glycoprotein primarily arise from acinar cells, and their concentration, and that of nonacinar proteins, tend to vary inversely with flow rate [53]. We investigated the possibility that phenytoin may bind variably to saliva proteins, by filtering saliva through dialysis tubing (molecular weight cut off 14,000) under reduced pressure, but there was no demonstrable binding.

3. Phenytoin concentrations in mixed saliva are independent of volume produced, intensity or duration of stimulation [48] and pH of saliva [45].

Phenytoin in renal failure

Patients in renal failure are known to respond satisfactorily to lower plasma phenytoin concentrations than patients with normal renal function [22, 23], which was believed to be related to depressed protein binding [21, 24]. It is not possible to predict free phenytoin concentrations from total plasma concentrations, and we therefore assessed the suitability of saliva as an index of free phenytoin (measured by ultrafiltration) in 17 epileptics with normal renal function, and in seven patients with end stage renal failure who required phenytoin to suppress convulsions accompanying metabolic encephalopathy or haemodialysis [28]. Plasma phenytoin concentrations varied widely between individuals, and the percentage of unbound drug was significantly higher in renal failure patients (16.6 ± 0.7) than in epileptics (7.8 ± 0.3). Saliva concentrations were 19.6 ± 0.9 per cent of total plasma concentration in the renal failure group, and 10.5 ± 0.4 per cent in the epileptics, which corresponds closely with the findings of other workers [43, 44, 54–58]. The relationship between saliva and plasma for both groups is shown in Figure 2. Although combined data show good statistical correlation (r = 0.93) patients with renal failure all fall above the regression line. When in these same patients, saliva is compared with plasma unbound phenytoin (Figure 3) the correlation is higher (r = 0.98) and there is much less scatter of individual points, indicating that saliva reflects unbound phenytoin in the presence or absence of normal protein binding. This makes measurement of saliva phenytoin more appropriate than plasma in patients with renal failure, and the same optimum range (4–9μmol/L in this laboratory), which is about one tenth of the normally accepted plasma range, is valid for all patients.

486

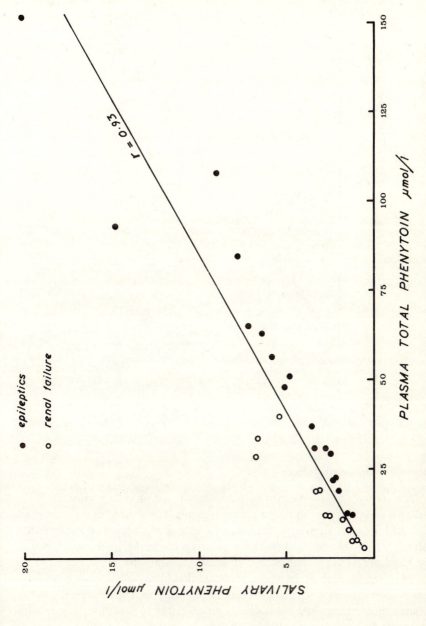

Figure 2. Saliva and plasma total concentrations in epileptics (●) and in patients with renal failure (○). (Reproduced by kind permission of the *Lancet*)

487

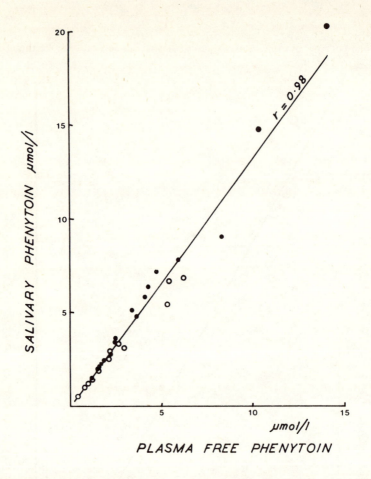

Figure 3. Saliva and plasma free phenytoin concentrations in epileptics (●) and in patients with renal failure (○). (Reproduced by kind permission of the *Lancet*)

Phenytoin-valproate interaction

We have recently been impressed by the increasing use of sodium valproate in combination with phenytoin. Our patients, particularly young children, were less impressed because valproate with a pK_a of 4.95 and consequent erratic secretion into saliva [59], necessitated plasma monitoring. It was previously established that valproate lowers plasma phenytoin while increasing the free fraction [35, 60–64]. Various authors, however, predicted that phenytoin displacement from plasma protein binding sites would result in increased hepatic clearance, lower plasma concentrations and consequently no alteration in phenytoin dose requirements [19, 64]. While monitoring both drugs in plasma samples, we soon noticed that plasma phenytoin concentrations did not reflect the clinical condition of our patients, many of whom exhibited clinical signs of cerebellar toxicity in the presence of low, or even subtherapeutic, plasma concentrations. We therefore studied the relationship between saliva, plasma unbound, and plasma total, phenytoin in patients receiving phenytoin with or without valproate, and the effect of valproate concentrations on phenytoin protein binding in vitro and in vivo [37].

In patients receiving phenytoin without valproate, we continued to find that saliva phenytoin concentrations were 10–11 per cent of corresponding plasma concentrations, and were significantly correlated (r = 0.96); in those receiving both drugs, the saliva:plasma ratio was higher (0.16 ± 0.04) and poorly correlated (r = 0.77, Figure 4). In patients in whom protein binding was also measured by ultrafiltration, the mean unbound fraction in the valproate group (0.1 ± 0.006) was higher than in patients receiving phenytoin only (0.072 ± 0.003). When saliva and unbound phenytoin concentrations are compared in these patients the two groups form a single population (Figure 5) showing that saliva bears the *same* close relation to unbound phenytoin (r = 0.97) in the presence or absence of valproate. The depression of protein binding is directly related to valproate

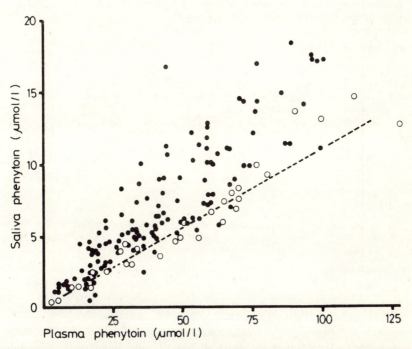

Figure 4. Relation between saliva and plasma phenytoin concentrations on 144 successive occasions in patients taking phenytoin and valproate (•) and in 31 controls (o) (r = 0.94 in control group, and slope = 0.11). (Reproduced by kind permission of the *British Medical Journal*)

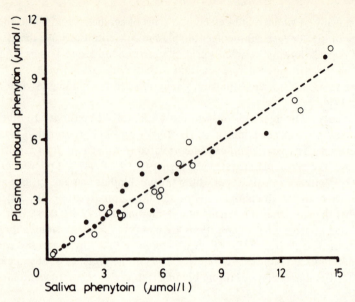

Figure 5. Relation between saliva and plasma unbound phenytoin concentrations in 19 patients taking valproate (●) and in 19 controls (○). (Reproduced by kind permission of the *British Medical Journal*)

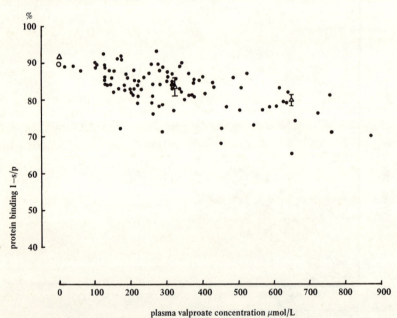

plasma valproate concentration μmol/L

Figure 6. The fall in saliva to plasma ratio with increasing valproate concentration in epileptic patients (●), closely corresponds to the depression of binding in vitro (△) using ultrafiltration of spiked pooled human plasma. In patients receiving phenytoin alone the s/p ratio (○) is consistent with previous findings

490

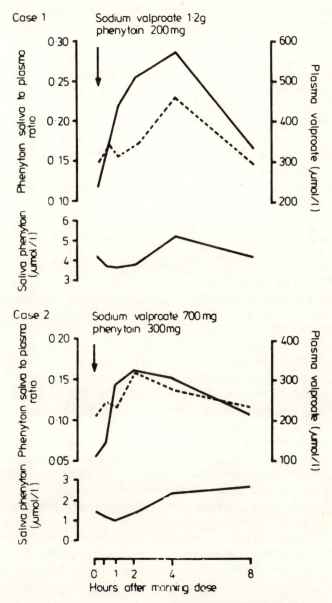

Figure 7. Phenytoin saliva to plasma ratio (dotted line), valproate concentration
(continuous line), and saliva phenytoin concentration in two patients studied for
eight hours after morning dose. (Reproduced by kind permission of the *British
Medical Journal*)

491

concentration (Figure 6) [65], but the correlation is too weak to allow accurate prediction of unbound phenytoin from a knowledge of plasma valproate concentration. Furthermore, hourly variations in plasma valproate concentration are rapidly reflected by hourly variations in free phenytoin fraction, and even concentration, and some individuals experience transient toxicity accompanying fluctuations of free phenytoin in and out of the optimum range (Figure 7) [66]. Such variations may be minimised by taking the daily requirement in divided doses, despite a possible sacrifice of compliance [67]. It is not uncommon for valproate to depress phenytoin binding from 90 per cent to 80 per cent or less, which effectively halves the upper and lower limits of the optimum range, and sole reliance on plasma phenytoin may suggest an inappropriate dose increment, resulting in worsening toxicity. When protein binding is depressed therefore, saliva phenytoin, which accurately reflects unbound phenytoin [43, 45, 52, 57, 68, 69], is essential.

Phenytoin in pregnancy

An important application of saliva rather than plasma anticonvulsant monitoring is found during pregnancy; many authors have reported that, with advancing pregnancy, a progressive decrease in plasma concentrations of anticonvulsants occurs associated with an increase in fit frequency *in spite* of receiving a constant daily dose [70–72].

Continuously changing physiology during pregnancy, such as decreased alimentary tract motility and absorption, increased drug clearance and volume of distribution, variable hormonal effects on metabolism due to changes in progesterone (an enzyme inducer) and oestrogen (a competitive inhibitor) concentrations, and the increasing drug metabolising activity of the fetus [73] have been said to contribute to the increased dose requirements [70–72].

In order to investigate the effects of pregnancy on protein binding we enlisted the co-operation of a 17 week pregnant primigravida who was taking a combination of phenytoin (300mg) and valproate (1200mg) daily, and who had previously been well controlled on these doses but had recently had one isolated seizure. At this time, plasma phenytoin concentration was 26.5µmol/L and, although the saliva concentration was effectively slightly higher (3.1µmol/L), it was also subtherapeutic. The plasma valproate concentration was however approaching the lower limits of the optimum range assumed to be appropriate for controlling seizures. Both anticonvulsants, were measured at monthly intervals thoughout this pregnancy.

A decrease in total plasma phenytoin and valproate concentrations, and a rising saliva : plasma ratio were observed (Figure 8). Phenytoin concentrations were never within the so-called therapeutic range, but saliva concentrations, which reflected unbound phenytoin concentrations, were almost always greater than 10 per cent of corresponding plasma concentrations, so that dosage adjustments made

492

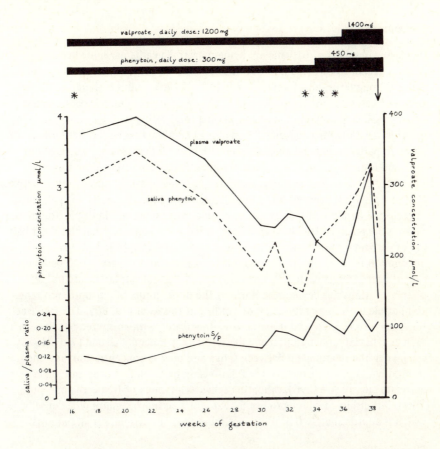

Figure 8. Changes in plasma valproate and saliva phenytoin concentrations and in saliva to plasma ratio, in a pregnant epileptic. * indicates seizures; ↓ indicates delivery. Initially one seizure occurred but three others preceded delivery when drug concentrations were at their lowest, and provoked a dose increase

using plasma phenytoin concentrations as a guideline would have been inappropriate. Initially our policy was to monitor anticonvulsant concentrations and maintain these within the optimum ranges, but this patient was so well controlled for most of her pregnancy, even when saliva phenytoin and plasma valproate concentrations were low, that we felt it unethical to prescribe higher doses of her anticonvulsants until, during the latter part of the last trimester, three isolated seizures occurred.

In contrast to our findings, Hooper and associates [26] did not find a decrease in protein binding throughout pregnancy and, although the albumin concentration correlated significantly with the saliva:plasma ratio [26] (r = 0.87), the correlation is too weak to be of any predictive value [31].

493

Carbamazepine

Increasing numbers of patients are being prescribed carbamazepine because its efficacy is said to be comparable to that of older anticonvulsants while the incidence of long term side effects is lower [43, 74–76], and it is therefore particularly advocated for use in children [77, 78]. We have studied the relationships between saliva, plasma unbound and plasma total carbamazepine concentrations in patients taking carbamazepine alone, or in combination with other anticonvulsants. In patients taking carbamazepine alone, the saliva:plasma ratio is about 0.25 and it does not differ significantly in patients on multiple drug therapy [79, 80], although the variation is greater. A range of saliva:plasma ratios between 0.25 and 0.37 has been reported by other authors [43, 57, 58, 81–85], but frequently the data presented are not separated into simple and multiple drug therapy making the results difficult to elucidate. It has been suggested that the short half-life of carbamazepine contributes to such variability [58, 82], and it is not uncommon for the peak and trough saliva:plasma ratio to vary by 20 per cent (unpublished observation). We have also found that saliva:plasma and unbound: plasma relationships cease to be linear at the upper limits of our optimum range compatible with some saturation of binding at this level [79, 86]. The free fraction may also be increased in patients co-medicated with antipyretic analgesics such as salicylate, phenylbutazone or steroids e.g. dexamethasone [79]. However, even when the relationship between saliva and plasma concentration, and the protein binding, are disturbed, the relationship between free drug and saliva correlate closely ($r = 0.96$), validating saliva as an index of free carbamazepine. This relationship enables us to use $6-12\mu$mol/L as our optimum range in saliva, which is approximately 0.3 of our optimum range in plasma, for all patients.

Phenobarbitone

Saliva phenobarbitone concentrations are approximately 38 per cent of corresponding plasma concentrations in this laboratory, which is consistent with findings from other laboratories [55,56,87,88] without adjusting for saliva pH [44,57]. We have found that saliva and plasma phenobarbitone concentrations correlate sufficiently well ($r = 0.94$) for saliva to be used when monitoring phenobarbitone therapy, and in some instances, for example with mentally retarded and aggressive, intoxicated patients, we find that collecting saliva is safer (for both patient and phlebotomist) than taking blood. We therefore use $15-35\mu$mol/L as our optimum range in saliva, corresponding to $45-110\mu$mol/L in plasma.

Primidone

In patients taking primidone, we find, in common with other workers [56–58, 87], that saliva concentrations approximate to plasma concentrations. Although the correlation between saliva and plasma is not high ($r = 0.88$), it is sufficiently strong

494

to validate saliva monitoring of this drug, especially in view of its limited use as a guide to therapy. One application of monitoring these drugs, however, is that the phenobarbitone:primidone ratio may be used as an index of compliance [89, 90]. We commonly find a phenobarbitone:primidone ratio of approximately unity in saliva (corresponding to 2.5:1 in plasma) in patients taking primidone regularly although, when other enzyme inducing agents (for example, carbamazepine) are taken in combination with primidone, this ratio may be increased slightly.

Anticonvulsants in pregnancy

In our experience, many women of child bearing age are prescribed phenobarbitone and/or primidone to control their seizures, and often the fetus is exposed to high concentrations of these drugs in utero. Phenobarbitone, particularly, is most frequently associated with withdrawal symptoms [91] and consequently convulsions and irritability in the neonate following delivery [92]. We were recently presented with a moderately well controlled mother (prescribed phenobarbitone 90mg, primidone 375mg, and carbamazepine 800mg daily, by another hospital) who was worried because her neurologist had advised her not to breast feed [93]. At this visit we measured anticonvulsant concentrations in maternal saliva, plasma and breast milk and in the baby's saliva. We found that maternal anticonvulsants were similar in breast milk and saliva on this and other occasions, but that the baby's saliva phenobarbitone concentration (14.8μmol/L) was approaching the therapeutic range (15–35μmol/L). Slow weaning from the breast was planned but following an abrupt decline in milk supply at seven months the baby presented with infantile spasms. The saliva phenobarbitone concentration of the baby declined dramatically to 6.7μmol/L and administration of phenobarbitone 30mg daily rapidly controlled the spasms. This dose of phenobarbitone was then gradually reduced with careful saliva monitoring.

With the readily available facility of anticonvulsant monitoring we not only encourage breast feeding in mothers receiving these drugs, but strongly support the view that it is positively indicated [94–102].

We have studied the relationship between maternal saliva and milk anticonvulsant concentrations in this patient and in two others receiving phenytoin alone.

TABLE I

		Number	Saliva:milk ratio ± SD
Phenytoin	Patient 1	7	0.66 ± 0.16
	Patient 2	8	0.46 ± 0.15
Phenobarbitone	Patient 3	6	1.09 ± 0.13
Primidone	Patient 3	6	1.56 ± 0.45
Carbamazepine	Patient 3	5	0.82 ± 0.26

Although we have found that the relationship between maternal saliva and milk concentration of phenobarbitone, primidone, phenytoin and carbamazepine are reasonably constant (Table I), neither of these measurements gives an estimate of the total dose the baby is absorbing [34, 103] or of the pharmacologically active concentrations in vivo [32, 33, 104]. We therefore routinely monitor saliva anti-convulsant concentrations of babies fed by mothers taking regular anticonvulsant medication.

Conclusion

We routinely use saliva to monitor all the common anticonvulsants except valproate. Good correlations between saliva and plasma drug concentrations in the absence of disturbed protein binding enable us to use the optimum ranges for saliva which are summarised in Table II. However, we have repeatedly found

TABLE II

	(Therapeutic range (μmol/L))	
	Plasma	Saliva
Phenytoin	40 – 80	4 – 9
Phenobarbitone	45 – 100	15 – 35
Primidone	25 – 55	25 – 55
Carbamazepine	20 – 40	6 – 12
Valproate	350 – 700	–
Ethosuximide	300 – 600	300 – 600

that saliva accurately reflects unbound drug concentrations [25, 37, 79] in the presence or absence of disturbed protein binding, and therefore the same optimum ranges are valid in all conditions investigated.

Saliva monitoring of anticonvulsants has numerous advantages; it is particularly useful when patients are housebound, live at inconvenient distances from the clinic, or when children are eager not to miss school, because they can, after instruction, collect their own samples at their convenience. We are aware of the possibility of direct drug contamination of saliva specimens particularly when tablets are not coated or available in capsule form (such as carbamazepine). We therefore always request that our patients either brush their teeth, eat a meal, or rinse their mouth thoroughly in the interval between drug ingestion and sampling [105, 106]. One frequent criticism of saliva monitoring is that it is inaccurate. Such a criticism does not validate plasma monitoring in the presence of disturbed protein binding. True, saliva concentrations are frequently lower than the corre-sponding plasma concentrations, but they are still above the lower limits of detection of many analytical techniques [87]. Furthermore, newer assay techniques such as HPLC and enzyme-linked immunoassays can provide reliable means of measuring low drug concentrations; good correlations between these methods and more traditional techniques such as GLC have been reported [58, 107–109].

There has been a recent surge of interest in the use of tears as a predictor of unbound drug levels. Piredda and co-authors [110] state that 'lachrymation is frequent in children' and that 'brisk tearing can easily be provoked by cigarette smoke or the sniffing of formaldehyde'. We are firmly convinced that collecting saliva is kinder, quicker, and less noxious.

Besides, we have no tears in our laboratory (Figure 9).

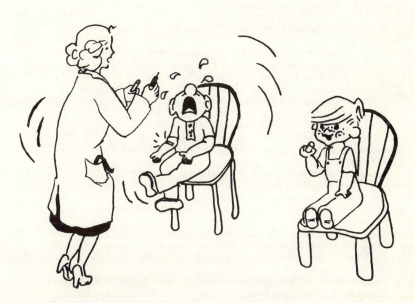

Figure 9. The child on the left has serum anticonvulsant monitoring and the child on the right, saliva monitoring

References

1   Dill WA, Kazenko A, Wolf LM, Glazko AJ. *J Pharmac Exp Ther 1956; 118:* 270–279
2   Svensmark O, Kristensen P. *J Lab Clin Med 1963; 61:* 501–507
3   Loeser E Jr. *Neurology 1961; 11:* 424–429
4   Vapaatalo H, Lehtinen L. *Europ Neurol 1971; 5:* 303–310
5   Bochner F, Hooper WD, Tyrer JH, Eadie MJ. *J Neurol Neurosurg Psych 1972; 35:* 873–876

6   Booker HE, Darcey B. *Epilepsia (Amst) 1973; 14:* 177–184
7   Eadie MJ, Tyrer JH. *Aust NZ J Med 1973; 3:* 290–303
8   Mawer GE, Mullen PW, Rodgers M, et al. *Br J Clin Pharmac 1974; 1:* 163–168
9   Ludden T, Allen J, Valutsky W, et al. *Clin Pharm Ther 1976; 21:* 287–293
10   Richens A, Dunlop A. *Lancet 1975; ii:* 247–248
11   Gannaway DJ, Mawer GE. *Br J Clin Pharmac 1981; 12:* 33–839
12   Kutt H, Wolk M, Scherman R, McDowell F. *Neurology 1964; 14:* 542–548
13   Reynolds E. *Proc Roy Soc Med 1975; 68:* 4–6
14   Birkett DJ, Graham GG, Chinwah PM, et al. *Med J Aust 1977; 2:* 467–468
15   Rambeck B, Boenigk HE, Dunlop A, et al. *Ther Drug Monit 1979; 1:* 325–333
16   Bergman U, Rane A, Sjöqvist F, Wilholm BE. *Ther Drug Monit 1981; 3:* 259–269
17   Lunde PKM, Rane A, Yaffe SJ, et al. *Clin Pharm Ther 1970; 11:* 846–855
18   Wallce S, Runcie J, Whiting B. *Br J Clin Pharmac 1976; 3:* 327–330
19   Gugler R, Shoeman DW, Huffman DH, et al. *J Clin Invest 1975; 55:* 1182–1189
20   Porter RJ, Layzer RB. *Arch Neurol (Chic) 1975; 32:* 298–303
21   Reidenberg M, Odar-Cederlöf I, Von Bahr C, et al. *New Engl J Med 1971; 285:* 264–265
22   Letteri J, Mellk H, Louis S, et al. *New Engl J Med 1971; 285:* 648–652
23   Odar-Cederlöf I, Borgå O. *Eur J Clin Pharmacol 1974; 7:* 31–37
24   Odar-Cederlöf I, Borgå O. *Clin Pharm Ther 1976; 20:* 36–47
25   Reynolds F, Ziroyanis PN, Jones NF, Smith SE. *Lancet 1976; ii:* 384–386
26   Hooper WD, Bochner F, Eadie MJ, Tyrer JH. *Clin Pharm Ther 1974; 15:* 276–282
27   Blaschke TF, Meffin PJ, Melmon KL, Rowland K. *Clin Pharm Ther 1975; 17:* 685–691
28   Olsen GD, Bennett WM, Porter GA. *Clin Pharm Ther 1975; 17:* 677–684
29   McColl KEL, Fletcher CD, Thomson TJ. *Lancet 1978; i:* 1201–1202
30   Ruprah M, Perucca E, Richens A. *Lancet 1980; ii:* 316–317
31   Perucca E, Ruprah M, Richens A. *Br J Clin Pharmac 1981; 12:* 276P
32   Ehrnebo M, Agurell S, Jalling B, Boreus LO. *Eur J Clin Pharmacol 1971; 3:* 189–193
33   Lund L, Lunde PK, Rane A, et al. *Ann NY Acad Sci 1971; 179:* 723–728
34   Morselli PL, Franco-Morselli R, Bossi L. *Clin Pharmacok 1980; 5:* 485–527
35   Patsalos PN, Lascelles PT. *J Neurol Neurosurg Psych 1977; 40:* 570–574
36   Fraser DG, Ludden TM, Evens RP, Sutherland EW. *Clin Pharm Ther 1980; 27:* 165–169
37   Knott C, Hamshaw-Thomas A, Reynolds F. *Br Med J 1982; 1:* 13–16
38   Chang T, Glazko AJ. *J Lab Clin Med 1970; 75:* 145–155
39   Breyer U, Villumsen D. *J Chromatog 1975; 115:* 493–500
40   Paxton JW, Rowell FJ, Ratcliffe JG, et al. *Eur J Clin Pharmacol 1977; 11:* 71–74
41   Schneyer LH, Young JA, Schneyer CA. *Phys Rev 1972; 52:* 720–777
42   Stephen KW, Speirs CF. *Br J Clin Pharmac 1976; 3:* 315–319
43   Troupin AS, Friel PN. *Epilepsia 1975; 16:* 223–227
44   Mucklow JC, Bending MR, Kahn GC, Dollery CT. *Clin Pharm Ther 1978; 24:* 567–5 567–570
45   Bochner F, Hooper WD, Sutherland JM, et al. *Arch Neurol 1974; 31:* 57–59
46   Koysooko R, Ellis EF, Levy G. *Clin Pharm Ther 1974; 15:* 454–460
47   Plavsic F, Culig J, Bakran I JR, Vrhovac B. *Br J Clin Pharmac 1981; 11:* 533–534
48   Paxton JW, Whiting B, Stephen KW. *Br J Clin Pharmac 1977; 4:* 185–191
49   Stephen KW, McCrossan J, Mackenzie D, et al. *Br J Clin Pharmac 1980; 9:* 51–55
50   Inaeba T, Kalow W. *Clin Pharm Ther 1975; 18:* 558–562
51   Hoeprich PD, Warshauer DM. *Antimicrob Agents and Chemother 1974; 5:* 330–336
52   Anavekar SN, Saunders RH, Wardell WM, et al. *Clin Pharm Ther 1978; 24:* 629–637
53   Mandel ID. *J Dent Res (Suppl) 1974; 53:* 246–266
54   Conard GJ, Jeffay H, Boshes L, Steinberg AD. *J Dent Res 1974; 53:* 1323–1329
55   Cook C, Amerson B, Poole K, et al. *Clin Pharm Ther 1975; 18:* 742–747
56   Schmidt D, Kupferberg HJ. *Epilepsia 1975; 16:* 735–741
57   McAuliffe JJ, Sherwin AL, Leppik IE, et al. *Neurology 1977; 27:* 409–413

58   Goldsmith RF, Ouvrier RA. *Ther Drug Monit 1981; 3:* 151—157
59   Gugler R, Von Unruh GE. *Clin Pharmacok 1980; 5:* 67—83
60   Jordan BJ, Shillingford JS, Steed KP. In Legg NJ, ed. *Clinical and Pharmacological Aspects of Sodium Valproate (Epilim) in the Treatment of Epilepsy 1975;* 112. Tunbridge Wells: MSC Consultants
61   Lecchini S, Gatti G, De Bernardi M, et al. *Il Farmaco Ed Pr 1977; 33:* 80—82
62   Berchou R, Lodhi R, Haidukewych D. In *Epilepsy International Symposium Abstracts, Vancouver BC, Canada, 1978;* 163
63   Monks A, Boobis S, Wadsworth J, Richens A. *Br J Clin Pharmac 1978; 6:* 487—492
64   Friel PN, Leal KW, Wilensky AJ. *Ther Drug Monit 1979; 1:* 243—248
65   Monks A, Richens A. *Clin Pharm Ther 1980; 27:* 89—95
66   Haidukewych D, Rodin EA. *Ther Drug Monit 1981; 3:* 303—307
67   Covanis A, Jeavons PM. *Devel Med Child Neurol 1980; 22:* 202—204
68   Vaida F, Williams FM, Davidson S, et al. *Clin Pharm Ther 1974; 15:* 597—603
69   Houghton GW, Richens A, Toseland PA, et al. *Eur J Clin Pharmacol 1975; 9:* 73—78
70   Mygind K, Dam M, Christiansen J. *Acta Neurol Scand 1976; 54:* 160—166
71   Eadie MJ, Lander CM, Tyrer JH. *Clin Pharmacok 1977; 2:* 427—436
72   Dam M, Christiansen J, Munck O, Mygind KI. *Clin Pharmacok 1979; 4:* 53—62
73   Krauer B, Krauer F. *Clin Pharmacok 1977; 2:* 167—181
74   Dalby MA. *Adv Neurol 1975; 11:* 331—344
75   Trimble M. In Roberts FD, ed. *Tegretol in Epilepsy. Proceedings of an International Meeting 1977;* 15. Basel: Geigy
76   Addy DP. *Br Med J 1978; 2:* 811—812
77   Gamstorp I. *Adv Neurol 1975; 11:* 237—248
78   O'Donohoe N. In Roberts FD, ed. *Tegretol in Epilepsy. Proceedings of an International Meeting 1977;* 10. Basel: Geigy
79   Knott C. In preparation
80   Kristenson O, Larsen HF. *Acta Neurol Scand 1980; 61:* 344—350
81   Chambers RE, Homedia M, Hunter KR, Teague RH. *Lancet 1977; i:* 656—657
82   Rylance GW, Butcher GM, Moreland T. *Br Med J 1977; 4:* 1481
83   Westenberg HGM, van der Kleijn E, et al. *Clin Pharm Ther 1978; 23:* 320—328
84   MacKichan JJ, Duffner PK, Cohen ME. *Br J Clin Pharmac 1981; 12:* 31—37
85   Paxton JW, Donald RA. *Clin Pharm Ther 1981; 28:* 695—702
86   Hooper WD, Dubetz DK, Bochner F, et al. *Clin Pharm Ther 1975; 17:* 433—440
87   Horning MG, Brown L, Nowlin J, et al. *Clin Chem 1977; 23:* 157—164
88   Pisani F, Oteri G, Diperri R. *Br J Clin Pharm 1981; 12:* 81—83
89   Reynolds EH, Fenton G, Fenwick P, et al. *Br Med J 1975; 2:* 594—595
90   Danhof M, Breimer DD. *Clin Pharmacok 1978; 3:* 39—57
91   Committee on Alcoholism and Addiction and Council on Mental Health. *JAMA 1965; 193:* 673—677
92   Erith MJ. *Br Med J 1975; 3:* 40
93   Knott C, Clayden G, Reynolds F, Fenwick P. In preparation
94   Shattock FM, Stephens DJH. *Lancet 1975; i:* 113—114
95   Addy DP. *Lancet 1976; ii:* 742
96   Leading Article. *Br Med J 1976; 1:* 1167
97   Downham MAPS, Scott R, Sims DG, et al. *Br Med J 1976; 2:* 274—276
98   Turner RWD. *Lancet 1976; ii:* 693—694
99   Barness LH. *N Engl J Med 1977; 297:* 939—941
100 Cunningham AS. *J Paediat 1977; 90:* 726—729
101 Jelliffe DB, Jelliffe EFP. *N Engl J Med 1977; 297:* 912—919
102 Tripp JH, Wilmers MJ, Wharton BA. *Lancet 1977; ii:* 233—236
103 Kaneko S, Sato T, Suzuki K. *Br J Clin Pharm 1979; 7:* 624—629
104 Hamar C, Levy G. *Clin Pharm Ther 1980; 28:* 58—63
105 Ayers GJ, Burnett D. *Lancet 1977; i:* 656
106 Paxton J, Foote S. *Br J Clin Pharmac 1979; 8:* 508—510
107 Castro A, Ibanez J, Dicesar JL, et al. *Clin Chem 1978; 24:* 710—713
108 Pesh-Imam M, Fretthold DW, Sunshine I, et al. *Ther Drug Monit 1979; 1:* 289—299
109 Couri D, Suarez del Villar S, Toy-Manning P. *J Analyt Tox 1980; 4:* 227—231
110 Piredda S, Monaco F. *Ther Drug Monit 1981; 3:* 321—323

51

PROGNOSTIC FACTORS IN SELECTING PATIENTS WITH DRUG RESISTANT EPILEPSY FOR TEMPORAL LOBECTOMY

C E Polkey

Introduction

The success of resective surgery for epilepsy is largely dependent upon the means used to select patients for operation, and this is certainly so in the case of the commonest of these operations namely temporal lobectomy. Provided the deep structures are removed, the success of the operation is not affected by the details of surgical technique which do however govern the occurrence of post-operative complications and the acquisition of pathological knowledge. This is less true of resections involving other cortical areas which may encroach upon eloquent areas or where electrocorticography may be more important in determining the extent of the resection.

The classical criteria for temporal lobectomy have been described in the past by Rasmussen [1] and by Falconer [2]. In essence they depend upon two broad principles, the first being the proof of a need for operation. The second is the demonstration of an electrical focus in the appropriate temporal lobe without evidence of a mass lesion, and with reasonable certainty that the remaining cerebral tissue is normal. From his experience of almost 300 temporal lobectomies, Falconer was able to show that if the resected temporal lobe contained a definite pathological lesion then there was more likely to be a good result from surgery [3]. Changes in available neuroradiological techniques have to some extent altered the population being presented for consideration of surgery as a means of treating drug-resistant epilepsy, as well as improving the detection of discrete lesions. This produces a dilemma of having to choose between those patients who should be offered operation because they have a discrete focal neurophysiological abnormality, although there is no overt evidence of a pathological lesion in the temporal lobe, and those in whom there is known to be such a lesion in the presence of less well localised neurophysiological abnormalities.

This chapter attempts to assess the value of the information available prior to operation in predicting the results of surgery. For reasons which will become clear later, no patient who fulfilled the classical criteria previously mentioned was refused operation and what is being proposed is a possible way of working out the likelihood of success.

Clinical material

The tradition of epilepsy surgery which Murray Falconer started at the Maudsley Hospital has continued and in a five year period from January 1976 until December 1980, 117 new patients were admitted for consideration of surgery for their epilepsy. The assessment was carried out by a multi-disciplinary team although the patients were admitted under the clinical supervision of the neurosurgeon. Interpretation of the results of various tests were made by each consultant and all the pathological examinations were carried out by one consultant neuropathologist. Among this group of patients, 63 were considered suitable for operation and 58 accepted surgery, of whom 46 (79%) underwent temporal lobectomy. A detailed account of this has been published elsewhere [4]. By the end of December 1981 the number of temporal lobectomies performed, using the 'en bloc' technique, had risen to 54 and the details of this group are shown in Table I.

TABLE I. Temporal Lobectomies. 1.2.76 – 1.2.82

28 males; 26 females		
25 left sided (10 LA) 29 right sided (5 LA)		
PATHOLOGY -	Mesial temporal sclerosis (MTS)	26 (48%)
	Tumours and hamartoma	16 (30%)
	Other pathology	6 (11%)
	Non specific	6 (11%)

However this chapter concerns two groups of 28 patients for whom an adequate follow-up is available. From Murray Falconer's material, commencing in 1976 and working backwards, 28 consecutive cases were selected in whom there was an adequate follow-up of at least four years, the longest follow-up being 11 years and the mean period of follow-up of this group was 6.1 years. The patients will be referred to as Group A. A further 28 consecutive patients were also selected from the 54 patients who had undergone temporal lobectomy since 1976. These patients were all followed for at least two years from surgery and some for more than five years, the mean length of follow-up being 3.4 years. This group will be referred to as Group B. Unfortunately there is an unavoidable small bias in the selection of both groups, which is more marked in the case of Group A, a bias that is in favour of patients with a good result. The reason for this is that patients whose fits persist, especially if they also have a personality disorder, tend either to become institutionalised or have an insecure base in the community and are thus less easy to trace.

The pathological lesions found in the temporal lobes resected are detailed in Table II. The distribution of lesions between the two groups differs, probably due to the small numbers of patients involved. The distribution of the pathological lesions in the 54 patients operated on since 1976 is similar to that described

TABLE II. Results of temporal lobectomy

	Group A			Group B		
Pathology	No.	%		No.	%	
MTS	17	61%		10	36%	
Other	6	21%		15	54%	
NS	5	18%		3	10%	
Results						
Gd 1	16	57%	68%	18	64%	78%
Gd 2	3	11%	improved	4	14%	improved
Gd 3	5	18%	32%	2	7%	22%
Gd 4	4	14%	not	4	15%	not

by Falconer and Taylor [5] but, although the proportion with mesial temporal sclerosis is the same, the number of tumours and hamartomas is slightly increased and the number with non-specific findings is reduced. The results of operations were graded according to the amelioration of their epilepsy using a simple scheme modified from one suggested by Jensen [6], and this is shown in Table III.

TABLE III. Temporal lobectomy — follow-up assessment

Grade 1 —	less than 5 fits in all	
Grade 2 —	75% better	
Grade 3 —	50% better	
Grade 4 —	Unchanged	
Grades 1 and 2 are considered a worthwhile result		

For pre-operative assessment a crude points system was used which has already been described [4]. It uses the four sources of evidence available pre-operatively, namely: clinical history of fits; neurophysiological investigations, usually comprising routine, sleep and pentothal-activated sphenoidal recording; psychometric

502

assessment and the neuroradiological studies. In the interest of brevity, details of the protocol for these investigations have been omitted; where necessary the Wada intracarotid amytal test has been used to determine hemisphere dominance and memory function. The neurophysiological investigations listed are the minimum carried out and more may be performed with changes in medication or sleep deprivation if necessary. Chronic stereotactic recording (SDEEG) was not undertaken. When the results of these four areas represent a localised, lateralised temporal lobe lesion then a high score is given. In dealing with the neuroradiological findings in group A it is necessary to compensate for the fact that CAT was not available. A positive scan has been allowed to those patients in whom there was a pathological lesion such as an hamartoma which subsequent experience has shown would have given a discrete CAT abnormality. Although a temporal horn which is dilated on AEG is often visible on CAT this has not been counted as a positive scan abnormality. The scheme is biased in that it allows a patient with a positive scan abnormality and an indifferent EEG to achieve the same score as a patient with a localised unilateral temporal EEG abnormality. The details of this scoring system are set out in Table IV. One can compare the

TABLE IV. Scoring of pre-operative selection criteria for temporal lobectomy

Criterion	Features	Points
Type of Fit	Aura, psychomotor attack	2
	Other complex seizure	1
	Generalised seizure	0
EEG Findings	Lateralised temporal abnormalities	2
	Unilateral widespread or minor bilateral abnormalities	1
	Multifocal, bilateral abnormalities	0
Psychometric Data	Appropriate verbal/performance and memory deficit	2
	Appropriate verbal/performance deficit	1
	No significant deficit	0
	Inappropriate verbal/performance deficit	1
	Inappropriate verbal/performance and memory deficit	2
Radiological Findings	Positive lesion	2
	Dilated temporal horn on AEG	1

scoring of the group with the longer follow-up (group A) with that of those with the shorter follow-up (group B) to see whether they followed similar patterns.

Results

In both groups the least number of points scored was one and the greatest was seven, with most patients scoring three or more. Because of the inclusion of the psychometric data, patients selected according to the classical criteria can score as little as one point. However, especially in relation to mesial temporal sclerosis, I believe that this is a valid indicator of damage outside of the temporal lobe to be removed, particularly when hemispheric dominance is taken into account. The results of operation for both groups are shown in Table II and it can be seen that they are reasonable. An average score can be calculated by totalling the points scored by all the patients with the same result from surgery shown in Table V. It can be seen that in both groups A and B a score above four usually has a good outcome whereas a score of less than four has a poor result. The same

TABLE V. Temporal lobectomy – scoring of pre-operative data

Result	Group A			Group B		
	No.	Points		No.	Points	
Gd 1	16	4.6		18	4.9	
			4.5			4.8
Gd 2	3	4.3		4	4.2	
Gd 3	5	3.6		2	2.5	
			3.6			3.2
Gd 4	4	3.5		4	3.5	

TABLE VI. Temporal lobectomy – distribution of points scored

Result	GD 1 + 2 (Improved)			GD 3 + 4 (Not improved)		
Score	A	B	Total	Total	A	B
1	0	0	0	2	1	1
2	1	1	2	1	0	1
3	4	3	7	3	2	1
4	5	3	8	7	5	2
5	4	9	13	2	1	1
6	3	5	8	0	0	0
7	2	1	3	0	0	0

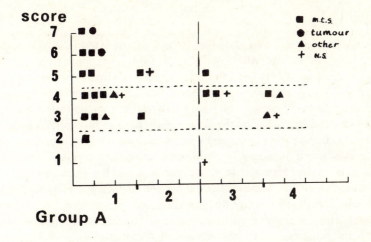

Group A

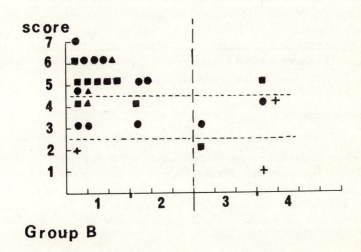

Group B

Figure 1. The points scored in the pre-operative assessment for each patient are compared with the results of operation. The pathology in each resected temporal lobe is indicated. The dotted lines indicate the areas where a good result is less likely. Group A comprises 28 patients operated upon by the late Murray Falconer, group B, 28 operated upon by the author

data, presented in a different form in Table VI, show that patients who score five or more have a high chance of being in Grade 1 or 2 whereas those who score only three or four have only an even chance of this, as illustrated in Figure 1.

Discussion

These results in no way invalidate the classical criteria used in selection for anterior temporal lobectomy. Although the result from operation is better when a positive pathology is found and this tends to be associated with higher scoring, as seen in Figure 1, a minority of patients in the reverse situation achieved a good result and this must represent selection purely on neurophysiological grounds. By careful consideration of all the pre-operative data we have been able, in 81 per cent of the 54 patients operated upon to date, to predict the presence of a pathological lesion subsequently confirmed at operation. In 60 per cent of these 54 patients we have been able to predict the nature of the lesion correctly.

The scoring system described here allows one to predict crudely the likelihood of success. It has the advantage that the assessment period is relatively easy to interpret. This is a complex and changing field. Any system of selection which relies upon simple tests must perforce deal disadvantageously with the more complex case. A number of methods are available to refine such a process. The use of chronic stereotactic recordings has been described by Crandall and his associates and the results of using this technique over a long period of time has recently been described by them [7,8] (see following chapter). In addition more sophisticated methods of scanning such a positron emission tomography (PET) [8], and CAT with subarachnoid metrizamide to outline structures at the tentorial hiatus [9], may make such decisions easier in the future.

Acknowledgements

As indicated this work is multi-disciplinary in nature and I am pleased to acknowledge the part played by my colleagues, Dr MV Driver in Clinical Neurophysiology; Dr RD Hoare and Dr J Dawson in Neuroradiology; Dr G Powell in the Department of Psychology of the Institute of Psychiatry and Dr I Janota in the Department of Neuropathology of the same Institute.

References

1   Rasmussen T. *Clin Neurosurg 1969; 16:* 288—314
2   Falconer MA. In Symon L, ed. *Operative Surgery. Neurosurgery. 3rd Edition 1979:* 315—322. London: Butterworth
3   Falconer MA, Davidson S. In Harris P, Mawdsley C, eds. *Epilepsy. Proceedings of the Hans Berger Centenary Symposium 1974:* Chapter 33, 209—214. Edinburgh: Churchill Livingstone
4   Polkey CE. *J Roy Soc Med 1981; 74:* 574—579
5   Falconer MA, Taylor DC. *Arch Neurol 1968; 19:* 353—361
6   Jensen I. *Acta Neurol Scand 1974; 52:* 354—373
7   Lieb J, Engel J, Gevins A, Crandall PH. *Epilepsia 1981; 22:* 525—538
8   Lieb J, Engel J, Gevins A, Crandall PH. *Epilepsia 1981; 22:* 539—548
9   Kuhl D, Engel J, Phelps M. *Acta Neurol Scand 1979; 72:* Suppl 538—539
10   Turner DA, Wyler AR. *Epilepsia 1981; 22:* 23—629

52

INDICATIONS FOR DEPTH ELECTRODE RECORDINGS IN COMPLEX PARTIAL EPILEPSY AND SUBSEQUENT SURGICAL RESULTS

P H Crandall, J Engel Jr, Rebecca Rausch

Progress in the surgical treatment of the partial or focal epilepsies has been entirely dependent on an accurate localisation of the epileptogenic cerebral cortex. British and Canadian neurologists, neurophysiologists and neurosurgeons are largely responsible for developing concepts of cerebral localisation and techniques leading to surgical treatment of seizures. Hughlings Jackson [1] from clinical observations recognised the significance of the focal spread of discharges through the cortex which was verified in the experimental studies of Sir David Ferrier [2]. From the time of Sir Victor Horsley in 1887 [3], through that of Otfrid Foerster and Wilder Penfield [4], the guiding principles of identification of the cerebral focus consisted of detection of gross *macroscopic* pathology (scarring, cysts, tumours or infectious lesions) and an adjacent cortex which, if stimulated electrically, would give rise to an aura or to a seizure, and that excision of this area was usually followed by cessation of attacks. Nearly everything we know concerning human cerebral functional topography resulted from their electrical mapping techniques [5].

After the introduction of electroencephalography in 1929 by Berger [6], the correlation of clinical seizure patterns and EEG recordings by Gibbs, Davis and Lennox in 1935 [7] and the utilisation of electrocorticography in 1935 by Foerster [8], the diagnosis of the seizure focus came to depend on the location of *interictal* epileptiform abnormalities.

Complex partial epilepsy has been found to be the single most common type of epilepsy affecting just under 40 per cent in one clinic's population [9]. Since epilepsy affects at least 1 in 200 Americans [10] and complex partial epilepsy is frequently not controlled by anticonvulsants, it appeared at one time that surgical treatment for this condition would be widely utilised. Indeed, interest in the surgical treatment of complex partial epilepsy peaked in 1954 and 1957 at the First and Second International Colloquiums on Temporal Lobe Epilepsy at Marseilles and Bethesda, respectively [11]. The safety and efficacy of anterior temporal lobectomy had been demonstrated in the world-wide literature [12], yet interest has waned and it continues to be the most under-utilised treatment in epilepsy and practised in only a few centres in the world.

Frederic Gibbs persuaded Percival Bailey to undertake anterior temporal lobectomy in 1948, based almost entirely on interictal electroencephalographic evidence [13] and clinical symptoms. The aetiology of this type of epilepsy was not known at that time because subpial suctioning surgical techniques were used and the hippocampal formation was not removed. After Murray Falconer developed an 'en bloc' technique of anterior temporal lobectomy, it was found that microscopic lesions were present in the mesial temporal lobes in the majority of these patients and that there was an important favourable prognosis in such patients [14,15]. Unfortunately, at that time, preoperative neuroradiological examinations disclosed the pathological substrate in very few patients. When the resected temporal lobe tissue appeared to be normal postoperatively, the prognosis for control of seizures was poor, so that an important objective for Falconer and his colleagues came to be the development of electrophysiological correlates of pathology to improve the surgical results in temporal lobe epilepsy in the Oslerian tradition [16].

The site of focal *ictal* onset of complex partial seizures was also found to be almost invariably in the limbic structures medial to the temporal lobe, as well as the pathological substrate after the development of long-term implanted electrode studies, monitoring techniques and ictal recordings [17—19]. Perhaps this is the reason that surface recordings and electrocorticography of interictal discharges, since these are recordings of secondary propagated discharges, were not as valuable as was once hoped. Depth EEG can select some patients with medically refractory epilepsy for surgical therapy who otherwise would not be candidates because scalp EEGs were not interpretable. Regarding the use of surgical treatment in 1967, Falconer wrote: "the selection of patients has been rigorous, and we estimate that only about one in nine persons (11%) referred for surgery fulfil (our) criteria" [20]. However, a recent review [21] of several series of depth electrode studies showed an increase in operative candidates of 36 per cent. Depth EEG can also alter surgical plans or prevent needless surgery by demonstrating different, multiple, or poorly defined foci. This amounted to 18 per cent of patients reported [21].

Materials and methods

This report is based on our UCLA experiences with 103 patients from 1961—77 who underwent depth electrode evaluation. We also discuss our criteria, in which depth electrode studies are not required, for other patients to receive surgical treatment. Criteria for acceptance into the programme at UCLA include the following: 1) a partial seizure pattern diagnosed on the basis of clinical or EEG findings, preferably with behavioural features at one time or another that suggest automatisms; 2) frequent seizure episodes that are resistant to adequate drug therapy and seriously interfere with daily life; 3) absence of evidence indicating progressive central nervous system disease or a space-occupying lesion (in the latter case depth electrode evaluation is not considered necessary and surgical treatment is determined according to the demonstrated lesion); and 4) absence of severe health problems, psychosis, or marked mental retardation.

Important preoperative factors for consideration

Age At the time of surgery, most of the patients were between the ages of 15 and 30; the youngest was 9 and the oldest 51. The onset of epilepsy was prior to the age of 9 in about half of the patients. The duration of epilepsy was never shorter than 3 years and longer than 10 years in the majority.

Our experience agrees with that of Lindsay, Ounstead and Richards [22], whose conclusions were derived from a study of 100 children followed for 29 years into adulthood. Ninety-five patients were divided into three outcome categories. Five patients died as children before the age of 15. Approximately one-third underwent spontaneous remission after anticonvulsant therapy and later were seizure-free, socially independent and were not receiving anticonvulsant medication. Approximately one-third were also able to support themselves socially and economically, but they were receiving anticonvulsants, were not able to support themselves and were considered to be totally dependent. They make three points. Uncontrolled complex partial epilepsy can be dangerous and has a significant mortality rate; on the other hand, it can be benign with spontaneous remission. These authors indicated the need for skilled review of the medical and social status of children about the age of 15 with partial complex seizures. For those who can reach full recovery, the withdrawal of drugs before the age of 15 is of great importance. When seizures continue into adolescence, full investigation with a view to possible neurosurgical treatment should be undertaken. These authors concluded that 'a major danger in caring for children with temporal lobe epilepsy is delaying operation for relief of seizures so long into adult life that social recovery has become impossible'.

In our experience the rehabilitation of younger individuals, particularly below 20–25 age group, has contrasted strongly with that of those patients over 30 years. In the latter group there is a high incidence of postoperative depression, need for psychotherapy, cyclic changes in emotional stability and memory problems. In fact in an older patient with a left-sided focus, surgical treatment may be contraindicated.

Aetiology and duration An aetiological history is not very important in determining prognosis except for a previous diagnosis of encephalitis after which the prognosis is poorer (5 patients). Fifteen patients had more than one aetiological factor recorded in their history. Perinatal injury (11 cases) and febrile convulsions (13 cases) were most common. No aetiology was recorded in six. In five cases, a family history of relatives presenting epileptic seizures was present and did not affect the prognosis, although the numbers are too small for statistical significance.

Psychological status This will be discussed below.
The UCLA Protocol is presented in Table I.

Phase I consists of those diagnostic tests which can be conducted in a medical neurological setting. These are listed as a set of tests of epileptic excitability and a set of tests of functional deficit. If there is a convergence of evidence from these tests indicative of an anterior temporal focus, a recommendation for anterior temporal lobectomy (Phase III) can be made with confidence, but all the tests are not of equal value. *Localisation on the basis of functional deficits alone should never be considered sufficient to recommend anterior temporal lobectomy since epileptic excitability must still be demonstrated in order to identify a lesion as epileptogenic.* The evolution of this protocol has been gradual since the beginning in 1961 (ie not all 103 patients received the entire set of tests) and the dates of application roughly approximate those of the references cited. During our most recent period approximately one-half of the patients from Phase I studies were recommended for Phase III. Therefore, the UCLA protocol does not call for depth electrode evaluation in all patients.

Phase I

1 Continuous scalp and sphenoidal telemetry during anticonvulsant withdrawal

Tests of epileptic excitability

a) Interictal spike analysis

The frequency and location of interictal spikes seen on routine EEGs as well as during scalp and sphenoidal telemetry were determined in all patients in this group by visual analysis of available EEG records and by a review of old EEG reports from UCLA and elsewhere. Since 1969 long-term telemetry has been used, first with a 4-channel and later with a 14-channel telemetry transmitter (Bio-Medical Monitoring Systems, Los Angeles). One or more prolonged baseline hard-wire recordings were made from all patients in order to survey the electrodes and choose the appropriate montages from the 10–20 International EEG system and indwelling sphenoidal electrodes. Electrodes were then attached to a lightweight telemetry transmitter which was secured to the patient's head with gauze bandage. Now twelve channels are used for EEG recording and two for time code data. Radio signals are received in a separate room and relayed to a 14-channel Ampex magnetic tape recorder. Analogue data are stored on tape, but all ictal and selected segments of

510

TABLE I

Requirements for admission to Phase I include frequent partial complex seizures by history and demonstrated failure of adequate doses of anticonvulsant medications. Usually routine evaluations including skull films, CT scan, and several EEGs have been carried out by this time.

Phase I (2 week hospital admission)

1 Continuous scalp and sphenoidal telemetry during anticonvulsant withdrawal

Tests of epileptic excitability

     a) Site of most frequent interictal spikes

     b) Autonomy of spike activity in sleep stages

     c) Thiopental activation of spikes

     d) Site of ictal EEG onset, sphenoidal and surface electrodes

Tests of functional deficit

     a) Baseline rhythms

     b) Decreased fast activity after barbiturates

     c) Intracarotid Wada test combined with angiography

2 Radiological procedures including CT scan,angiography and pneumo-encephalography

3 Psychological and/or psychiatric evaluation

4 Neurosurgical Consultation

Phase II (4 week hospital admission)

1 Continuous SEEG telemetry with sphenoidal electrodes during anticonvulsant withdrawal

2 EEG analysis

Tests of epileptic excitability

     a) Site of most frequent interictal spikes

     b) Ictal EEG onset

     c) Autonomy of spike activity in sleep stages

     d) Thiopental activation

Tests of functional deficit

     a) Baseline rhythms

     b) Decreased fast activity after barbiturates

     c) Elevated AD thresholds after electrical stimulation

Phase III

1 Surgery

2 Tissue for routine histology, EM, Golgi preparation

interictal data are also transferred to paper for visual analysis utilising a 16-channel Grass Model 6 EEG machine.

A Sony video camera continuously recorded the patient's behaviour, and this was stored on a Panasonic videotape recorder simultaneously. (We have used time-lapse and real-time methods). A time code generator displayed actual clock time digitally every second on the EEG so that behavioural and electrical events could be precisely correlated. In order for an electrical event to be considered the origin of a behavioural seizure, it was necessary that the event preceded the ictal behaviour as observed on videotape.

Monitoring was continued 24 hours a day for approximately two weeks during Phase I. Montages were periodically varied to best display the electrical phenomena observed and to sample all derivations. Anticonvulsant medications were generally tapered during this period but were rarely completely withdrawn. The goal was to obtain recordings of several seizures of a spontaneous nature. The only provocative measure used was sleep deprivation. Ictal events were identified for study in several ways: 1) patients were under continuous observation from staff either directly or via video monitors placed at the nursing station so that unusual behaviour could be noted; 2) to indicate an aura or the beginning of a seizure, the patient had a signal button to push which called the nurse and also placed a mark on the EEG; and 3) telemetry tapes were randomly searched to obtain samples of interictal activity and subclinical electrical seizure discharges.

b) Autonomy of spike activity in sleep stages

In a limited number of patients the all-night sleep records were segmented into four stages: waking, light sleep, deep sleep, and REM sleep. The rate of spike activity was observed to estimate the autonomy of spike activity [23].

c) Thiopental activation of spikes or attenuation of barbiturate-induced fast activity

During EEG monitoring, 25mg of thiopental was injected intravenously every 30 seconds until the corneal reflex was abolished [24,25]. The patient was then allowed to wake up. The EEG was visually analysed for activation of focal spike activity as well as for focal attenuation in barbiturate-induced fast activity. A 50 per cent decrease in amplitude of fast activity at one sphenoidal electrode 50 per cent of the time was considered to be a significant attenuation (Figure 1).

d) Site of ictal EEG onset, sphenoidal and surface electrodes

During Phase I, scalp recordings were made with gold disc electrodes applied with paste or, for telemetry, with collodion according to the International 10–20 System. Each sphenoidal electrode consisted of 15 braided 50-gauge stainless steel wires, coated with Teflon and bared for 1mm at the tip. These were threaded through a 3.8cm, 22-gauge hypodermic needle and

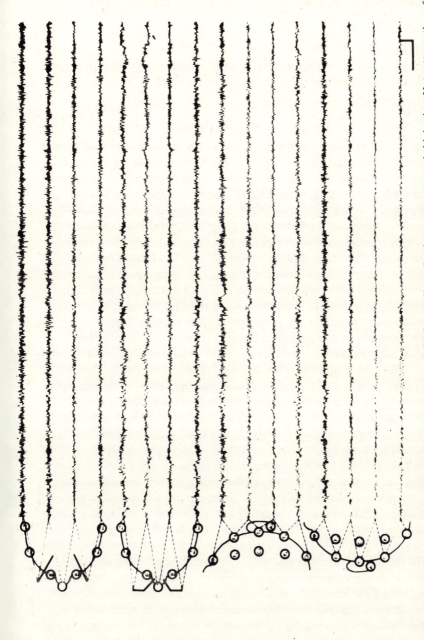

Figure 1. Simultaneous sphenoidal, nasopharyngeal and scalp EEG recordings after intravenous pentothal injection. Note attenuation of low voltage fast activity recorded at the left sphenoidal electrode (channels 3 and 4), but not at right sphenoidal (channels 1 and 2) or at nasopharyngeal or scalp recordings. Pathology was hippocampal sclerosis. Calibration 1 sec, 100 μV

inserted according to the technique described by Pampiglione and Kerridge [26] . These electrodes were well tolerated. Initial ictal EEG recordings were sometimes well-defined but later were usually obscured by muscle artifact.

Tests of functional deficit

a) Baseline rhythms

Focal abnormalities of normal baseline rhythms are rarely seen during scalp EEG recordings but, when present, are highly significant

b) Decreased fast activity after barbiturates — see 1c above

c) Intracarotid Wada test — combined with angiography

Usually this test is performed near the end of the period of evaluation or prior to operation, ie, after a definite decision has been made for surgery and it is necessary to ascertain hemispheric dominance for language [27] or, more importantly, memory function [28,29] . The most frequent pathological substrate in complex partial epilepsy is hippocampal sclerosis which in 80 per cent of cases is primarily unilateral [30] ; such patients are dependent on one hippocampal formation for memory processing. An induced transient global memory deficit, following pharmacological blockade of one hemisphere, correlates with the presence of an epileptogenic lesion in the contralateral temporal lobe. Other deductions from this test include 'pathological shifting' of language dominance from left to the right hemisphere, which has been related to an epileptogenic lesion in the left temporal lobe.

Before injection of sodium amytal in the internal carotid artery catheter, baseline measurements are made of the patient's language and memory functions to serve as a comparison for drug-related behaviour changes. Immediately prior to injection, the patient is asked to count aloud while bilateral grip strength is continuously assessed. Over a 4—6 sec period, 125mg of sodium amytal in 10cc of saline solution is injected into one internal carotid by a transfemoral cannula. Each hemisphere is infused, with at least a 30 minute delay between injections. EEG is simultaneously recorded for correlation of drug effects with the continuous performance task described below. Within seconds after the injection, EEG slowing, contralateral hemiparesis and cessation of counting are seen. If the hemisphere is not dominant for language, the patient resumes counting within seconds. If the language dominant hemisphere has been injected, marked aphasia is immediately apparent, varying from mutism to perseverative speech. Initial aphasia testing is carried out in the first minute after injection. The exam assesses expressive and receptive language skills and includes naming, reading, and responses to simple commands. Following this, a continuous measure of selective language skills (ie naming, reading) and short-term memory functions of verbal and non-verbal material is obtained for 10 minutes. At the end of the continuous performance task, a grand recognition test of previously presented items provides

514

an assessment of retrograde amnesia. EEG and positive contrast studies are made to aid in the determination of spread and duration of drug effectiveness.

2 Radiological procedures

Focal structural lesions are rarely demonstrable in radiological procedures. An asymmetric smaller middle cranial fossa, elevated petrous ridge or calcification can be seen sometimes in plain films or X-ray CT scans. Calcification can indicate an indolent tumour such as oligodendroglioma or astrocytoma. Other lesions are hemangioma calcificans, parasitic disease or tuberous sclerosis. Pneumoencephalography is less often used now but a dilated temporal horn related to hippocampal sclerosis may not be revealed by X-ray CT scans with present-day technology. An arteriovenous malformation is occasionally revealed by angiography since many of these patients have seizures and not necessarily episodes of haemorrhage.

3 Psychological and/or psychiatric evaluation

Neuropsychological testing is an important part of the presurgical evaluation and includes a number of tests sensitive to dysfunction of the temporal lobes as well as extratemporal areas. Standardised batteries, such as the Halstead-Reitan Neuropsychological Test Battery, have not proved to be useful in detecting subtle cognitive deficits in patients with complex partial seizures of unknown aetiologies [31]. A comprehensive neuropsychological evaluation, which includes measures of language, sensation, perception and motor skills, as well as selective tests particularly sensitive to temporal lobe dysfunction (i.e. verbal and non-verbal short-term memory tests, dichotic listening tests, etc) provides useful diagnostic information regarding the areas and extent of brain dysfunction.

The most reliable neuropsychological measure of lateralisation of temporal lobe dysfunction is obtained by comparing a patient's performance on verbal and non-verbal short-term memory tests. The immediate and delayed recall of logical prose, associative learning, and visual-reproduction subtests of the Wechsler Memory Scale [32], and the Rey-Osterrieth draw and recall test [33]. A verbal memory deficit (independent of other confounding neuropsychological deficiences) is usually associated with dominant temporal lobe epileptogenic lesions. A comparable deficit in remembering material not easily verbalised (ie, line drawing) associated with an epileptogenic lesion in the non-dominant temporal lobe [34,35]. Interpretation of the neuropsychological profile is dependent upon knowledge of the hemispheric organisation of language; this is provided by the intracarotid sodium amytal test.

Phase II

1 Continuous SEEG telemetry during anticonvulsant withdrawal

The indications for stereo-electroencephalography are as follows. Only

515

patients who appear very likely to benefit from surgical treatment should be selected for this procedure; it should not be used for the diagnosis of 'mixed' seizure disorder other than secondarily generalised seizures which may accompany complex partial epilepsy. When Phase I telemetry reveals a high incidence of bilaterally synchronous epileptiform EEG discharges, patients are not usually considered for further studies, even if the ictal onset is well localised, since this has been associated with an absence of pathological changes in the resected temporal lobe and a poor surgical outcome.

When the clinical diagnosis is clearly complex partial epilepsy but the battery of tests of Phase I is inconclusive, depth electroencephalography (SEEG) offers a great diagnostic advantage. SEEG is most frequently employed when: 1) bilateral independent fronto-temporal interictal discharges are present; 2) EEG recorded ictal onsets of partial complex seizures are well lateralised but equally prominent in extratemporal and temporal regions; 3) EEG recorded ictal onsets of partial complex seizures are well localised to one temporal lobe but confirmational evidence of focal functional deficit is missing or conflicting; 4) EEG recorded ictal onsets are clearly localised to one temporal lobe but other studies and/or the behavioural seizures suggest an extratemporal lesion; or 5) Phase I evaluation indicates a lesion in one temporal lobe which may extend further posteriorly than the standard anterior temporal lobectomy allows.

There are some general contraindications which relate to the safety of SEEG recordings over a number of weeks. These exclude patients who have serious multiple illnesses, active infections, or are otherwise poor surgical risks (eg, patients with diabetes mellitus who are prone to infection), as well as those with skull defects which would make electrodes unstable. In Phase I studies our patients are closely observed for emotional instability or psychiatric disorders which would not allow them to tolerate this procedure, which is also not advisable in children under the age of 10, patients with intelligence quotients below 70, or patients with severe memory disorders. Care is taken to ensure that each patient has a full understanding of the purposes and the risks involved.

Stereotactic depth electrode procedure

Patients admitted for Phase II SEEG telemetry have depth electrodes stereotactically implanted into mesiotemporal and frontal structures. Since limbic system epilepsy is invariably, and frontal lobe epilepsy commonly, bilateral the implantation of electrodes is bilateral and symmetrical. Our electrode arrays are also arranged to survey a wide region since the epileptogenic zones are never highly focal. Bipolar electrodes are inserted in a transverse approach through the middle and inferior temporal gyri. A multilead electrode is inserted through the inferior frontal gyrus along the inferior frontal lobe to end in the gyrus rectus, and another through the superior frontal gyrus to end in the supplementary motor cortex. The latter electrodes have been used only since 1977 and

516

mainly in patients who have a prominent motor pattern in their observed attacks during Phase I. The temporal approach has fewer blood vessels than the frontal approach. Stereotaxic operations under general anaesthesia are performed using the Todd-Wells apparatus and teleroentgenograms to reduce magnification of X-ray images (14 feet target-film distances). The anatomical target is centred in the X-ray beam (AP and lateral) to reduce errors due to the divergence of X-rays.

The stereotaxic coordinates are derived from two Talairach atlases. Temporal lobe structures are referenced to an axis on the temporal horn and midline [36]. Neocortical areas according to Brodmann are identified in relationship to the anterior-posterior commissural axis and the midline [37]. The ventricular landmarks are demonstrated after the supine patient's head is fixed in the stereotaxic apparatus by making a ventriculogram. A combination of gas (nitrous oxide-oxygen) for superior ventricular parts and about 4–5cc of water-soluble contrast medium has been found to be useful to render these ventricular landmarks in sharp images. The contrast medium is injected into the trigone of the lateral ventricle from a lateral approach plotted with the aid of the preoperative pneumo-encephalogram of Phase I studies. Particular attention is paid to the position of arteries and veins by means of the preoperative angiograms. It is also necessary in some cases with atrophy to plot positions by direct imaging rather than the stereotactic maps. Such sulci can be demonstrated by subarachnoid injection of gas. The arc system is flexible enough to allow many angles of approach to be selected.

The twist drill holes in the direction of the targets are drilled by a special fluted drill, which allows bone to be drilled without penetrating the dura and thus the cortex with its vessels. The dura mater is opened by coagulation. The supports of the electrode arrays are self-tapping hollow screws, which provide solid fixation as well as guidance for both insertion and withdrawal of electrodes. A cap with inserts seals and fixes the electrode in place.

Electrodes in the temporal bone are bonded together into an aggregate plate using methylmethacrylate above the scalp to ensure stability. Insulated nail electrodes distributed according to the International 10–20 System (except the occipital and frontopolar leads) are used to survey the cortical areas of the convexities. Electrodes for the frontal lobes are secure due to the thickness of the skull in these regions. Recordings from surface and depth electrodes have been quite free from artifacts. After the completion of the studies the electrodes are removed under general anaesthesia; the cement is drilled away from the head of each screw, each electrode extracted through the screw and then the screws are removed.

In the postoperative period these patients are usually ambulatory within two days of the implantation procedure. The electrodes are non-painful as long as they are rigidly secure much the same as skull tongs. Throughout the study

517

period the patients head is kept in a sterile head dressing which is changed weekly at which time a sterile cleansing and shaving is carried out.

2 EEG analysis of Phase II

Tests of excitability

a) Site of most frequent interictal spikes

The same monitoring technique is used as described before. Interictal discharges in the depth are much greater in amplitude, frequent, independent, and always have been found bilaterally even in patients with unilateral scalp interictal discharges. Thus interictal spike data were analysed in more detail with a computer. Automatic spike detection was carried out off-line on all-night sleep recordings on a PDP-12 minicomputer, utilising an assembly language computer programme (COUNTR) [38,39] for which spike recognition variables had previously been optimised by comparing its performance with that of human observers.

b) Ictal EEG onset

Two ictal EEG patterns were found to be the most important criteria to recommend anterior temporal lobectomy with a good prognosis. A focal type onset fulfilled Jackson's hypothesis. In these circumstances (Figures 2a and b) the seizure discharge can be seen to originate in one, or possibly two, single sites well before any clinical manifestations (as long as 35 sec), propagate to nearby sites, and perhaps eventually appear in the contralateral limbic sites, although reaching these sites in unison [40]. Bilateral spread in the limbic sites coincided with automatism and change in consciousness.

A regional focal onset (Figure 3) consists of high-amplitude discharges appearing simultaneously in all limbic sites of one side, again preceding any clinical manifestation other than an aura and spreading to the opposite side with the same effect. This suggests the possibility of a much larger volume being involved at the time of initiation or that a different focal origin has spread to these sites. The prognosis for seizure relief is nearly as good as for focal-type onset.

Because of the rhythmicity of the ictal discharge and freedom from artifacts an automatic seizure detector could be used in depth electrode studies which called the nurse and printed out the clock time for later searches of the tapes [41].

c) Autonomy of spike activity in sleep stages

In agreement with the findings of Gentilomo et al [23] the autonomy of interictal epileptiform activity was much more frequent in depth electrode recordings than those made from the surface. Possibly this is explicable by the electrodes' location in the primary epileptogenic zone in which interictal discharges tend to be constantly active.

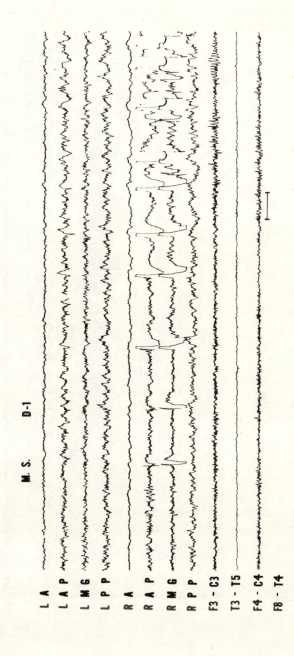

Figure 2a. Focal type ictal onset in depth electrodes begins with polyphasic spike and wave discharges in the right anterior pes hippocampi and mid parahippocampal gyrus with later spread into F3-C3

519

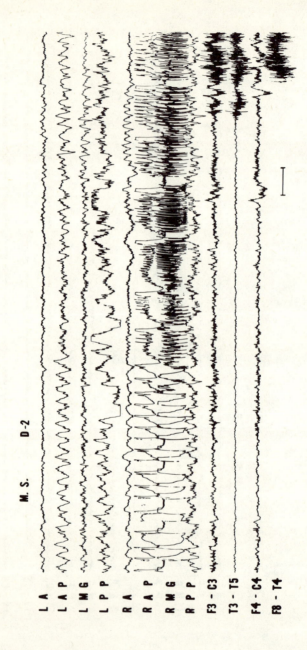

M. S.   D-2

L A
L A P
L M G
L P P
R A
R A P
R M G
R P P
F3 - C3
T3 - T5
F4 - C4
F8 - T4

Figure 2b. SEEG recording is continuous with 2a. Bilateral rhythmical discharges are seen in the limbic system leads which were associated with automatism. Muscle artifacts seen in superficial cortical leads are due to chewing movements of the patient. (Note R=right; L=left; A=amygdala; AP=anterior pes; MG=mid parahippocampal gyrus; PP=posterior pes hippocampi; calibration 1 sec, 1000μV)

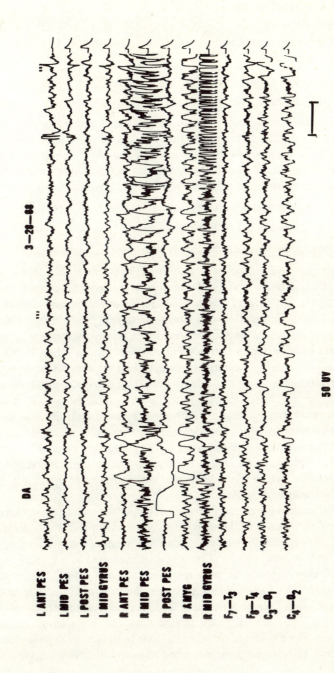

Figure 3. Regional onset of spontaneous seizure in right (R) depth sites. High amplitude discharges appear in all of the right depth areas except the posterior pes hippocampi. Ictal discharge spreads secondarily to left depth sites. Calibration 1 sec. Sensitivities are set differently (rear margin of each channel) in depth leads for the sake of readability

521

d) Thiopental activation

Interictal spike discharges may be activated by thiopental perfusion but it has been less common, although our experience dates only to a limited number of patients since 1977.

Tests of functional deficit

a) Baseline rhythms

An attenuation of normal rhythmic activity was recorded from the temporal depth more commonly than from the surface. In our experience, when encountered, it has always been on the side of resection. Bipolar chain linkage montages were often required to demonstrate attenuation of baseline rhythms, and appears to be an accurate test of localised decreased function.

b) Decreased fast activity after barbiturates

This generally coincided with the above test.

c) Elevated after-discharge thresholds after electrical stimulation

We have previously reported in a study of 30 patients [42] that electrical stimulations at limbic system sites may provide useful information to correlate with the pathological substrate. These 30 patients consisted of 20 with hippocampal sclerosis, five with hamartomas, one neoplasm and four with no apparent lesions. Comparisons were made between anatomical sites, operated and non-operated structures and different disease states. It was found that patients with hippocampal sclerosis had higher after-discharge thresholds in structures on the operated side (p=0.015). The patients with lesions other than hippocampal sclerosis were found to differ from those with hippocampal sclerosis in that there were no differences between their diseased and non-diseased structures. This correlates with experimental studies that show that neuronal density is a critical factor in the production of an after-discharge [43,44]. Electrode sites chosen for stimulation have bilateral temporal lobe representation, which allows hemispheric comparisons of thresholds. The order of site stimulation is random.

The threshold for eliciting an after-discharge for each site is determined by electrical stimulation of the individual concentric bipolar depth electrode in increments of 1.0ma, from 2ma up to a maximum of 5ma, or until an after-discharge is elicited. Electrical current is administered by a specially constructed current-regulated, patient-isolated stimulator [45], which generates symmetrically biphasic pulses with a pulse duration of 1msec, a train duration of 12 sec, and a frequency of 60Hz. The maximum charge density is $55.5C/cm^2$. We have continued to find thresholds for after-discharges to be *higher* (ie after-discharges are *more difficult* to obtain) in the hippocampus containing the epileptogenic lesion and related mesial temporal sclerosis.

Complications of depth electrode procedures

(103 consecutive procedures, 1961—1977)

Infection was a complication in five patients. In three instances this was superficial scalp infection which cleared after removal of the electrodes. In one case there probably was a cerebritis demonstrated by a 'ring shadow' on CT scans which also cleared after electrode removal and an extended period of antibiotic treatment. One case of transient meningitis after electrode removal occurred. Bleeding was a complication in four patients. In three instances it arose from a superficial cortical vessel which was easily managed as the exact site was evident and no neurological deficit ensued. In one case in 1964 a death occurred due to massive haematoma from puncture of the posterior cerebral artery. There has been no instance of a late complication due to depth electrode implantation.

Anterior temporal lobectomy

Indications A definitive set of criteria for the surgical therapy of complex partial epilepsy cannot be derived incorporating the studies discussed in this report or others. Each patient is unique and must be evaluated according to the peculiarities of his or her own case. Our point, however, is that each patient's case can be better characterised by tests of epileptic excitability and tests of functional deficit and that this will permit more patients to receive successful surgical treatment.

If all evidence of surface-recorded epileptic excitability, including site of ictal onset, and evidence of decreased function agree, it may not be necessary to risk depth electrode investigations. When surface evidence of epileptic excitability and decreased function conflict, however, depth electrode implantation is essential, not only to identify the site of seizure origin but it is likely to provide more certain evidence of focal functional deficits than studies from surface recordings. The most reliable and predictive tests continue to be the focal or regional ictal onset patterns from depth electrode studies. In general, focal onsets appear to indicate that the electrode tip is near the epileptogenic lesion, while regional onsets seem to represent epileptiform activity propagated from other than the recording sites. The differentiation between primary and propagated ictal discharges remains a problem, and sampling errors from the necessarily limited electrode array may result in false localisation.

Ideally, all seizures should originate in one area of the brain and confirmatory tests should reveal focal dysfunction in the same area. In practice, a few seizures originating contralateral to the presumed epileptogenic lesion (especially if these seizures are atypical and/or occur perhaps as drug-withdrawal attacks) are not considered a contraindication to surgery since patients with such findings often do well [46]. In our experience to date, when SEEG recorded ictal onset has been localised to one temporal lobe but confirmatory tests suggest the focus may lie, in part or entirely, outside the usual 'en bloc' resection, intraoperative electrocorticography is then necessary to define the abnormality better.

Results

The anterior temporal lobectomy used in this series was the 'en bloc' technique devised by Murray Falconer [15]. The outcome of 59 patients who represented 57 per cent of the series is given in Table I. Forty-five patients (76%) had substantial benefit with regard to control of seizures.

TABLE II

1961 – August 1977 (to # 103)

103 patients underwent depth electrode evaluation (6.4/yr)
59 (57%) had anterior temporal lobectomy (3.7/yr)
40 (78% of complete specimens) had structural lesions
20 (34%) are seizure free ⎫
12 (20%) have had rare seizures ⎬ 76% benefited
13 (22%) have worthwhile improvement
14 (24%) have not benefited
14 (14%) other procedures
30 (29%) no surgery

Twenty patients are completely free of seizures causing alteration of consciousness (some patients have had auras, usually in the first postoperative year). Twelve patients have had rare seizures, no more than twice a year (generalised in eight cases, complex partial in three and partial elementary in one). Thirteen patients (22%) had a worthwhile reduction in seizure frequency, with free intervals of over a month or more (generalised seizures in two, and complex partial in 11). Fourteen patients (24%) have either had no relief from surgery or have had a disabling complication. Eight patients continue to have seizures, six patients have one or more serious neurological deficits.

It will be noted that 30 patients (29%) were not recommended for anterior temporal lobectomy or any other surgical procedure. Most of these patients had a preoperative diagnosis of complex partial seizure disorder but ictal recordings disclosed generalised discharges at the time of ictus. Three patients had demonstrable multifocal seizures from ictal recordings. Fourteen patients [14%] had surgical operations other than anterior temporal lobectomy. It will be recalled that Falconer could recommend anterior temporal lobectomy to 11 per cent of patients referred to him [20]; in this series 57 per cent of patients could be referred to undergo anterior temporal lobectomy as a result of the tests described, and the plans for surgical therapy were changed in a further 14 per cent.

524

There was no mortality in the 59 patients with anterior temporal lobectomy. Three patients have a permanent contralateral hemiparesis which mainly disabled their upper extremity and also included homonymous hemianopia. Three patients showed a mild motor impairment, one with hand tremor and another with hemianopia and third nerve impairment (these patients had seizure relief and are not considered to be seriously disabled). One patient required a shunt procedure for the relief of hydrocephalus developed postoperatively. Two patients have significant memory disturbance but not a global amnestic syndrome.

Conclusion

Our group of patients can be characterised as especially difficult problems, drug-resistant cases, complex electrographic abnormalities and long duration of seizures — yet approximately two-thirds of our patients have been recommended for specific anterior temporal lobectomy or other surgical treatment with results equally as good as those obtained by pre-1960 criteria. With more recent use of the complete battery of tests, especially to include more tests of focal cerebral dysfunction, outcome with respect to seizures has greatly improved. Over 80 per cent of patients operated upon since 1977 are now seizure-free and only one has not benefited [47]. The principal goal of the use of depth electrode studies and the tests of functional deficits is to make surgical treatment of complex partial epilepsy available to a large number of patients and, conversely, to spare some patients from a major operative procedure which would not be sucessful.

Acknowledgments

This research was supported by Grant NS 02808 from the National Institutes of Health. The authors are indebted to the members of the staff and investigators in the UCLA Clinical Neurophysiology Program and the UCLA Brain Research Institutes for their assistance. Luigi Ravagnati MD collected some of the outcome data. We are grateful to Sasha Biletsky for preparation of the manuscript.

References

1   Jackson JH. *Western Riding Lunatic Asylum Med Reports 1873; 3:* 315–339
2   Ferrier D. *Western Riding Lunatic Asylum Med Reports 1873; 3:* 30–96
3   Horsley V. *Brit Med J 1887; 1:* 863–865
4   Foerster O, Penfield W. *Brain 1930; 53:* 99–119
5   Penfield W, Jasper H. *Epilepsy and the Functional Anatomy of the Human Brain 1930;* 896
6   Berger H. *Arch f Psychiat 1929; 87:* 527–570

7   Gibbs FA, Davis H, Lennox WG. *Arch Neurol and Psychiat (Chicago) 1935; 34:* 1133–1148
8   Foerster O, Altenburger H. *Dtsch Z Nervenheilk 1935; 135:* 277–288
9   Gastaut H, Gastaut JL, Goncalves e Silva GE, Fernandez Sanchez GR. *Epilepsia 1975; 16:* 457–461
10   Commission for the Control of Epilepsy and Its Consequences: Plan for Nationwide Action on Epilepsy. *DHEW Publication No (NIH) 78–311: 1978:* 314–343. Washington DC, Department of Health, Education and Welfare
11   Baldwin M, Bailey P. *Temporal Lobe Epilepsy 1958;* 581. Springfield Ill: CC Thomas
12   Jensen I. *Acta neurol Scand 1975; 52:* 354–373
13   Bailey P, Gibbs FH. *JAMA 1951; 145:* 365–370
14   Falconer MA, Serafetinides EA. *J Neurol Neurosurg Psychiat 1963; 26:* 154–165
15   Falconer M. In Rob C, Smith R, eds. *Operative Surgery 1970; 14:* 142–149. Butterworths
16   Engel J Jr, Driver MV, Falconer MA. *Brain 1975; 98:* 129–156
17   Talairach J, DeAjuriguerre J, David M. *Presse méd 1952; 28:* 605–609
18   Crandall PH, Walter RD, Rand RW. *J Neurosurg 1963; 20:* 820–840
19   Bancaud J, Talairach J, Geier S, Scarabin JM. *EEG et SEEG dans Les Tumeurs Cérébrales et L'epilepsie 1973;* 351. Paris: Édifor
20   Falconer MA. *NZ Med J 1967; 66:* 539–544
21   Spencer SS. *Ann Neurol 1981; 19:* 207–214
22   Lindsay J, Ounstead C, Richards P. *Develop Med Child Neurol 1979; 21:* 285–298
23   Gentilomo A, Colicchio G, Pola P et al. In Levin P, Loella WP, eds. *Sleep 1975;* 444–446. Basel: Karger
24   Kennedy WA, Hill D. *J Neurol Neurosurg Psychiat 1958; 21:* 24–30
25   Engel J Jr, Driver MV, Falconer MA. *Brain 1975; 98:* 129–156
26   Pampiglione G, Kerridge J. *J Neurol Neurosurg Psychiat 1956; 19:* 117–129
27   Wada J, Rasmussen T. *J Neurosurg 1960; 17:* 266–282
28   Milner B, Branch C, Rasmussen T. *Trans Amer Neurol Assoc 1962; 87:* 224–226
29   Blume WT, Grabow JD, Darley FL, Aronson AE. *Neurol 1973; 23:* 812–819
30   Margerison JH, Corsellis JAN. *Brain 1966; 89:* 499–530
31   Matthews CG, Klove H. *Epilepsia 1967; 8:* 117–128
32   Wechsler D, Stone CP. *Wechsler Memory Scale 1945.* New York: Psychological Corp Publishers
33   Osterreith P. *Arch Psychol 1944; 30:* 206–356
34   Milner B. In Purpura DP, Penry JK, Walter RD, eds. *Advances in Neurology 1975; 8:* 299. New York: Raven Press
35   Russell EW. *J Consult Clin Psychol 1975; 43:* 800–809
36   Talairach J, David M, Tournoux P. *L'exploration Chirurgical Stereotaxique du Lobe Temporale dans L'epilepsie Temporale 1958;* 136. Paris: Masson et Cie
37   Talairach J, Szikla G. *Atlas du Telencephalon 1977;* 225. Paris Masson et Cie
38   Lieb JP, Joseph JP, Engel J Jr et al. *Electroencephalogr Clin Neurophysiol 1980; 49:* 538–557
39   Lieb JP, Woods SC, Siccardi A et al. *Electroencephalogr Clin Neurophysiol 1978; 44:* 641–663
40   Walter RD. In Brazier MAB, ed. *Epilepsy, Its Phenomena in Man 1973;* 99–119. New York: UCLA Forum in Medical Sciences No 17, Academic Press
41   Babb TL, Mariani E, Crandall PH. *Electroencephalogr Clin Neurophysiol 1974; 37:* 305–308
42   Cherlow DG, Dymond AM, Crandall PH et al. *Arch Neurol 1977; 34:* 527–531
43   Pinsky C, Burns BD. *J Neurophysiol 1962; 25:* 359–379
44   Segal M, Ledercq B. *Can J Physiol Pharmacol 1965; 43:* 685–697
45   Babb TL, Mariani E, Sneider KA et al. *Neurol Res 1980; 2:* 181–197
46   Engel J Jr, Rausch R, Lieb JP et al. *Ann Neurol 1981; 9:* 215–224
47   Engel J Jr, Troupin AS, Crandall PH et al. *Arch Neurol;* In press

53

EMPLOYABILITY

R L Masland

Among the social problems of persons with epilepsy, unemployment is paramount. World-wide figures, even in 1976, showed an unemployment rate from 10–20 per cent; the estimated figure in the USA was 22 per cent. Studies of one selected group of epileptic volunteers revealed that while 19.5 per cent were listed on the labour force as unemployed, 33 per cent were actually not working. Equally important is that among epileptic workers, many are denied promotion because of limitations imposed by reason of their disability.

The causes of unemployment of persons with epilepsy are complex. The most obvious is fear of injury. In an unpublished survey of employers [1], it was observed that few would employ persons known by them to have had a generalised seizure within a year. However, the US Social Security Administration considers an individual totally disabled only if he has major motor seizures at a frequency of one per month, or over – or minor seizures occurring more frequently than once weekly. The discrepancy between the attitude of employers and that of the Social Security Administration points to an obvious basis for social distress.

However, much evidence suggests that the seizures themselves are only one factor in the unemployment of epileptic persons. An analysis by Denerll et al [2] reveals that when employed and unemployed epileptic persons were compared, the unemployed had lower intelligence and a higher incidence of psychopathology, but little difference in seizure type. They were more likely to show subtle impairment on neurologic examination. The authors concluded that 'Social adaptive abilities appeared to be as important as seizure control, and perhaps even more important in the final outcome'. More recently this conclusion has been supported by Batzell et al [3] and Dodrill et al [4] who have developed a psychosocial inventory for epilepsy. This inventory – the Washington Psychosocial Seizure Inventory (WPSI) – evaluates family background, emotional adjustment, interpersonal relations, vocational adjustment, financial status, acceptance of seizures, and medical factors. This inventory, as well as the Minnesota Multiphasic Inventory (MMPI), have both been found to have a high correlation with employability [5,3]. There is also a high correlation between these judgment scales and the presence of underlying neuropsychological deficits [6]. Freeman and Gayle [1] found that among a group of epileptic clients of a rehabilitation programme, only one-third had obtained full-time employment. The best rehabilitation results were with high school graduates who were given a college education. The interplay of all these factors is highlighted by a multi-institutional study in Japan [8] (Table I).

TABLE I. Factors influencing social adjustments [8]

Factor	% with normal social adjustment
Frequency	
≥ 1/day	46
≥ 1/month	67
≥ 1/year	83
Intellectual Deficit	
None	87
Mild	25
Severe	5
Personality Disturbance	
None	80
Mild	40
Severe	14

Regardless of these findings, the importance of the seizure itself as a bar to employment cannot be overlooked. Emlen and Ryan [7] have observed a very significant relationship between seizure frequency and employment. Educational factors were also important (Tables II and III).

Given these complex and interrelated inhibitory factors in employment, what measures can be expected to overcome them? To be realistic, the most significant will be an improvement in the overall level of employment. No matter what we do, the handicapped person is bound to be at the bottom of the list on the rolls of the unemployed. I am no economist, but I am concerned that there must be preferable ways of curing inflation than by putting people out of work.

Next, we must make a vigorous effort to ensure that every epileptic child has a full educational opportunity. For him, superior education is a must. He must be prepared to compete in a job market where he is likely to be excluded

TABLE II. Factors influencing employment [7]

Seizure Frequency	% not employed
1 or more generalised convulsion/year	50.0
1–4 psychomotor/year	50.0
5 or more psychomotor/year	48.2
Less than one psychomotor/year	33.3
Less than one generalised convulsion/year	23.1
5 or more minor seizures/year	20.9
Less than 5 minor seizures/year	13.4

TABLE III. Factors influencing employment [7]

Educational Level	% not employed
Less than High School	42.9
13–15 years school	41.9
High School graduate	36.2
College graduate	18.2

from work involving manual or physical activities. Legislation in the USA mandates that every handicapped child must receive a full and appropriate education. For many with epilepsy, this involves special consideration. In a large study of 524,000 children in the Chicago school system, 16 per cent of those with epilepsy were receiving special educational services [12]. In Italy [13], 17 per cent were failing. In England [14] only one-third of a group of epileptic children were making satisfactory progress. Stores and Hart [15] discovered that especially epileptic boys with focal epilepsy were likely to suffer from specific reading disability.

What these figures mean is that every epileptic schoolchild should be carefully monitored for learning problems, and should receive counselling, support and special assistance if he begins to fail. For him, a successful educational experience is crucial.

But regardless of education, many people with epilepsy require help to obtain employment. The experience of the Training and Placement Service (TAPS) sponsored by the Epilepsy Foundation of America (EFA) has demonstrated that such help must include at least two components. The first is improvement of attitude and in job-seeking skills. Embittered by illness and adverse social experiences, many epileptic applicants are hostile and suspicious. Inexperienced in the technique of interview, they are quickly rejected in the process of applying for work. Their approach can be improved by interaction with others in self-help groups, by special instruction, and by practice interviews.

The other component is in actual job-finding effort on the part of the vocational or rehabilitation programme. Employers will hire epileptic applicants if they can be assured of appropriate referrals. It is also desirable for the referral agency to maintain continued contact with their employed clients to assure that the failing candidate will be supported or removed if necessary.

The receptiveness of employers in the USA has been further enhanced by legislation that makes it illegal to deny employment to a qualified applicant because of a disability. The crucial question is, 'For what type of work is an epileptic applicant qualified?' The answer clearly depends upon the nature of the epilepsy. The EFA has developed an interview guide, the purpose of which is to define the important characteristics of the person's epilepsy. A profile is being developed, and this profile is being correlated with the many different jobs and environments which make up the spectrum of employment. The salient features, aside from the frequency of diurnal attacks, are:

1 Does the individual have a generalised attack with falling and without warning? Such an individual cannot work where falling might result in serious injury.

2 Does the individual have absence of consciousness with automatic behaviour? Here also the individual is not safe to work near dangerous equipment or moving machinery.

3 Does the individual have a consistent aura? If such an aura is of sufficient duration to make it possible for him to seek safety, many otherwise hazardous positions are acceptable.

4 Does the attack consist only of brief loss of consciousness without falling or automatic behaviour? Such an individual can occupy any position that does not require constant vigilance.

5 Is the individual conscientious and reliable in behaviour and compliance to medical regimen? This imponderable personal factor is still one of the most important in suitability for employment.

In considering the appropriateness of employment, several principles deserve consideration. Employment is an important personal and social objective. An individual with epilepsy is always subject to risk or injury, whether at home or at work. For the sake of working, it is justifiable for him to be exposed at work to hazards similar to those at home.

In evaluating the work place, note that if a place of work is not safe for the persons with epilepsy it is not entirely safe for any employee. Sands [10], in a study of compensation claims, discovered that more persons have been injured by accidents due to sneezing than by those resulting from seizures. Risch, in his Epihab factory, claims that standard safety equipment is sufficient protection

TABLE IV. Accident ratios of medically impaired drivers

Condition	California[1] 1	Oregon[2]
Lapses – including epilepsy	2.0	1.8
Lapse – unspecified		2.1
Epilepsy		1.3
Other physical impairments	2.8	
Neurological impairments		1.5
Diabetes	1.8	1.7
Vascular disease	1.6	1.1
Alcohol abuse	1.7	
Drug abuse	1.0 (2.6)	
Mental illness	2.1	1.1

[1] Waller [9], rate per mile; impaired/control
[2] Oregon [10], % drivers having accident; impaired/others

for any epileptic worker. In the final analysis, however, in each instance there is the question of a risk-benefit ratio. The person with epilepsy is inherently at some increased risk for injury or loss of work time. He will be employed only if either there is social pressure for his employment, or he has some superior skill to provide him with a competitive advantage. Under these conditions, some additional risk is tolerable.

Unfortunately, we have almost no data regarding the actual work record of persons with various profiles of epilepsy. Such facts are sorely needed. One source of relevant data is the performance record of epileptic drivers. There is no more

TABLE V. Accident ratios during prior years[1] for drivers with lapses according to how reported. Rate/1.0 million miles

	Rate	Ratio
Control	0.181	1.0
Self report	.149	0.8
Dept Health morbidity	.280	1.5
Doctor's report	.443	2.4
Law enforcement	.926	5.1

[1] California [11], 1978
The above data are derived from a small sample. Later reports with a larger sample indicate that the accidents of self reporting epileptic drivers are in fact considerably higher than those of the control population.

hazardous pursuit than driving an automobile. In the USA, persons subject to lapses of consciousness may drive if they report themselves free of seizures for a year. Such drivers have an accident rate which is 1½–2 times that of the average driver (Table IV). As might be expected, even here the accident rate appears to be determined more by the degree of reliability of the subject than by his epilepsy (Table V). That such an increased risk is considered socially acceptable is evidenced by our tolerance of equally unfavourable driving records of other definable subgroups of the population.

It is unfortunate that at this time we do not have risk/benefit ratios more specific to employment in the various occupations. It is hoped that at future conferences such data may become available. Only then can we approach a prospective employer with facts with which to balance his or our own prejudices.

The issue of employment was a topic for discussion at the meeting of Epilepsy International in London in August 1982; the specific question of the employment record of persons with various types of epilepsy will be the subject of a special symposium being organised in association with its meeting in Washington in 1983.

References

1   Freeman JM, Gayle E. *Epilepsia 1978; 19:* 233–239
2   Denerll Rd, Rodin EA, Gonzales S et al. *Epilepsia 1966; 7:* 318–329
3   Batzell LW, Dodrill CB, Fraser RG. *Epilepsia 1980; 21:* 235–242
4   Dodrill CB, Batzell W, Queisser HR et al. *Epilepsia 1980; 21:* 123–135
5   Dikmen S, Morgan SF. *J Nerv Men Dis 1980; 68:* 236–240
6   Hermann DP. *Epilepsia 1981; 22:* 161–167
7   Emlen AC, Ryan R. *Unpublished 1980*
8   Okuna T, Kumashiro H. *Epilepsia 1981; 22:* 35–54
9   Waller JA. *N Engl J Med 1965; 273:* 1413–1419
10   Oregon State Board of Health. *Automobile Driving and Chronic Disease 1967*
11   California Department of Motor Vehicles. *Medically Impaired Drivers. An Evaluation of California Policy 1978; Report No 67 (SB2033)*
12   Myklebust H. *Report of the Commission for the Control of Epilepsy and its Consequences 1977; 2:* Part 1, 474–490
13   Passaglia P, Frank-Passaglia L. *Epilepsia 1976; 17:* 361–366
14   Holdsworth L, Whitmore K. *Develop Med Child Neurol 1974; 16:* 746–758
15   Stores G, Hart J. *Develop Med Child Neurol 1976; 18:* 1705–1716
16   Sands H. *Personal communication 1960*

54

EPILEPSY AND DRIVING

J F Taylor

It is extremely difficult, where any major trauma is involved, to determine whether a road traffic accident is due to epilepsy. If there is any autopsy evidence of a brain lesion, it is entirely a matter of conjecture whether a seizure occurred prior to or after impact. Any precipitate collapse at the wheel whilst driving at speed normally results in death of the driver. Having considered the matter in the light of autopsy reports, my conclusion is that there is no way in which we will determine the part that epilepsy plays in road traffic accident driver fatalities.

However, in those road traffic accidents where trauma is not extreme and the driver survives, we do have an opportunity to investigate. In collaboration with a voluntary reporting system from police in Great Britain it has been possible to investigate 1,300 road traffic accidents leading to damage to persons and property where collapse at the wheel appears to have been the cause of the event, the driver surviving. In this survey 38 per cent of accidents were on account of witnessed grand mal convulsions. Blackouts NAD accounted for some 23 per cent of survivors collapsing at the wheel, insulin therapy was responsible for 17 per cent, whilst all forms of heart conditions in aggregate accounted for only 10 per cent and strokes etc only 8 per cent. Excluding first seizures, 70 per cent of the people collapsing at the wheel due to epilepsy had failed to declare their condition in relation to their driving licence; 12 per cent of the accidents were on account of a first seizure.

Specific legislation in relation to seizures and driving invariably applies to a person who has a continuing liability to seizures and not to the solitary convulsion case. The prognosis of isolated seizures in adult life has been well documented and perhaps most recently by Cleland et al's survey at Newcastle General Hospital [1]. Cleland and his associates investigated the subsequent prognosis in 70 patients who suffered an isolated seizure in adult life. Thirty-nine per cent of the cases subsequently developed epilepsy and the chances at the end of one year of recurrence were 4 to 1 but at the end of two years the risk of subsequent epilepsy fell to 15 to 1. A similar recurrence rate was established in the survey by Johnson et al [2] which reviewed 77 naval enlisted men. The figures suggest that a patient with a solitary seizure and negative EEG findings might be advised to resume driving 12 months after initial seizure whilst those with a positive EEG would be best advised to wait for two years before resuming driving.

Looking now at driving and the law, both British and international, the general pattern across the world is that, in the Eastern block, people who suffer from epilepsy are prohibited from driving and the same situation obtains in Italy and Spain. However, the average freedom from attacks period before driving is allowed to commence in most countries is now approximately two years. Britain and West Germany have allowed a concession to people who have established a pattern of regular attacks asleep but other countries do not do this.

Looking at international proposals, in 1975 the United Nations published a Draft Agreement [3] setting down minimum medical standards for the international exchange of driving licences. Later the standards in that Agreement were adopted by the EEC as a Draft Directive for the introduction of a Common Community Driver's Licence. These draft agreements both distinguished between the ordinary driver's licence valid for driving motorcars and light commercial vehicles which falls into category Group 1 and the Group 2 licence which comprises the heavy goods (HGV) and public service vehicle (PSV) licence. Both the EEC Draft Directive and United Nations Draft Agreement say that driving permits for Group 1 shall neither be granted nor renewed to applicants or drivers suffering from epilepsy but that domestic legislation may provide that, subject to competent medical opinion, permits may be granted to persons suffering from epilepsy in the past but who have been free from attacks for a long time (eg at least two years). So far as Group 2 licences are concerned, that is the HGVs and PSVs, driving permits shall neither be granted nor renewed to applicants or drivers who suffer or who have suffered in the past from epilepsy. This distinction, between HGV and PSV drivers on the one hand and ordinary motor vehicle drivers on the other, should be explained.

In the first place, heavy goods vehicles' weights have been progressively increasing over the years. In the UK, there are now proposals for a maximum laden weight of 40 metric tonnes gross.

The speed of HGVs has been progressively increasing. Before the Second World War the speed restriction on HGVs was 20 mph, but these vehicles can now travel at 70 mph. The combination of speed and mass produce a velocity which, in the circumstances of a sudden collapse at the wheel, do substantially more damage than can an ordinary motor vehicle. In fact the British national road accident statistics for 1980 show that, for each mile travelled, heavy goods vehicles were responsible for 70 per cent more deaths than car drivers although, due to their greater protection in heavier vehicles, the HGV drivers themselves had a lower death rate than car drivers.

534

If one is considering epilepsy as a cause of collapse at the wheel, then clearly the more hours spent at the wheel the greater the risk of collapse. My survey suggested that the average private motorist spends approximately half an hour per average day at the wheel of his vehicle whilst the HGV and PSV driver spends 12 times this time per working day. Thus the risk of a seizure actually occurring at the wheel is enhanced in the HGV/PSV driver by about 12 times.

With public service vehicles, the bus driver working in urban and city areas approaches queues of people up to 100 or more times per working shift, so that any collapse at the wheel could lead to serious consequences to the public. Long distance bus drivers usually have to work to very tight schedules and there is an incentive in these circumstances to continue driving, even sometimes in spite of warning symptoms. Heavy goods vehicles carry a wide variety of cargoes, from anything as benign as a load of hay to the most dangerous chemical cargoes.

British domestic legislation is currently under review. The Honorary Medical Advisory Panel that advises the Government in relation to epilepsy and driving have recommended that there should be a straight two years freedom from attack period before commencing driving in this country, and indeed this is the situation that pertains in most of the western world. The current law in Britain in relation to the heavy goods vehicle driver and public service vehicle driver is that any attack since attaining the age of three precludes licensing for these vehicles. The Honorary Panel have suggested that the age of five would be more appropriate to cover late febrile convulsions.

Much is said about the inflexibility of legal bar regulations. There has been much heart searching and serious consideration has been given to the thought of deprescribing epilepsy. The great advantage of an absolute bar is that it takes the decision concerning whether or not a person is fit to drive in relationship to epileptic attacks out of the clinical, patient/doctor relationship and into the field of parliamentary legislation and the courts. The Honorary Medical Advisory Panel have felt great concern about iatrogenic seizures resulting from considered advice that a patient should either reduce or discontinue anti-convulsants. In this context it is well worth bearing in mind the risks. Juul-Jensen [4] in 1964 showed that about half of those who had their anti-convulsant drugs discontinued because they had been attack free for two years, started to have attacks again. Clearly if the patient with epilepsy needs and wants to drive, it is important to protect him by chemical therapy. If one could postulate a situation where the iatrogenic or special circumstance fit could be exempt from the regulations by medical certification, then one can imagine the considerable abuse that would ensue. I do not think we can seriously challenge the view that doctors are generally in the position of having to certify on the basis of the history as given by the patient. Bearing in mind the hardship that can occur with loss of licence, including livelihood, on account of iatrogenic and special circumstance fits, the Panel decided overall that it would be right to reduce the seizure free period from three to two years.

One welcomes the fact that discussion has commenced concerning the Pearson Commission Report on compensation and proof of negligence. British third party motor insurance is compulsorily payable only on proof of negligence. A driver who collapses at the wheel due to an epileptic seizure is not normally held to be negligent. Some years ago the Medical Defence Union had a case where a doctor completing an HGV medical certificate did not declare on the form that his patient had suffered an attack of epilepsy since attaining the age of three. Subsequently, driving in pursuance of the heavy goods vehicle licence, the patient suffered an attack at the wheel and did substantial damage to a Sussex cottage. In consequence, the owners of the cottage sought compensation from their house insurers and they in turn sought compensation from the third party motor insurers who refused liability. Subsequent enquiries revealed that the doctor had deceived the Licensing Authority and, in Medical Defence Union language, the matter of the doctor's negligence was resolved by an out of court settlement by payment of a substantial sum.

Alcohol withdrawal seizures do present a 'Catch 22' situation. A 39 year old heavy goods vehicle driver had his first initial seizure six years ago and some 36 hours after a binge. His seizure occurred at the wheel of his HGV and, in consequence of the law, he lost his licence. However on investigation in hospital it was explained to him that he did not suffer from epilepsy, that he had only had a solitary seizure, and that if anything his problem was one of alcohol. He therefore eventually took the law into his own hands and decided to drive a heavy goods vehicle without a licence, and in consequence caused the death of a pedestrian by suffering a second seizure some 36 hours after a birthday party in which he consumed a quantity of spirits. The 'Catch 22' situation for these unfortunate people is that the withdrawal seizure happens at a time when usually the blood alcohol is below the prescribed legal limit in Great Britain of 80mg.

Epileptic risks following craniotomy presents a special problem in driving. The Honorary Medical Advisory Panel, having reviewed the latest epidemiological data, have suggested that six months should elapse after a major supratentorial craniotomy before driving is resumed. In cases of cerebral abscess, meningioma or aneurysms of the middle cerebral artery or associated with intracranial haematomas, the period of waiting should be 12 months. Up to the present time the Panel have felt constrained to advise that supratentorial major craniotomy should preclude HGV or PSV driving.

It is perhaps prudent to mention comparative mortality rates between different forms of transport. The risk of being killed per 100 million kilometres travelled by lorry is 4 times that of by rail, by car 7 times that of by rail, and by the motorcycle rider 162 times that of by rail, whilst the pillion passenger has a risk of being killed of 281 times that of travelling by rail. Clearly if your daughter has a boyfriend who suffers from epilepsy and who rides a motorcycle, she should be permanently banned from travelling on his pillion.

At the beginning of this chapter, it was stated that there was great difficulty in determining the part that epilepsy plays in road traffic accidents. Recently there has been a survey of over 2,000 road traffic accidents in East Berkshire involving nearly 4,000 drivers. This survey took place over a period of some four years and involved a substantial portion of the M4 motorway. Despite fog, snow, ice and all sorts of adverse environmental conditions, only two and a half per cent of these accidents were considered absolutely to be due to the conditions of road and environment. Vehicle defects as the sole cause, accounted for only two and a half per cent of the accidents. Interestingly enough one-third of those defects were due to defective tyres, one-third defective brakes and the rest miscellaneous defects but, overall, the road user came out as being absolutely and solely responsible for 65 per cent of the accidents, in the majority of which there was multifactorial aetiology, the different causes interacting. This survey follows closely the results of a similar one in Indiana.

In 1978 19 persons died per average day due to road traffic accidents at an estimated national cost of £4½ million. Despite this, Great Britain comes out top in relation to the least number of car user deaths per 100 million car kilometres travelled.

In conclusion, epilepsy is responsible for an unquantifiable number of road traffic accidents in a relatively small population of people with epilepsy, many of whom do not declare their condition when applying for a driving licence.

References

1   Cleland PG, Mosquera I, Sheward WP, Foster JB. *Br Med J 1981; 283:* 1364
2   Johnson LC, De Bolt WL, Long MT et al. *Arch Neurol 1972; 27*
3   United Nations (Economic Council for Europe). *Agreement on Minimum Standards for the Issue and Validity of Driving Permits (APC) 1975 (Geneva)*
4   Juul-Jensen P. *Epilepsia 1964; 5:* 352–363

55

SPECIAL SCHOOLING FOR CHILDREN WITH EPILEPSY

Zarrina Kurtz

Before the turn of the century most children with epilepsy in Great Britain did not go to school at all and remained largely uneducated. In 1893 the Charity Organisation Society estimated the prevalence of school-age children with epilepsy to be 2–3 per 1,000 and found that very few such children were at school [1]. The Society saw this as the beginning of an almost inevitably sad downhill path through life for children with this condition: " The life of many an epileptic may soon be told. As a child, he is not educated. As a young man, he fails to obtain employment, or, obtaining it with difficulty, he keeps it only on sufferance. As years advance, and strength decreases, he retires to the workhouse or to the asylum." However, from 1890 onwards, the needs of children with marked disabilities of all kinds began to be recognised and the first special schools and classes were organised within the framework of universal education.

The Elementary Education Act of 1899 permitted school boards, as they then were, to make provision for the 'defective and epileptic child'. Although the enhanced rate of grant was payable for this special provision, 10 years later, only 133 out of 327 local education authorities were using their powers under the Act [2]. A subsequent Act in 1918 converted these powers into a statutory duty, but only one special school for children with epilepsy had been built by an Education Committee: Manchester's Soss Moss residential school opened in 1911. By that time schools had however been opened at several of the 'colonies' for epileptics, which had been founded by philanthropic organisations in response to the recognition that the Poor Law system was failing to cope adequately or appropriately with the needs of disabled people. Their main inspiration for these developments in England came from a village for epileptics started in 1865 by the Rhineland and Westphalian provincial mission committee at Bielefeld in Germany.

Schooling for children in the epileptic colonies was first set up in 1899 at Lingfield in Surrey by the Christian Union for Social Service. In 1957, patients were exchanged between Lingfield and the Chalfont Centre for Epilepsy in Buckinghamshire and Lingfield Hospital School came into being, catering solely for children and the largest of the schools for epilepsy. St Elizabeth's School in Hertfordshire was opened by an Order of Catholic nuns, Daughters of the Cross of Liège, in 1903. The David Lewis colony near Manchester set up its own school in 1914 although, from 1905 until Soss Moss was opened nearby, it had admitted children under an arrangement with Manchester Education Committee. The Maghull Homes in Liverpool had provided day schooling for some time before opening a residential school in 1908. Finally, the second local authority school was opened in 1951 by Lancashire School Health Service at Sedgwick House near Kendal in Cumbria in response to the 1944 Education Act which required education authorities to provide for pupils who suffer from 'any disability of mind or body'.

In 1928, a census of epileptics in Surrey [3] showed that 20.2 per cent of children of school age were attending residential schools for epileptics and 24.5 per cent of educable children were attending no school at all. The schools of epilepsy did not admit 'feeble-minded' and 'imbecile' children, except Lingfield which received educable children sought out from the imbecile wards of the workhouses. In 1932 it was decided that the accommodation at Lingfield should be given to those most likely to benefit from the education and treatment provided, and a policy of not admitting children with an IQ below 60 was followed for the next 25 years. Probably all children with epilepsy were not offered schooling until April 1971 when the 1970 Education Act came into force and all children including those with severe handicaps became the responsibility of local authority education departments.

These six residential schools form the provision specifically for epilepsy in children in England and Wales. Originally, custodial care rather than education was offered. Except for the Chilton school, the schools are situated in beautiful open countryside and a regular open-air life with sensible wholesome diet was felt to be very healthy for children suffering from fits, especially if they came from poor, crowded homes situated in the city slums. Dr William Alexander, Medical Superintendent of the Maghull Homes, commented in 1889 [4] that "the epileptic (child) is spoiled by the almost inevitable partiality of his parents; the mind, already debased more or less by the disease, becomes still worse regulated by indulgence." For this reason also, the care offered in these boarding schools was regarded as highly beneficial. Children living in any part of the country may attend any one of the schools, and enter and leave at any stage of their school careers.

The children attending the six residential schools now form only a small proportion of all children with epilepsy, most of whom are educated in ordinary schools. Estimates of the prevalence of epilepsy in children of school age are notoriously difficult to make. In 1969, the Reid report, 'People with Epilepsy' [5] suggested a figure of 8 per 1,000 based on several different surveys carried out in Great Britain. From information based on rigorous definition of cases of epilepsy in children from the National Child Development Study [6], when they were 11 years old, a probably closer estimate of 4–5 per 1,000 was made; this would mean about 30,000–40,000 school-age children in Great Britain. Of the 64 children identified as having epilepsy at 11, 59 were followed up to school-leaving age at 16. Table I shows that 22 of these were receiving special education of some kind, but only four were attending one of the six residential schools for epilepsy.

TABLE I. Type of school attended by 16 year olds with epilepsy in the National Child Development Study

	Type of School	Number of Children
	Ordinary	37
	ESN (M)	11
	ESN (S)	4
Receiving special education	Physically Handicapped	2
	Special Class in a Comprehensive School	1
	Residential School for Epilepsy	4
	Total	59

As a result of recommendations made in the Reid report, the children attending the six residential schools for epilepsy were the subject of a special study [7] commissioned by the Department of Health and Social Security and the Department of Education and Science. Figure 1 shows where the schools are and the number of children in each in 1977. The committee set up under the chairmanship of Dr John Reid was the third to consider services for people with epilepsy since the beginning of the National Health Service in 1948, but the first to consider health, welfare and other services together, recognising the important inter-relationship of social and clinical factors in epilepsy. The Committee reported that children with epilepsy were inadequately provided for medically and educationally and were at a disadvantage socially.

The committee made two main recommendations: that the diagnosis, assessment, treatment and continuing care of people with epilepsy should be provided by multi-disciplinary teams each consisting of relevant specialists such as a neurologist, paediatrician, psychiatrist, psychologist, social worker and health visitor: that a number of special centres should be set up where the comprehensive assessment and management of people with complicated epilepsy could be carried out; these would contain a specialist neurological and neurosurgical unit

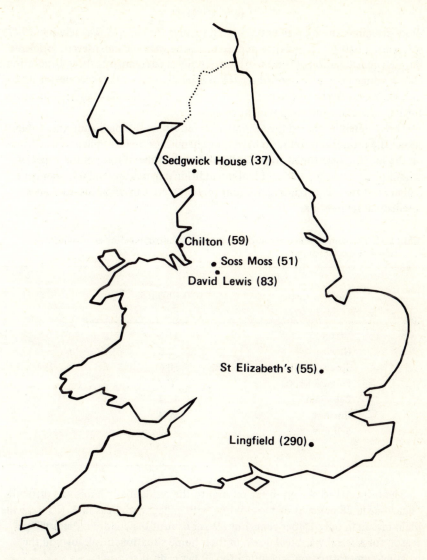

Figure 1. Map of England and Wales showing where the special schools for children with epilepsy are sited and the numbers in each, in January 1977

and a residential unit so that observation could take place under as near to normal daily living conditions as possible and the residential component of a special centre for children should be a special school. The Reid committee recommended that the way in which these services were developing should be reviewed after about five years.

As a result of these recommendations with regard to children, a study of all those attending the six residential special schools for epilepsy was set up in 1977, recognising that this population represents those with the most severe problems but that consideration of these will highlight the needs of many others. In addition, all the young people who left these schools in 1972 and 1977 were personally interviewed by the author to find out about their medical and social circumstances, further education and employment.

The children attending the schools suffered from multiple handicaps. Table II shows the proportion found to have other handicaps besides epilepsy, as defined on the medical assessment form completed at the time of referral for a special school place. Only 5.6 per cent had no additional handicaps and 65.6 per cent had at least two. The major conditions present were behaviour disorder and intellectual retardation.

TABLE II. Problems found on medical assessment of children before admission to residential special school

Problem area	Children %
Vision	11.5
Hearing	2.6
Speech and language	30.6
Physical health	27.7
Behaviour	72.2
Intellect	66.4
Self care	21.0
	n = 575

The principal reason given for referral to the residential schools was difficult behaviour in 28 per cent of the children with epilepsy whereas their fits were the main reason in only 15 per cent. For 39 per cent of the children, the principal reason for referral was breakdown in their home situation; breakdown in the existing school situation accounted for 29 per cent of referrals.

It was found that a high proportion of the children (21%) had parents who were widowed, divorced or separated and, although about half of these had remarried or were living with another partner, the percentage of single parents was higher than that found in the national census of 1971 (7.1%). In addition, the number of children in care of the local authority was over six times the national average. There was little difference between national figures and those for the children in the six special schools for fathers's employment status and social class, but only half as many mothers were employed as was found nationally. These children came from large families with an average of 3.4 children, not

542

necessarily from completed families; the national average was 2.4. Thirty-eight per cent of the families had four or more children compared with 9 per cent nationally. Family problems such as financial difficulty, marital disharmony, difficulties with employment or conditions of work, parental chronic mental or physical ill health, involvement with the police and bad housing conditions were recorded for 60 per cent of the children and half of these had more than one problem.

Results from a previous study of children admitted to Lingfield in 1963 [8] showed that IQ levels were little different from those found in the schools as a whole in 1977, but the prevalence of behaviour disturbance had risen from 63 per cent to 72.2 per cent and the proportion coming from disturbed home backgrounds had risen markedly from 20 per cent to 60 per cent.

Although it is well known that the many difficulties these children face must require careful assessment and Reid specifically recommended that no child should be admitted to a special school until he has been 'fully investigated, medically and socially as well as educationally', it was found that only 25 per cent of the children had been fully assessed in this way. If comprehensive medical assessment had been carried out, frequently this was several years before referral for special school placement; otherwise medical assessment on referral was done by a local authority medical officer who had little previous knowledge of the child and often insufficient experience of epilepsy. Children admitted after 1976, when new forms for assessment for special education were introduced, were more likely to have had psychological and educational assessment than before.

Requests for placement at the residential special schools are being made when children are older than previously, 50 per cent of requests now being for children aged 13 years or older. Thirty-three per cent of children in the schools had attended ordinary schools previously but 60 per cent had already received some form of special educational treatment. Children with more severe intellectual retardation and behaviour disturbance were admitted at younger ages and tended to remain at the schools for longer periods. The average time spent at the schools is becoming longer; Reid reported that approximately half the children admitted stay for less than two years whereas, in 1977, it was found that less than a quarter of children had been discharged within two years over the previous five year period. Over two-thirds of the children stay until they are 16.

It has been found that children with seizures who attend ordinary schools may well have more problems with learning and behaviour and that some children are more at risk than others: boys with epilepsy are particularly predisposed to behavioural difficulties; persistent left temporal spike discharge on the EEG appears to be associated with reading retardation, inattentiveness, emotional dependence and, in boys, other types of disturbed behaviour, especially overactivity [9]. In addition, it was found that those taking phenytoin were more likely to show poor reading skills and impaired attentiveness and there was other evidence that drug treatment contributes to behaviour problems.

543

The epileptic children attending ordinary schools in the National Child Development Study achieved mean scores in reading and maths tests which were not significantly different at the 5 per cent level from the scores of the rest of the cohort. However, only three of those receiving special education were regarded as having enough ability to cope with everyday reading needs. These children were much more likely to be having fits still in their 16th year (59%) than those attending normal schools (22%). It has been suggested that children educated at normal schools may have an intrinsically different form of epilepsy from those at special schools. Certainly, those with mainly nocturnal fits and those whose fits are well controlled by drug treatment are more likely to attend ordinary schools, as are those whose epilepsy is uncomplicated by intellectual retardation or physical handicap such as cerebral palsy. In the National Child Development Study, those at special schools were more likely to have clear-cut organic brain abnormalities than those in normal schools; in the residential special schools for epilepsy it was found that 52 per cent of the children had secondary epilepsy whereas, in unselected samples, about a third have secondary epilepsy.

The proportion of those leaving the residential special schools who go on to do any further education or training is low (40%), particularly when some form of education beyond normal school age would seem desirable for these young people who are likely to be immature emotionally and socially. The follow-up study carried out in 1979 showed that 30 per cent of the school-leavers were already in residential care, and only 24 per cent were employed; the other young people were either attending an adult training centre (19%) or doing nothing at home (21%). In 1928, the Medical Superintendent of Lingfield followed-up children who had left between 1919 and 1927 [10], and found that 42 per cent were in residential care, 28 per cent were wholly or partially self-supporting and 14 per cent were at home unemployed. The annual death rate was 3.7 per cent; in 1979 it was one per cent.

These fifty years have seen improvement in survival but, even considering that children at the schools for epilepsy are now more severely disabled than in the 1920s, the long-term outcome shows little real change. The young people who might have been in residential care previously are now living at home but may well not even have a place at an adult training centre. There is reluctance even to admit children to residential care in the form of a special school. The boarding schools are now usually regarded as places of last resort for the most difficult cases whereas, when they were established, they seemed to offer the most desirable type of care. There has also been a shift in their emphasis from primarily medical care to more specific educational measures. Although medical deficit is the label giving eligibility for this type of provision, educational disadvantage from a variety of causes is the reason for which it is sought. As long ago as 1905 [11] it was recognised that those with obvious 'feeble-mindedness' and fits would be identified and would receive special treatment, but concern was expressed that milder degrees of disability might pass unnoticed by teachers who usually initiate the requests for the medical assessment that is necessary before referral takes place. The members of the Royal Commission also recognised that 'feeble-mindedness' with or without fits could be managed in the same way, and the Reid committee also felt that children with epilepsy who needed residential care should be placed according to their primary handicap which would very rarely be their fits.

Epilepsy is not a homogeneous condition with regard to its aetiology or its manifestations. Special schooling must encompass provision for a whole range of problems. Fits per se do not require a specific educational approach but close medical supervision and sensitive adjustment of medication to balance their control with a minimum of side effects. This should be carried out whatever type of schooling the child is receiving. Medical assessment must be sufficiently expert to be useful as a baseline for comparison with the findings of further assessments. Educational difficulties should be sought for and tackled more actively in normal schools. Comprehensive assessment of the condition of any child with problems is essential and should be made at definite intervals during the school years. Because complicated epilepsy may well be a life-long condition, these children need to be under the supervision of their local services and should receive appropriate special schooling as near to their homes as possible. Residential schooling will be required for those with the most severe and intractable problems and should be provided in local establishments for children with a variety of medical, educational and social problems. The length of time spent in residential care should be varied to suit the requirements of each child and his or her family. These recommendations are in line with those made by the Warnock Committee in 'Special Education Needs' in 1978 [12]. In addition, there should be several residential schools as part of special centres specifically for epilepsy in different parts of the country. These should undertake the short-term investigation and management of children with the most complicated problems and act as centres for training and research with regard to epilepsy.

Acknowledgments

I would like to thank the Department of Health and Social Security for their financial support and Professor A E Bennett for his helpful advice.

References

1 Charity Organisation Society. *The Epileptic and Crippled Child and Adult – Suggestions for Better Education and Employment 1893*. London: Swan Sonnenschein and Co
2 *Annual Report for 1909 of the Chief Medical Officer of the Board of Education 1910:* 152. London: HMSO
3 A Census of Epileptics in Surrey. *Lancet 1928; ii:* 568
4 Alexander W. *The Treatment of Epilepsy 1889:* quoted in 1 op cit
5 People with Epilepsy. *Report of Joint Sub-committee of the Standing Medical Advisory Committee and the Advisory Committee on the Health and Welfare of Handicapped Persons 1969*. London: HMSO

545

6   Ross EM et al. *Br Med J 1989; 2:* 207–210
7   Kurtz Z, Bennett AE. *Report to the Department of Health and Social Security 1981*
8   Richman NF. *The Prevalence of Psychiatric Disturbance in a Hospital School for Epileptics. 1964.* Unpublished thesis submitted as part of an examination for the academic DPM. London
9   Stores G. *Develop Med Child Neurol 1978; 20:* 502–508
10 Tylor Fox J. *Lancet 1928; ii:* 545–547
11 *Royal Commission on the Care and Control of the Feeble-minded, etc 1905.* London: HMSO
12 *Report of the Committee of Enquiry into the Education of Handicapped Children and Young People 1978.* London: HMSO

56

SPECIAL CENTRES

R H E Grant

In this chapter, I propose to discuss the wider implications of a special centre for epilepsy rather than the strictly limited definition of the so-called Reid Report published in 1969 [1] although the importance of that excellent Report in the future development of services for people with epilepsy cannot be overemphasised.

Throughout the centuries, the 'falling sickness' has occupied a position of some importance if surviving medical writings are a reliable indication. Lennox [2] has calculated that 2.6 per cent of all the Hippocratic writings are concerned with epilepsy compared with the 1959 edition of Cecil's Medicine, which contained only 0.5 per cent about epilepsy. The major contribution by Hippocrates was to dissociate epilepsy from the concept of possession by evil spirits but, unfortunately, his hypothesis was largely ignored by the medical fraternity for some 2000 years. Because of the widespread ignorance and prejudice over the centuries, the person with epilepsy has had more than his fair share of adversity and, although much improved, this state of affairs still exists today.

Gradually, the kindlier elements of society provided places where people with epilepsy could escape from a hostile world intolerant of their condition. It seems that the earliest recorded expression of this was at the end of the fifteenth century when a 'hospice for epileptics' was established by monks at the Priory of Saint Valentine at Rufach, in Alsace. With the spread of Christianity over the previous millenium, people had come to expect help from saints and relics, and some saints lent their names to the disease and became its patrons [3]. It is likely, at least initially, that fear of epilepsy as a contagious disease may have been a prominent consideration, as well as philanthropy. In 1773 the Bishop of Würzburg established a home for people with epilepsy, and this survived for many years. By the nineteenth century, the practice of putting insane people in chains was discontinued and, because epileptics had often been confined with the insane, this was of benefit to them as well. In general, it was only from the time of Pinel (1745–1826) in France, and the Tukes, in England, that people with epilepsy confined to institutions became the object of systematic medical attention [3]. In 1815, Esquirol made a strong plea for the establishment of special divisions for epileptics, but the reason for this plea is interesting. Esquirol thought that the sight of an epileptic attack might be sufficient to make a healthy person epileptic, and even more so for the mentally deranged! About 1850 it became the practice in England to confine epileptics to separate wards in lunatic asylums and, when this segregation had become an established fact, the logical sequence was a demand for special institutions for people with epilepsy.

In Britain this demand began to be fulfilled from 1860, when the National Hospital for the Paralysed and Epileptic was opened in Queen Square, London. In Germany, in 1867, four people with epilepsy were taken into custodial care by a pastor in a farmhouse outside the town of Bielefeld. In 1872, Pastor Friedrich von Bödelschwingh took over what became the institution of Bethel, which, in some respects, is now one of the leading special centres for epilepsy in the world. This was followed in 1882 by the colony at 'Meer en Bosch' in Heemstede, The Netherlands, and The Filadelfia Colony in Dianalund in Denmark. In England, the first special institution for epileptics was established at Maghull, near Liverpool. This was followed by the Chalfont Colony for Epileptics in Buckinghamshire in 1894, due to the efforts of a lady called Miss Burden-Sanderson who had visited Bethel with a group of friends in 1891. When she returned to England, an appeal was launched so successfully that, within six months, the National Society for the Employment of Epileptics (later the National Society for Epileptics) was formed, and a pilot scheme was started at Skippings Farm, Chalfont St Peter, and named the Chalfont Colony. The David Lewis Epileptic Colony, near Alderley Edge, Cheshire, was opened in September 1904 under the Trust Deed of Mr David Lewis, who founded a department store now widespread in the north of England. Altogether, some 17 homes or institutions for people with epilepsy developed in Great Britain between 1888 and 1933, with one in Scotland, the Colony for Epileptics, Bridge of Weir, founded in 1902 (Epilepsia 2nd Series 1: 1937–1940).

Meanwhile, in the United States of America, similar developments were taking place initially at Gallipolis, Ohio, in 1891, followed the next year by a colony at Sonyea, New York State. Ultimately, 14 institutions were developed in various States, which, by 1933, provided a bed capacity of 10,342. Today, only the New Castle State Hospital, in Indiana, survives. Basically, these and many other 'colonies' developed to provide a haven of retreat from an increasingly industrialised and hostile world, and were originally intended to provide custodial care for many years, or for life. To this end, they were largely self-supporting communities and it is significant that many of the centres in Britain, Europe and the USA were deliberately established away from the urban areas of industry and employment. They performed a much needed service that most of society had neglected but, by the middle of this century, a new role was necessary.

Present trends

In England, during the 1950s, two reports concerning people with epilepsy were published. The first concerned the special welfare needs of epileptics [4] ; amongst many recommendations, it was advised that separate accommodation should be provided in the epileptic colonies for (a) the 'low grade', (b) the 'difficult' and (c) those requiring short-term stabilisation. Of more importance was the subsequent report of the Cohen Committee [5] which recommended that the epileptic colonies should be as much therapeutic as custodial, and that they should be concerned with the rehabilitation of patients, ultimately returning them to a normal life in the community.

Very little action was taken over the more fundamental recommendations of these two reports, and it was not until the Reid Report [1] that progress began to take place. The proposals have been well summarised by Dr Reid himself [6]. Of a total of 56 recommendations, 12 concerned the epileptic colonies and the proposed new concept of special centres, but the Report contains much wider implications and recommendations concerning the general management and care of people with epilepsy.

Meanwhile, progress was being made elsewhere, particularly in Europe and the USA. In France, a day hospital specifically for epileptics was established at Créteil, near Paris [7]. In The Netherlands, in conjunction with the Instituut voor Epilepsiebestrijding, outpatient clinics and special centres for epilepsy had been established, not only at Heemstede, but in other parts of the country [8]. In Norway, a country which had never had epileptic colonies, a bill was passed in the Norwegian Parliament, in 1970–1971, for the further development of the care of epileptics in that country, based on the developments in Britain [9]. Up to then there had been one National Hospital for Epileptics, the Statens Sykehus for Epileptikere, at Sandvika, which is associated with the department of neurology at Oslo University. In Denmark, the Filadelfia Colony remained functional at Dianalund, and the Danish Epilepsy Association founded a day centre for severely handicapped people with epilepsy in a suburb of Copenhagen [10]. In the United States of America the general trend had been to close the epileptic colonies and replace them with institutions and training schools for the mentally retarded, the concept being that epileptics with psychiatric illness should be admitted to psychiatric institutions and those with severe brain damage and mental retardation should be placed in hospitals for the mentally subnormal. This arrangement did not appear to deal with people whose predominant problem was epilepsy. However, one colony remained; the Indiana Village for Epileptics was established in 1905, and was primarily intended for long-term custodial care. In 1955, the name of this institution was changed to New Castle State Hospital, and the emphasis was changed to intensive medical treatment, rehabilitation and return to the community. In addition, an outpatient service was provided for people with epilepsy. Later, The National

549

Institute of Neurological and Communicative Disorders and Stroke (NINCDS) established five Comprehensive Epilepsy Programmes, or centres of excellence with the function of providing a service of diagnosis, treatment and rehabilitation. They were also charged with developing an educational service for professional and lay groups, and sponsoring and co-ordinating clinical and social investigations concerned with epilepsy. There are now four Comprehensive Epilepsy Programmes sponsored by the NINCDS in the USA, situated in Augusta (Georgia), Seattle (Washington State), University of California and the University of Minnesota in Minneapolis. Other programmes continue at the University of Virginia in Charlottesville and in Portland, Oregon.

The next development in the USA occurred on July 29th 1975, when, under Public Law 94-63, The Commission for the Control of Epilepsy and its Consequences was established, under the Executive Direction of Dr Richard L Masland of Columbia University, New York. The four-volume report was sent to the President at the White house on August 1st 1977 [11]. The first volume is similar to, but considerably longer than, the Reid Report in England and Wales. Out of 418 recommendations, the Commission included nine on the development of a Comprehensive Epilepsy Service Network with the Comprehensive Epilepsy Programmes acting as supra-regional special centres. It was envisaged that this network would be fully established by 1982.

The establishment of special centres in England and Wales

The Reid Report, on which the present Special Centres in England and Wales are based [1,6], stressed that, with good co-ordination between family doctors and the hospital and local authority services, the vast majority of people with epilepsy could be given a high standard of care in the community, based on a multi-disciplinary approach. It was recommended that special epilepsy clinics should be extended and should be situated at district general hospital level as well as in regional neurological and neurosurgical centres. Furthermore, they should not be in isolation, but rather as parts of appropriate departments, such as neurology, psychiatry or paediatrics. It was, nevertheless, recognised that however good these services turned out to be, there still remained a small but significant number of people with epilepsy who required even more specialised attention because of continued seizures, and also those who required medical supervision under ordinary living and working conditions. The concept of 'Special Centres' was introduced and it was recommended that they should comprise the following:

1 A hospital neurological and neurosurgical unit containing all the necessary facilities for diagnosis and treatment, which today would include CAT brain scan and serum anti-epileptic drug monitoring.

2 A residential unit to which *appropriate* people with epilepsy could be

admitted for a period of further treatment, after an established diagnosis and assessment has been made. The word 'appropriate' is stressed because the danger was clearly seen that such residential components might become dumping grounds of convenience, in the same way that part of the epileptic colonies had been used during the first half of the twentieth century.

The ideal concept is that special centres should be purpose-built, with residential and workshop components in close proximity to the neurological department, but it was realised that this would involve heavy capital expenditure. It therefore suggested that the residential component might be situated in an existing epileptic colony, or psychiatric unit, provided that the need for assessment and rehabilitation could be separated from the long-term care function. It was also considered essential that full social work support and workshop facilities should be available. The Reid Report, based on experience in The Netherlands, suggested that some five or six regional centres should be established in England and Wales. Since 1972, there have been two centres recognised by the Department of Health for adults. The special centre at Chalfont Colony was designated as the National Hospital – Chalfont Centre for Epilepsy, administered jointly by the two respective organisations and opened with a 45-bed unit. In the north of England, the Special Centre for Epilepsy at Bootham Park Hospital, York, was designated. In fact, the latter was an ongoing development of the Neuropsychiatric Unit established in 1966 as a 20-bedded unit in Bootham Park Psychiatric Hospital already staffed by a multi-disciplinary team [12]. In addition, there is a 'special centre' at The David Lewis Centre for Epilepsy, in association with the North West Regional Health Authority.

It is frequently argued that people with epilepsy should not be segregated as this might reinforce the feeling of being special, and outcast, and might cause neurotic reaction. Like Meinardi [8], it is my daily experience that this argument is not correct except in a very few cases and has, in any case, not been formally substantiated. I think the centres have a useful part to play in the management of a proportion of people with epilepsy, and that this will continue for a long time, but it is likely that they have not yet been used to their full potential.

The present state of special centres. Their role in the management of epilepsy

The following functions should be considered an integral part of a special centre for epilepsy, regardless of the country:

1 Comprehensive assessment of the patient is of paramount importance. This includes a detailed neurological, neurophysiological and psychiatric examination and assessment by a clinical psychologist. This is closely followed by a full social assessment, including educational, domestic and employment problems. Experienced social workers are mandatory in this respect. The

551

majority of the work should, of course, have been carried out in the epilepsy clinic, but I agree strongly with Parsonage [12,13] who has found that a significant proportion of patients admitted to the special centre have, in fact, turned out not to have epilepsy at all. This particularly applies to those patients with outpatient records weighing at least 1 kg and heavily marked with the words 'known epileptic'. This label requires highly critical considera-tion.

The advantages of the residential component of a special centre are several. Paramount of these is the fact that repeated and detailed observation of seizure patterns can be made by staff experienced in the finer nuances of seizures. Clini-cal observation may be supplemented, when necessary by the more sophisticated techniques of intensive monitoring [14–16]. Such observation can be carried out in an environment much closer to normality than the sterility of a hospital ward and this, in itself, can help towards a more realistic appraisal of the epi-leptic state.

2 Control of seizures with the minimum of side effects is also fundamental, and admission to a residential special centre should be considered in all patients who have failed to respond to seemingly adequate treatment as outpatients. The uncertain relationship between the type of epilepsy and medication often demands lengthy trials of different drugs, especially in those slow to achieve steady-state blood levels. A higher rate of compliance with treatment can be obtained and serum drug level monitoring can be carried out much more frequently than in outpatients. It is common to find that patients are taking several drugs, many of which may be interacting with each other, and that reduction of medication is not only necessary, but beneficial [12]. Clearly, this can often be done on an outpatient basis, but by no means always, particularly in those cases where there is doubt about correct administration of treatment.

3 Social adjustment. It cannot be denied that many people with epilepsy have considerable difficulty with social relationships, both within the family situ-ation and also the community. Social rejection of epileptics appears to be widespread, even in so-called advanced societies [17], and this may be more marked than in the case of mental illness or ethnic minorities. Bagley [17] suggests that this may be largely, or at least in part, responsible for the in-creased prevalence of behaviour disorders in the epileptic population. I believe there is a great deal of truth in this because, in the accepting environment of a special centre, some behavioural abnormalities disappear without the need for change in medication. Admission to the residential component of a special centre can often lead to considerable improvement in social adjust-ment in a relatively short time. Indeed, this also happens in the main epilepsy centres (updated colonies), provided that appropriate individual accommoda-tion is provided and independence encouraged, in spite of the apparent para-

552

dox of segregation mentioned by Meinardi [8].

4 Management of associated disorders. These are usually psychiatric and require appropriate treatment. Depressive states usually respond well to treatment, but long-standing personality disorders may require a longer period of residential treatment than is appropriate in a special centre, and referral to a longer-term centre for epilepsy may be required.

5 Occupational training is essential. Many of the patients admitted to a special centre have a history of problems with employment — sometimes simply because of seizure frequency, but often for multi-factorial reasons. The main need appears to be simply to get back into a daily working routine. The actual occupation is of less significance, but it must be seen as meaningful and constructive to the patient and, if possible, relevant to prospective employment in the community. There are advantages in an industrial workshop environment, either in a special centre itself or within reasonable reach by public transport. In the workshop, a more accurate assessment of seizure type and frequency is possible than in many other situations. In addition, the patient's abilities, attitude to work, time-keeping, flexibility, relations with 'management' and peer groups can be repeatedly assessed, and appropriate guidance given when necessary.

6 Rehabilitation must be the ultimate aim of all special centres, and can only be achieved if the foregoing factors are properly managed. It is clear that a multi-disciplinary approach is essential and regular case conferences between all personnel involved should be held on each patient. It is also important to ensure that those patients requiring longer-term treatment in a centre or hospital for epilepsy, should be transferred as soon as possible, when it is certain that no further improvement can be achieved. This point was stressed in the Reid Report [1] paragraph 112, and is one advantage of having the residential component of a special centre within the campus of a main centre for epilepsy.

During the patient's stay in the special centre, every effort should be made to eliminate dependence on 'the system' with minimum restrictions on social activities, consistent with medical needs. In fact, many of the patients admitted to a residential centre have been subjected to various forms of overprotection for many years and find a relaxed, informal, non-hospitalised environment very beneficial. The minimum of 'nursing' techniques should be applied and, although there must be a structure of discipline, it should be unobtrusive.

Contact with the community, and especially family, must be maintained, and this can be most effectively supervised by experienced social workers, whether the patient is in the residential component or being treated as an outpatient. Good communication is vital — a facility notoriously denied to members of the medical profession. If the patient is in residence and already has employment, the employer should be contacted immediately and an outline of the therapeutic programme explained. Employment for some people with epilepsy is difficult enough as it is, without running the risk of losing it because of a treatment which is supposed to help. Liaison with a Disablement Resettlement Officer (DRO) particularly interested in epilepsy is important, but not always easy to achieve. The DRO must be involved early on in the assessment of those patients who have not been employed for some time, but who appear to have reasonable prospects after treatment. Attendance at an Employment Rehabilitation Centre may be advisable before returning straight to open employment.

Finally, arrangements must be made for continued supervision for those patients discharged from the residential centre. The ideal is for this to be done from the neurological or other outpatient component of the special centre – at least, for a period of time – to ensure that improvement is maintained. It is important that this should be done with the co-operation of the patient's family doctor who is, and should remain, the first line manager of the person with epilepsy.

7 Research programmes should be included whenever possible, particularly linked with the appropriate university department. The extent of such programmes will obviously depend on the resources, both financial and temporal, of the individual centres but, at the very least, could include short-term clinical trials of anti-epileptic drugs, both new and established. However, it is not only drug treatment that needs evaluation, because there is no doubt that some people with epilepsy are not only handicapped by the occurrence of seizures but by social problems, failure to work at adequate speed, neurotic behaviour etc, and the environment of a special centre is suitable for the investigation of such factors.

8 Teaching is another function of a special centre so that greater appreciation of the problem of epilepsy can be achieved at all levels of training. Although primarily directed at the personnel of the special centre itself, it should include sessions for other groups, such as visiting doctors, medical students, social workers, disablement resettlement officers and youth employment officers and, if possible, employers. Last, but by no means least, members of the patient's family can be included in some discussion groups to ease the transition of the patient back to the community.

At the present time, Epilepsy International is compiling a directory of epilepsy centres throughout the world, based on the following broad definition [18]:

"An epilepsy centre is an organisation or institution with a multi-disciplinary staff, including both medical and para-medical specialities, recognised as a leader in its catchment area in its ability to provide the newest diagnostic and treatment services, education at both professional and non-professional levels and knowledge about referral sources in related services such as:-

schooling, vocational rehabilitation, legal and social services, residential, transition, and respite care services."

It is likely that there will be considerable national and regional differences, and the type of patient catered for will also vary, but any attempt to collate the services offered in different parts of the world is to be welcomed.

Provision of longer-term accommodation

The Reid Report [1] envisaged that the special centre should have facilities for those people with severe epilepsy, whose seizures cannot be adequately controlled, and who require longer-term accommodation purely on account of this. However, the accommodation for this purpose should be in a separate part of the residential unit. Furthermore, if sited in one of the main centres (colonies), the needs of the patients must be recognised as being different from the long stay resident who is there for other reasons, mainly custodial care. Dr and Mrs Laidlaw, formerly of Chalfont Centre for Epilepsy, Buckinghamshire, eloquently describe the need of those people with epilepsy who, *very nearly but not quite,* can manage on their own, who are employable but break down under external environmental stresses, who, given just a little bit of support, can be most successful [19]. The philosophy of today is that disabled people should be '*maintained* in the community' but this assumes that the community is first willing, and secondly able, to carry out this function. Very often it is not, and the patient becomes '*contained'* in the community with increasing isolation, frustration and no real opportunity for achievement, however limited. Thus, although apparently maintained in the community, one feels that this is more for the convenience of doctors and social workers, who can then pass on to the next problem. The Laidlaws suggest therapeutic communities for people with epilepsy, but correctly stress that the attitude within such a community must be radically different from that of the original colonies. I think it *is* practical to form a limited number of such units within the structure of a main centre for epilepsy, but it is not easy because of entrenched attitudes, mostly on the part of senior staff, from previous decades. At the present time, however, this might offer an alternative and better solution to the problem of some people with epilepsy than merely existing, unemployed and forgotten, in a so-called open community that neither cares nor understands the problems peculiar to the condition.

At The David Lewis Centre we have started a project which approximates to the Laidlaws' concept, although there are still many deficiencies. One of the existing buildings in the main centre has been completely refurbished to modern standards, exceeding the quality of most university accommodation, including individual bedrooms with a high standard of furnishing. There is accommodation for 19 patients, two of whom share a large double room. This is a mixed sex house and is run on the principle of a minimum support group with only one full time staff member supported by the senior social worker, and directly responsible to myself. There is no night staff and no real 'supervision' —only guidance. The patients who are admitted must agree in writing to take responsibility for themselves, collect, store and prepare their own food and be entirely responsible for their medication, which is obtainable on prescription from the nearby town, and not from the Centre's pharmacy. No member of staff is allowed to enter the unit except by invitation, and this includes medical and nursing staff. Originally, it was anticipated that all patients would be discharged within 12—18 months but this criterion has now been relaxed, and it is possible that some patients will remain there for several years. In addition there is accommodation for a further 17 patients in four domestic houses previously occupied by staff, including the Resident Physician. These patients are entirely responsible for themselves, with the minimum of staff intervention only on specific request. Although most of these patients work in the Centre workshops or at other occupations, some are in normal employment in the local community. Obviously the latter is the ideal for all, but it is likely to be limited in practice, because of the general unemployment problem and the geographical situation of the Centre in relation to public transport. Nevertheless, after only two years' experience, we are taking active steps to accommodate patients in ordinary domestic houses previously allocated to key staff. It is also intended to purchase one or two houses in one of the local towns to provide a genuine controlled 'half-way house' facility.

The principle of these minimum support groups is to remove the 'medical model' as far as possible, giving medical advice only on the specific request of the individual patient, although regular reviews of the epileptic state are carried out in the usual way in the clinic. In this way, we hope to provide small communities within a main centre for epilepsy, which will fill a need for those people who 'very nearly but not quite' can manage on their own to cope with the 'falling sickness'.

The special needs of children

The general indications for the establishment of special centres for children with epilepsy are broadly the same as for adults with an important difference — namely that they should be based on firm educational principles. Learning difficulties of one kind or another are common in epileptic children, and it is important that teachers are aware of these and able to deal with them. Some of the problems are related to the underlying cerebral damage that is responsible for epilepsy, and the effect of medication also has to be taken into account. Problems at school are not necessarily due to seizures and they can occur in children whose seizures are well controlled. For example, the attitude of the teacher can be important if the teacher does not understand epilepsy and believes that the child is slow or inattentive, or just plain lazy, or is simply frightened that the child may have a seizure in the classroom and disturb the routine. The reaction of peer group children can also provide considerable problems. Whitmore and Holdsworth [20] in their investigation of children with epilepsy attending normal schools, found that 42 per cent of these children were described as 'markedly inattentive' with unsatisfactory educational progress. The various descriptions applied to these children included lethargic, absent-minded, sleepy, doped, lacking in concentration or otherwise unresponsive. Stores [21] has emphasised the difficulty of the exact definition of 'inattentive' but agrees that the concept is of great clinical and educational importance in children with epilepsy.

Faced with these and many other problems, it is hardly surprising that some children with epilepsy make sub-optimal progress at school. Few authorities would disagree with the general policy in the United Kingdom of educating all children, including those with disabilities of all kinds, in normal schools whenever possible. Nearly forty years ago, the following statement was made in the British Parliament by Mr Chuter Ede, the Parliamentary Secretary for Education, during a debate on the Education Bill, 1943, which subsequently became the Education Act 1944:

"May I say that I do not want to insert in the Bill any words which make it appear that the normal way to deal with a child who suffers from any of these disabilities is to be put into a special school where he will be segregated. Whilst we desire to see adequate provision of special schools, we also desire to see as many children as possible retained in the normal stream of school life."

(Hansard Vol 398, Col 703, 21 March 1944)

Forty years later, the continuing need for special and residential education for children with disabilities, including epilepsy, is recognised in the recent 'Warnock Report' [22] and of course in the earlier Reid Report [1].

In the United States of America, the Commission on the Control of Epilepsy and its Consequences came to the same conclusion with strong emphasis on education in normal schools but, perhaps, went to the extreme in that no positive recommendation was made for the establishment of special schools or centres specifically for children with epilepsy [11]. A survey of special education in Denmark [23] revealed that only 30 children with epilepsy, out of a total of 129,734 children receiving special education, were in special schools specifically for epilepsy, in spite of an earlier plea for special institutions for epileptic children [24]. In The Netherlands, there are no schools specifically designated for children with epilepsy as such, but children admitted to the Instituut voor Epilepsiebestrijding in Heemstede, are educated during their period of investigation. Almost all these children have multiple handicaps. In 1972 Siegenthaler reported that 200 of a total of 1000 beds in the four centres for epilepsy in Switzerland were for children, and the concept appeared to be similar to that in the United Kingdom [25].

Present status of special centres for children in England and Wales

At the present time there is only one officially designated special centre for children with Epilepsy at the Park Hospital, Oxford [26], to which children of all ages are referred with problems of diagnosis, seizure control and educational and behavioural difficulties. In addition, there are five residential schools which cater specifically for children with epilepsy*. Of these, two (David Lewis and Lingfield) come nearest to the concept of special centres, and it was envisaged by the Reid Report [1] that, as the services for epilepsy developed, there would be an increasing need for short-term admissions for assessment and stabilisation of epilepsy. Subsequently, this was supported by the Warnock Report [22]. Paragraph 8, 14, of this Report reads as follows:

> "We see a need for another kind of resource centre, also based in a special school, which would be developed in collaboration between local authorities and would specialise in relatively rare or particularly complex disabilities such as severe visual, hearing or physical disabilities, severe speech or language disorders, severe epilepsy and severe conduct disorders.
> Centres of this kind would provide facilities for specialist assessment, short- and long-term day and residential education and specialist advice and support to teachers and pupils in other schools as well as to other professionals. They would also be places where parents of children with the same type of disability could meet together."

It was recognised that some special schools already carry out these functions, to which I would add the words ". . . at least in part." With the present economic climate in Britain, I think it likely that special services for children with epilepsy will be concentrated in two or three of the existing residential schools. As I have already indicated, the basic principles for admission and management are the same as for adults, with the addition of a formal educational structure. These need not conflict with the wider need for special education of the child with epilepsy who has severe seizures requiring a combination of medical treatment, education and care beyond the combined resources of the family and day school, or when learning difficulties or other barriers to educational progress are so severe that the whole life of the child needs to be under continuous and consistent medical and educational control.

The outcome of special centre treatment

The long-term centres (colonies)

Throughout their history of about 100 years, the epileptic colonies satisfied a very real need which had not been adequately provided for since the origins of man. They served their residents and the community well. Some of them were

---

* Chilton House School, The Maghull Homes, Maghull, Lancs. David Lewis School, David Lewis Centre, Alderley Edge, Ches. Lingfield Hospital School, Lingfield, Surrey. Sedgwick House School, Nr Kendal, Cumbria. St Elizabeth's School, Much Hadham, Herts.

well in the forefront of medical treatment in their day and provided opportunities for the study of epilepsy on a formal basis; for example, William Aldren Turner's classic book was based partly on work carried out at the Chalfont Colony, Buckinghamshire, England [27]. In spite of the fact that they were institutions, the attitudes within were often quite liberal and unrestrictive. In his annual report dated November 1911, Dr Alan McDougall, the first Director of the David Lewis Colony, Cheshire, England, wrote:

> "It is seven years since this Colony began its work. Those years have taught us this: that unless misunderstood and improperly treated, the epileptic is a pleasant and very likeable person. The troublesome features that many of them show at the time of admission have arisen less from the disease than from the mishandling that the patient has received in the past from those most anxious to help him . . . they must be allowed to run some risk; to protect them completely from risk would be to promote mental and physical degeneration and early decay."

The majority of patients admitted to these colonies improved so long as they remained resident, but detailed analysis of the long-term outcome is impossible. I believe they did their job well until the wind of change began to affect the approach to epilepsy in the last two or three decades.

The modern special centres

There are considerable difficulties in the evaluation of the results of treatment in special centres in Europe and the USA — largely because insufficient time has elapsed since their inception, and little has been published in the medical literature. Review of *Cumulative Index Medicus* from 1973 through 1978 reveals a total of only 29 papers concerned with rehabilitation in epilepsy over the six-year period, and none of these concerned special centres. Parsonage [12] has reported his experience in an English Centre for Epilepsy shortly after its official designation as a National Special Centre for Epilepsy, although the survey covered the period 1966–1972 and concerned patients with a range of neuropsychiatric disabilities. During 1972 a total of 133 patients with epilepsy were seen at the Special Centre, 79 outpatients and 54 inpatients. Of the latter, 40 had psychiatric handicaps in addition to their epilepsy, including impaired intellect in 15 and personality disorders in 14; seven patients had affective disorder and four psychosis. The average duration of treatment in the residential special centre was two months for males and three months for females; two patients required five months' treatment and one nearly seven months to stabilise the epilepsy.

The final outcome in Parsonage's series of 54 inpatients is interesting. Twenty-one (38%) returned to employment or resumed education at school or university and four were suitable for sheltered employment or residential training courses. Thus 25 (46%) of the total had good prospects after discharge from the centre.

559

On the other hand, 23 (42.5%) were unemployable, usually because of impaired intellect or personality disorder. Only two of the total 54 patients failed because of uncontrolled epilepsy. In general, those who were employed before admission to the Special Centre were able to return to work but those previously unemployed remained so after discharge. This experience was confirmed in a later report by Parsonage [13] and he also drew attention to the significant number of patients admitted to the Centre with a diagnosis of epilepsy who were subsequently shown not to be suffering from the condition. In 1975 this proportion was 24 per cent.

My own experience at the David Lewis Centre is similar. A total of 200 patients have been admitted to the small twelve-bedded residential 'special centre' since 1973. The duration of stay has ranged from 1—46 weeks with a mean of 18.5 weeks. The higher average duration of treatment compared to Parsonage's series is partly accounted for by the fact that some patients admitted for assessment were then 'abandoned' by relatives and sponsoring authorities and the process of transferring them to alternative accommodation was lengthy. The staffing ratio is also lower than at the Special Centre in York. Of the 190 patients discharged, just under half were placed either in open employment, sheltered workshops or residential training establishments. One in four patients were considered totally unemployable, usually because of intellectual retardation, and 15 per cent were assessed as requiring longer-term residential treatment in the main centre. The remaining patients had very indefinite futures and I have not classified them. Twelve patients (6%) who had been treated for up to ten years were found not to have epilepsy at all. No figures are available for long-term follow-up.

Morgan and Bennett [28] have recently reported the results of a survey of residential care in epilepsy centres (updated colony) and remedial care in Special Centres for Epilepsy. The latter section is based on studies at the National Hospital — Chalfont Centre and the Special Centre for Epilepsy at Bootham Park Hospital, York, and includes a follow-up study of a sample of patients after discharge. In the first three years of operation of these two designated centres the average annual admission rate was 121 patients with a significant re-admission rate of 16 per cent. The ratio of men to women was 3:2. The great majority were between the ages of 16 and 35 years and only about 17 per cent were 'economically active' and employed. Two-thirds of the patients had physical and and/or psychiatric disorders in addition to epilepsy and nearly half had an intelligence quotient below 85. In other words, the population was fairly typical of 'the more difficult epileptic'.

Study of 428 patients showed that two-thirds of the patients at York remained at the Centre for less than three months, while at Chalfont two-thirds stayed for more than three months; this was accounted for by different forms of organisation and objectives. Seizure control was improved in 52 per cent of males and 69 per cent of females, and it was significant that the highest rate of improvement was in those patients staying in the Centres between three and five months, suggesting that there is an optimum period of stay beyond which little further seizure control is achieved. The rate of improvement in psychiatric disorders was much lower, being only about one-fifth overall. However, there was a significant difference between the two centres because improvement in psychiatric disorders was higher in York (males 23%, females 61%) than in Chalfont (males 18%, females 13%).

Of the 428 patients, 321 (75%) were finally discharged to their homes and the remainder to a variety of residential establishments including epilepsy centres (updated colonies). It was eventually possible to interview 211 of the 321 patients in their own homes, almost always with their 'key helper'. There was an average interval of about two years since discharge from the special centre. The degree of seizure control was, not unexpectedly, difficult to quantify and the data must be considered with caution, but the overall assessment was that 59 per cent of the patients were better from the point of view of seizure control, 15 per cent were worse and 26 per cent were unchanged. Ninety-two of the patients had been admitted to hospital on at least one occasion since their discharge from the special centre, 10 per cent of them because of status epilepticus. Overall one-third of the admissions to hospital were related to the epilepsy. An alarmingly high 25 per cent reported no medical supervision whatever. Social disadvantage was evident in about one-third of all the patients. However, the employment situation of the patients has improved when compared with the position prior to admission to the special centre, and 32 per cent of both male and female patients were employed at the time of interview. Improvements were also found among the 76 men and 64 women interviewed who had been classified as not economically active at their first admission.

The patient's subjective view of their own stay at the special centre is interesting. Overall, 67 per cent of the patient said that it had been helpful in some way, 26 per cent were equivocal and 7 per cent said it actually made them worse. Enthusiasm amongst the 'key helpers' (usually family) was less obvious. Although only about half felt that the patient's stay in the special centre had been helpful to the family, none reported that it had been unhelpful. Twenty per cent felt that the patient's admission to a special centre had been beneficial because it 'provided a break', but on the other hand as many as 16 per cent were dissatisfied with staff. However, the authors stress that the 'key helpers' were interviewed in the presence of the patients and their answers might have been restrained.

Morgan and Bennett conclude that both epilepsy centres (updated colonies) and special centres do have a continuing role in the foreseeable future and that there is a complementary relationship between the two. They feel that a total of four special centres would be adequate to serve the needs in England and Wales. Furthermore, they suggest that no patient should be admitted to an epilepsy centre for medium- or long-term care unless he or she has undergone a period of assessment in a special centre. Their report is the most comprehensive document ever written on special services for people with epilepsy in this country.

My personal opinion is that whatever interpretation may be placed on this report, there are, and probably will be for some time to come, a proportion of people with epilepsy who can *only* be adequately assessed in a special centre for epilepsy because of the need for a multi-disciplinary approach by professionals who are dedicated to the problem. Dedication to the problem of epilepsy may be an old-fashioned concept, but in few conditions in medicine is it more appropriate. Many of the patients admitted to special centres have never been properly assessed by the ordinary medical services available. I believe the Special Centres for Epilepsy will be with us for quite a long time to come.

References

1   Department of Health and Social Security and Welsh Office. *People with Epilepsy (Report of a joint sub-committee of the Standing Medical Advisory Committee on Health and Welfare of Handicapped Persons) 1969.* London:HMSO
2   Lennox WG. *Epilepsy and Related Disorders 1960.* Little, Brown and Company
3   Temkin O. *The Falling Sickness. A History of Epilepsy from the Greeks to the Beginnings of Modern Neurology 1971 2nd Edn.* Baltimore and London: The Johns Hopkins University Press
4   Ministry of Health. *Welfare of Handicapped Persons. The Special Needs of Epileptics and Spastics 1953; Circular 25/53.* London: HMSO
5   Ministry of Health Central Health Services Council. *Report of the sub-committee on the Medical Care of Epileptics 1956.* London: HMSO
6   Reid JJA. *Epilepsia 1972; 13:* 211–217
7   Vidart L. *Annales Medico-psychologiques 1966; 124:* 343–367
8   Meinardi H. *Epilepsia 1972; 13:* 191–197
9   Henriksen GF. *Epilepsia 1972; 13:* 199–204
10   Lund M, Randrup J. *Epilepsia 1972; 13:* 245–247
11   US Department of Health, Education and Welfare. *The Commission for the Control of Epilepsy and its Consequences 1978 DHEW Publication No (NIH);* 78–276. Bethesda, Maryland: Public Health Service, National Institutes of Health
12   Parsonage MJ. In Harris P, Mawdsley C, eds. *Epilepsy: Proceedings of the Hans Berger Centenary Symposium 1974; Chapter 46.*Edinburgh, London and New York: Churchill Livingstone
13   Parsonage MH. *2nd South African International Conference on Epilepsy 1976*
14   Grant RHE. *Irish Medical Journal 1980; 73 Suppl:* 7–11
15   Penry JK, Porter RJ. In Penry JK, ed. *Epilepsy: 8th International Symposium 1977;* New York: Raven Press
16   Stores G. In Stott FD, Raftery EB, Sleight P, Golding L, eds. *Proceedings of the 3rd International Symposium on Ambulatory Monitoring 1979.* London: Academic Press
17   Bagley C. *Epilepsia 1972; 13:* 33–45
18   Cereghino JJ. *Advances in Epileptology 1982.* New York: Raven Press In press
19   Laidlaw J, Richens A. *A Textbook of Epilepsy 1976; Chapter 10.*Edinburgh, London and New York: Churchill Livingstone
20   Whitmore K, Holdsworth L. *Spastics Society Study Group on Medical Aspects of Children with School Difficulties 1971.*Durham
21   Stores G. *Dev Med Child Neurol 1973; 15:* 376–382
22   *Special Educational Needs Report of the Committee of Enquiry into the Education of Handicapped Children and Young People 1978.* London: HMSO
23   Jørgensen IS. *Special Education in Denmark 1979.* Copenhagen: Det Danske Selskab
24   Lund M. *Epilepsia 1972; 13:* 219–220

25   Siegenthaler M. *Epilepsia 1972; 13:* 221–224
26   Stores G. *Advances in Epileptology 1982.* New York: Raven Press In press
27   Turner WA. *Epilepsy – A Study of the Idiopathic Disease 1907. Facsimile edn.*
      New York: Raven Press
28   Morgan JD, Bennett AE. *The Development of Services for Epilepsy in the 1970s.*
      Report to the Department of Health and Social Security 1980

57

HEALTH EDUCATION AND EPILEPSY

A G Craig

The debate surrounding the practice of polypharmacy has non-clinical relevance as well. What has come to be called 'health education' related to epilepsy has arisen more by accretion than by design, and suffers from 'polypharmacy' in the shape of a plethora of 'paper pills' containing exhortations and directions about being a 'good patient.' It is therefore not surprising that that other perennial clinical problem — non-compliance — also has parallels outside the clinical sphere, especially as multi-professional approaches to the individual with seizures gain in popularity [1].

Many patients fail to comply with professionally written directions, however attractive the coating on the 'paper pill.' The added sophistication of patient-education videotapes and other media may bring marginal improvements over printed materials, but is still not a remedy for the problem. It would be naive, however, to blame patients entirely for this seemingly 'wilful' disregard of advice offered by those who 'know best' about epilepsy [2,3]. Non-compliance is not amenable to simplistic explanations and, in seeking an answer for this and other problems related to health education and epilepsy, it is useful to look outside the clinical domain. Similar problems confront the practice of health education elsewhere, and strategies which are being evolved to meet them may be transferable to the epilepsy setting [4–6].

While our gaze is fixed on this wider perspective, it would also be productive to examine the attitudes that doctors and other professional helpers take towards epilepsy. These attitudes determine the quality of professional/patient communications, which in turn underpin the whole therapeutic relationship. This is a weak area generally [7] and, where epilepsy is concerned, the picture can be quite dismal [8,9]. Lack of empathy can erode an otherwise well-intentioned relationship with the patient and weaken its potential for health education [10]. This might be overcome if professional helpers were during their training made aware of patients' attitudes towards epilepsy [11]. Such awareness coupled

564

with the skills of constructive counselling would be a very appropriate vehicle for effective health education [12,13]. Sadly, too many of our future health care providers are still not exposed to this element in their training.

A thorough consideration of the areas just outlined would require far more space than one chapter, so that the present chapter will confine itself to a closer examination of a typology of health education concerning epilepsy, and offer some reflections from this schematic view of the subject towards the larger problems already mentioned.

It requires to be said more frequently than usually happens, that health education is neither simply an adjunct to medical procedures, nor relevant only to those of the population who have yet to join the ranks of people with disabilities. In the comprehensive view of the World Health Organisation:

> "the focus in health education is on people and action. In general its aims are to persuade people to adopt and sustain healthy life practices, to use judiciously and wisely the health services available to them, and to take their own decisions both individually and collectively, to improve their health status and environment." [14]

This view of health education concentrates on change and behaviour, and rests on an understanding of 'health' as the ability of a system (whether an individual or a community) to adapt its equilibrium as a response to change, either endogenous or exogenous in origin. It is therefore well suited to a condition such as epilepsy, which manifests itself as episodic impairments of neurological capabilities. What health education within the epilepsy setting seeks to do is to help the individual attain an *optimum* level of functioning rather than strive towards some absolute state of physical and mental wellbeing [15]. The active participation of the person with seizures, and his family if possible, is crucial to the success of this type of undertaking.

A recently suggested typology for general health education [16] can be applied to epilepsy health education with interesting results [17]. From this can be identified at least three main approaches to the subject, and each is examined in detail below.

Epilepsy Health Education: A Typology

Type One

Objective:	maximum patient compliance with a treatment regimen
Mode of operation:	giving selected information to achieve compliance
Locus of control:	external to patient; doctor in control
Programme:	presentation of 'facts' and implications of diagnosis

Method:	medical authority stresses 'right' ideas and actions and condemns deviations
Resources:	doctor talking, plus printed information
Evaluation:	informal/anecdotal
Modifications:	low success rate may produce 'victim blaming' and a devaluation of health education itself

Type Two

Objective:	preventive problem solving for 'good patients'
Mode of operation:	giving selected information to achieve remediation
Locus of control:	external to patient; multiprofessional 'experts' in control
Programme:	recognising/reporting problems (patient's role), leading to problem solution (professional role)
Method:	persuasion/counselling of patient to adopt 'right' attitudes and actions and guidance of professional helper
Resources:	multi-media patient education/one-to-one and group work in hospital and community settings
Evaluation:	patients' attitudes and behaviour measured by professionals
Modification:	efforts to increase efficiency of materials and techniques to meet professionally-set 'success' criteria

Type Three

Objective:	optimum functioning by patient/treatment partnership with professional helper
Mode of operation:	provides conceptual understanding as a framework for thinking, feeling, and doing by patient in relation to epilepsy
Locus of control:	internal to patient/shared with 'experts' who may not be health professionals
Programme:	alternatives to a 'medical model' of epilepsy
Method:	patient-centred learning techniques and agenda setting, with professional guidance

Resources:	'self help groups', health education games and simulations, assertiveness training
Evaluation:	parallel patient and professional measurements of 'success' criteria
Modification:	away from 'illness management' towards 'health maintenance' by the 'self empowered' patient and his family

Discussion

Type One health education in epilepsy is probably the most prevalent type on offer in all countries, and reflects the traditionally pre-eminent role of the medical profession in controlling access to health information. It relies on authority models and the doctor-patient relationship vehicle to transmit pre-selected information with compliance as the objective. Within the 'medical model' of epilepsy, this is seen as 'good patient' behaviour [18]. Examples of this approach to health education abound, and two from different cultures are given below:

A Spanish example

Health education for the child with epileptic attacks consists of the exploration and frank discussion of his attitudes. In this way, it is possible to modify standards of behaviour which, until then, were conditioned by lack of information, mistaken advice, and by prejudices of every kind.

....

In our experience, a short pamphlet aimed at the relatives of epileptics . . . has been shown to be very useful among families of less favoured classes, and totally useless among the semi-marginal population located in the suburbs with an insufficient literacy and cultural level [19].

Education sanitaria y epilepsia, 1978

An American example

Since understanding is so essential and the problems presented by lack of awareness — particularly in taking medication — are so great, educational efforts of the physician need to be reinforced.

One technique for reinforcement would be development of
specific educational modules....which the physician could
'prescribe' for the patient and the family [20].

Plan for Nationwide Action on Epilepsy, 1978

No one should doubt the sincerity behind these two statements, but the
approach advocated is not likely to achieve the level of results hoped for by the
authors. Reliance on a strictly 'educational' style of providing information and
hoping it will automatically lead to 'right actions' is naive, especially when the
information takes a printed form only. If doctors see themselves, as in the
American example, as literally 'prescribing' such health education as part of
the treatment regimen, the way is open to non-compliance of a fundamental
kind. Even where apparently successful, such 'fact giving' may take little regard
of the patient's aptitudes and circumstances, the quality of his existing health
knowledge, and other factors from the physical and social environments which
influence health behaviour. Type One health education is ill-suited to recognise
and overcome such barriers when they lead to non-compliance.

Clinicians should query simplistic reasons for non-compliance and avoid
'victim blaming'. Failure may stem from the patient's perceptions of shortcomings in the doctor's role, since it is easy to discover from general reading that
there are still many debates around issues of recognition and management of the
condition. Not complying with a set of medical instructions may be a form of
'testing out' of the relationship with the practitioner. Better communications
rather than exhortations and more 'paper pills' might help resolve this situation;
otherwise, a lower than expected success rate may lead to a devaluation of the
whole health education undertaking [15].

Type Two health education also deals in information selected by a professional
helper, but the objective is remedial and preventive rather than bald compliance,
and the leading figure in the relationship with the patient may not necessarily be
a doctor. Sometimes 'good patients' encounter problems with treatment or other
aspects of life, and their professional helpers will be called upon to devise solu-
tions once the problems are recognised and reported. Central to the achievement
of this, is a productive professional/patient relationship. This recent advice to
French doctors on the subject applies across all national boundaries.

> ... to dedramatise the situation, the doctor ought to explain
> the condition of epilepsy and his treatment of it; he ought
> to listen to the patient and his family, and establish a dialogue
> particular to each set of circumstances. He ought to interest
> himself in schooling, employment and emotional problems,
> and if necessary remove any feelings of guilt.... He should never
> forget that his 'medical explanation' will always be 'interpreted'
> by his hearers in their own particular way [21].

Epilepsies et Epileptiques, 1980

Remedial health education in such an atmosphere of professional empathy has a much greater chance of success than mere information giving. Counselling provided to mothers about the recognition and reporting of medication side-effects is one obvious area for Type Two health education which has shown successes [22]. It has been suggested that some families of children with epilepsy may show a more autocratic structure making the family more proficient at problem solving [23]. This, plus the central role the mother often plays in families with a handicapped child, may explain why Type Two health education is so compatible with the professionally-set 'success' criteria [24].

Both Type One and Type Two health education are more *in* epilepsy than *about* it. They derive their coherence from a medical model where management of epilepsy is undertaken by health professionals who also set the criteria for 'success'. Though Type Two is more likely to produce results encouraging to the professional worker, both types share a weakness which can affect even carefully constructed programmes. This weakness is the small amount of attention which may be paid to factors influencing patient behaviour outside the medical model of epilepsy. Behaviour has many predisposing, enabling and reinforcing elements, and patients are not 'empty buckets' waiting to be filled with the information selected for them by their professional helpers [25]. It is encouraging to note, therefore, that some Type Two programmes are being modified by means of the 'health belief model' in their planning stages so that they are relevant to the complex of beliefs, attitudes, knowledge and perceptions which are the motivators of patient behaviour [26,27]. Health education input on this basis is more likely to be of lasting use to the patient as well as rating high on the professional's criteria for 'success' [28].

Type Three epilepsy health education is rather different from the first two types on several counts. It originates from an awareness by the professional helper that problems related to treatment may arise because of dissonance between the medical mode of epilepsy and the evaluations placed by individuals and the community on 'being epileptic' [29]. This type is not primarily concerned with 'fact giving', but with patient-generated understanding and the development of coping skills which increase self-esteem and help the individual to act in a more 'self-empowered' manner in aspects of life beyond those identified as 'medical' ones [30].

Sharing direction with the professional helper in the treatment programme is something that is increasingly talked about. The growth of information technology alone may mean that 'the distribution of power and control between patient and doctor will . . . be radically shifted towards a new equilibrium. The patient will be capable of making choices which are more informed than we now believe either possible or prudent' [31]. It should be stressed, however, that the internal 'locus of control' Type Three health education uses does not imply competition between patient and his professional helpers, but partnership. It seems clear that persons who feel they have more control over their own lives, as opposed to

569

feelings of relative powerlessness, may be more motivated to follow medical directions. This seems to happen because they perceive their own interests as lying in the same direction as compliance with those instructions [32]. The encouraging thing from the health educationist's standpoint, is that it appears to be possible to teach people to improve their sense of internal locus of control in ways which also improve levels of self-esteem [33] and thus increase the ability of some individuals to 'withstand the attitudes of persons in their surroundings . . . and also interpret the reactions of others more positively than those with lower degrees of self-esteem' [34]. Self help groups, use of games and simulations, and various forms of assertiveness training — though they at first may not appear to be traditional forms of health education — may provide the basis of awareness, attitudes and skills from which patients are self-motivated to acquire the sort of 'facts' which the Type One view of health education seeks to impart at the outset [35].

Conclusion

Despite advances in the 'state of the art', our present level of knowledge means that we must still accept Gowers' view that 'the ultimate course of epilepsy can never be foreseen' [36]. Including appropriate health education in what is made available to people living with seizures is one relatively cheap and effective way of helping patients and professional workers progress together towards a clearer understanding of what the future may hold in individual cases.

References

1   Hermann BP. *A Multidisciplinary Handbook of Epilepsy 1980.* Springfield, Ill: CC Thomas
2   Buchanan N. *Br Med J 1982; 284:* 173–174
3   Haynes RB, Taylor DW, Sackett DL. *Compliance in Health Care 1979.* Baltimore: Johns Hopkins University Press
4   Anderson DC, Perkins ER, Spencer NJ. *Who Knows Best in Health Education 1979.* Nottingham: University of Nottingham
5   Tones BK. *J Inst Health Educ 1981; 19(4):* 110–115
6   Tones BK. *R Soc Health J 1981; 101(3):* 114–117
7   Byrne PS, Long BEL. *Doctors Talking to Patients: A Study of the Verbal Behaviour of GPs Consulting in their Surgeries 1976.* London: HMSO
8   Beran RG, Jennings VR, Read T. *Epilepsia 1981; 22:* 397–406
9   Beran RG, Sutton C. *Br Med J 1981; 283:* 674–675
10   Lance JW. *Med J Aust 1977; 25:* 907–908
11   Beran RG, Read T. *Clin Neurol 1980; 17:* 59–69
12   Betts TA. *Bulletin of the Royal College of Psychiatrists 1980 (Dec).*
13   Baron J. *Counselling 1981; 38:* 26–29
14   World Health Organisation. *Planning and Evaluation of Health Education Services 1969 (Technical Report Series No 409).* Geneva: WHO
15   Craig AG. *Br J Clin Pract.* In press
16   Draper P, Griffiths J, Dennis J, Popay J. *Br Med J 1980; 281;* 493–495
17   Craig AG. In Dam M, Gram L, Penry JK, eds. *Advances in Epileptology: XIIth Epilepsy International Symposium 1981;* 179–182. New York: Raven Press

18   Burkitt A. In Clark J, ed. *Readings in Community Medicine.* Edinburgh: Churchill Livingstone In Press

19   Claramunt F, Herrero P, Lacampre M et al. In *La Epilepsia: Diagnostico Y Asistencia 1978;* 81–85. Madrid: SEREM

20   Commission for the Control of Epilepsy and its Consequences. *Plan for Nationwide Action on Epilepsy 1978; 1:* 133–146. Washington DC: USDHEW Publication No (NIH) 78-276

21   *Epilepsies Et Epileptiques 1980;* 142. Paris: Ligue Francaise Contre L'Epilepsie

22   Shope JT. *Patient Counselling and Health Education 1980; 2(3):* 135–141

23   Ritchie K. *J Child Psychol Psychiat 1981; 22:* 65–71

24   Wilkin D. *Caring for the Mentally Handicapped Child 1979.* London: Croom Helm

25   Green LW. *Health Education Monographs 1974; 2 (Suppl 1):* 43–64

26   Becker MH. *The Health Belief Model and Personal Health Behaviour 1974.* Princetown, New Jersey: Slack

27   Shope JT. In Hermann BP, ed. *A Multidisciplinary Handbook of Epilepsy 1980;* 199–223. Springfield Ill: CC Thomas

28   *Health Education 1981.* Portland, Oregon: Epilepsy Center of the Good Samaritan Hospital & Medical Centre

29   West PB. *Sociol Rev 1979; 27 (4):* 719–741

30   Hopson B, Scally M. *Lifeskills Teaching 1980.* London: McGraw-Hill

31   Marinker M. *J Roy Coll Gen Practit 1981; 31 (230):* 545

32   Wallston BS, Wallston KA, Kaplan GD, Maides SA. *J Consult Clin Psychol 1976; 44 (4):* 580–585

33   Lefcourt HM. *Locus of Control 1976.* New Jersey: Lawrence Erlbaum Associates

34   Ekermo E. In Janz D, ed. *Epileptology: Proceedings of the Seventh International Symposium on Epilepsy (West Berlin) 1975;* 96. Stuttgart: Georg Thieme

35   Report of the first National Epilepsy Self-Help Workshop. In *Epilepsy Self-Help Newsletter 1981; 3 (1):* 1–15. Evanston, Ill: Northwestern University

36   Gowers W. *Epilepsy and Other Chronic Convulsive Diseases 1901(2 Edn):* 302. London: J & A Churchill

571